MW00535440

Leading health experts praise *Nature's Secret Nutrient*™...

"I love this incredible book. Well done and easy to understand, it's clearly the work of great investigative spirits. Nature's Secret Nutrient is about miracles, which happen in your life only when you open up, so open up this book and open up to life. Miracles will happen!"

Wim Hof, The Iceman; author, *The Wim Hof Method*

Φ

"A masterpiece. By uncovering the universal key to health, healing, and beauty, Dr. Friedman & Matthew K. Cross have unlocked a "secret" formula that can help us transform each area of our lives so that quality longevity is within the reach of every human being. This book deserves a Nobel Prize in Medicine."

Ann Louise Gittleman, M.S., C.N.S., bestselling author, *The Fat Flush Plan*

Φ

"For millennia scientists have noted significant mathematical relationships that seem to optimize function. In this landmark book, these relationships have been extended to optimizing our lifestyle. Obviously, we are all genetically unique, so one size does not fit all. However there are limits beyond certain mathematical relationships where performance drops. This book provides an excellent starting point to retake control of your life by finding and honoring those limits. I Strongly Recommend It."

Dr. Barry Sears, bestselling author, *The Zone*

Φ

"If Leonardo da Vinci and Thomas Edison were alive today, they would no doubt be impressed to see how Dr. Robert D. Friedman and Matthew K. Cross have ingeniously utilized the Golden Ratio in the pursuit of health and longevity."

Michael J. Gelb, bestselling author, *How to Think Like Leonardo DaVinci*

Φ

"The key to improving and maintaining health is to approach the challenge from all sides. This book is genius because it does exactly that. It considers all the angles in a unique and proactive manner that will work wonders for those willing to apply its secrets."

Dennis Schumacher, M.D., body, mind & wilderness medicine expert

Φ

"A seminal work which can lead to a renaissance of well-being for the reader. Cross & Friedman show how the Golden Ratio can impact every aspect of your life in powerful ways that seem miraculous."

Dr. Phil Nuernberger, author, *The Warrior Sage*

Φ

"I've been in the health & fitness industry for over 30 years and Nature's Secret Nutrient is one of the most comprehensive resources I've ever seen. It's simple, thought-provoking and covers all the basics to live a life of optimal health & happiness! The thing I like most about your book is its balance and hierarchy of needs. I recommend this book to everyone who wants to lead a life with more energy, better health and VITALITY! Well done—This is an Excellent Book!"

Chris Johnson, author, *OnTarget Nutrition*

Nature's Secret Nutrient

Discover the Golden Ratio for Vibrant Health, Performance & Longevity

Robert D. Friedman, M.D.
Matthew K. Cross

www.NSNpower.com

The goal of life is to make your heartbeat match
the beat of the universe, to match your Nature with Nature.

Joseph Campbell

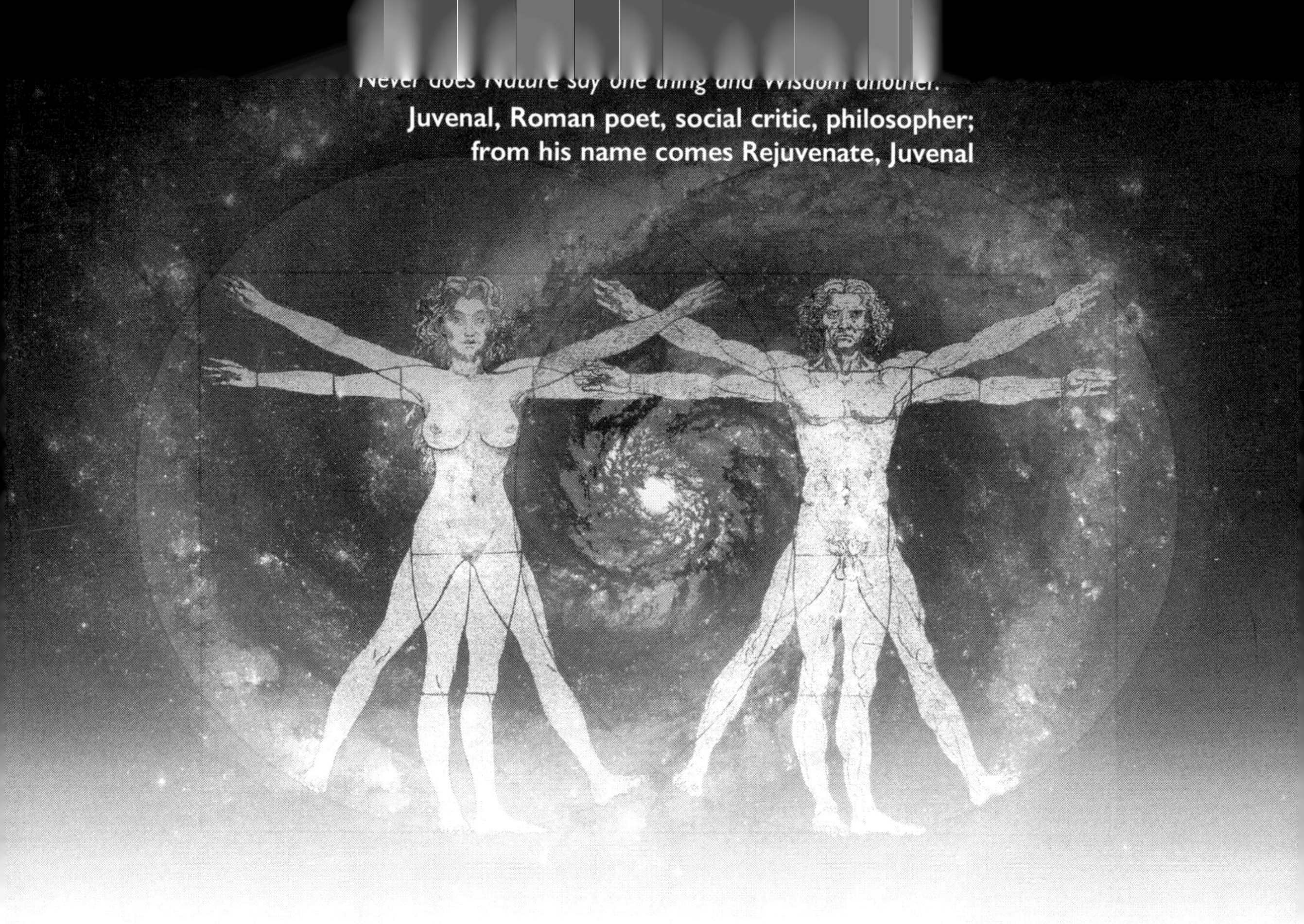

Never does Nature say one thing and Wisdom another.
Juvenal, Roman poet, social critic, philosopher;
from his name comes Rejuvenate, Juvenal

NSN: Nature's Intelligence (NI) in Action

Nature's Secret Nutrient/NSN may sound like a new high-potency vitamin, yet it's simply the core principle of Nature's Intelligence/NI in action (NI being the strongest antidote to AI/Artificial Intelligence). By mirroring Nature through easily integrating her prime code carriers into your life—the Golden Ratio & Fibonacci Sequence—*you have the potential to reset and restore your system to its prime zone state of optimal health, performance and maximum longevity—for free!*

Due to life's inherent personal and environmental stresses, your DNA can become damaged over time—resulting in dysfunction, disease, the degenerative condition known as aging—and premature death. If these genetic changes are ameliorated or reversed your DNA can be restored to the pristine, ageless state it had at birth. By applying the Golden Ratio to your daily lifestyle activities through easy to apply "P℞escriptions"—which take just minutes or seconds to do—you generate the magic elixir known as Nature's Secret Nutrient/NSN. The NSN system is a totally original and natural approach that anyone can use to access the elusive Fountain of Youth. It's simply a matter of learning and applying Nature's Intelligence in your daily life—and reaping the great rewards in store for you.

Dedication

To our parents, Maxine & Jerry (Robert's) and
Jan & Matt (Matthew's) for the gift of life, their loving wisdom
and support and for helping us tap our genetic potential and
strive to live healthy, joyful, meaningful lives and make a difference.

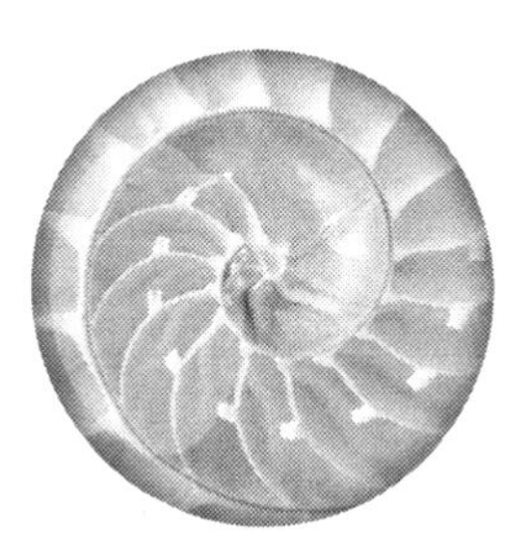

Buckminster Fuller explained to me once
that because our world is constructed from
geometric relations like the Golden Ratio
or the Fibonacci Series, by thinking about
geometry all the time, you could organize and
harmonize your life with the structure of the world.

Einar Thorsteinn, innovative Icelandic
Golden Ratio architect

DISCLAIMER ~ NOTA BENE

The information, recommendations and/or products in this book are not meant to diagnose, treat or cure any disease or medical condition. None of the statements in this book, including those accompanying any of the concepts/practices/products featured in this book have been evaluated by the U.S. Food and Drug Administration. Before beginning or following any of the nutritional recommendations, exercise protocols, training techniques, health improvement or any other health-related suggestions described in this book please consult your physician or health care professional. The reader assumes 100% total responsibility for any/all interpretations they may have and/or actions they may take and/or not take and/or results they may enjoy as a result of reading this book. Neither the Publisher nor the Authors are liable for any loss, injury, damage or misunderstanding of any kind which may occur from any interpretation and/or application of any of the information within this book.

The quotes and data featured within this book are from numerous sources, and are assumed to be accurate as quoted in their original and/or previously published formats. While every effort has been made to verify the accuracy of the featured quotes or data, neither the Publisher nor the Authors can guarantee or be responsible for their perfect accuracy. All websites, URLs and telephone numbers within this book are assumed yet not guaranteed to be accurate at time of publication, knowing that websites may be modified or shut down and URLs or telephone numbers changed without notice. Therefore the Publisher and Authors are not responsible in any way for the content contained in and/or missing/modified within any web site featured within this book.

The authors' insights/conclusions presented within this book are theirs alone, and, however provocative or mind-expanding they may be, may not be endorsed by any of the people, companies or organizations referenced within this book. The reader should know that this book is intended to be a holographic, gestalt approach to understanding and applying the principles explored within it. The authors are thus not responsible for any improvement, however small or great, in the reader's condition or for any sense of enlightenment or wonder that might result from reading, enjoying and/or applying the principles explored in this book—only the reader can improve and/or heal themselves.

This book is available at quantity discount.
Contact Hoshin media at: info@HoshinMedia.com

Book design produced+directed by Matthew K. Cross; genius design insights from Robert D. Friedman, M.D. and design+production mastery from Tom Reczek, www.RZKdesign.com

This book is a completely re-engineered, revised & expanded version of *The Golden Ratio Lifestyle Diet*.

Published in the United States of America by: **Hoshin Media Company • ISBN: 978-1-939623-05-8**
P.O. Box 13, New Canaan, Connecticut 06840 USA • Tel. +1.203.322.1456 • www.HoshinMedia.com

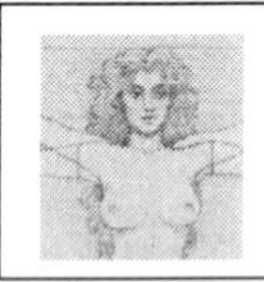

Special acknowledgement to artist Chloe Hedden for her masterful rendition of the commissioned *Divine Code Vitruvian Woman*.
Visit: www.ChloeHedden.com

The single most important biological structure,
the DNA molecule, is in PHI [Golden Ratio] *proportion.*

Stephen McIntosh, integral theorist

Contents

(i) = *INFOGRAPHIC*

ⓘ = *INFOGRAPHIC*

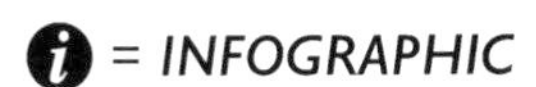
= INFOGRAPHIC

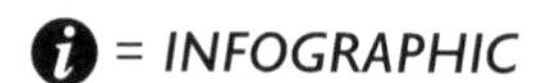
(i) = INFOGRAPHIC

ⓘ = *INFOGRAPHIC*

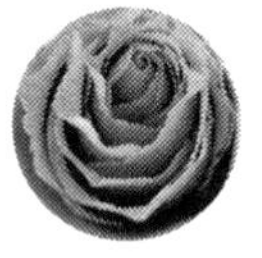

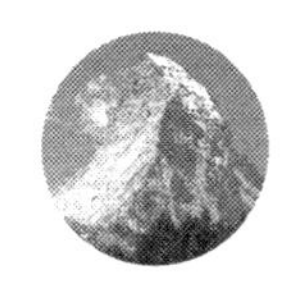

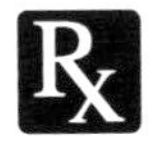

(i) = *INFOGRAPHIC*

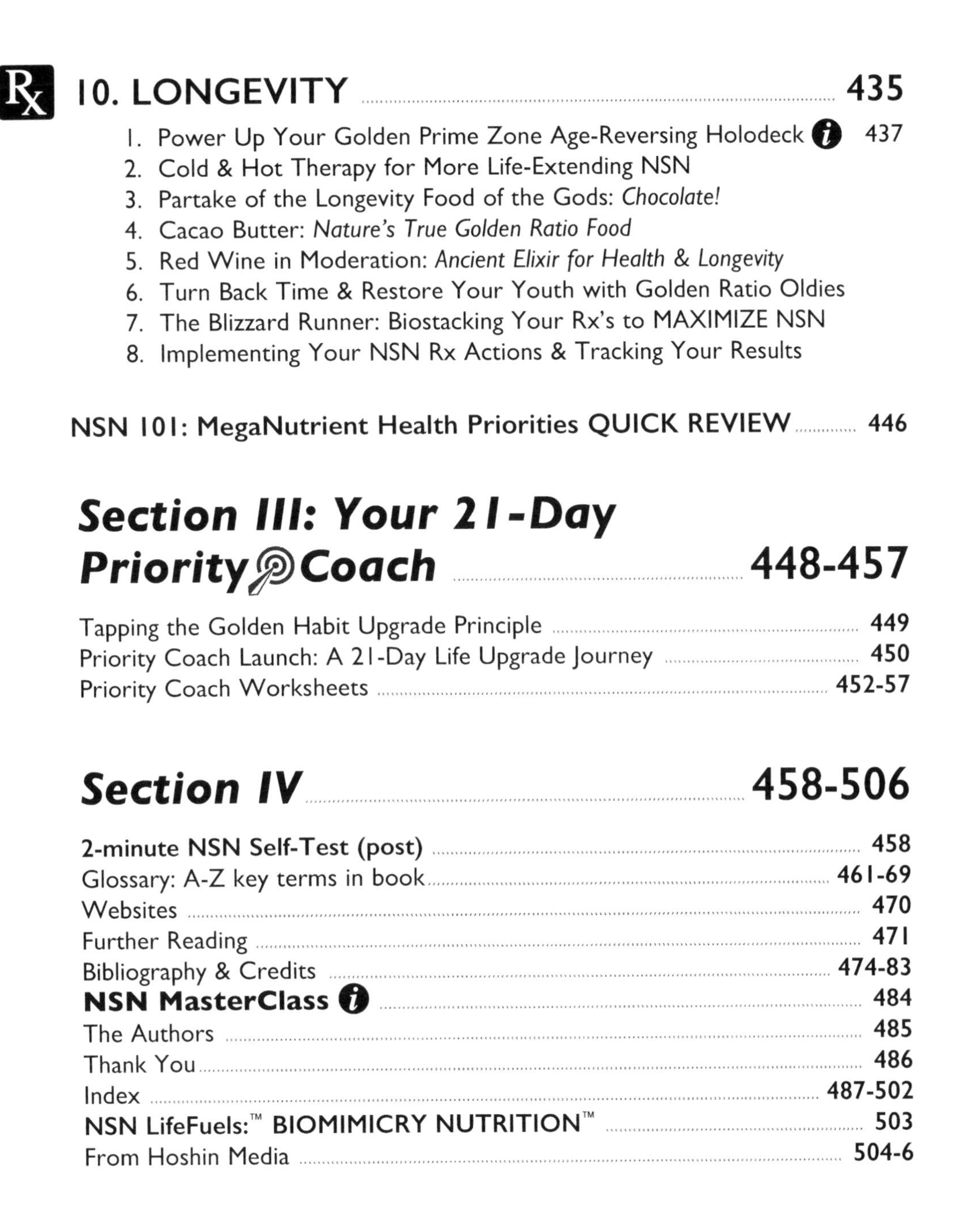

> *The best chemist* [and healer via NSN/Biomimicry] *is Nature.*
> **Dr. Siyaram Pandey, cancer research pioneer**

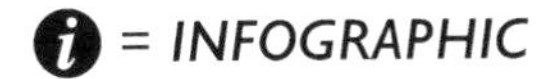
= *INFOGRAPHIC*

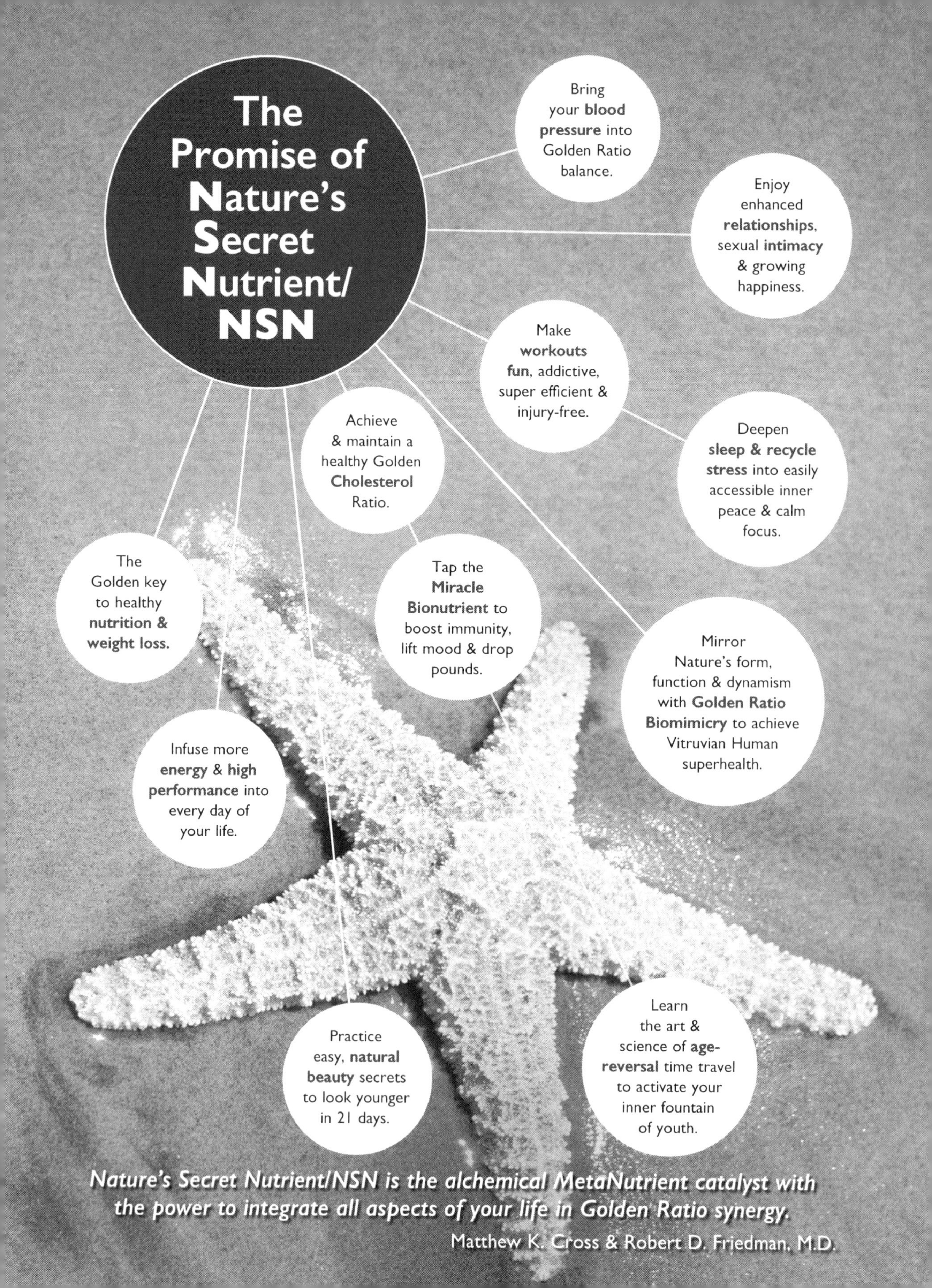

The Promise of Nature's Secret Nutrient/ NSN

Bring your **blood pressure** into Golden Ratio balance.

Enjoy enhanced **relationships**, sexual **intimacy** & growing happiness.

Make **workouts fun**, addictive, super efficient & injury-free.

Deepen **sleep & recycle stress** into easily accessible inner peace & calm focus.

Achieve & maintain a healthy Golden **Cholesterol** Ratio.

The Golden key to healthy **nutrition & weight loss.**

Tap the **Miracle Bionutrient** to boost immunity, lift mood & drop pounds.

Mirror Nature's form, function & dynamism with **Golden Ratio Biomimicry** to achieve Vitruvian Human superhealth.

Infuse more **energy** & **high performance** into every day of your life.

Practice easy, **natural beauty** secrets to look younger in 21 days.

Learn the art & science of **age-reversal** time travel to activate your inner fountain of youth.

Nature's Secret Nutrient/NSN is the alchemical MetaNutrient catalyst with the power to integrate all aspects of your life in Golden Ratio synergy.

Matthew K. Cross & Robert D. Friedman, M.D.

Authors' Welcome

Socrates called it the Heavenly Pattern, which anyone can discover,
and once they have found it they can establish it in themselves.

John Michell, geometer & author of *How The World Is Made*

Would you like to dramatically increase your daily energy, vitality and performance? Restore a former state of higher health? Address a health concern of a chronic or serious nature? Maybe you just want to live long, strong and prosper... If you answered yes to any or all of the above, we have GREAT NEWS for you. This book reveals a fundamental health and healing secret of the Universe, one that Mother Nature uses for the growth and enhancement of all life. We know it as the Golden Φ Ratio—and this is the first book in history to apply this alchemical formula for your transformation to PEAK health, performance and longevity. The Golden Ratio generates a powerful yet invisible MetaNutrient (*Meta: above, beyond*) called Nature's Secret Nutrient/NSN.

NSN is the ultimate MetaNutrient—and can be ingeniously distilled and extracted from your daily life MegaNutrient categories: *Breathing, Hydration, Sleep, Sunlight, Nutrition, Posture, Exercise, Detox, Happiness, Beauty & Relationships.* The result? A master catalyst for optimizing *all* facets of your health and life. Via **Golden Ratio Biomimicry,**™ NSN restores your alignment and resonance with Nature—the absence of which is the root cause of the 3 D's: *Dysfunction, Disease & premature Death*. It's Nature's unseen gift to humanity; with NSN you get Nature—*the most powerful health and healing alliance ever known*—back in your corner. NSN is the golden key for accessing the maximum quality and quantity of life potential encoded in your DNA. The inspiration for this health, performance and longevity breakthrough comes from countless Golden Ratio geniuses—ancient and modern masters including Pythagoras, Plato, Leonardo da Vinci and Albert Einstein. They knew the vast power of the Golden Φ Ratio and expressed it in their historic artistic and scientific works, which continue to impact our world today. This book takes up where they left off, bringing the power of the Golden Ratio into your hands in the form of Nature's Secret Nutrient. As you'll discover, modern medicine and science are just now beginning to validate the astonishing health and performance optimizing powers of the Golden Ratio. This paradigm leap in health is Nature's ultimate biohack—an ingenious, super-effective life quality and longevity catalyst. We celebrate your emerging vitality as you discover and activate your free gift of the Universe's greatest health and healing secret.

Robert D. Friedman, M.D. & Matthew K. Cross

The 5 Core Principles of **N**ature's **S**ecret **N**utrient

1.
The **Golden Ratio is Nature's Biomimicry Design Code** for NSN: The master health, healing and longevity system.

2.
NSN is the MetaNutrient catalyst emerging when our **Micro, Macro & Mega Nutrients** are tuned to the Golden Ratio.

3. The **Hoshin North Star Process™ sequences** the prime MegaNutrient priorities impacting health, performance & longevity.

4. **NSN Action Rx's** transform Golden Ratio Principles into Practices to help you **Become Your Own Doctor.**

5. The innovative **Priority Coach System** makes lifestyle upgrades & habit transformation easy & effective.

The power of the Golden Ratio to create harmony arises from its unique capacity to unite different parts of a whole, so that each preserves its own identity and yet blends into the greater pattern of a single whole.

György Dóczi, *The Power of Limits*

Section I: Introduction & Knowledge Base

Doctors of the future will use Nature's Secret Nutrient/NSN as the guiding principle for optimal care of the human frame, as the basis for nutritional therapy, and as a new scientific paradigm for understanding the cause and prevention of disease.
Robert D. Friedman, M.D. & Matthew K. Cross, inspired by Thomas Edison

Congratulations! **You're holding the first and finest book of its kind in history.** The Nature's Secret Nutrient/NSN system is a revolutionary, Golden Ratio Biomimicry-based approach for stepping *out* of Dysfunction, Disease and premature Death—and *into* PEAK Health, Healing, Happiness, Performance and Longevity. NSN supports a paradigm shift in responsibility for your health from the medical system to YOU. The NSN system is based on Biomimicking Nature's timeless healing wisdom, future-edge medical nutrition science and physiology and transformational business strategy. **The resulting synergy reveals a potent, natural biohack—a more enjoyable and efficient path to maximum life quality and quantity.** Whatever your health aim or concern, you'll be equipped to apply Nature's Secret Nutrient/NSN for increased immunity to disease, while simultaneously manifesting your birthright of vibrant health, happiness and long life.

But First Things First: We challenge you to reclaim the primary power and responsibility for your health & healing. By activating NSN, you'll have the opportunity to take a giant step towards becoming your *own* doctor, in the spirit of the original root of the word Doctor: ***Teacher*.** You'll learn to teach yourself, harness and share the core elements of NSN and extract its essence in support of your own health and longevity. The Action Rx's in the NSN system cost little or nothing to implement. There are no expensive health care plans, dangerous drugs, extreme diets, or specialists to consult—with the exception of consulting yourself and the greatest healer known—Nature. By learning how to harness Nature's Secret Nutrient, you'll be empowered to take greater command of your health and life, an increasing must in modern times. Another key to becoming your own doctor can be found by pulling back the curtain around the commonly misunderstood word *Diet*. For many, Diet conjures up thoughts of deprivation, struggle and failure. Yet the root of the word Diet actually contains a great treasure (of similar interest is the word *Physician*, the Latin root of which is *Physica—Things Relating to* ***Nature***). In fact, the word Diet was originally used by classical medical pioneers such as Hippocrates to describe our *total* Mode or Way of Life.

NOTE: Throughout the book look for the Φ PHI symbol denoting the Golden Ratio (1.618 : 1.0 or 62 : 38) point between any two parts/measures.

The Three-Part Synergy of the Nature's Secret Nutrient/NSN System

Parts 1, 2 & 3 combine to align you with the Golden Ratio for maximum NSN generation.

In PART 1–Principles, you'll discover:

Φ The Golden Ratio Biomimicry Code behind Nature's Secret Nutrient/NSN.

Φ How sequencing the relative priorities of the NSN MegaNutrients amplifies their power: Breath, Hydration, Sleep/Sunlight, Nutrition, Posture, Exercise, Detox, Happiness, Beauty/Relationships and Longevity.

In PART 2–Practice, you'll learn:

Φ How to turn PART 1 (Principles) into Practices via **NSN Action Rx's**—potent cross-reinforcing health prescriptions that can be activated in 5 minutes or less; some in just 30 seconds. Look for the **Time to BeneFIT** Stopwatch.

In PART 3–Performance tracking, you'll harness:

Φ The **Priority Coach** self-empowerment and feedback system that equips you to turn your chosen **NSN Action Rx's** into consistent Practices. This system is a proven focus and momentum booster, takes only 3 minutes a day and is available in either paper format or downloadable app.

Thus your Diet—your *Mode of Life* or *Way of Daily Living*—encompasses everything you do in your everyday life, not just what you eat. Lifestyle is actually the most accurate synonym for the all-encompassing meaning behind the modern limited definition of Diet. In fact, many other key elements of your daily Diet/Lifestyle—beyond what you eat—have every bit as much (and even more) impact on your total health, healing, vitality and longevity. These include Nature's Secret Nutrient's key priority MegaNutrients—*Breathing, Hydration, Sleep/Sunlight, Posture, Exercise, Detoxification, Happiness, Beauty/Relationships*—and yes, *Nutrition*. By restoring the broader, proper application of the word Diet, you can take new actions to upgrade the quality and quantity of your life.

This expanded definition of Diet is the key to the powerful, easy-to-follow health enhancement system which will transform your life, one simple step at a time. Recapturing the responsibility and meaning behind these key words—*Doctor/Teacher and Diet/Lifestyle*—leads to optimal weight and body composition, vibrant health, magnetic beauty and maximum longevity. Let's take a quick tour of Nature's Secret Nutrient's unique attributes and power.

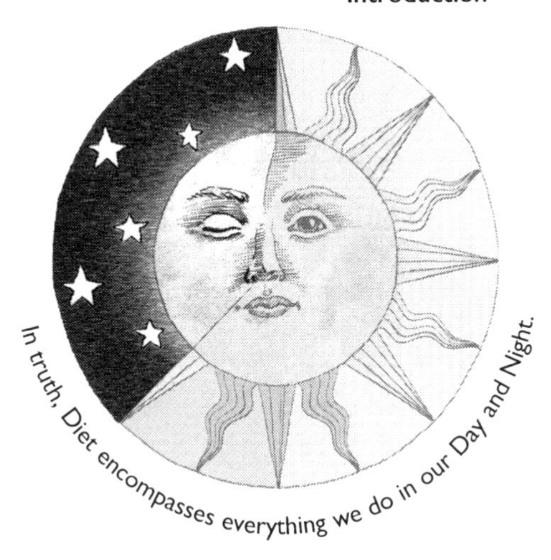

In truth, Diet encompasses everything we do in our Day and Night.

The Golden Ratio & Fibonacci Sequence: Nature's Secret Nutrient/NSN's Biomimicry Code

The single most important biological structure,
the DNA molecule, is in PHI [Golden Ratio] *proportion.*
Stephen McIntosh, integral theorist; author of *The Golden Mean Book*

Across history, great artists, architects and scientists utilized the Golden Ratio to bring harmony, beauty and power into their work. Geniuses such as Plato, Da Vinci and Einstein were much inspired by it. Yet no one has integrated this golden principle into the fields of health and longevity ...until now. The Golden Ratio has remained hidden in modern times, although it's an open secret, clearly seen in the workings of the Universe and in the human body. We've taken the next step and distilled the Golden Ratio into an easily usable **Meta**Nutrient: NSN. This **Meta**Nutrient is **Biomimicry** in action—the bridge through which we can align with and directly access the greatest health and healthing force ever known: *Nature.* The Golden Ratio, also known as Phi, Φ or ϕ, is a fundamental principle underlying the structure and movement of energy and matter throughout the universe. It's the Master Code that blueprints the universe at every level—including the total form and function of the human body. When applied to anything, the Golden Ratio supports greater beauty, efficiency and harmony. It fosters a special unity and healthy synergy and is a catalyst for cultural evolution—the creativity, genius and inspiration underlying the arts, architecture, science and spirituality which advance humanity. A key reason anyone is successful at anything, even though they may not know why or may attribute it to other causes, is that they've applied Golden Ratio principles in some way in whatever they think, make or do. Mounting evidence points to the reason that we consider anything to be good, true or beautiful is that it awakens and delights our innate Golden Ratio nature. In this book we'll show you how this golden principle can be easily tapped to transform your health, performance and longevity. Nature utilizes an intriguing number series which frames the Golden Ratio throughout all creation. First introduced to the West in master mathematician Leonardo Fibonacci's classic book, *Liber Abaci* (1202) and later named in his honor, the infinite Fibonacci Sequence is formed by adding one number to the next, beginning with 0, as shown here:

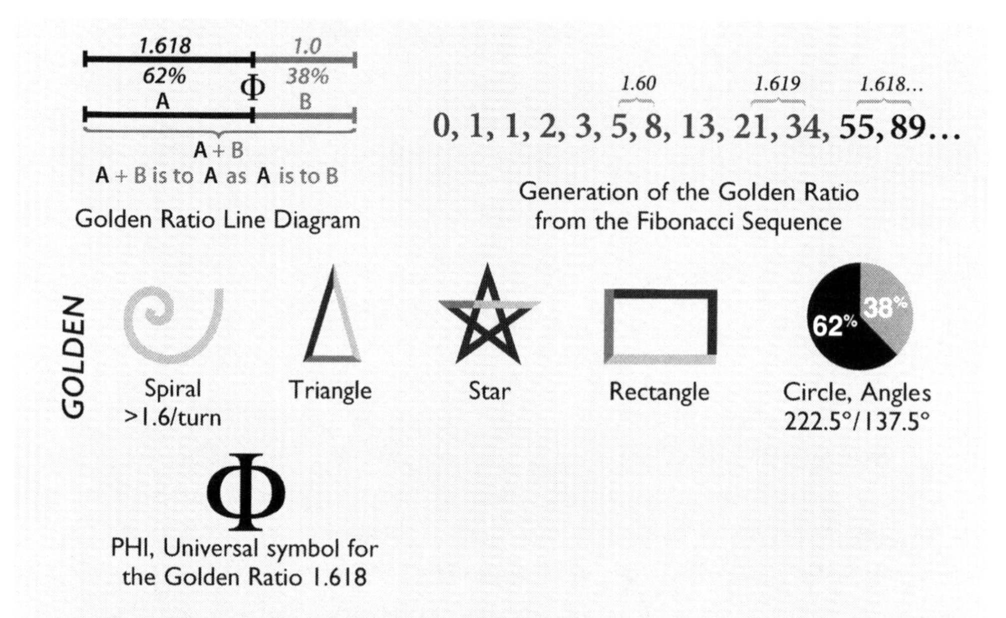

The Golden Ratio & Fibonacci Sequence: Key Visible Facets *(also see infographics, pgs. 42-45)* Line diagram (*top L*) of the prime Golden Ratio formula: *A small part in relation to a large part in the same ratio as the large part is to the whole.* The Fibonacci Sequence (*R*) shows how the Golden Ratio/1.618 first appears in the ratio of adjacent Fibonacci Sequence numbers 55–89. Second line shows 2-D depictions of the Golden: Spiral, Triangle, Star/Pentagon, Rectangle & Circle/Angle. Bottom: PHI/Golden Ratio symbol, two 3-D representations of the Golden Ratio in two Platonic Solids, the icosahedron & dodecahedron. These orbs are geometrical approximations of a sphere, constructed with core geometrical building blocks: triangle & pentagon.

Golden Ratio Pulse: Nature's Heartbeat

The Golden Ratio (Phi, Φ or ϕ) is a special, infinite value, closely related to the Fibonacci Sequence and very close to the ratio of its successive numbers. Graphing the ratios of adjacent numbers in the Fibonacci Sequence, we see that they converge on the Golden Ratio: 1.618... The ratios actually "dance" around the Golden Ratio, with the first ratio *lower* than 1.618 and the next ratio *higher* than 1.618, ad infinitum. This is Nature's way of honing-in on the elusive Golden Ratio, which doesn't actually exist in our 3-dimensional reality, as it's an infinite or irrational number, like Pi (π, 3.14...).

Either way we arrive at two special numbers that approximate the Golden Ratio: 1.618, or 0.618 if you invert the ratio. The Golden Ratio is an ideal—like perfection, we're always striving for it, even if we may never reach it. It's akin to a guiding North Star, calling us to our higher potential. The Golden Ratio pulse graph (below) shows how progressive Fibonacci Ratios converge ever-closer towards the Golden Ratio. The numbers expand in the Fibonacci Sequence pulse above and below the ethereal Golden Ratio, like a divine heartbeat in search of perfect rhythm. To maximize efficiency and harmony, all living systems—from atoms to galaxies, from DNA to the human heartbeat—have built-in homeostatic, balance-seeking mechanisms which gravitate towards and around the Golden Ratio 1.618:1. Constantly changing circumstances invariably introduce chaos and turbulence into our lives and thus our biological systems. A healthy cellular response always returns us towards Golden Ratio balance, whose symptoms we clearly recognize as vibrant health, performance and long life.

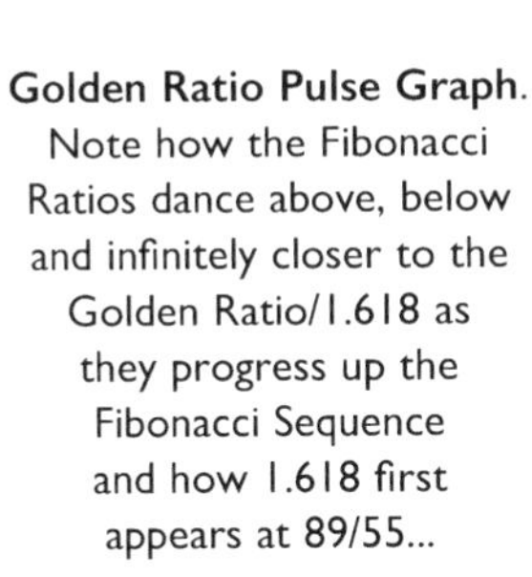
Golden Ratio Pulse Graph. Note how the Fibonacci Ratios dance above, below and infinitely closer to the Golden Ratio/1.618 as they progress up the Fibonacci Sequence and how 1.618 first appears at 89/55...

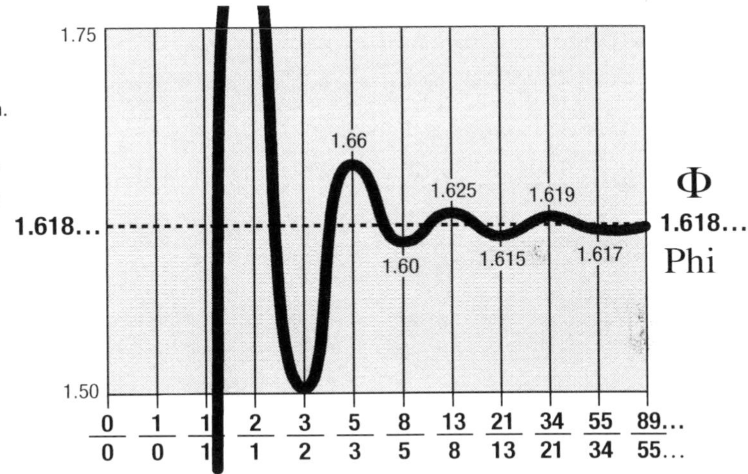

NSN: The Unified Field Theory & Practice of Optimal Lifestyle Nutrition

Nature's Secret Nutrient/NSN is a true **Meta**Nutrient *(meta: above, beyond)* —**the philosopher's stone of nutrition**. It's in a class all its own, different from anything discovered before in the fields of nutrition, science or medicine. At its core, NSN is an innovative application of the Golden Ratio—Nature's secret elixir—that will lift your health, performance and enjoyment of life to PEAK levels. To understand what NSN, the true **Meta**Nutrient is, let's first review the 3 other more basic categories of nutrients:

Φ **Micro**Nutrients: the vitamins, minerals, enzymes, catalysts & co-factors found in all foods, required in *small amounts* for all biochemical processes in your body.

Φ **Macro**Nutrients: the carbohydrate, protein, fat & fiber components of food. Required in *large amounts* to build and maintain tissues as well as fuel and regulate metabolism and other physiologic functions. Carb, Protein and Fat as **Macro**Nutrients are a subset of total Nutrition, explored in depth in chapter 4.

Φ **Mega**Nutrients: the ubiquitous yet underrecognized lifestyle nutrients required in *very large amounts* which support **Micro** and **Macro**Nutrients. We extract **Mega**Nutrients from Nature's hidden-in-plain-sight environmental abundance and daily lifestyle activities. For example, everyday we need to breathe around 10,000 quarts of Air and drink at least 2 or more quarts of Water. It's hard to equate Sleep in terms of milligrams or grams, yet 8–9 hours is a lot and definitely belongs in this category. Likewise, Posture, Exercise, Detox, Beauty, Relationships, Happiness and Inner Peace—all of which have never been considered as "dietary" nutrients—may not be quantifiable in standard nutritional terms, yet nevertheless also fall squarely into the category of **Mega**Nutrients. *The simple truth is, we need to satisfy our daily **Mega**Nutrient requirements in order to reach our full health potential and live a vibrant, long life.*

Φ **Meta**Nutrient is Nature's Secret Nutrient/NSN, which can only be obtained by applying Golden Ratio proportions to fine-tune the consumption of the above three nutrient classes. When you consume a Golden Ratio of any **Micro**, **Macro** or **Mega**Nutrient, your entire physiology shifts into a higher state of

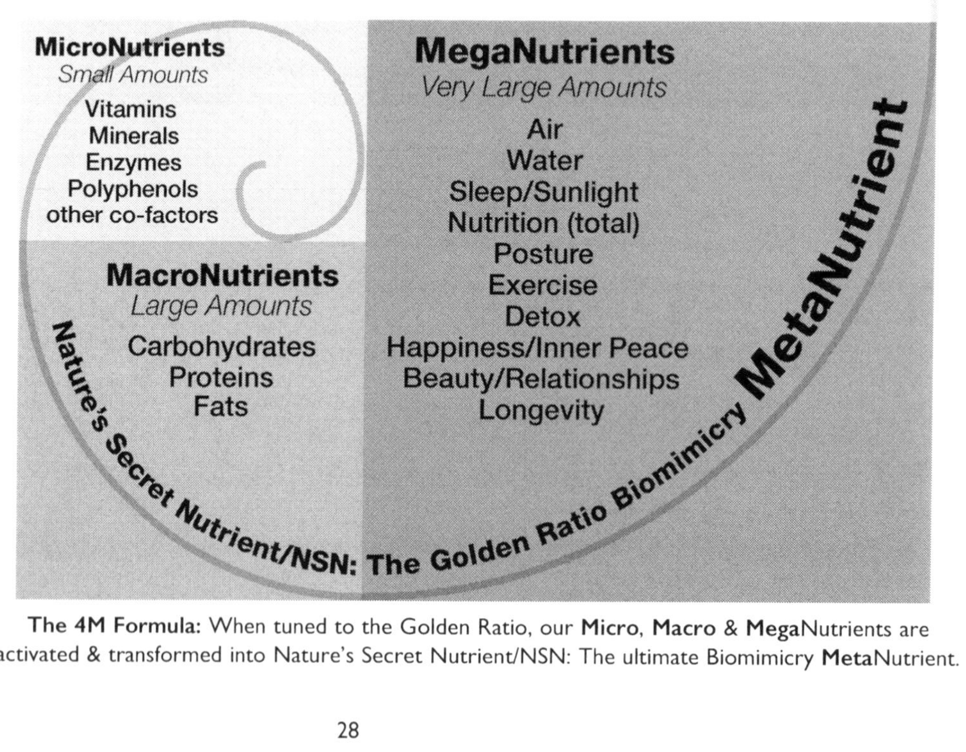

The 4M Formula: When tuned to the Golden Ratio, our **Micro**, **Macro** & **Mega**Nutrients are activated & transformed into Nature's Secret Nutrient/NSN: The ultimate Biomimicry **Meta**Nutrient.

operating efficiency and vitality. By biomimicking the Golden Ratio imprints found throughout Nature, **Micro**, **Macro** and **Mega**Nutrients produce a special elixir known as Nature's Secret Nutrient—a **Meta**Nutrient matrix that *amplifies and potentiates the healing power of Nature in your body and life.*

The Golden Ratio is a prime optimization signal being broadcast 24/7 throughout the universe. *It's the master organizing and integration principle of life, health and harmony*—and this book is the first in history that equips you to amplify and infuse this signal into your life. Once you experience the power of NSN, you'll want this vital **Meta**Nutrient with you always. You'll recognize it to be as important for vibrant health as any other essential nutrient like vitamins A, B, C, D or E. Just as these vitamins are key catalysts for multiple biochemical processes, NSN is the unseen yet vital master catalyst for health, healing, performance and longevity. NSN's Biomimicry MetaNutrient system fulfills the promise of the **Unified Field Theory & Practice of Optimal Lifestyle Nutrition.**

Goldilocks & The True Meaning of *Just Right*

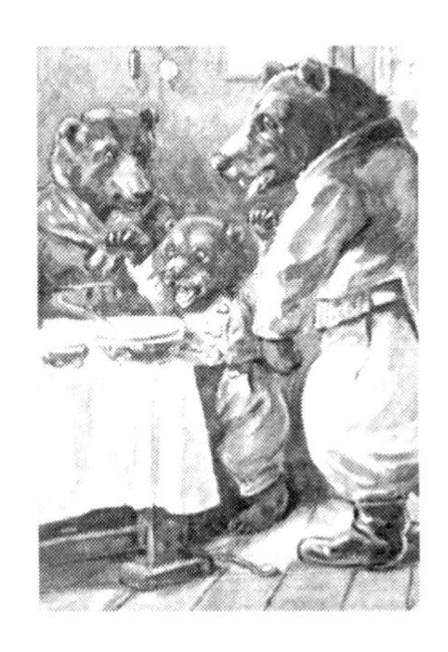

A playful way to understand Golden Ratio balance is by revisiting the childhood fable *Goldilocks and the Three Bears.* This classic tale can be reinterpreted in a way you've never considered—as a metaphor for healthy Golden Ratio balance. As you remember, Goldilocks entered the 3 Bears' house while they were away. Papa Bear, Mama Bear and Baby Bear each had their own customized bowl of porridge, chair and bed. Goldilocks made herself at home, sampling each bowl of porridge, each chair and finally each of the 3 beds. As she tasted the porridge, the first bowl was too hot, the 2nd bowl too cold—but the 3rd bowl was *just right.* A similar scenario occurred when she sampled the chairs and finally the beds, before she found the chair and bed that were *just right.* Goldilocks is repeatedly giving the reader the message of *ideal balance,* yet in a metaphorical way—and with a hidden twist. All fairy tales are metaphorical, containing layers of deeper meaning, with clues to their understanding often hidden in plain sight. Goldilocks is searching for the perfectly balanced porridge, chair and bed, i.e., she's looking for the ones that are *just right.* If we shift our perception of what she appears to be saying and look at her quest through Golden Ratio eyes, we come to a new, expanded understanding of what *just right* actually means. Seen from this perspective, Goldilocks is hinting through a double entendre that perfection is not simply *just right,* but actually *just right of center.* "Center" is of course what we commonly know as the

Golden Ratio/NSN: The Ultimate Biomimicry Health-Hack

Biomimicry is when somebody discovers a property in Nature and applies it to human problems. Nature has already solved every single problem facing humanity. We can turn this world [and our health] *around using Biomimicry as our model.*

Jay Harman, inventor and author, *The Shark's Paintbrush: Biomimicry and How Nature Is Inspiring Innovation*

Biomimicry/Biomimetics is the preeminent science for emulating the efficiency, harmony and success of Nature. Prime Biomimicry examples include: Bird➔Airplane, Human Brain➔Computer, Whale➔Submarine, Thistle➔Velcro, Plants➔Drugs. Activating Golden Ratio Biomimicry via the NSN system aligns the form and function of your body with Nature for optimal health, happiness, performance and longevity.

50% dividing or balance point of a line or any quantity or quality. Yet by moving "*just right of center,*" we move from a static 50% halfway point to the dynamic 62% Golden Ratio point of unity, harmony, efficiency and "*rightness.*" This is the hidden, magic answer to Goldilocks' (Goldi–locks) embedded riddle and in the case of our lives, the Golden Key to unlock vibrant health, performance and longevity Goldilocks' quest for perfection, whether in a bowl of porridge, a chair or a bed, is at its core a powerful archetypal image that subconsciously reminds us of the quest for the Golden Ratio and NSN in our daily lives. Contrary to popular belief, "perfect balance" is often not found at the 50% halfway point of measure—but at the 62% Golden Ratio point of dynamic balance that feels just right, as revealed in this simple description of the Golden Ratio:

In the classical division of a line into two segments, there's only one possible point that divides the line into two segments where the ratio of the longer to the shorter segment is proportional to the ratio of the entire segment to the longer.

It's the point of *dynamic* balance that divides the line into segments that are not too long and not too short, but *just right.* It's not at the 50% division point of the line —|— It's at the Golden Ratio 62% division point —|— that this "just rightness" is revealed. *Nature chose this specific asymmetrical ratio as her dynamic design template throughout all creation.* We see the Golden Ratio across the cosmos, from spiral galaxies & solar systems to everywhere on Earth, in all life forms, all the way down to DNA and sub-atomic levels.

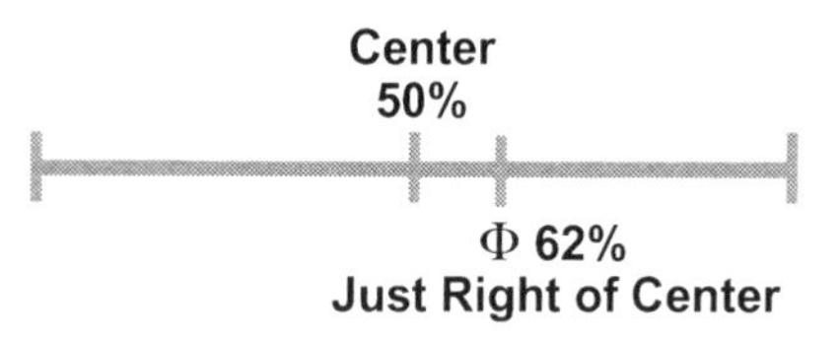

Difference between a static 50% ratio and the dynamic "*just right of center*" 62% Golden Ratio (see line diagram, p. 26).

Getting Adequate Sleep: A Classic Example of *Just Rightness*

To reiterate, the Golden *just right* zone is not necessarily at the 50% division mid-point —|— of any measure or volume; instead, it's at the 62% division —|– point. *This is a critical distinction when considering Golden Ratio balance, for only at this dynamic point range does Nature's Secret Nutrient become available.* In all of the 10 NSN priority drivers of health and longevity, we're identifying these same *just right* Golden Ratio balance points, where all of our physiologic systems are functioning at peak efficiency. Golden Ratio balance gives us the key to opening the lock that leads to just-rightness in *all* facets of our lives.

As a prominent example, let's look at healthy Sleep, one of NSN's top priorities for regeneration and rejuvenation. A 50% split between waking and sleep is unrealistic, as it would result in 12 hours of both wakefulness and sleep. However, a Golden Ratio between waking and sleep would be somewhere around 15 hours of wakefulness and 9 hours of sleep. In today's world, 9 hours of sleep might sound overly luxurious. Finding the proper ratio isn't as easy as it might sound, due to the stresses of modern life. In our fast-paced info/tech age, we're rapidly trending away from Golden Ratio balance. A leading indicator of this imbalance is a recent Gallup poll showing that 40% of Americans are sleep deprived. This societal trend towards sleep deficit has become epidemic, leading to negative ripple effects in too many areas of health and life.

As a society we're just like Goldilocks, looking for a comfortable bed to sleep in to get some much needed sleep. After some trial and error, Goldilocks finds a bed that's just right and immediately falls asleep. However, much to her surprise, she's rudely awakened by the 3 Bears and scurries away, barely escaping with her life. The Bears represent the many distractions and misplaced priorities that can keep us from getting an adequate quantity and quality of restorative sleep. Like Goldilocks, we may *bearly* escape with our lives after months and years of chronic sleep deprivation. The NSN system offers many simple tips and tools that can safely and surely lead you back to a Golden Ratio range of waking to sleep. **First and foremost is seeing what your current waking/sleep ratio is and then making the necessary adjustments to bring you back into Golden Ratio range.** The general trend away from Golden Ratio balance and towards poor lifestyle habits makes daily conscious atunement with the Golden Ratio vitally important. Learning to harness the Ratio via Nature's Secret Nutrient, even from something as simple as a bed and your sleeping time in it, should be considered a critical tool essential for everyone desiring to survive and thrive in the 21st century and beyond.

Hoshin North Star for Health = ***NSN Priorities Sequence***

The secret to your success is in the **sequence** *of your priorities.*

Matthew K. Cross

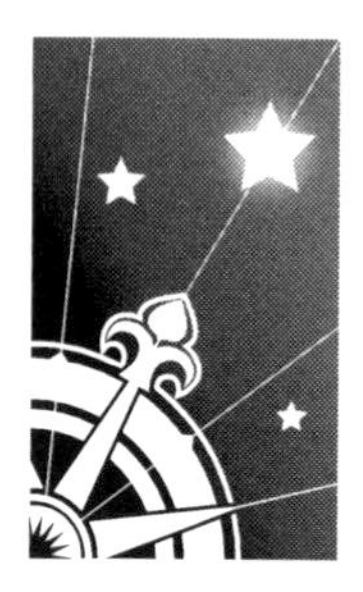

Hoshin (*way of the shiny compass needle in Japanese*) is a master strategic planning process which supports optimal prioritization of the success factors towards achievement of any goal. Due to the complex nature of many opportunities and challenges, the means to identify and act on the key success factors isn't always clear. Hoshin has the near-miraculous ability to clarify *and* sequence the most important priorities influencing any subject—including health and longevity. Using Matthew Cross' next-generation Hoshin North Star Process,™ aka the Hoshin GPS,™ (**G**reat **P**erformance **S**ystem) we determined the optimal priority sequence for activating NSN's health and longevity drivers. In simple terms, we were able to rank the relative priority of each of the health and longevity drivers in this book. Although *all* of the drivers are important and work synergistically, the top-ranked drivers cannot be neglected if we want to optimize our health and longevity. Hoshin was originally inspired by the Einstein of Quality, **Dr. W. Edwards Deming**, the primary architect of Japan's miraculous post-WW II economic recovery. By strategically prioritizing the vital attribute of quality with respect to products and services, *Deming engineered the greatest business success story never told:* the creation of trillions of dollars in ever-growing value across the entire spectrum of business and industry worldwide. Today, Hoshin guides world-leading organizations such as Toyota, Honda, 3M and Proctor & Gamble. It's also a cornerstone of co-author Matthew Cross' Fortune 100 and personal growth and transformation work. The Hoshin GPS is the foundational prioritization instrument for sequencing the chapters in this book, as well as the exercises in the Action Rx's and the 21-day Priority Coach™ System. In order to create and support optimal health and performance with utmost efficiency and impact, it's vital to determine and follow the relative priorities of

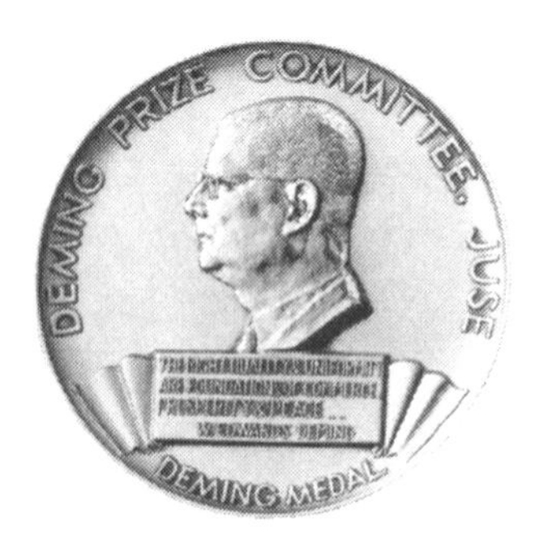

(*L*) **The Deming Prize**, in honor of Dr. W. Edwards Deming (1900-1993), is awarded to companies and individuals recognized as having made major contributions to the advancement of quality.
(*R*) **Hoshin Kanri** (Japanese characters), inspired by Dr. Deming, is the master blueprint behind the Hoshin North Star Process™ which was used to determine the optimal priority sequence for NSN's prime health and longevity drivers.

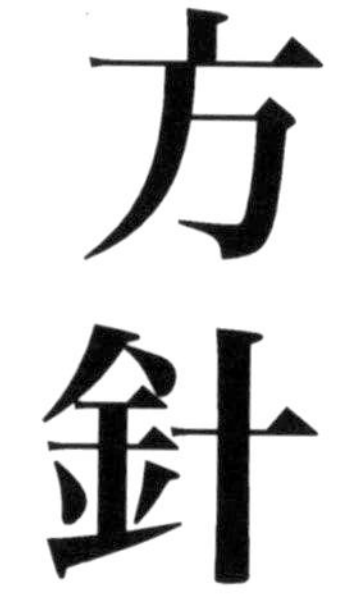

the key drivers involved. As Dr. Deming said, ***It is not enough to just do your best or work hard. You must know what to work on*** [and in what best order].

The Hoshin North Star™ process, as applied to this book's prime focus,

Φ **Identified** and defined the priority, life-driving **Mega**Nutrients necessary for achieving, maintaining and enjoying optimal health, performance & longevity;

Φ **Revealed** the best, *sequenced prioritization* of these **Mega**Nutrient life/health drivers for most effectively implementing the Nature's Secret Nutrient system.

Key priorities we identified as vital health and longevity **Mega**Nutrients are:

Nutrition • Exercise • Hydration • Posture • Happiness
Sunlight • Sleep • Breathing • Beauty • Relationships • Detox

All of these factors are clearly essential. We wanted to know which were the key foundational factors, deserving greater consideration—*and in what prioritized order for greatest cross-reinforcing impact.* Before we reveal the results of our Hoshin GPS analysis, take a moment and review the above key factors underlying great health and longevity. **Which would *you* rank as the top 4 influences? List your 1-4 answers here:**

My Top 4 Health Priority Drivers:

1. ______________________ **3.** ______________________

2. ______________________ **4.** ______________________

What questions did you consider to determine your top 4 priorities? The criteria we used to determine the priorities and their optimal sequence came from the Hoshin GPS process. Here are two key questions that gave us critical insight into their sequence:

Φ ***Which category is more Causal or Foundational in relation to the others?***

Φ ***How long can a person Survive or Thrive without it?***

Decoding The Top Priorities of Great Life Quality+Quantity

SPOILER ALERT: Read no further until you've chosen YOUR top 4 priority drivers above. Done? OK, in a moment take a look at the Hoshin GPS FAR Pyramid™ (**F**oundation, **A**ction, **R**esults) on the next page. Like Abraham Maslow's Hierarchy of Needs Pyramid,

Vitruvian Man & Woman Know the Secret of the NSN Sequence

You can reclaim the inherent genetic potential in your DNA to elevate your life quality and quantity to that approaching the ideal human: **Vitruvian Man/Woman**. With innovative NSN technology, you can become the best version of yourself via a next-generation form of gene sequencing. For geneticists, it's now possible to edit defective genes with a process called CRISPR/Cas9. This high-tech method can repair defective DNA segments by deleting and inserting the correct gene sequences at the exact defect location. "Incurable" diseases will soon vanish, much like small pox and other previously deemed incurables.

The NSN lifestyle technology in these pages is similar to gene editing, yet easy and low-tech. Imagine the 10 NSN health drivers in this book as rungs on a Golden DNA ladder. In molecular DNA, rungs on the ladder are composed of base pairs: A–T & G–C. Various combinations of base pairs are translated into proteins our body needs for all functions. Yet if there's a mistake in the DNA code—*if even one code letter is deleted or* ***out of sequence***—faulty proteins are produced, leading to poor functioning and even genetic diseases. Likewise, if your 10 NSN health drivers aren't sequenced and supported in the best order, you won't function at peak efficiency. If even *one* lifestyle driver is deleted or out of sequence, you're risking loss of power in that driver—which impacts all other drivers, compromising optimal functioning and longevity.

With the Hoshin North Star Sequencing Process used in this book, you correctly sequence the 10 fundamental lifestyle drivers for peak health, performance and longevity. Leonardo da Vinci envisioned the ideal human in his iconic *Vitruvian Man*, one who's genetically intact and has mastered the art of quality living. **With proper lifestyle sequencing**, you'll become an ideal human and reclaim your vibrant Vitruvian nature and greatest potential.

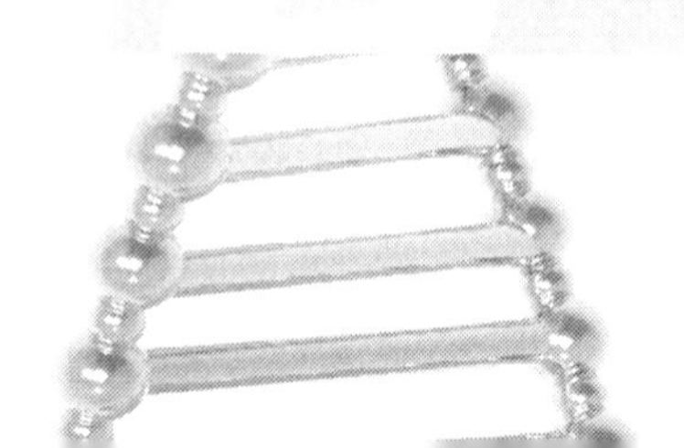

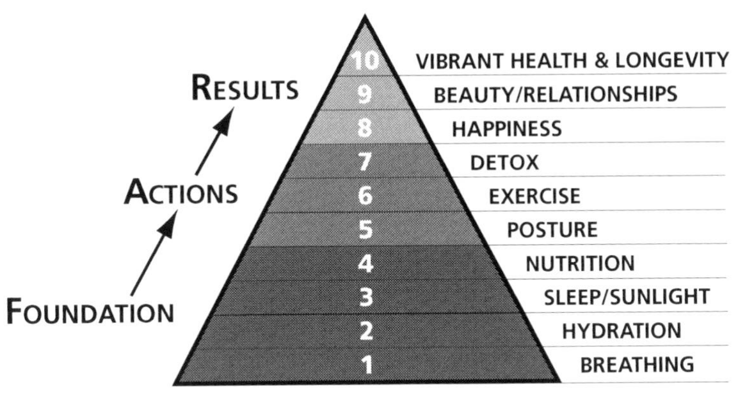

Hoshin GPS Bottom-up FAR Pyramid™ for Vibrant Health. As in Maslow's Pyramid, the Hoshin GPS FAR Pyramid™ highlights the fact that the lower **Mega**Nutrient priorities need to be satisfied in a sequential, bottom-up manner (**F**oundation–**A**ctions–**R**esults) in order to achieve and enjoy peak health and longevity.

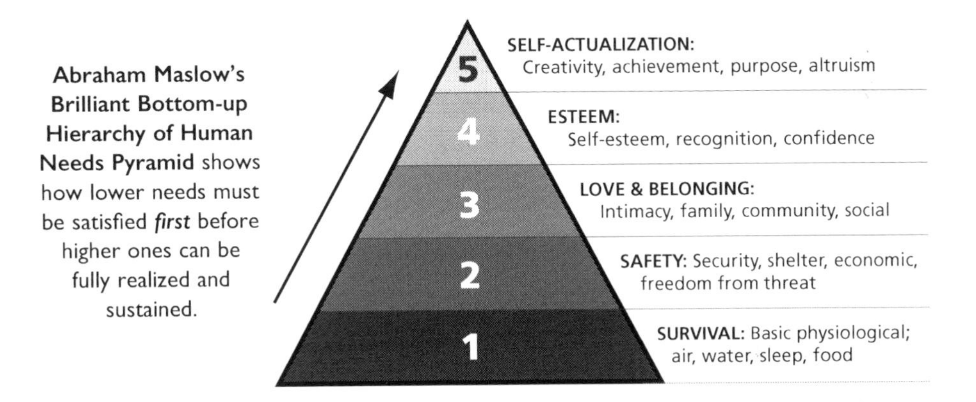

Abraham Maslow's Brilliant Bottom-up Hierarchy of Human Needs Pyramid shows how lower needs must be satisfied ***first*** before higher ones can be fully realized and sustained.

the **FAR** Pyramid graphically illustrates our optimal sequence of the key health and longevity priorities. Note that the sequence we arrived at is a direct reflection of our perspective, research and questions. You may come up with alternative prioritizations, depending on your perspective. Breathing is clearly the #1 health MegaNutrient, as death results from mere minutes of deprivation, yet some people can go 4 days or more without water before succumbing to dehydration. Sleeplessness becomes metabolically and cognitively deranging after just a few days, although some people can stay awake up to 10 days without dying. In fact, sleep is so essential that it ranks as our #3 lifestyle factor for health—surprisingly coming before nutrition and exercise, as people with adequate fat stores can go without food for months, and so on. *The remaining categories are all important for human life, yet are less essential to survive and thrive in the shorter term.*

By validating how essential the optimal sequence of breathing, hydration, sleep, sunlight, nutrition, posture, exercise and detox are for short-term health, we can extrapolate across the long-term to months, years, decades—a lifetime. Imagine how life-enhancing these same factors can be if *consciously* nurtured and cultivated, in the best prioritized

Foundation	Actions	Results
1. Breathing **2.** Hydration **3.** Sleep/Sunlight **4.** Nutrition	**5.** Posture **6.** Exercise **7.** Detox	**8.** Happiness **9.** Beauty/Relationships **10.** Vibrant Health & Longevity

Nature's Secret Nutrient's Hoshin GPS FAR (Foundational, Actions, Results) sequence for optimal health and longevity. Note that there is always overlap and cross-reinforcing integration between priority drivers.

sequence. Obviously, none of these life factors exist in a vacuum. All are at once singularly important, interrelated and continually cross-reinforcing one another. Air is a vital nutrient in its own right; at the same time it's clearly a vital thread woven through every other factor. Adequate hydration is necessary for proper respiratory function and oxygen uptake, while both adequate hydration and good respiratory function are necessary for refreshing, restorative sleep, and so on. When the optimal sequence of your vital health and longevity priorities is supported, it creates an exponential ripple effect resulting in *all* of the priorities being cross reinforced and enhanced over time. As the NSN Phi Musketeers would say, it's *All for One, One for All and All for All!*

It may be a surprise to see that Nutrition and Exercise were not in our top 3. However, our top 3 factors were revealed in relation to the strategic Hoshin GPS questions we posed. Alternative rankings are possible, if you ask different starting questions. Nutrition and Exercise are the two prime focus points of the majority of health-conscious people and of course the multi-billion dollar weight-loss and fitness movements. **Yet when sequenced through the Hoshin GPS process with our focus, the positions of Nutrition and Exercise came in at #4 and #6, respectively.** They are nevertheless obvious vital health factors interconnected with all others. In the race to monetize people's obsession with their weight and appearance, many foods, supplements, diets, exercise equipment and health programs are touted to achieve quick-fix cure-alls. Perhaps this is why there's been far less focus to-date on proper breathing, hydration, sleep, sunlight, posture and detox, relative to sound nutrition and exercise. Yet insufficient or poor quality of any of the other NSN **Mega**Nutrients—oxygen, hydration, sleep, sunlight, posture, detox—are under-appreciated yet key causal factors related to most all sub-optimal health and disease conditions, as well as compromised lifespan. A good Hoshin analogy is a combination lock code: *ALL numbers MUST be*

Like a combination lock, **all** health priorities must be lined up in the ***proper sequence*** to open the vault to healthy longevity. NSN is the master "Open Sesame" vitality password.

in the proper combination sequence or the lock will not open. Even if you have all the right numbers, if just ONE is out of sequence, no deal. The Hoshin GPS process confirms the optimal sequence of priorities to focus on for best results, both short *and* long term. To fully unlock their power and potential, ***all*** priorities must be properly supported by the foundational priorities preceding them. The secret to unlocking NSN's power is aligning the top health and longevity priorities in their optimal sequence. Once the top healthy longevity factors were prioritized, we could then group them into 3 key, simple categories for powerful implementation. Refer to the Hoshin GPS **FAR** Pyramid™ (**F**oundation, **A**ction, **R**esults) diagram opposite to see how our top health and longevity factors are prioritized for effective implementation. The **FAR** sequence holds great power when followed, which is why it guides the chapter sequence in this book and is used as a basis for the NSN Action Rx's and **Priority Coach** System.™

The First 15% Success Principle

The beginning is the most important part. **Plato**

The Hoshin GPS also reveals The **First 15% Principle**, which states that 85% of the results in any endeavor live in the First 15% or front-end of the journey; *that the foundation for success is in the beginning stages.* A little added early focus on the First 15% will produce greater results. It's similar to the 80/20 rule, in that it assures you're working on the right things in the right order to best launch any effort. In terms of NSN drivers, the First 15% suggests that if you could only work on two of the top drivers you'd get greatest impact from initially working on Drivers 1 & 2: **Breathing and Hydration**. That said, we recommend that you select at least one Rx from each of the 10 Rx chapters to fully support your success. The First 15% mirrors the beginning of a golden spiral, from a tiny start point unfolding to infinity. Get it right on the front end and the back end tends to fall into place; get it wrong and... well, you get the idea. Sony executive Teruaki Aoki's perfectly summed up the power of the First 15%: *If you do right in the upstream, the downstream will be much easier.* The First 15% helps you work

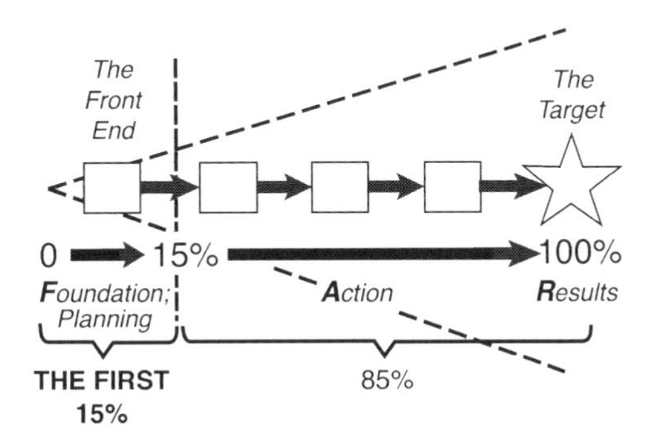

85% of the results are in the First 15% of the process. Better focus on the First 15%—*the front-end of any endeavor or process*—sets the stage for sustained progress, habit upgrade and long-term success.

smarter on the front end towards your aim, revealing the best first-things-first for success. It's like how an airline pilot carefully reviews his preflight checklist—*in sequence*—before taking off, to assure a safe flight. A great immediate and practical example:

To set a strong foundation for the day ahead, you need to build a strong First 15%—*the first 2 hours after waking*. What you do in those first 2 hours determines 85% or more of the success in your day. So review the first 6 NSN Drivers and aim to support each of the 6 in the first 2 hours of your day: **1.** Breathing: 5-8 Golden Ratio breaths. **2.** Hydration: 1-2 glasses of pure water within five minutes of waking. **3.** Sleep/ Sunlight: After a good night's sleep, synchronize your biological clock (biorhythms) with a 3-minute facial sun-bathing exercise (eyes closed). **4.** Nutrition: Have a Golden Ratio Zone (40/30/30 carb/protein/fat) breakfast. **5.** Posture: In a mirror, check spinal alignment from both front and side views. **6.** Exercise: Warm up for your day with easy exercise/stretching for 10+ mins.

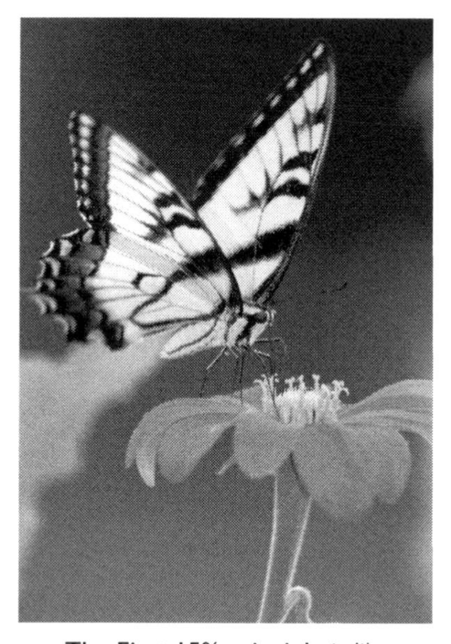

The First 15% principle is like the butterfly effect from chaos theory: *Small changes in the beginning of a process can create massive downstream effects,* e.g., the flapping of a butterfly's wings in Africa can cause a hurricane in Florida. **Likewise, small NSN habit changes can result in massive health, performance and longevity upgrades over time.**

The Hoshin GPS prioritizing process integrates the First 15%, as seen in how it revealed the optimal 1-10 chapter sequence of the NSN drivers in this book. We've applied the First 15% principal throughout the book to help you establish new healthy habits to activate NSN in your life, e.g., the Rx sections are organized so that the key First 15% Rx's start off each of the 10 Rx sections.

NSN Foundation, Actions, Results System: FAR

FOUNDATION: Knowledge Base. The core Foundation of this book is in the introduction and first 10 chapters, which provides the key NSN principles. With this Foundation in place you can successfully proceed to the Actions and Results sections, along the FAR sequence. The knowledge base **Foundation** supports the NSN **Action** Rx's—which become consistent habits via the Priority Coach system—to manifest the desired **Results** of peak health, performance and longevity.

ACTIONS: NSN Rx's. The Actions which activate Nature's Secret Nutrient are called Action Rx's. These are easy, targeted "prescriptions" that help you extract the essence of NSN, whether from the air you breathe, the food and water you consume, your exercise routine, posture or a great night's sleep. **Action Rx's are simple practices that tune your MegaNutrient sources to the Golden Ratio, the ultimate MetaNutrient.** You'll select a few Action Rx's to start. For example, an easy/effective NSN Breathing Rx has you inhale to a count of 3/exhale to a count of 5 for a few minutes daily (the ratio between Fibonacci numbers 3 and 5 results in a Golden Ratio of inhalation to exhalation). Your whole physiology elevates towards Golden Ratio balance via this practice. All NSN Action Rx's revolve around the principle of aligning with Nature's master Golden Ratio guidance system to extract maximum NSN. Again, it's like lining up the right numbers on the combination to the vault of vibrant health—with NSN, the lock opens. NSN applied is the secret "Open Sesame" password for maximum vitality. The good news for those who disdain math is that you won't need to do any calculations to do the Action Rx's.

Tracking Daily RESULTS: Your 21-Day Priority Coach. The Results of your Action Rx's are charted in the **Priority Coach** system over an initial 21-day period. This easy-to-use habit upgrade system keeps you focused on your daily health and performance priorities and activates NSN in your daily life and triggers an ongoing upgrade in your *whole life.* **Priority Coach** is featured in the back of the book as a paper version and as a smartphone app.

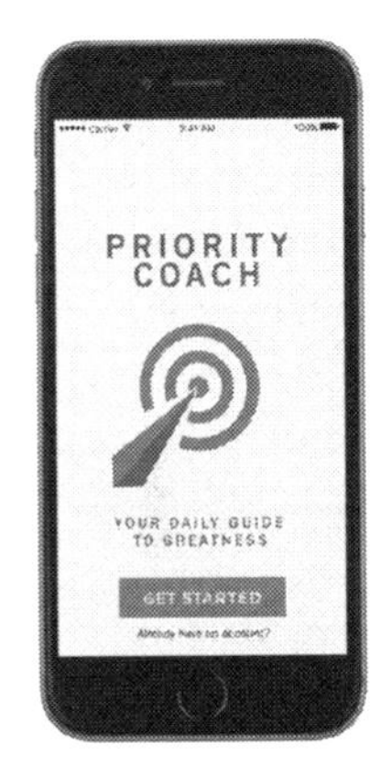

Priority Coach makes it fun and super easy to stay focused on, track and share your progress on your chosen top Action Rx's.

Congratulations for stepping up into the elite club of NSN pioneers!
You'll carry this secret of peak health, performance and longevity with you always. Following the sage advice of Thomas Edison, you'll step into the role of a *Doctor of the Future* by using NSN as the guiding principle for best care of your frame and as the basis for sound health, healing and nutritional therapy. NSN will become a new working paradigm you'll use for understanding the cause and prevention of disease—as well as for supporting your greatest health and happiest life journey.

Golden Ratio/NSN: Nature's Biomimicry Keys for Maximum Efficiency & Performance (*ⓘnfographics on next 2 page spreads*)

The two Golden Ratio infographics ahead show myriad Ratio examples across a vast spectrum. Nature and humanity utilize the Ratio for efficiency, beauty and strength in both form and function. The infographics reveal the Ratio's ubiquity and the vast potential Nature's Design Code infuses into health, performance and longevity. This Secret of the Ages is unveiled for the first time for your benefit.

The GoldenΦRatio (Phi Φ, 1.618...) is a mathematical construct, an irrational number without end (like Pi ϖ, 3.14...). It can't be expressed as a fraction, as its decimals repeat infinitely; it's thus mathematically impossible to pin the GoldenΦRatio down. Like perfection, it exists as a useful ideal only, a North Star guiding us in perfection's direction. Yet Nature and her creative offspring Homo sapiens found an elegant way to resolve this enigma: real-world approximations of the Golden Ratio via Fibonacci Ratios—ratios between successive numbers in the Fibonacci Sequence: 5:3, 8:5, 13:8, 21:13, 34:21, 55:34, 89:55, etc. Progressive Fibonacci Ratios reveal ever-closer approximations of the GoldenΦRatio 1.618. **For practical ease, the GoldenΦRatio & Fibonacci Ratio are used interchangeably in this book; NSN is a functional synergy of the two**.

Throughout history, innovative geniuses such as Albert Einstein and Alan Turing (father of modern computing & AI) were intrigued by the Fibonacci Sequence's predictive role in growth, patterns and form throughout Nature, e.g., the Sequence's über-efficient sunflower seed phyllotaxis distribution. These geniuses surmised that by mimicking Nature's use of Fibonacci Ratios, they could obtain multifaceted advantages in their pursuits. Herein lies the rub: not all humans make the intuitive, evolutionary jump allowing them to see and use this priceless gift of Nature. Skeptics question/attack the validity of the Ratio's application to human endeavors, saying it's just coincidental mathematics in Nature; that any evidence for its human value is fanciful thinking. Another criticism is that the Ratio, Nature's Universal Design Code, is not fully tested and thus an empty theory with nothing behind it. The Ratio's ubiquity isn't debatable to open minds; it's abundantly seen on Earth as well as across the Universe. With countless life forms embodying Fibonacci Ratios and Spirals, alignment with this Golden constant must carry a vital survival advantage. Charles Darwin's famous quote inspires us to ponder how the Ratio might imbue such evolutionary advantage:

It Is Not the Strongest of the Species that Survive, but the Most Adaptable.

Due to the Ratio's ubiquity in countless life forms, alignment with it clearly bestows a key advantage, helping them adapt, evolve and thrive into the present. We see evidence in the adaptation of animate forms to Earth's current conditions and in how inanimate forms like spiraling hurricanes, ocean waves and galaxies shape as they move through time and space. Adaptation and alignment to the Golden Ratio is described by Dr. Ronald Sandler as *Nature's Path of Least Resistance and Maximum Efficiency and Performance*. In other words, it's far easier to sail with the wind at your back vs. against it. This is precisely what innumerable life forms have done as they've evolved through eons of trial and error, validating that alignment with the Ratio is a super-efficient strategy to adapt to and master life's ever-changing circumstances. The art and science of **Biomimicry**—using Nature's form, function and patterns for innovation and problem solving—elegantly validates this premise. Broad scientific research confirms what we've suspected about the Ratio's adaptive and energetic advantages for decades. Six notable examples of scientists who've published serious research on Fibonacci Numbers and Golden/Fibonacci Ratios offers further validation:

- Φ **Jean-claude Perez, Ph.D.** discovered that *DNA coding utilizes the Fibonacci Sequence & Golden Ratio*. Together with Nobel Prize winner and HIV discoverer, **Professor Luc Montagnier** (1932-2022), they showed that the Corona virus SARS-Cov-2 lacked Fibonacci & Golden Ratio harmonics and thus was not a natural bat mutation transferred to humans, but a synthetically manipulated lab creation.
- Φ **Dr. Hanno Ulmer**, et.al. discovered that in well individuals a Golden Ratio between systolic and diastolic blood pressure *confers decreased mortality risk over time*.
- Φ **R. J. Tamargo, M.D.** and **J. A. Pindrik, M.D.** discovered *Golden Ratio relationships between the skull's cranial bones*. This compliments the brain's Golden Spiral shape and corresponding delta/theta/alpha/beta brain waves in Golden Ratio.
- Φ **Jasper Verguts, M.D.**, et.al., discovered that *the uterus is in 1.6 Golden Ratio height to width proportion* at peak fertility (ages 16-21).
- Φ **Dr. Ronald Sandler** discovered that by aligning training & resting cycles to Fibonacci Ratios, *peak performance is virtually guaranteed*—without injury or burnout.

Why wait decades for more research before using Nature's most powerful synergy agent *today*? Why not be *ahead* of the curve and herd and do what every life form on Earth has been doing for eons: use the Golden Ratio/NSN as the ultimate **Biomimicry Biohack**—the ultimate survival, evolution and transformation codex. Who *wouldn't* want to align with this life-enhancing principle, joining millions of fellow life-forms partaking of the free, vitalizing elixir that is NSN.

The Golden Φ Ratio

The Fibonacci Sequence is the Mathematical* [Biomimicry] *Code to Nature... It's a mathematical sequence that the whole universe is based on.

Joe Rogan, podcaster, comedian & ESPN host

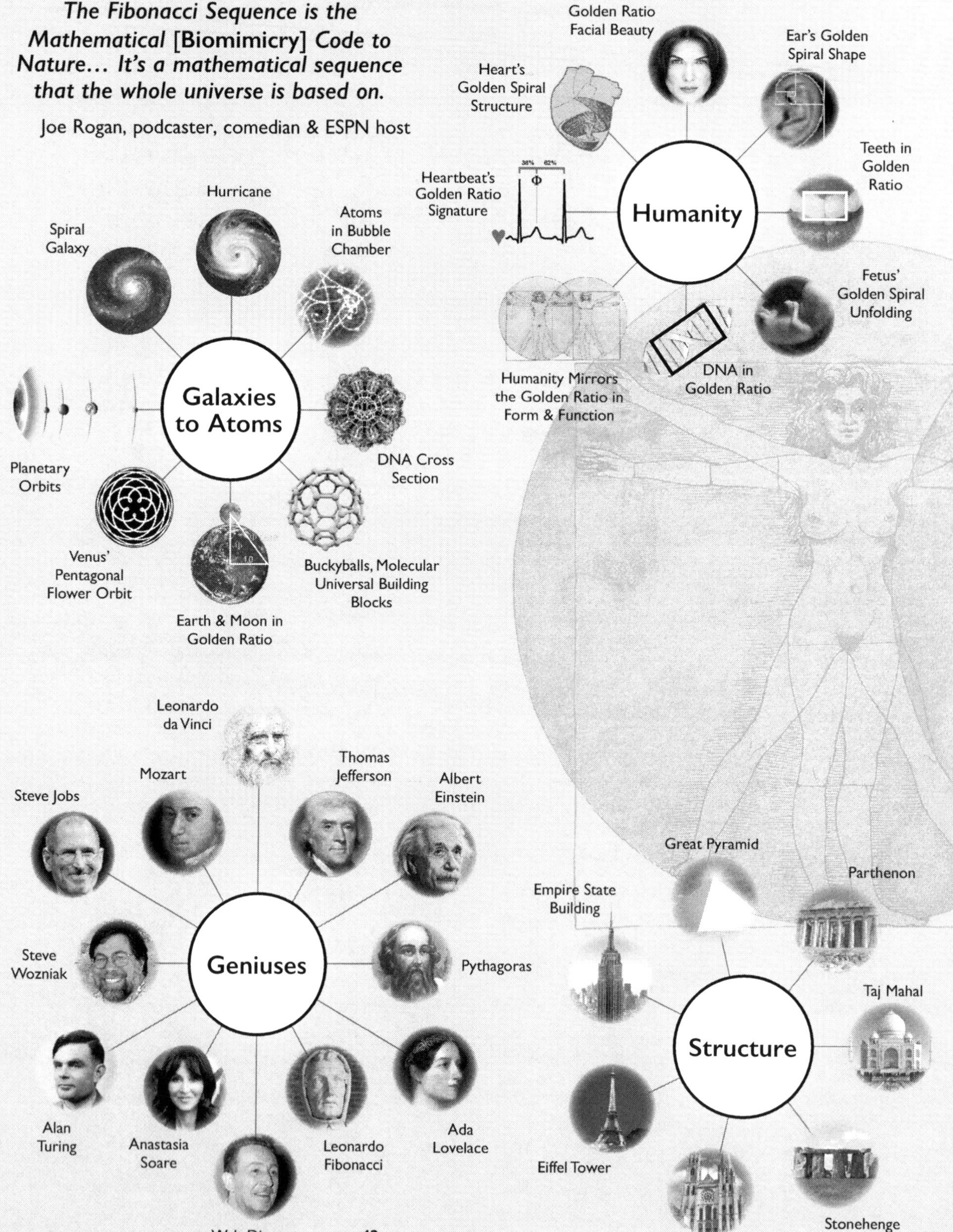

Throughout the Universe

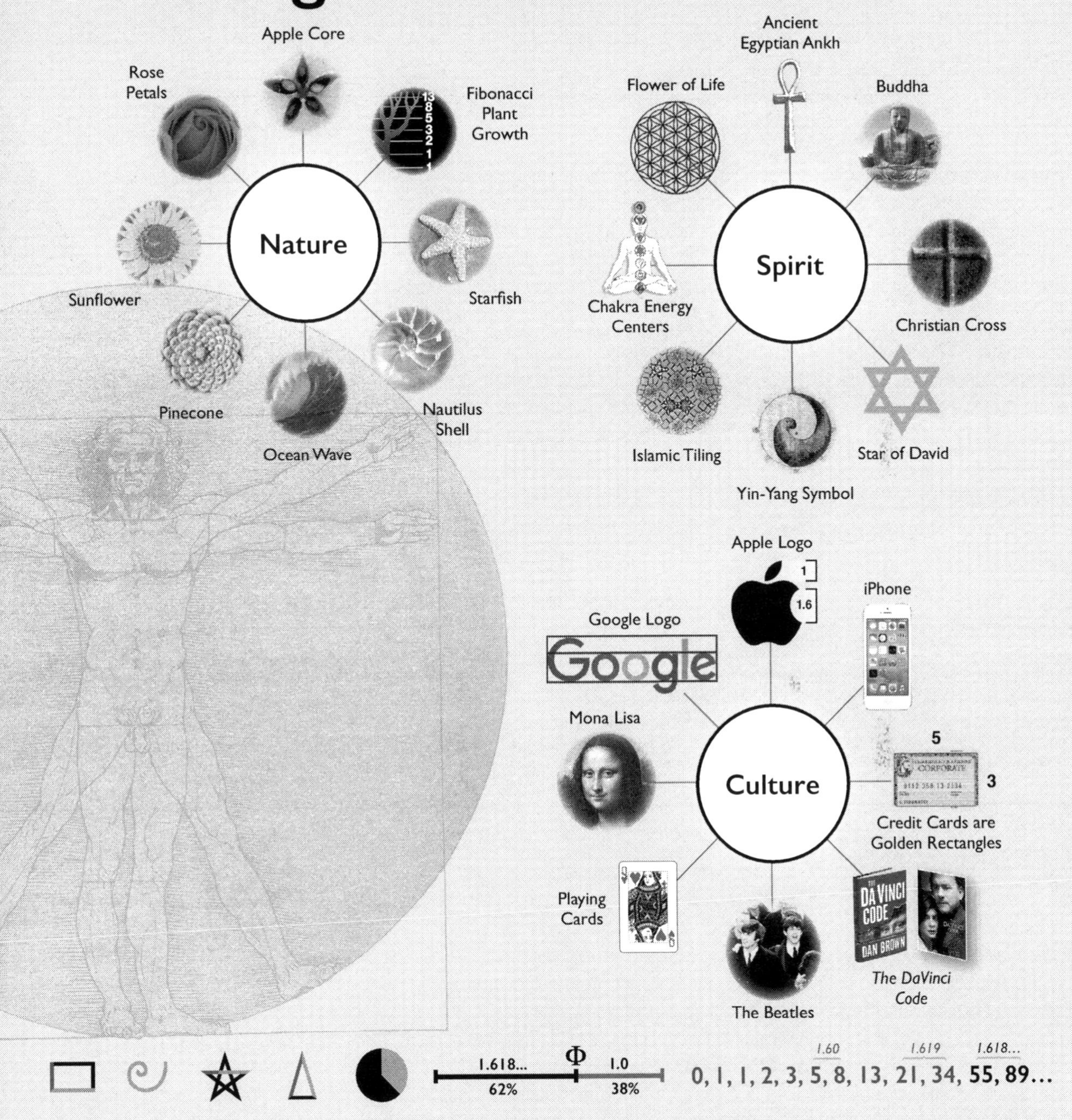

The Golden Ratio and Fibonacci Sequence are the fundamental principles behind the structure and movement of energy, life and matter in the Universe. They're two facets of Nature's master design code, defining a beautiful, super-efficient relationship or ratio between any two parts or objects, ***where the whole is greater than the sum of its parts.*** Mathematically known as the ratio of 1.618 to 1, this special relationship can be appreciated by looking at the infinite ways the Golden Ratio is expressed, from galactic to atomic, throughout Nature and humanity. The Ratio can be seen as beauty and efficiency in the structure and function of man, in culture, art, architecture, science and spirituality. The Golden Ratio was the secret ingredient inspiring geniuses like Pythagoras, Da Vinci, Einstein and others to manifest works that fueled the Renaissances, ancient and modern, that continue to drive humanity's evolution. To learn more, see the authors' companion book ***The Golden Ratio & Fibonacci Sequence***.

The Golden Φ Ratio Form

The Golden Ratio is the Basis of All Life and All Growth.

David Wilcock, author of *The Synchronicity Key*

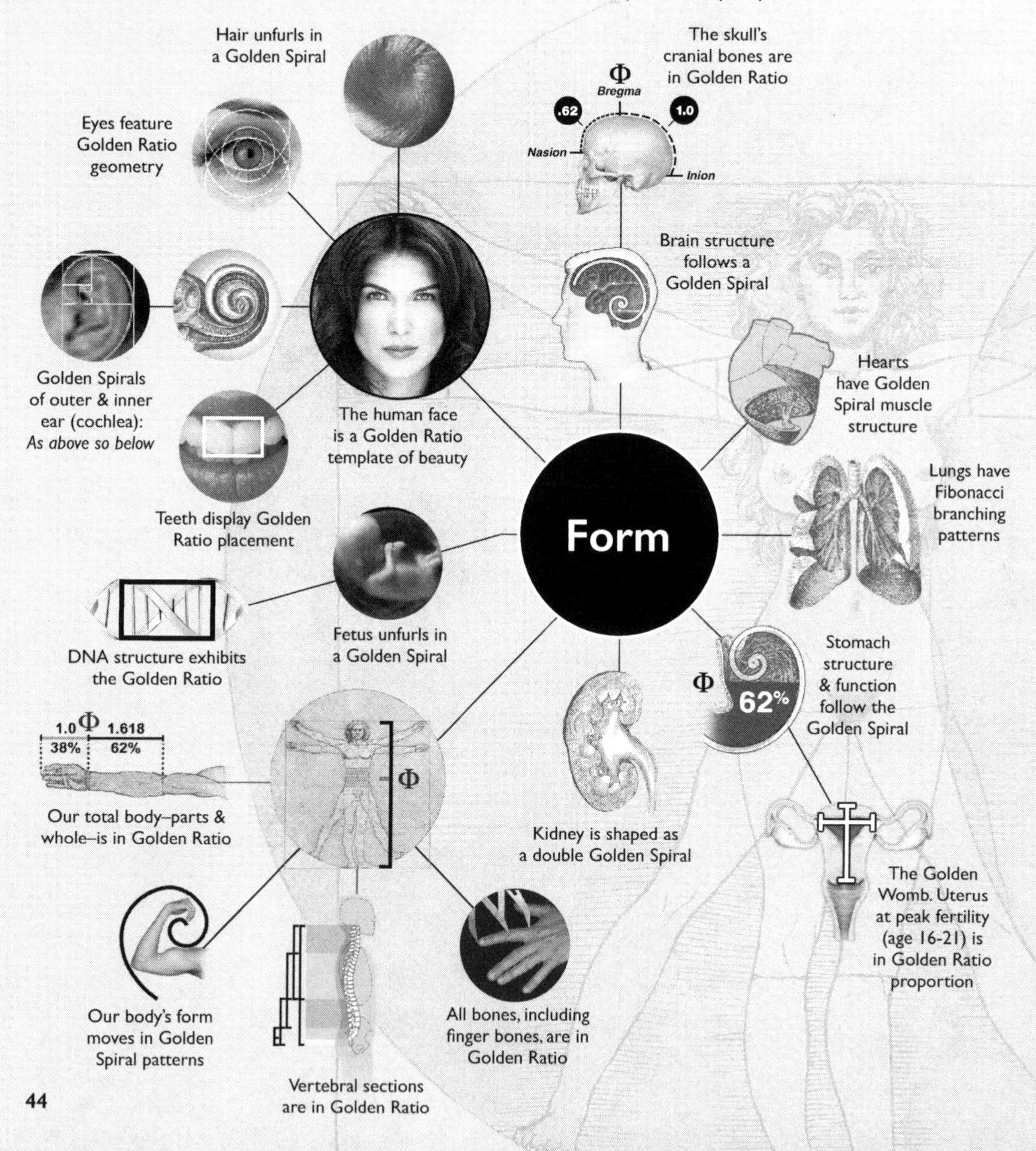

Hair unfurls in a Golden Spiral
The skull's cranial bones are in Golden Ratio
Φ
Bregma
.62
1.0
Nasion
Inion
Eyes feature Golden Ratio geometry
Brain structure follows a Golden Spiral
Hearts have Golden Spiral muscle structure
Golden Spirals of outer & inner ear (cochlea): *As above so below*
The human face is a Golden Ratio template of beauty
Lungs have Fibonacci branching patterns
Form
Teeth display Golden Ratio placement
DNA structure exhibits the Golden Ratio
Fetus unfurls in a Golden Spiral
Stomach structure & function follow the Golden Spiral
Φ
62%
1.0 Φ 1.618
38% 62%
Φ
Our total body–parts & whole–is in Golden Ratio
Kidney is shaped as a double Golden Spiral
The Golden Womb. Uterus at peak fertility (age 16-21) is in Golden Ratio proportion
Our body's form moves in Golden Spiral patterns
All bones, including finger bones, are in Golden Ratio
Vertebral sections are in Golden Ratio

The number of Golden Ratio-based human form and function design elements is astounding. These multiple Golden Ratio factors create an exponential effect, supporting the Ratio's unity function: *bringing parts together into a greater harmonious whole.* For example, your skeletal system has Golden Ratio relationships between one bone to the next, both in your long bones and spine. These fractal relationships allow your bones and muscles to move synergistically in Golden Ratio expression—the Golden Spiral. The Ratio is hard *and* soft-wired throughout your body, all they way down to your DNA, which guides the growing fetus to unfurl in a Golden Spiral. This spiral is also clearly visible in many organ shapes, including your ears, stomach, kidneys, heart muscle and even your brain's shape.

& Function of Humanity

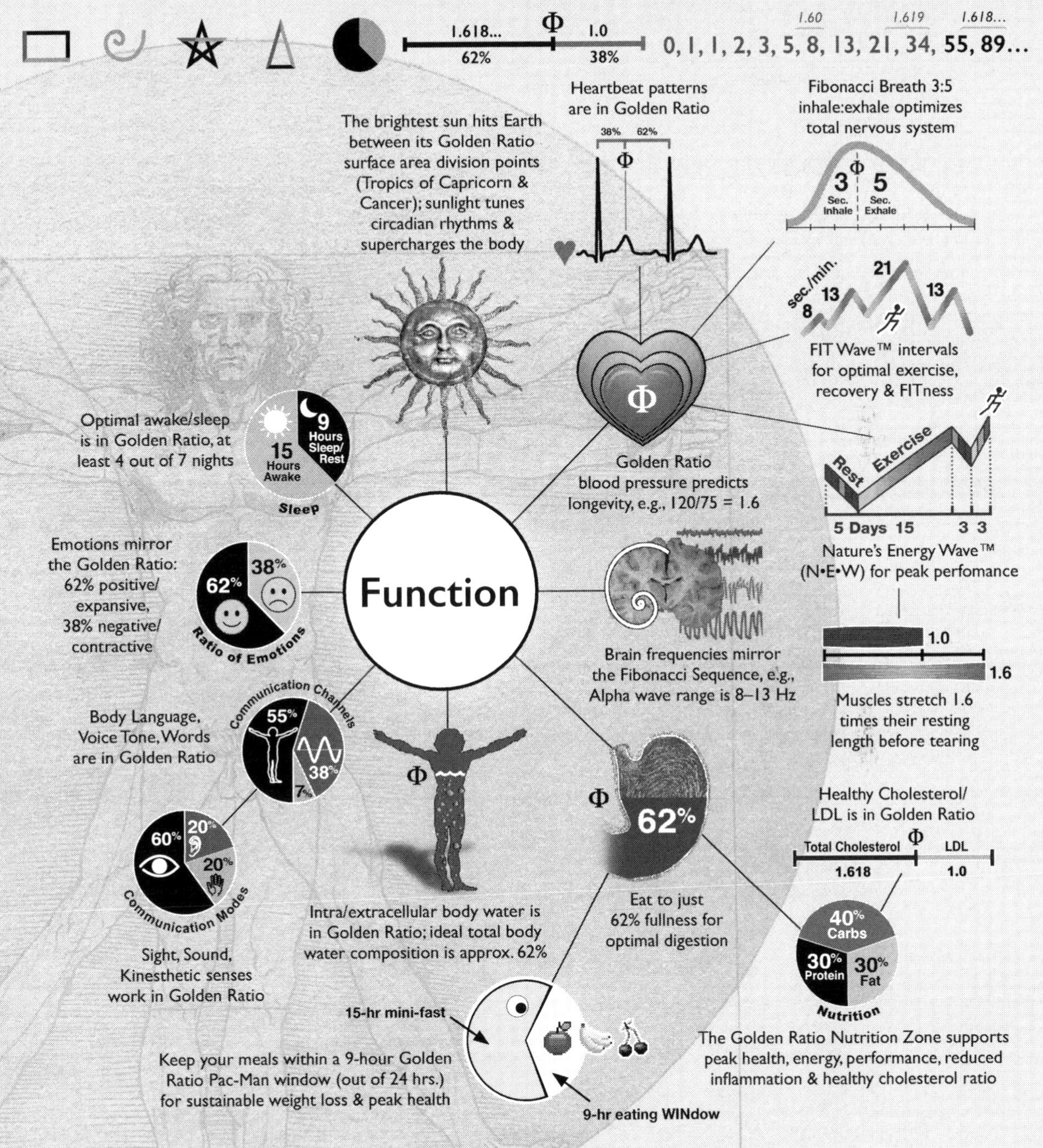

1.618...
Φ
1.0
62%
38%
1.60
1.619
1.618...
0, 1, 1, 2, 3, 5, 8, 13, 21, 34, 55, 89...
The brightest sun hits Earth between its Golden Ratio surface area division points (Tropics of Capricorn & Cancer); sunlight tunes circadian rhythms & supercharges the body
Heartbeat patterns are in Golden Ratio
38%
62%
Φ
Fibonacci Breath 3:5 inhale:exhale optimizes total nervous system
3
Sec. Inhale
5
Sec. Exhale
sec./min.
8
13
21
13
FIT Wave™ intervals for optimal exercise, recovery & FITness
Φ
Optimal awake/sleep is in Golden Ratio, at least 4 out of 7 nights
9 Hours Sleep/ Rest
15 Hours Awake
Sleep
Golden Ratio blood pressure predicts longevity, e.g., 120/75 = 1.6
Rest
Exercise
5 Days 15
3 3
Nature's Energy Wave™ (N•E•W) for peak perfomance
Emotions mirror the Golden Ratio: 62% positive/ expansive, 38% negative/ contractive
62%
38%
Ratio of Emotions
Function
Brain frequencies mirror the Fibonacci Sequence, e.g., Alpha wave range is 8–13 Hz
1.0
1.6
Muscles stretch 1.6 times their resting length before tearing
Body Language, Voice Tone, Words are in Golden Ratio
Communication Channels
55%
38%
7%
Φ
Φ
62%
Healthy Cholesterol/ LDL is in Golden Ratio
Total Cholesterol
Φ
LDL
1.618
1.0
60%
20%
20%
Communication Modes
Sight, Sound, Kinesthetic senses work in Golden Ratio
Intra/extracellular body water is in Golden Ratio; ideal total body water composition is approx. 62%
Eat to just 62% fullness for optimal digestion
40% Carbs
30% Protein
30% Fat
Nutrition
15-hr mini-fast
Keep your meals within a 9-hour Golden Ratio Pac-Man window (out of 24 hrs.) for sustainable weight loss & peak health
9-hr eating WINdow
The Golden Ratio Nutrition Zone supports peak health, energy, performance, reduced inflammation & healthy cholesterol ratio

All of these Golden Ratio-designed structures support your body parts and organs to function with maximum efficiency and health. Your essential life functions—from heartbeat to optimal breathing and sleep cycles—are all Golden Ratio aligned. It infuses your perceptive senses including sight, sound and feeling. Even your ideal body percentage of life-giving water is around 62%. By **Biomimicking** Nature you align more with the Golden Ratio, enjoying more energy, health and longevity. Once you infuse your daily activities with Nature's supreme health principle, the invisible Golden Ratio factor—Nature's Secret Nutrient/NSN—becomes your *secret regeneration agent.* This book is your golden key to NSN, the master health, performance and longevity elixir. Further explanation of the pictures and data shown is found in the authors' full-color companion book, ***The Golden Ratio & Fibonacci Sequence***.

2-minute NSN Self-Test (post)

This easy self-test quickly reveals where you stand today regarding the health priority MegaNutrients of the NSN system, to set up simple steps to rapidly upgrade your health, performance and longevity.

1. Rate yourself on the 0–4 frequency scale (top of opposite page) on your frequency **today** living the key NSN health and longevity practices.
2. Be honest and non-judgmental when rating yourself. Note your lowest scored items and commit to **raising them higher in the weeks ahead**.
3. When done, tally your score. Give lowest scored items a "*".
   Great News! *The lower your total score, the more you can improve in the coming weeks,* as you practice key elements of the NSN system.

Note your lower scored items and commit to raising the score on a select 1–3, *by even one point higher in the weeks ahead.* Challenge yourself: *this is one game you're guaranteed to win.* By learning and applying the Golden Ratio Biomimicry principles by which Nature operates, you'll ignite the power of the NSN Rx's to transform your health, happiness, performance and longevity. We recommend that you repeat this self-test on page 459, *after* you complete your initial 21-Day Priority Coach program. You'll undoubtedly see positive progress between your *before* and *after* scores.

Decode Your Results

85+: GREAT	You're doing really well. Aim for the top by closing any gaps to peak health, happiness, performance and longevity.
71–84: GOOD	You're on track—yet why not kick it up a notch? Are you ready to feel your best *and* live long and strong?
56–70: FAIR	You're hanging in there… yet why just hang? Step up to the plate, select the vital 1-3 biggest gaps to close and ***go for it.***
41–55: RISKY	This is your Life Wake Up Call. Will you answer the call?
40 or less: HELP!	You *do* want to ***keep*** enjoying the miracle of THIS life, don't you? If so, it's time to get serious—**Now.**

Deploy the *Triangulation Of Fire* principle: circle 3 of your lower scored items to focus on for the next 21 days. Select the appropriate Rx(s) from the NSN Action Rx section to lift your 3 chosen lower scored items. Re-test and compare your before and after scores in 21 days.

Self-Score	← LESS		FREQUENCY	MORE →	
	0	1	2	3	4

On a DAILY basis I: *Ch.*

		Ch.
1. ______	Breathe with awareness, taking deep breaths throughout my day.	1
2. ______	Drink at least 1 large glass of pure water upon arising.	2
3. ______	Use filtered pure water for drinking.	
4. ______	Keep my urine in the pale yellow to clear range—no darker than Chardonnay.	
5. ______	Get between 7.5–9 hours quality sleep at least 4 nights a week.	3a
6. ______	Take a relaxation break or short nap to recharge & reset once a day.	
7. ______	Get outdoor sunlight on my face for a few minutes soon after arising.	3b
8. ______	Have a healthy breakfast within 3 hours of arising (a quality smoothie counts).	4
9. ______	Eat only about two-thirds full at meals.	
10. ______	Include SuperFoods in my diet, e.g., greens, berries, chia seeds, ginger, turmeric, kelp, green tea, dark chocolate, red wine, fish oil, nutritional yeast, spirulina, probiotics, etc.	
11. ______	Maintain a trim abdomen (a vital health & longevity indicator).	
12. ______	Am mindful of my posture during the day, keeping my spine relaxed & tall.	5
13. ______	Exercise 3–4+ times a week.	6
14. ______	Include strength, endurance & flexibility training in my regular exercise regimen.	
15. ______	Have a well-formed, easy bowel movement at least once daily.	7
16. ______	Do regular detox, e.g., deep breathing, exercise, sauna sweating, colon/liver cleansing.	
17. ______	Experience joy, happiness and satisfaction as my predominant emotions.	8
18. ______	Practice daily meditation, centering, presence, prayer and/or mindfulness.	
19. ______	Consistently enjoy my work.	
20. ______	Am happy with my ratio of work to free time.	
21. ______	Express gratitude daily (e.g., for my body, my life & the good people & things in it).	
22. ______	Use only non-toxic/organic cleansers & moisturizers on my face & skin.	9
23. ______	Am happy with my romantic life.	
24. ______	Connect regularly with positive people I care about who care about me.	10
25. ______	Have an inspiring, energizing purpose in my life.	

Total

Breathing: #1 driver for robust health & longevity

What do people & cars have in common? Both require **oxygen, the master catalyst** to ignite & burn their fuel.

Low energy? Deep breathing of healthy air ignites your **cellular engines** (mitochondria), generating ATP—the universal energy molecule.

The **Golden Ratio breathing** technique—breathe in to 3, breathe out to 5—is an easy way to access Nature's Secret Nutrient/NSN.

Your breathing & heart function are both **guided & harmonized** by the Golden Ratio.

What is the #1 predictor of human longevity? High **Vital Capacity** (VC)—the volume of a full breath out.

Low cellular oxygen is a major cause of disease, resulting from polluted air, poor posture & shallow breathing.

You're only as good as your last breath—so **make each breath count**. Breathe with awareness to live with awareness. Breath is Life!

Your lungs are designed with multiple Golden Ratios for **greater efficiency**.

Learning how to extract NSN from your breath is the #1 secret to a long and robust Life.

Robert D. Friedman, M.D. & Matthew Cross

1

Breathing

Oxygen is the giver of life.

Otto H. Warburg, M.D.,
biochemist & Nobel Prize winner

Breathing. It's our first act upon entering the world and our last upon leaving. Yet even though our breath (like our heartbeat) is the continuous pulse of our entire life, so often we breathe with *zero* conscious awareness—resulting in insufficient, shallow breathing over time and chronic hypo (low) oxygenation. This leads to accelerated aging, subpar performance, lower life quality and premature death, with often chronic disease along the way (most diseases thrive in low oxygen/ anaerobic environments). ***Remember, you're only as good as your last breath.*** This means you can step right back into healthy breathing with your next breath. To top it off, the ancients taught that the life-giving oxygen we breathe is also imbued with prana (life force). Perhaps best of all, *breathing is still free!* In this chapter, we'll explore the profound power of increasing the quality and quantity of oxygen intake in your daily life, with the vast power of Nature's Secret Nutrient—the Golden Ratio—as your super-charging life guide for maximizing MegaNutrient #1.

So let's begin by taking, through your nose, a nice deep b r e a t h ....

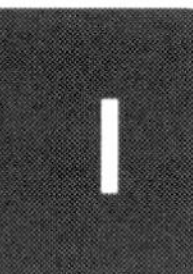

ABC's of Healthy Breath & Circulation

Most everyone is familiar with the ABC's of CPR (Cardio-Pulmonary-Resuscitation): Airway, Breathing, Circulation. These are the life-saving techniques used in cases of cardiac arrest or other life-threatening emergencies. Since these three critical aspects of maintaining life are of the utmost importance in an acute situation, it stands to reason that they might also be important (although overlooked) factors in supporting life in every moment. These automatic, unconscious functions of breathing and blood circulation are critical factors in either manifesting peak health—**thriving**—or struggling along with less than optimal wellbeing—**surviving**. Your health and longevity is dependent on a cardiopulmonary system (heart and lungs) that can harmoniously handle constant activity and stress from birth to death. Nature's Secret Nutrient can expand the range and efficiency in which your heart, lungs and circulatory system function. Breathing and circulation are intimately connected via the Golden Ratio—and in good health they work together in perfect harmony. Without good respiratory function, a good cardiovascular system isn't of much value, and vice versa. Since breathing is the number one driver in the Nature's Secret Nutrient hierarchy, it's imperative to take full advantage of this critical energizer and life giver. **If there's one thing that you take away from this book, let it be the knowledge of how to access and amplify the Golden Ratio through your breath**. Our bodies have set up an ingenious anatomical and physiological leverage system by harnessing the Golden Ratio. This system can be activated via the simple act of taking deep, conscious breaths tuned to the Golden Ratio, as shown in the Fibonacci/Golden Ratio Breath on p. 53. *Breath Is Life*, as yogi/lifestyle coach Gurumarka Khalsa notes. We can enhance both the quality and quantity of our lives by breathing consciously, enriching our breath often with Nature's Secret Nutrient.

Your Vital Capacity (VC): #1 Predictor of Longevity

He lives most life whoever breathes most air.

Elizabeth Barrett Browning

Through the Hoshin North Star process, breathing was determined to be driver #1 and thus the vital foundation for optimal health and longevity. Not surprisingly, there is key corroborating data from longevity science supporting this premise. **Your Vital Capacity (VC) is a measurement of how much air you can breathe out, after a maximal inhalation.** As it turns out, *VC is also the #1 predictor of life span and longevity.* By looking at the relationship between Vital Capacity and age, we are immediately drawn to one of the most important studies ever performed in the field of

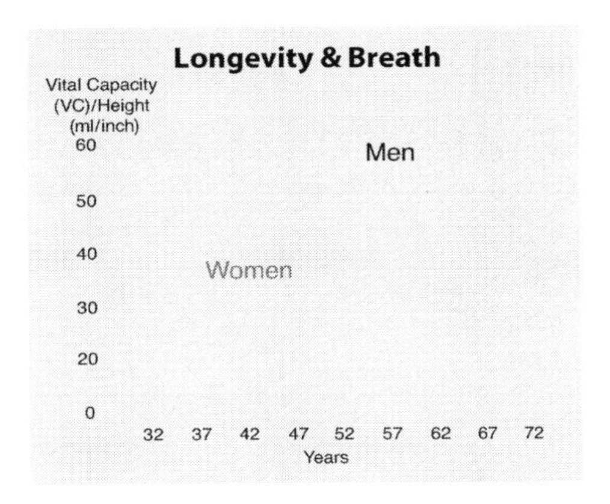

Vital Capacity (VC) decreases with age and is the #1 predictor of life span and longevity. VC is the amount of air that can be exhaled after a full inhalation and can be increased with Golden Ratio breathing techniques. (Framingham Study, 1948-68; after Walford: *Beyond the 120 Year Diet;* originally from Kannel/Hubert, 1982)

longevity. The Lung Capacity Graph above is adapted from the renowned Framingham Study and shows that Vital Capacity VC) decreases in direct relationship with age in both men and women. By continuously investing in growing your Vital Capacity, you can effectively increase your longevity quality *and* quantity. With this singular direct measure, an accurate prediction can be made about any individual's remaining lifespan. Longevity researcher **Roy Walford, M.D.** noted the importance and inference of this relationship:

> *People with low VC for their age did not live as long on the average as those with high VC, and as we have learned, predictability is the most important indicator that a biomarker is measuring true 'functional' age.*

"Functional" age is your true physiological age as opposed to your chronological age. For example, if you were 50 with a low Vital Capacity, we could extrapolate from the data above and predict that your true functional or physiologic age would be much older. We'd want to then intervene with some key Nature's Secret Nutrient Action Rx's to see if we could lower your functional age. Not surprisingly, many studies have documented that Vital Capacity can be increased and presumptive functional age lowered through mindful deep breathing exercises such as yoga and meditation, with an emphasis on breathing through your nose vs. your mouth. The mechanism for increasing your Vital Capacity includes improving chest expansion and strengthening respiratory muscles via effective practices such as NSN Lung Yoga (see Rx 2, p. 307).

Golden Ratio Anatomy of Your Lungs

The anatomic structure of your lungs also follows the Golden Ratio. Indeed, your breath moves in spiraling wave motions as it travels through your Golden Ratio-designed airways, mirroring the wind and water currents found in Nature. The asymmetrical nature of your anatomy, including your lungs, follows the Fibonacci Ratios embedded in your anatomic structure. We need to re-envision ourselves as not being just 50/50 beings. Left and right asymmetry gives rise to the spiraling, dynamic energy that animates us. Indeed, you have left and right lungs that are divided into segments that reflect the Fibonacci Sequence: your left lung has 2 lobes and your right lung has 3 lobes. Remember that 2 and 3 are numbers early in the Fibonacci Sequence: 0,1,1,**2**,**3**,5,8,13… Not only do the lobes of your lungs reflect the Fibonacci Sequence, your bronchial tubes do, as well. As Robert Prechter, Jr. describes in *Pioneering Studies in Socionomics (2003),*

> *In the early 1960s, Drs. E.R. Weibel and D.M. Gomez meticulously measured the architecture of the lungs and reported that the mean ratio of short to long tube lengths for the fifth through seventh generations of the bronchial tree is 0.62, the Fibonacci ratio. Researchers Bruce West and Ary Goldberger have found that the diameters of the first seven generations of the bronchial tubes in the lung decrease in Fibonacci proportion.*

This precise Fibonacci branching pattern allows for a huge amount of surface area for the exchange of O_2 and CO_2. The surface area of the alveoli—the tiny air sacs at the end of each bronchiole—would be the equivalent of slightly less than **half the surface area of a singles tennis court**. Even more amazing is the fact that there are close to 620 miles of capillaries surrounding the alveoli to facilitate efficient air exchange (note that the number 620 is a multiple of the rounded Golden Ratio of .618 or .62).

NSN Biomimicry Medicine: Tapping Nature's Prime Life Principle

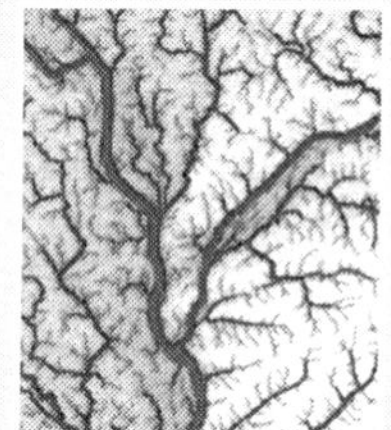
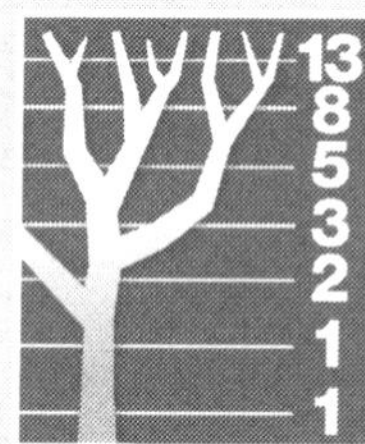

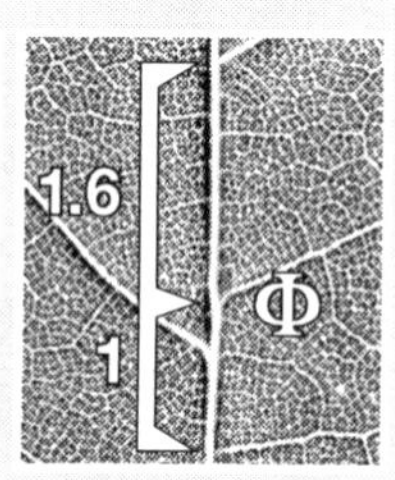

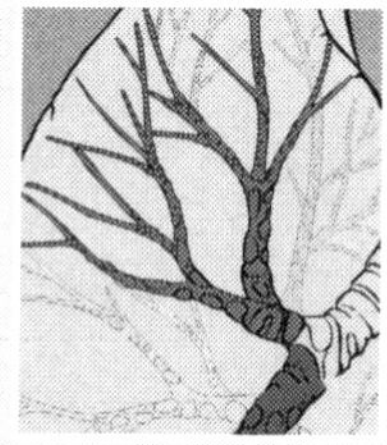
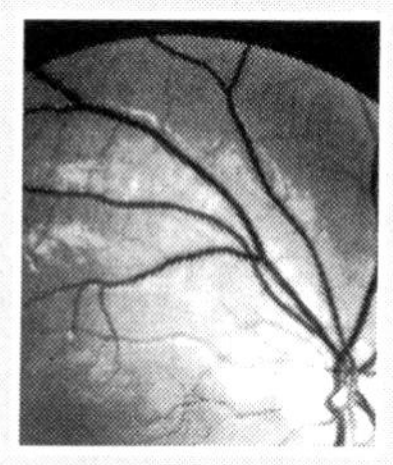

(*L–R*): 1. River branching. 2. Tree/Plant branching w/ Fibonacci ratios. 3. Leaf veins w/ Golden Ratios optimize plant respiration. 4. Lung bronchial branching. 5. Circulatory system branching (retina).

The ubiquitous Golden/Fibonacci Ratio branching pattern is evident across all living systems. Through the evolutionary process, Nature biomimics herself through Golden Ratio fractal scaling, aka the *As Above/So Below principle*. This self-similar branching pattern reflects Nature's timeless quest for *the most efficient path* to deliver life force via air, water and nutrients in living systems. Utilizing NSN Rx's, we can consciously biomimic Nature by integrating Golden Ratio principles into our daily lives. This is the first time in history that this revolutionary approach, NSN & Biomimicry Medicine, has become available for achieving peak health, performance and longevity.

1

Beyond Oxygen: The Fibonacci Golden Ratio Breath Calms & Charges Your Body/Mind in Seconds

An easy, powerful way to optimize your oxygen (O_2) uptake and carbon dioxide (CO_2) exchange is by using a 3 second inhalation to 5 second exhalation ratio. This 3:5 ratio sends a strong Golden Ratio signal reverberating through your body, upgrading your physiology to a more integrated and harmonious level. Breathing through your nose vs. mouth is recommended, as it filters the air and activates and synergizes brain, body and mind.

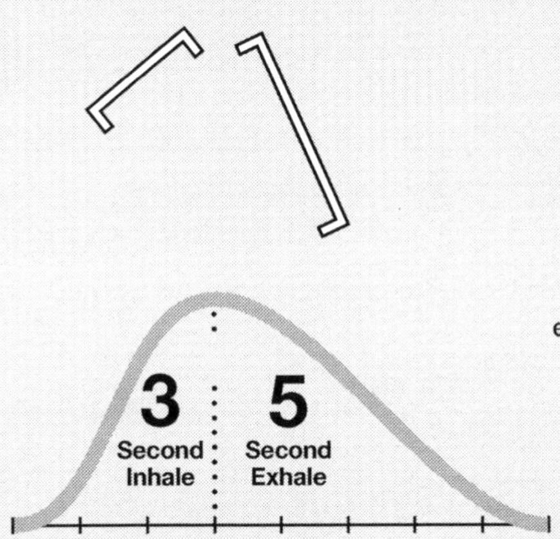

In addition to having 2 left lobes and 3 right lobes, your lungs display bronchial segment lengths in Fibonacci/Golden Ratios, resonating down to the alveolar level (alveoli are the tiny air sacks at the end of each bronchiole).

Breathing is NSN's #1 health, performance & longevity driver, so if you only had time for *one* exercise to enhance your total health, the Fibonacci/Golden Ratio Breath would be it. **The breath is simple: inhale to 3... exhale to 5.....** Exhalation decreases heart rate, through parasympathetic nerve activation; conversely, inhalation increases heart rate. It's the Golden Ratio differential between inhalation and exhalation that enhances Heart Rate Variability (HRV), balances your nervous system and fills you with profound calmness and vibrant energy. A pulse monitor shows an immediate heart rate drop during exhalation (the 5 second exhale in a 3:5 breath). As your lung capacity increases, try moving to higher Fibonacci Breath Ratios, e.g., 5:8, 8:13, for greater vitality & equanimity. To enhance O_2 & CO_2 exchange and enjoy an added boost, pause for 3, 5 or 8 seconds at the top & bottom of each breath. Breathe especially deeply in remote, natural settings where the air is higher quality, ionically charged and pure. See Breathing Rx 1, p. 305 for more information on putting this principle to work.

Golden Ratio Lung Physiology

Each of the top categories in the Nature's Secret Nutrient has built within it a detoxification phase in order to maintain Golden Ratio balance of intake and output. In the case of breathing, the number-one driver, your lungs bring in fresh oxygen, while at the same time releasing carbon dioxide—CO_2. The exhalation phase of breathing not only gets rid of carbon dioxide, it also helps to regulate our vital acid/alkaline balance. Without adequate respiration, not only will our cells be starved of oxygen, but there will be a backup of metabolic acids, causing adverse health effects.

The rate of breathing is of course dependent on whatever our activity demands are at any given time. We continuously sense both oxygen and CO_2 levels. When we're exercising, we breathe faster and when we're at rest we naturally breathe slower. Our body's Divine intelligence has the ability to dynamically change in response to the demands of the moment. With each heartbeat, blood delivers oxygen (O_2) and absorbs carbon dioxide (CO_2) at the cellular level and reverses the process in our lungs. A dynamic interaction between lung and heart activity (breathing and circulation) is required for efficient cellular respiration to occur. At rest, a general rule of thumb is that the ratio of respirations (breaths) to heartbeats x 10 approximates the Golden Ratio of 1.618:

(Respirations ÷ Heartbeats) x 10 = 1.6 Φ

For example, a person with a respiratory rate of 12 breaths per minute and a resting heart rate of 75 beats per minute will have this ratio:

12 ÷ 75 x 10 = 1.6 Φ

This Golden Ratio of respiration to heart rate may not hold during intense exercise or if one crosses the anaerobic threshold, yet the natural Golden Ratio pulse will reestablish itself during the recovery phase. Where most people get into trouble is when they're at rest and tend to *hypo*ventilate or under-breathe. Over-breathing or *hyper*ventilation is a less common, temporary occurrence and is typically caused by anxiety. Under-breathing or hypoventilation is usually exacerbated by poor posture, where rounded shoulders and a caved-in chest inhibit deep and adequate respirations. When one isn't breathing deeply enough, acidity develops in the blood which then forces the kidneys to get rid of the excess acids. Over time, this stress moves even deeper into one's physiology, putting stress on endocrine glands and even dips into mineral buffers in your bones to keep the acid/base balance in your blood normal. The wisdom of your body is programmed with many different physiological Golden Ratio set points (homeostasis/rheostasis).

Your body is constantly striving to keep all of your physiologic set points in Golden Ratio balance, including O_2/CO_2, acid/base, blood sugar levels, hormones, blood pressure, temperature, hydration, etc.

> *For breath is life, and if you breathe well you will live long on earth.*
> **Sanskrit Proverb**

Extreme Hypoventilation: David Blaine's World Record Breath Hold

Natural Golden Ratio respiratory set points can be artificially changed through training, as in the case of certain athletic endeavors. *The Oprah Winfrey Show* was the stage for the 4/30/08 world record breath-hold by Houdini-inspired magician David Blaine. Blaine demonstrated his skill for Assisted Static Apnea: the length of time a person can hold their breath *after breathing pure oxygen.* Blaine's record-setting time? An amazing 17 minutes, 4 seconds, shattering the previous record of 16 minutes, 32 seconds set by Peter Colat. Blaine was able to suppress his instinctual respiratory impulse long enough to set a new world record. David Blaine utilized a technique called air gulping, where he was able to increase the amount of oxygen he could take in to his lungs and thereby hold his breath longer. We don't need to go to that extreme to increase our respiratory capacity. What we're after is simply making sure that we don't hypoventilate and that our lungs are well ventilated with oxygen and that the CO_2 doesn't build up in our system. The most efficient way to do that is by taking full, deep breaths, both inhalation and exhalation. There is a lot of leftover air in our lungs at the end of each breath that we can expel by squeezing our abdominal muscles. Getting rid of that stale air is

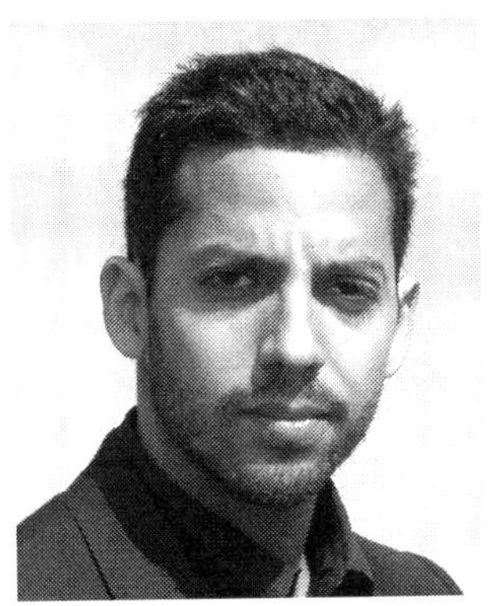

David Blaine, world-renowned magician, illusionist and record-setting breath holder.

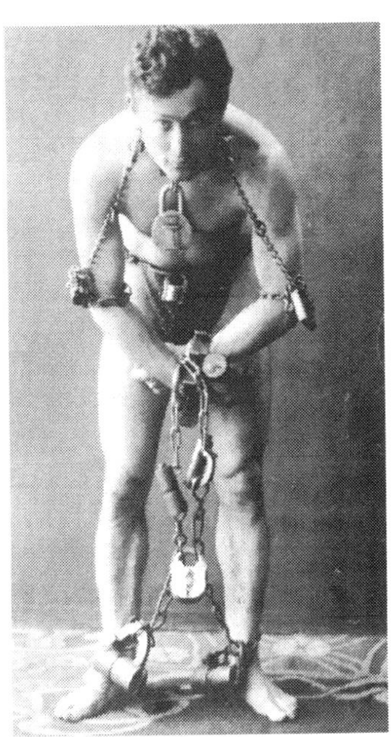

Legendary escape artist and magician Harry Houdini in 1899. Houdini was the *inspiration* for many of David Blaine's death-defying feats, including his 2008 record-setting breath hold.

the only way to make room for the next breath of fresh air. Practicing Lung Yoga (in the Rx section of this book) is a simple and effective way to get rid of stale air and build your lung's Vital Capacity. There is only one difference between David Blaine's willed apnea and the average person's shallow breathing or hypoventilation: Blaine's respiratory suppression was intentionally trained, while the average person's lack of respiratory drive is largely unconscious and exacerbated by factors like poor posture, polluted air and inactivity. Even though Blaine suffered no apparent ill effects from his stunt, the average person over time will suffer many low-grade symptoms like fatigue, malaise and poor mental and physical performance resulting from poor breathing habits. Hypoventilation and decreased oxygen levels can also set the stage for many chronic, degenerative conditions. These facts ought to inspire us all to become conscious, mindful deep breathers as opposed to breathing shallowly on autopilot.

Stig Severinsen: Superhuman Breath-Holder

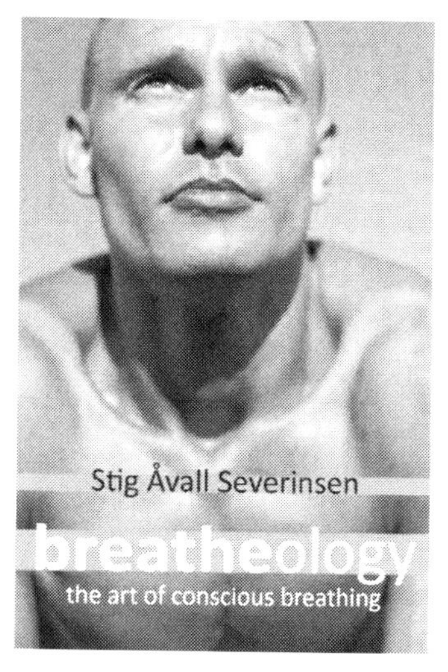

World-record breathholder and freediver Stig Severinsen, on the cover of his book *Breatheology: The Conscious Art of Breathing.*

Danish world champion breath-holder and diver Stig Severinsen set a *Guinness World Record* in May, 2012 with an astounding assisted static apnea breath-hold of 22 minutes, eclipsing David Blaine's 17:04 set just a few years earlier, live on *Oprah*. Stig was able to accomplish this feat by using his own version of Lung Yoga—which he calls *Breatheology*—to expand his lungs and thereby retain more oxygen. Regarding his remarkable lung expansion, Stig commented in a *60 Minutes* interview,

> *I have quite big lungs...8 plus liters. Because of this training, I can pump in more air and reach about 14 liters.*

Expanding the lungs as much as Stig does is impressive, but could it be dangerous? We know that muscle tissue can lengthen to a Golden Ratio of 1.6 times its resting length before tearing, according to myofascial release pioneer Aaron Mattes (see Ch 6 Exercise). Just like muscle tissue that can tear with over-stretching, lung tissue can rupture like an over-filled balloon with too much air. For a simple example, if we assume Stig's 8-plus liters pre-training air volume to be 8.6 liters, that would give a perfect Golden Ratio increase in lung volume when compared to the post-expansion volume of 14 liters (14 ÷ 8.6 = 1.62). Stig's comment about expanding his lung volume to 14 liters from 8 plus liters makes us

Stig's Emergency Air Pollution Avoidance Technique

At times, it can be quite appropriate to hold your breath. If you're behind the exhaust of a bus or truck, it is the most natural thing in the world for me not to breathe. Some may think this is stretching it a bit far, yet when you consider the amount of particle pollution we are exposed to every day in cities, it is not totally crazy.

Stig Severinsen, world record freediver & breath holder; author of *Breatheology*

realize that he had very likely reached his extreme of lung expansion possible without rupturing or tearing his lungs. Although dangerous, his Golden Ratio lung expansion was also the critical biohacking factor that allowed him to access vast yet latent physiologic reserves, enabling his superhuman performance. The lung Vital Capacity graph on p. 51 reveals that increased lung volume is directly correlated with longevity—yet there are profound short-term benefits as well. People from all walks of life have shown dramatic and rapid improvements in health and performance from learning the science of breathing and breath-holding. Stig has retired from competitive pursuits and now focuses on teaching Breatheology or as they say in Danish—*Andedraet* (pronounced "on-ah-drot"). **According to Stig, the Danish understanding of breathing is often translated as "regulating the spirit," or breathing as a bridge to spiritual and life growth and evolution.** Breathing science has always had a spiritual connection, e.g., the ancient sanskrit word for air, *prana*, speaks of the vital life energy air carries and imparts through the breath. When we examine more closely the word Breatheology, we see that it's composed of four parts: Breath/Breathe, Theo, and -ology. The expanded meaning is the **Study of Breath as the Connecting Thread to God.** So, refining the breath or "regulating the spirit" is what Stig is really teaching his students through his Breatheology technique and philosophy. Stig was once asked what the human limit to breath-holding might be. He answered that it was probably around 30 minutes. His prediction moves ever-closer to reality, as his own assisted static apnea world record has since been eclipsed by 3 people: Goran Colak, 23:01 (June 2014), Aleix Segura, 24:03 (February 2016) and current *Guinness World Record* holder Budimir Šobat, a 55-year-old free diver from Croatia with a time of 24:37 (March 2021). Stig set the under-ice swim record of 250 feet/76.2 meters in April 2013, exceeding Iceman Wim Hof's previous world record by 47.6 feet/14.5 meters (see Ch 10 Longevity).

Stig retired from chasing under-water breathing records after his 2013 under-ice world record. Although we don't yet have long-term data on the health of professional breath-holders, Stig likely surmised that there was a high potential of brain damage with

Dr. Roy Walford: Caloric Restriction, Oxygen Malnutrition & The Danger of Out Of Order Priorities

Dr. Roy Walford, M.D. (1924-2004) lived to the unripe old age of 79, just slightly above the average life expectancy for U.S. males. He was one of the world's most brilliant life extension scientists, with over 340 published articles. Dr. Walford's research showed that simply cutting the caloric intake of laboratory mice in half doubled their expected life span. The Biosphere 2 experiment gave him the opportunity to put caloric restriction to the test on himself and his crew when food stores ran unexpectedly low. When the Biosphere crew severely restricted their calories, they had amazing improvements in their blood pressure, blood sugar and cholesterol levels.

Yet the obvious question is: *If caloric restriction is so great, why didn't Walford live to 90, 100 or beyond?* The answer is revealed when Walford's entire protocol is viewed through the perspective of the Nature's Secret Nutrient health hierarchy. **The prioritization sequence of our health drivers is of the utmost importance.** While Walford's main focus was on health and longevity driver #4/Nutrition, he severely compromised the quality and quantity of his Air (driver #1, breathing). **Since the prioritization of his lifestyle drivers was literally "out of order" (i.e., *not working*),** Dr. Walford suffered the consequences and ended up dying of a neuro-immune disease—ALS, aka Lou Gherig's disease.

The tragic irony of Walford's untimely death is that not only did he practice caloric restriction, but due to the unforeseen circumstances that developed in the Biosphere, Walford was also forced to practice oxygen restriction as well. Oxygen levels in the Biosphere dropped from around 21% oxygen to 14.5%. While such a spartanesque approach can in fact be beneficial from a nutritional standpoint, it can be deadly when applied to health driver #1, Breathing. Even being the brilliant scientist that he was, Dr. Walford still had a critical blind spot—in not fully honoring the life-sustaining importance of breathing air with sufficient oxygen content. If *any* of the vital health and longevity drivers are out of sequence, this can not only produce inefficiency in your physiology and metabolism—the results can be fatal. The synergistic increase in life force and immune system strength, which arises with the correct prioritization and sequencing of health and lifestyle drivers in conjunction with Golden Ratio balance, is the true healthy life extension therapy.

continued apneic (suspension of breathing) stresses. Like any great athlete who performs and then retires at the top of their game, Stig gracefully exhaled his last competitive breath, echoing the wisdom of country music legend Kenny Rogers in *The Gambler*:

You've got to know when to ***hold*** *'em; know when to fold 'em…*

The Golden Oxygen Ratio

Your brain is, on average, less than 3% of your body's weight, yet it uses more than 20% of your body's oxygen. As you become aerobically fit, you double your capacity to process oxygen.
Michael J. Gelb, author of *How to Think Like Leonardo da Vinci*

Oxygen is the predominant element found in the human body, at a Golden Ratio level of about 62% of total body weight (the remaining 38% is largely composed of a combination of carbon, hydrogen, nitrogen, calcium, phosphorous, potassium and other trace minerals). This is one of the prime reasons it's the #1 NSN MegaNutrient, in addition to it being a moment-to-moment life necessity. Interestingly, oxygen is also the predominant element in the Earth's crust. Oxygen is the primary research focus of **Ed McCabe**, pioneering oxygen researcher and author of *Flood Your Body With Oxygen*. He convincingly argues that a prime factor of all diseases and degenerative conditions, including cancer and AIDS, is oxygen deprivation. Why? Most, if not all, of these diseases thrive in an *anaerobic* (low or no-oxygen) internal environment. As McCabe points out:

The air we breathe today is reported to have only about 21% oxygen. The other 79% is mostly nitrogen... We have shortness of breath when the oxygen level drops into the teens, and below 7% oxygen we cease to live... Allowing for pollution in the cities, our society as

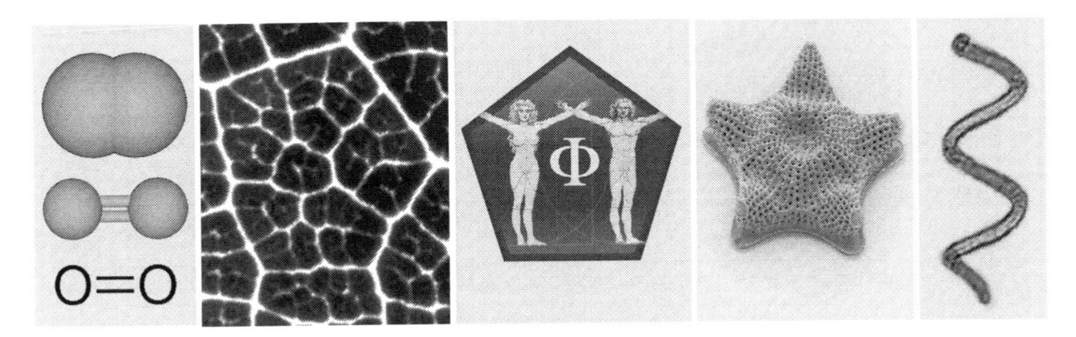

The majority of the Earth's atmospheric oxygen or O_2 (*1*) is produced by plants and phytoplankton, many of which have Golden Ratio/pentagonal structure. Leaf closeup (*2*). NSN Biomimicry Medicine logo (*3*). Star Diatom plankton, source of diatomaceous earth (*4*). Phytoplankton Spirulina (*5*) has a Golden Ratio 62% protein by weight and also a protein : carbohydrate ratio of 1.62:1.

1

The Biosphere 2

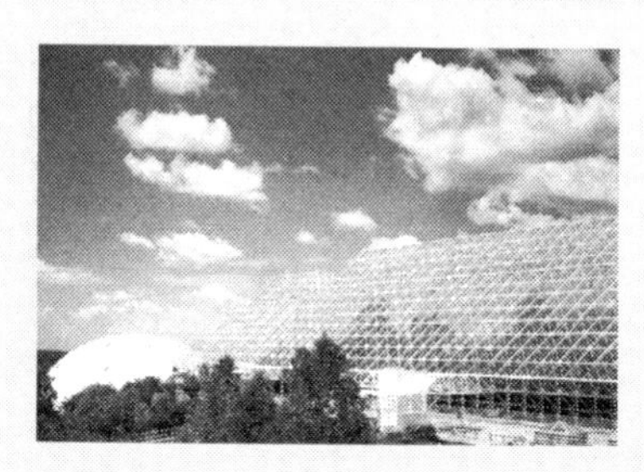

The Biosphere 2 (Biosphere 1: Earth) is a closed ecosystem in Oracle, Arizona that looks like a giant greenhouse. Its first mission, from September 1991 through September 1993, was composed of eight people including team leader Roy Walford, M.D. The plants inside Biosphere 2 didn't produce enough oxygen to keep up with the crew's oxygen needs; as a result of the constant deficit, oxygen levels fell from 20.9% to 14.5% after the first 16 months. Dr. Walford eventually developed ALS (Lou Gherig's disease) resulting from the prolonged oxygen deprivation.

a whole has allowed so much pollution to accumulate, and so much of the environment to be destroyed, that our available oxygen commonly drops below 21% in the air, depending upon the location sampled. This physical machine we walk around in was designed to exist here on the planet within an atmospheric sea full of high-level fresh oxygen...

McCabe's analysis takes on an ominously prophetic tone in light of Beijing's first-ever smog red alert (three consecutive days of severe, choking smog) in December 2015 which closed schools, grounded cars and forced people to stay indoors. While 1.4 million people in China die prematurely from air pollution yearly, severe air pollution is not isolated to China—an estimated 3.3 million people die yearly from air pollution worldwide, a figure forecasted to double to 6.6 million by 2050. This clearly poses a serious risk for life on earth if this trend of increasing poisoned air continues.

> *Peak oxygen is the problem—not peak oil.*
> *Oxygen levels in many cities are as low as 10%,*
> *creating functional frontal lobotomies in the population.*
> **William Deagle, M.D.**

For optimum health and mental functioning, our physical bodies need that Fibonacci number of 21% (or more) oxygen. Oxygen deprivation over a long period of time is documented to have many deleterious effects. Thomas H. Maugh II, *Los Angeles Times* staff writer describes in Biospherian Roy Walford's obituary the serious effects of the oxygen deprivation Walford experienced during his time as a Biospherian:

Before ALS caught up with him, he stood 5 feet, 8 inches and weighed 134 pounds. He had a bodybuilder's physique, the product of workouts at a local gym. He got an inadvertent chance to test his theories in humans when he became a member of the Biosphere 2 team. Biosphere 2 (Biosphere 1 being Earth itself) was a $150 million, 3 acre, glass-enclosed structure built to determine whether humans could live in a self-sustaining environment on another planet. Walford, then 67, was by far the oldest member of the team. The next-oldest was 40; the rest were about 30. Soon after they were sealed inside in 1991, they realized that they couldn't grow enough food for a normal diet. Walford convinced them to adopt a near-starvation regimen: vegetables and a half-glass of goat's milk daily, meat or fish once a week. They didn't exactly flourish, but they did get healthier. Men lost nearly 20 percent of their body weight; women about 10 percent. Their blood pressure, blood sugar, cholesterol and triglyceride levels all fell by at least 20 percent to extremely healthy levels.

The team members also exhibited an increased capacity to fight off illnesses, such as colds and flu. But levels of nitrous oxide—produced by microorganisms in the soil and normally broken down by sun-light—rose to dangerously high levels, and the crew suffered periods when the oxygen level in the Biosphere was unusually low. Walford later speculated that both problems caused the death of brain cells. 'I remember, when I would talk to him while he was in there, his voice would be slurred, and he would say he would bump into things while he was walking because he was light-headed,' said his Daughter, Lisa Walford. 'The disease started in the Biosphere, even though I wasn't aware of it at the time,' Roy Walford told The Times. 'You can see it on the videos. I was getting a little bit wobbly.'

Solar Malnutrition of the Biospherians

As the story above illustrates, physiologic deprivation factors of the Biospherians included low oxygen tension and decreased caloric intake, among other factors. A key—yet neglected—essential variable was the effect of decreased UV sunlight radiation coming through the Biosphere's glass shell. According to an *Engineering and Construction* review by Zabel, et.al., *the glass used consisted of double-layered, laminated, heat-strengthened glass, with a plastic layer sandwiched between the two glass sheets.* Over the experiment's length, it's quite certain that the triple-layer solar shield decreased the sunlight UV required to produce vitamin-D (solar nutrient) to such an extent that it became a critical factor in the failing health of the Biospherians, especially Dr. Roy Walford.

Oxygen concentration has varied throughout Earth's geologic cycles. It seems logical, as can be inferred from Ed McCabe's oxygen research and Roy Walford's story, that for optimum health and mental functioning our physical bodies need a higher level of oxygen than is found in much of the air we breathe today. Chronic shallow breathing can result in lowered cellular O_2 levels, suboptimal nutrient assimilation and incomplete cellular detoxification, not to mention impaired mental and emotional function. The air we breathe is also charged with vital life energy or *prana*, as the ancients called it. One of the scientific correlates of prana is the measurable healthy negative-to-positive ion ratio and quantities. Balanced, ample levels of negative and positive ions and prana are found in natural environments such as mountains, oceans, rivers and are particularly strong near waterfalls. Man-made waterfalls or fountains simulate Nature's pranic and ion charge and are a good place to recharge your vital energy when you can't get out in Nature. It's vital scientifically and energetically that we consciously upgrade both the *quantity* (Vital Lung Capacity) and *quality* (pranic charge; optimal amounts and balance of negative and positive ions; living in cleaner air environments) of every breath we take. Let's drop down from the anatomic and functional levels to the biochemical level of breath. In order to extract energy from our food, we need a sufficient constant supply of oxygen. The two major pathways of energy production are known as *aerobic* (requiring oxygen), and *anaerobic* (without oxygen). Aerobic respiration is much more efficient than anaerobic. This efficiency is reflected as comfort when you are exercising at a comfortable rate. We all know the lactic acid burn when we cross from aerobic metabolism into anaerobic. Once the "red-line" is crossed, the inefficient anaerobic metabolism can't be sustained for very long.

> *Cancer, above all other diseases, has countless secondary causes. But, even for cancer, there is only one prime cause. Summarized in a few words, the prime cause of cancer is the replacement of the respiration of oxygen in normal body cells by a fermentation of sugar.*
>
> **Otto H. Warburg, M.D., biochemist & Nobel Prize winner**

Breathing (O_2) ➡ ENERGY (ATP) ➡ Health ➡ Performance ➡ Longevity

Vital Capacity (VC) decreases with age—and is the #1 predictor of longevity. *VC is the total amount of air exhaled after a full breath.* How does ↑ Vital Breath Capacity relate to ↑ PEAK Health, Performance and Longevity? **It's all about generating energy at the cellular level.** After food is eaten, digested and transported to your cells, it's burned/combusted *in the presence of oxygen*, generating **ATP**

(Adenosine TriPhosphate). ATP is called *the universal energy molecule* because all cells use ATP to fire their metabolic processes. In an *As Above, So Below* relationship, the more oxygen your lungs breathe in, the more oxygen is available for your cells to breathe in. Your lungs act as a bellows, enabling you to fan the metabolic flames of energy production. The deeper and more efficiently you breathe, the greater the rate of cellular combustion and ATP production. The more ATP that's produced the more efficiently all cells function—and efficient cellular operation over decades leads to both greater health *and* greater longevity. By becoming proficient and dedicated to the regular practice of Golden Ratio Breathing (3 second inhale to 5 second exhale, p. 53), you strengthen

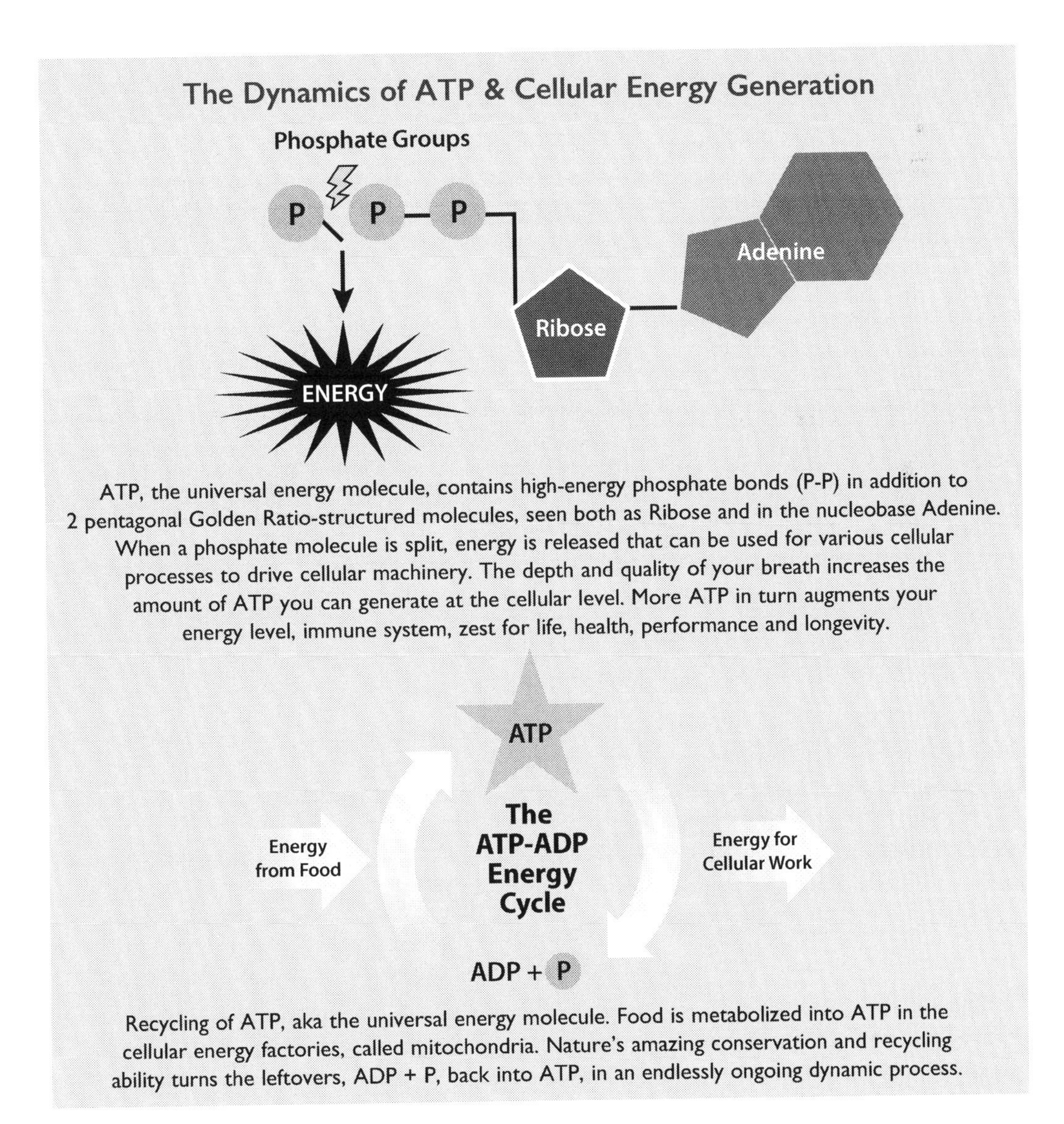

ATP, the universal energy molecule, contains high-energy phosphate bonds (P-P) in addition to 2 pentagonal Golden Ratio-structured molecules, seen both as Ribose and in the nucleobase Adenine. When a phosphate molecule is split, energy is released that can be used for various cellular processes to drive cellular machinery. The depth and quality of your breath increases the amount of ATP you can generate at the cellular level. More ATP in turn augments your energy level, immune system, zest for life, health, performance and longevity.

Recycling of ATP, aka the universal energy molecule. Food is metabolized into ATP in the cellular energy factories, called mitochondria. Nature's amazing conservation and recycling ability turns the leftovers, ADP + P, back into ATP, in an endlessly ongoing dynamic process.

your body's unseen yet most important respiratory muscle—**your diaphragm.** A stronger diaphragm enables the oxygen catapult to fully load and deliver more oxygen to your trillions of cells—conversely, more CO_2 can be exhaled with a stronger diaphragm. Better breathing efficiency and expanded lung capacity naturally translates to greater ATP production, creating a self-reinforcing cycle of optimal metabolism, steady energy and better overall health. While many people *breathe too little and eat too much* (key factors contributing to dysfunction, disease and premature death), the great news is that when you reverse this pattern—**when you breathe deeper and more robustly and eat in more moderation**—you generate more ATP and get more energy from the food you eat. So breathe a little more, eat a little less and move towards the Golden Ratio, where you experience high energy and robust health as your normal state of being.

> *BREATHE—it's for free, it's life, it's GOOD!*
> **Iceman Wim Hof, master teacher of how to access superhuman powers through the breath & cold therapy (see Ch 10 Longevity)**

Secrets of Barometric Pressure: mini-Hyperbaric Oxygen Therapy (m-HBOT)

Historically, people report worsening in various medical conditions coinciding with low atmospheric barometric pressure changes, e,g., many people with arthritis may experience low barometric pressure with increased pain and swelling in their joints, while the average person often experiences low barometric pressure with a sense of fatigue, lethargy, apathy & listlessness. Conversely, sunny days with clear skies and higher barometric pressure are notable for reports of physical improvement in many conditions as well as an enhanced sense of wellbeing. People wonder why on some days they feel better than others for no apparent reason. Even though diet, sleep schedule, stress levels, etc., may not change, many have never considered that fluctuations in barometric pressure may be responsible. We rarely notice the barometric pressure that surrounds us, much like a fish swimming in the ocean doesn't notice that it's wet.

However oblivious we are to barometric pressure changes, it nevertheless exerts such a strong effect on our health that the medical field learned decades ago how to harness it for its healing effects. **H**yperbaric **O**xygen **T**herapy (**HBOT**) was first used medically over a century ago to treat divers with decompression sickness (the bends). Since then, hyperbaric chambers have been found to be very useful in the treatment of infections, radiation injury, burns, wound healing, cancer, neurologic conditions and many other conditions where driving more oxygen into the cells is conducive for healing. **An apt metaphor is the simple act of inflating a bicycle tire.** It's possible to increase

Golden Ratio Barometric Pressure Performance Graph

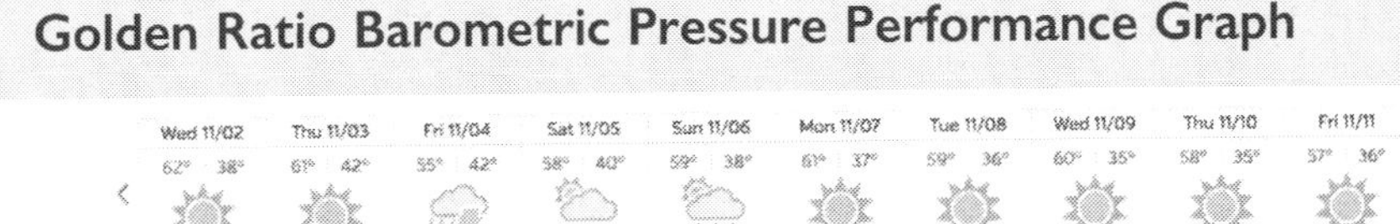

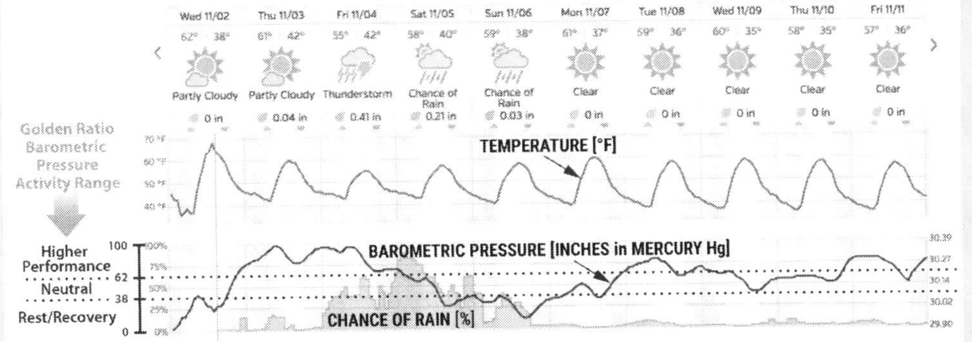

Adapted from wunderground.com

Data gleaned from 10-day weather forecast graphs can enable you to predictively schedule best days to optimize athletic performances or any important life activities. The barometric pressure graph line shows that high atmospheric barometric pressure occurs before and after thunderstorms (rain indicated by the shaded histogram). On the left of the graph is a 0-100 scale denoting the *Chance of Rain* (%). We can also use this 0-100 scale to mark barometric Golden Ratio divisions of 38% and 62%. Barometric pressure of 62% or above (**m-Hyperbaric Oxygen Therapy** range) is where our cells are pressurized with more oxygen and is the most advantageous time to turn in an optimal performance, whether on the job, in the field or in any area of life. Conversely, the best time for rest/recovery is generally when barometric pressure is 38% or below. The area between 38% and 62% is a more neutral barometric zone when you can do moderate activity or baseline training. By balancing activity and rest/recovery days around Golden Ratio barometric fluctuations, another Golden opportunity to generate NSN is easily available.

the performance of a bicycle simply by increasing tire pressure to an ideal, higher level. With higher tire pressure the bicycle moves over the road with decreased effort by the cyclist and easier steering control and handling. If the tire pressure is too low however, it necessitates more energy output by the rider and steering will be sluggish and squishy. Likewise we can see that on high-pressure barometric days, the atmosphere is effortlessly driving more oxygen into our cells. The result is high performance in all areas of life—wherever the rubber meets the road. To take advantage of this natural oxygen charging phenomenon, all we need to do is synchronize, as possible, our workouts or events requiring high performance with increased barometric pressure days. Elite athletes take advantage of high and low atmospheric pressure, but in a different way.

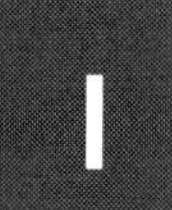

They use altitude to modulate oxygen tension; one method is to train at high altitude (low pressure) and then take advantage of competition at sea level (high pressure), where the oxygen tension is higher. Others will train at sea level routinely to get higher oxygen delivery to their cells and get a higher workout performance.

> *If you follow your breath, you lose all limitation.*
> **Kathryn Sanford, yoga teacher**

Taking advantage of altitude differentials is effective for many athletes and has resulted in numerous peak performances and records. Although it's difficult to access altitude differentials in our busy lives, Nature offers us an easy way that's free-of-charge. By attuning ourselves to day-to-day barometric pressure fluctuations, we can determine the days that offer us access to our own personal **m**ini-**H**yperbaric **O**xygen **T**herapy (**m-HBOT**). All we need to do is to learn how to decipher simple weather graphs that are available on many internet weather sites. High barometric pressure days deliver extra oxygen into our cells, *resulting in increased cellular energy production (ATP) and higher performance days.* Conversely, low pressure days result in lower oxygen tension at the cellular level and are better allocated as healing and *rest/recovery days*. Strategically scheduling active days and recovery days in synchrony with barometric fluctuations presents a golden opportunity to better flow with Nature's cycles. We can "load the catapult" on stormy days and be ready to spring forward on the next sunny days.

In this first chapter we've explored the universality and vital importance of oxygen and how critical breathing deeper and more robustly—tuned to the Golden Ratio—is to our health, performance and longevity. It's interesting that another of the top success factors in the Nature's Secret Nutrient system has long been touted as being universal as well. Specifically, the second-highest priority MegaNutrient in the NSN system, Water, is known as the *Universal Solvent*, as we'll explore in the next chapter...

Remember, you're only as well ***Oxygenated*** *as your last* ***BREATH***. So breathe consciously, in Golden Ratio: Inhale to 3... Exhale to 5..... Practice NSN Lung Yoga daily: inhale a few extra sips of air at the top of a full in-breath & exhale a few extra puffs of air at the end of a full out-breath. Feel the powerful surge of life-giving oxygen/prana as it circulates through your entire body.

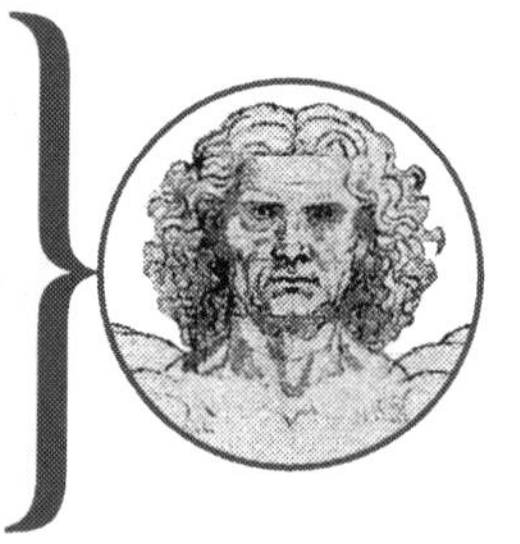

Why Oxygen is NSN's #1 MegaNutrient: It's Woven into *All* Subsequent Health, Performance & Longevity Drivers.

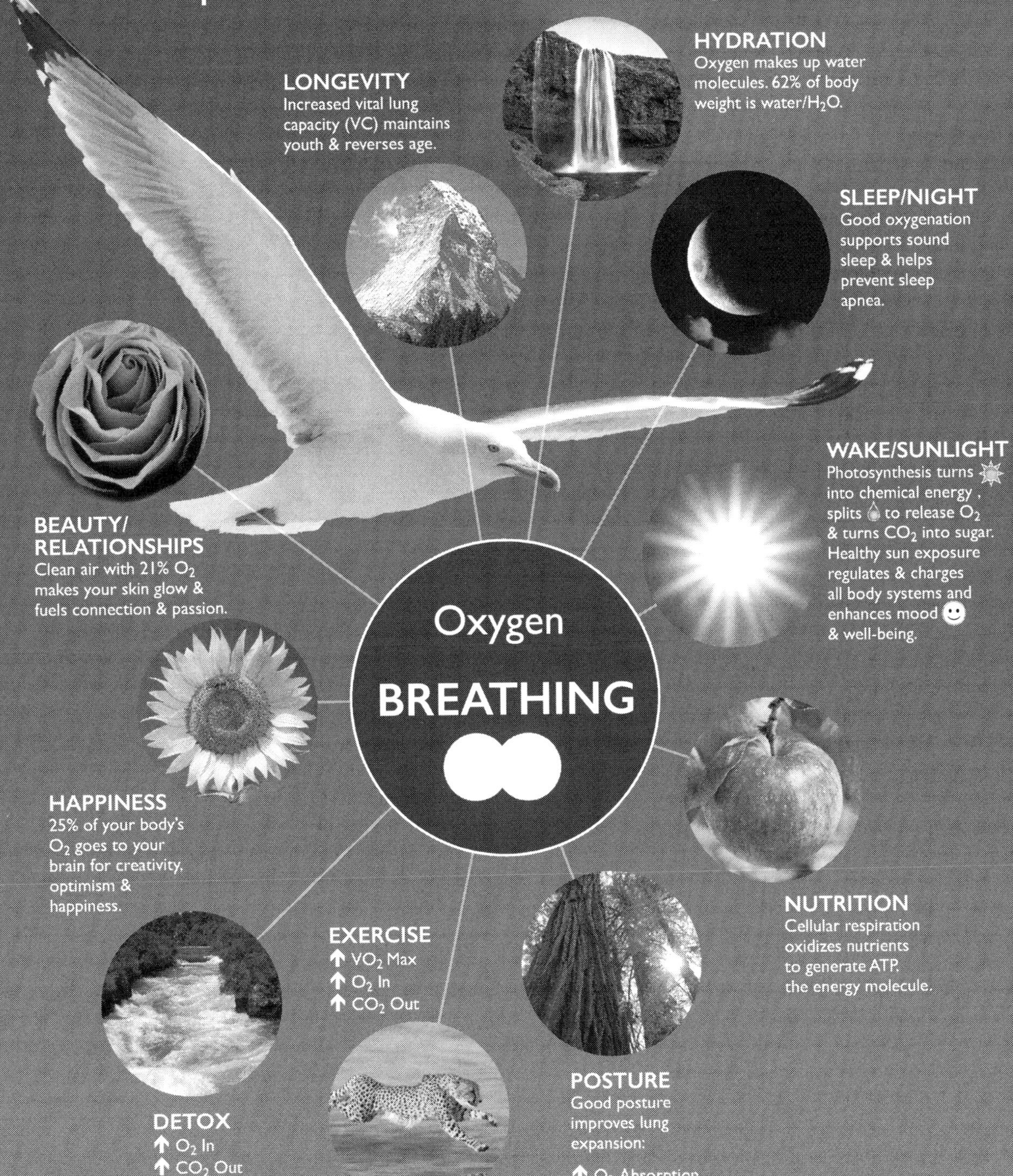

LONGEVITY
Increased vital lung capacity (VC) maintains youth & reverses age.
HYDRATION
Oxygen makes up water molecules. 62% of body weight is water/H_2O.
SLEEP/NIGHT
Good oxygenation supports sound sleep & helps prevent sleep apnea.
WAKE/SUNLIGHT
Photosynthesis turns into chemical energy, splits to release O_2 & turns CO_2 into sugar. Healthy sun exposure regulates & charges all body systems and enhances mood & well-being.
BEAUTY/ RELATIONSHIPS
Clean air with 21% O_2 makes your skin glow & fuels connection & passion.
Oxygen
BREATHING
HAPPINESS
25% of your body's O_2 goes to your brain for creativity, optimism & happiness.
NUTRITION
Cellular respiration oxidizes nutrients to generate ATP. the energy molecule.
EXERCISE
↑ VO_2 Max
↑ O_2 In
↑ CO_2 Out
DETOX
↑ O_2 In
↑ CO_2 Out
POSTURE
Good posture improves lung expansion:
↑ O_2 Absorption
↑ CO_2 Release

Breathing is Health Priority Driver #1, as mere minutes without Oxygen (O_2) results in death. Chronic Oxygen deficiency/poor breathing prevents optimal health, energy and performance and is an associated factor in many diseases. Breathing is the gateway bringing O_2 into the body and ushers out Carbon Dioxide (CO_2). It's the basis of the prime NSN Rx: **The Fibonacci/Golden Ratio Breath: 3 second inhalation... 5 second exhalation.....** This infographic shows how O_2 is woven through all health drivers, linking them together in a synergistic whole.

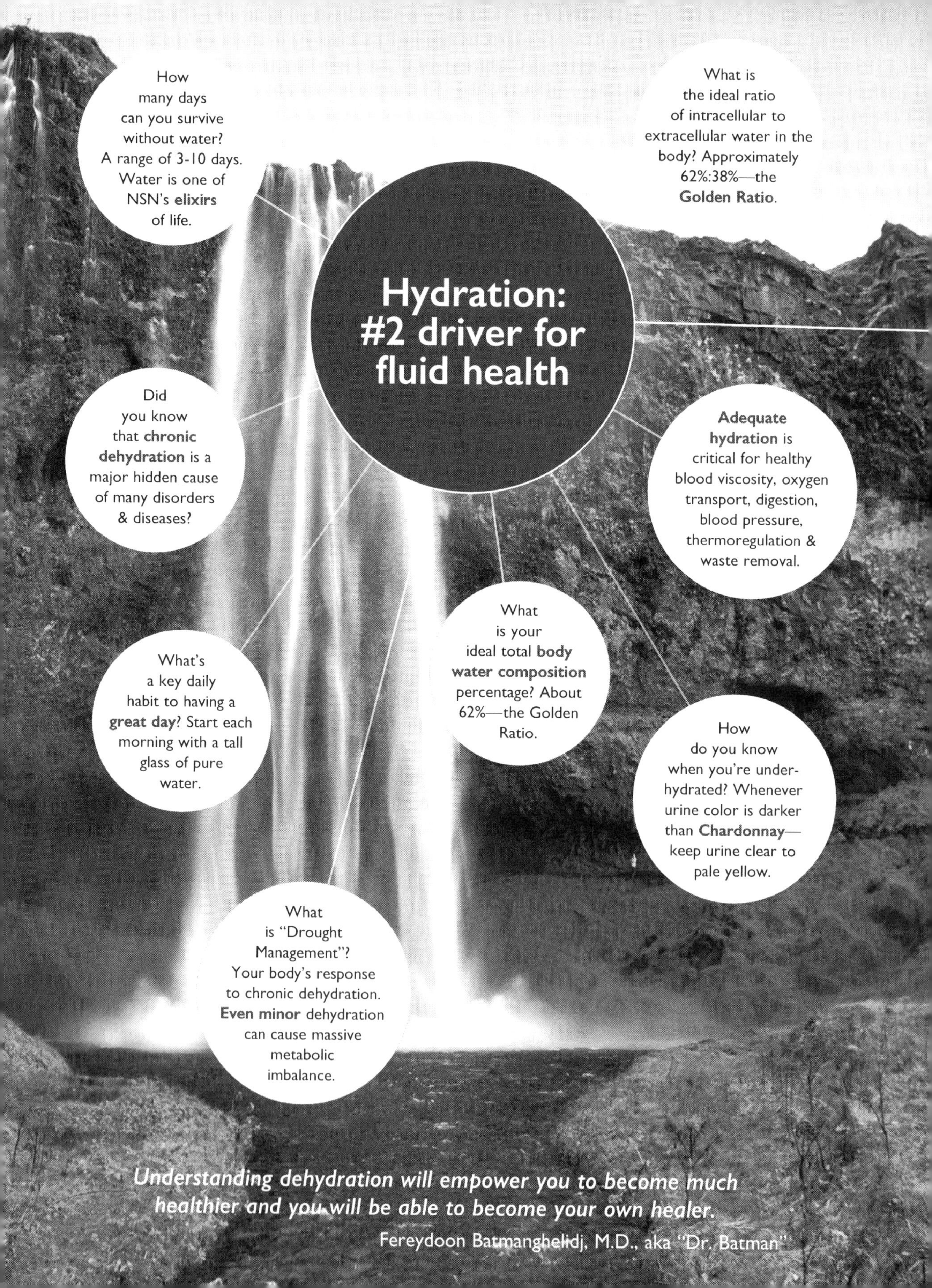

Hydration: #2 driver for fluid health

How many days can you survive without water? A range of 3-10 days. Water is one of NSN's **elixirs** of life.

What is the ideal ratio of intracellular to extracellular water in the body? Approximately 62%:38%—the **Golden Ratio**.

Did you know that **chronic dehydration** is a major hidden cause of many disorders & diseases?

Adequate hydration is critical for healthy blood viscosity, oxygen transport, digestion, blood pressure, thermoregulation & waste removal.

What is your ideal total **body water composition** percentage? About 62%—the Golden Ratio.

What's a key daily habit to having a **great day**? Start each morning with a tall glass of pure water.

How do you know when you're under-hydrated? Whenever urine color is darker than **Chardonnay**—keep urine clear to pale yellow.

What is "Drought Management"? Your body's response to chronic dehydration. **Even minor** dehydration can cause massive metabolic imbalance.

Understanding dehydration will empower you to become much healthier and you will be able to become your own healer.

Fereydoon Batmanghelidj, M.D., aka "Dr. Batman"

2

Hydration

Water is the Driver of Nature.

Leonardo da Vinci

Humans can only survive without water for a few days without increasingly compromised functioning and ultimately death. Throughout our evolution, we've had to either develop water conservation strategies or live with a water source close by. We didn't evolve like camels that can go several weeks without water or kangaroo rats that can go 3+ years. We humans require a constant pure water intake to survive *and thrive.* Unless we can maintain our Golden Ratio fluid balance through regular water intake, our functioning, health and performance will be compromised short-term, leading to increasingly compromised health and longevity long-term.

We can harness water's magical ability to act as a universal solvent to keep us hydrated—*supercharged with a potent synergy of hydrogen and oxygen*—transport nutrients for metabolic processes, support detoxification and temperature regulation and purify and inspire body, mind and soul. As elite athletes know, even a 2% drop in fluid levels dramatically affects performance on all levels. We need a radical paradigm shift in our appreciation of the moment to-moment importance of the role that water—NSN MegaNutrient #2—has in preventing chronic dehydration, maintaining optimal health and performance and enhancing longevity.

2

Dr. Batman to the Hydration Rescue

You are not sick, you are thirsty. Don't treat thirst with medication.

Fereydoon **Batman**ghelidj, M.D.

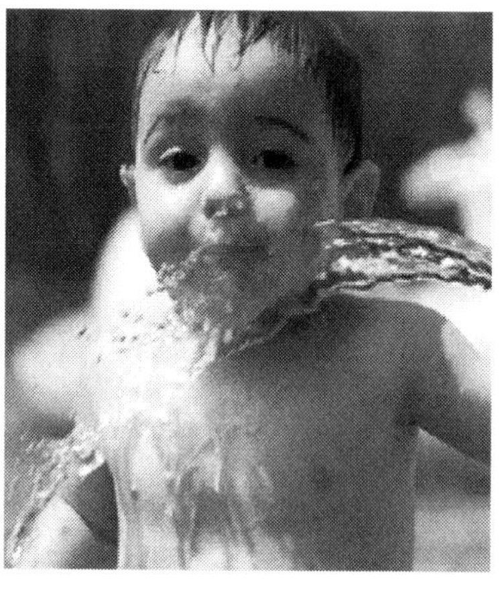

Water is driver #2 in the Nature's Secret Nutrient system.

In acute dehydration our bodies divert water away from organs and tissues like skin, muscle and the gut to vital organs like the brain, heart and kidneys in order to sustain life. If we accept the reality of chronic dehydration, then those same survival mechanisms get activated, yet in slow motion, therefore going unnoticed. This was the revolutionary insight of Iranian physician Fereydoon **Batman**ghelidj, M.D. (1931–2004). Through his years of research, he hypothesized that most of the so-called chronic diseases of modern life were in actuality the body's attempt at "drought management." The disease manifestations are merely the body's attempt to stop dehydration by different adaptation mechanisms in different tissues. Dr. Batmanghelidj proposed the following partial list of functional ailments and pathologies directly stemming from dehydration:

allergies	*dry eyes*	*hypertension*
asthma	*dry skin*	*kidney stones*
autoimmune diseases	*emotional/mental issues*	*low back pain*
excess blood thickening	*fibromyalgia*	*low energy*
cancer risk	*gout*	*migraines*
cholesterol imbalance	*headaches*	*obesity*
chronic fatigue	*heartburn*	*osteoporosis*
colitis	*heart disease*	*pain of various causes*
constipation	*hormonal imbalance*	*poor performance*
diabetes	*hot flashes*	*rheumatoid arthritis*

It might initially sound outlandish that chronic dehydration could be a factor in all of the above problems, yet theoretical mechanisms are explored in Dr. Batmanghelidj's books, including *Your Body's Many Cries for Water*. One prominent example of chronic dehydration is in the case of "essential" hypertension: high blood pressure of unknown cause. Blood pressure is controlled by a symphony of neural and hormonal feedback mechanisms. Normally, blood pressure in the arterial system is high enough to perfuse the capillary beds all the way down to the cellular level. Adequate blood pressure is necessary for multiple vital reasons: to deliver oxygen and nutrients to the cells; to remove waste and simply to maintain consciousness, e.g., you'll often get light-headed if you stand up too fast because your brain isn't receiving enough blood. The body's intelligence regulates blood pressure to accommodate water fluctuations on a moment-to-moment basis. In acute and sub-acute scenarios, dehydration usually results in low blood volume and low blood pressure—hypotension. That may be the case in acute and sub-acute conditions of dehydration, but Dr. Batmanghelidj proposed a fascinating theory of what happens to people in a chronically dehydrated state. Although it may take months or years to arrive at a prune-like state, if the total body water deficit is not replaced, the vascular system has no choice but to compensate by remaining in overdrive for organ perfusion, thereby creating what is known as hypertension or high blood pressure—**in addition to potentially dangerous blood thickening, which can lead to clots.** The treatment seems simple—recognize the chronic dehydration state and give the patient water—the opposite of what is normally done to patients with hypertension. They are prescribed diuretics and medicines that dilate the blood vessels, treatments which only exacerbate the dehydration, leaving the patient feeling drained and without energy. It's amazing that such a simple substance like water could be *both* the cause of disease and the cure, depending on the circumstances. This is a profound example of how the simple power of water has been overlooked by mainstream medicine. Although this scenario doesn't take into account other factors involved in hypertension such

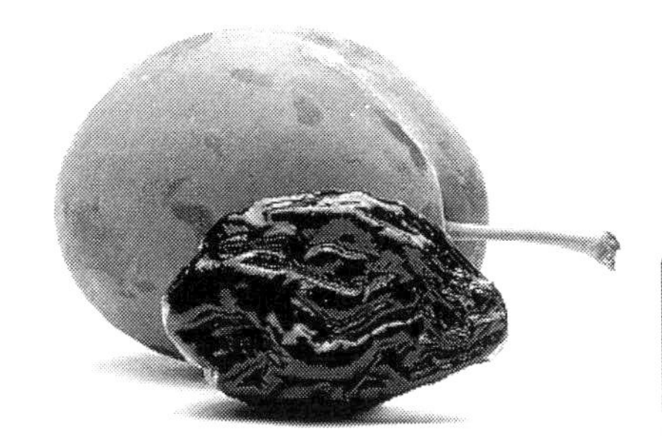

Juicy plum or dried prune—your hydration determines which one you resemble. *Get juicy!*

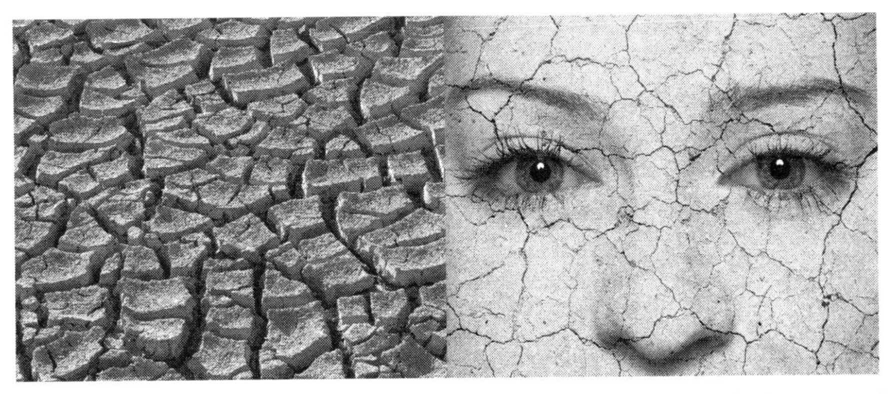

A dried lake bed, skin of the Earth (*L*) reflects what can happen to our skin (and our internal environment) with chronic dehydration—and excess sun exposure (*R*). Remember to stay well hydrated, moisturize and get adequate yet not excessive sun exposure.

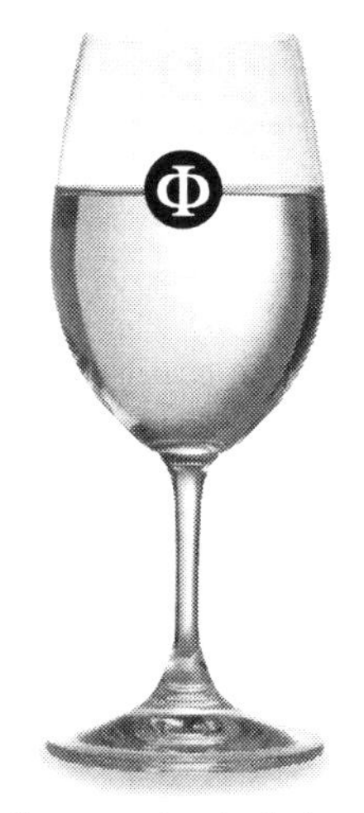

If your urine is darker than Chardonnay, you are very likely dehydrated.

as arterial stiffness, cardiac or kidney conditions or various endocrine effects, *it may in fact explain the cause of "essential" hypertension in many people.* In drought management, your body uses various mechanisms to shunt water into critical organs and tissues first, replenishing the remaining tissues and organs in a prioritized hierarchy. The specific manifested ailment is but a compensatory mechanism for the underlying problem: *Dehydration.* **Dr. Batmanghelidj says that doctors have mistakenly focused all of their attention on the *solute* (drugs and medications) instead of the *solvent* (water)—** This revolutionary yet sane way of viewing our physiology is Copernican in its impact on both medical thinking and healthy longevity. The medical worldview considers so-called diseases as actual entities in and of themselves, *unaware that the causal mechanism might be something as simple and as easily remedied as dehydration.* Yet this makes perfect sense when you consider the fact that the exquisite Golden Ratio balance and efficiency of your entire physiology is thrown off when you're dehydrated—whether acutely or chronically. Knowing how the Golden Ratio manifests at different scales, we can surmise that the same process that's going on in acute dehydration could also be going on over the more extended timeframe of chronic dehydration. Total body water and the Golden Ratio of intracellular to extracellular water becomes imbalanced when you're dehydrated. **Adequate hydration daily/hour-to-hour is absolutely critical for a multitude of vital life functions, including:**

- Φ Maintaining normal blood viscosity: ***blood can abnormally clot if it gets too thick*** (a key reason ample hydration is CRUCIAL on long plane flights).
- Φ Facilitating plasma transport of oxygen, CO_2, nutrients and waste products: water helps dilute the blood to make it easier to transport nutrients and waste.
- Φ Hydrolyzing & breaking down nutrients for easy, thorough absorption.
- Φ Maintaining vascular hydrostatic pressure: keeping your blood pressure at the right level to perfuse all vital organs including your heart, brain and kidneys.
- Φ Maintaining adequate urine flow: perfuses your kidneys with enough blood to generate adequate urine to remove waste products.

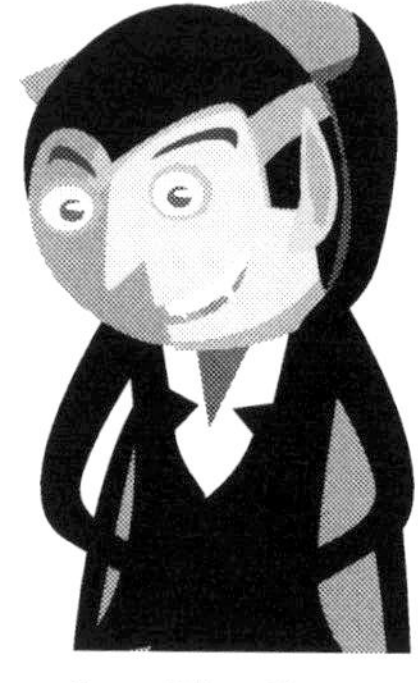

Even The Count knows how important proper hydration is for healthy blood viscosity to avoid clotting.

Φ Thermoregulation through perspiration, respiration and shunting of blood from extremities to core, or vice-versa: helps keep your body at the right temperature for optimal metabolism.

The orthodox medical establishment has not yet embraced Dr. Batmanghelidj's hypothesis. Yet his paradigm jump in medicine aligns perfectly with the precepts of Nature's Secret Nutrient—Water being the #2 driver in the NSN health hierarchy—especially when we consider the *full* impact adequate water has on health and longevity.

Top 2 Hydration Rules: Chardonnay & Drink *Before* You're Thirsty

The critical factor in the development of chronic dehydration is the remarkable fact that our thirst impulse doesn't accurately reflect our need for water. This is even truer as we age—an older individual's thirst reflex becomes extremely *dampened* and should not be relied upon to monitor fluid needs. We need to cultivate other strategies to preempt dehydration, such as evaluating our skin texture, seeing if we have dizziness on standing and of course, checking the color of our urine. Unless your urine is very light yellow or clear, you need to drink until it clears. Complicating matters is the fact that regular consumption of dehydrating beverages like tea, coffee and alcohol tend to make us run water deficits. We can temporarily have clear urine after drinking coffee or tea, yet later on our urine will become more concentrated and thus darker.

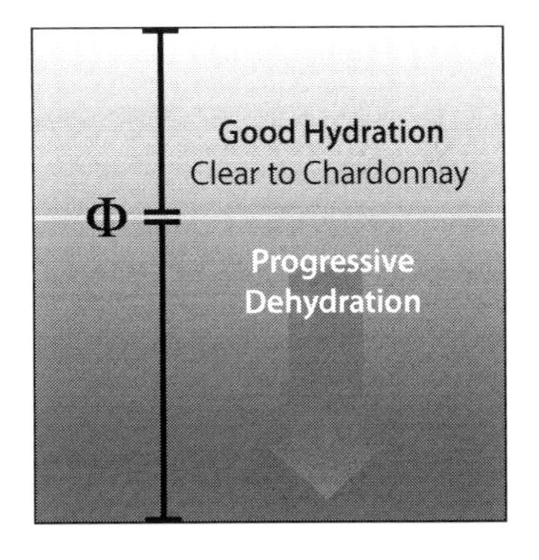

The Golden Ratio Urine Color Chart shows your relative hydration status: Φ and above indicates good hydration; below PHI indicates progressive dehydration. Note: Kidney, bladder or systemic diseases, B-vitamins & some drugs can change urine color & invalidate this test.

The key here is that pure water alone is always the best hydrator. You can surmise that if you have any of the above noted ailments, you are probably dehydrated. Since our bodies are like sponges, the uptake of water into the deep intracellular compartments of our tissues can actually take days or even weeks to replenish—so regular, ample water consumption needs to become a way of life. You can begin approaching your ideal body composition and physiology by simply drinking more water. You can also focus on building more water-containing tissue—muscle—while at the same time decreasing your body's percentage of fat. There are many easy methods for accomplishing the twin goals of increasing lean muscle mass while decreasing body-fat in Ch 4 Nutrition and Ch 6 Exercise.

Water & Golden Ratio Body Composition

Some people are afraid of heights. Not me, I'm afraid of widths.

Steven Wright, humorist

Idealized Golden Ratio Human Body Water Composition Label Facts	
Body Water %	
Men, ages 25-34	**62%**
Women, ages 25-34	**62% (-5 to -8%)**
Intracellular/Extracellular Water Distribution %	
Intracellular Water %	**62%**
Extracellular Water %	**38%**

What a body water composition label might look like for an ideal human.

Imagine that your body had a nutritional content label. A typical label would include percentages of the three **MacroNutrients: Protein, Fat and Carbohydrates**. While this can show the nutritional value of energy bars, it's not practical for *Homo Sapiens*, or the rapidly increasing American overweight species, *Homo Fatruvius*. America has become one of the most overfed, overweight yet undernourished countries in the world, with a way out-of-ratio fat to lean body mass. Along with this growing girth has come elevated rates of heart disease, cancer, arthritis, autoimmune and Alzheimer's disease. How could you determine the optimal values of your body's nutritional label? Scientists have developed various techniques called Body Composition Analysis (BCA) to determine amount of fat and fat-free mass. Total body fat is made up of subcutaneous fat (*fat under the skin*), visceral fat (*fat around organs*) and brain & nerve fat. The remainder of your body is

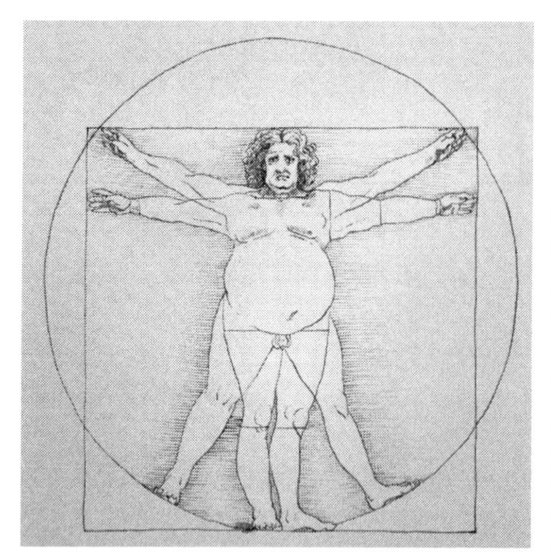

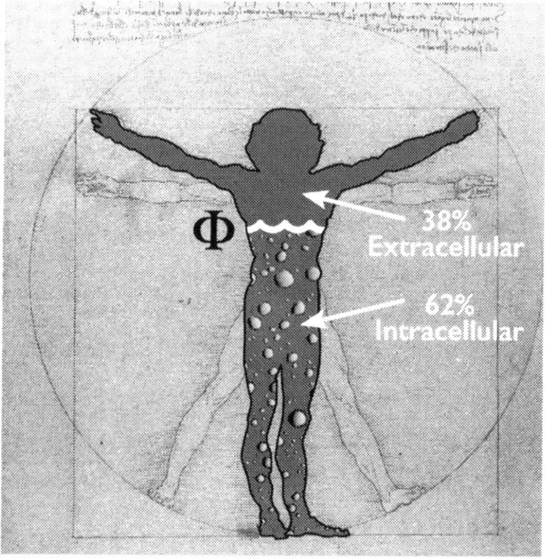

(*L*) Homo Fatruvius or *Fatruvian Man*, with increased body fat % & excessive waistline. Excess body fat means lower muscle and body water %. (*R*) Homo Vitruvius (*Vitruvian Man*), with ideal lean body mass and a 62% Golden Ratio total body water composition. He also has a 62:38 Golden Ratio intracellular-to-extracellular water balance. ***Your Waistline is Your Lifeline,*** Jack LaLanne, aka The Godfather of Fitness.

Body Water Percentages at Different Periods of Life

Fetus	~94%
Infants	~75%
Adults	~62%
Elderly	~50%

Body water percentage is a constantly changing parameter. Healthy adult humans in the prime of life have a Golden Ratio percentage range of body water.

lean body mass—muscle, bone and organ tissue. Several methods reveal body composition, e.g., thanks to Archimedes' principle, we can submerse a person in a tank of water and measure the water displacement (*known as Underwater Hydrostatic Weighing/UHW*). Since densities of fat and lean body tissue differ, percentages of body-fat and lean body mass can be precisely calculated. A simpler method—skin fold calipers—is used to measure subcutaneous fat thickness at different points, e.g., back, waist, arms, legs. With these values body-fat % and lean body mass estimates can be made. An advanced method is called *body composition analysis* through Bioelectrical Impedance Analysis (BIA), where a weak electrical current is passed through the body. Since fat and muscle (lean body mass) conduct electricity at differing rates, the percentages of each can be determined. It's difficult to get a Golden Ratio handle on the ideal fat % you'd want on your Body Composition Label; typical recommendations for ideal body-fat percentages range from 8-19% for men (age 20-39) and 21-33% for women (age 20-39). Both ranges lack clear Golden Ratio dynamics, yet there's another way of viewing Body Composition that provides key data for aligning with the optimal Golden Ratio range.

Viewing Body Composition from the Perspective of Water % vs. Fat %

BioDynCorp.com features data obtained from bioelectrical impedance testing which points directly to Golden Ratio relationships in healthy body composition. If we look instead at *body water percentage*, surprising results reveal exactly where you'd want your body composition to be for maximal physiologic functioning, e.g., **in the men's 25-34 age group, body water percentage measures 61.4%, within .4% of the more exact 61.8% Golden Ratio**. This is uncanny, yet not surprising, as Golden Ratio relationships are ubiquitous throughout the body. In this 25-34 age range males are at their physiologic prime, functioning and performance-wise. Body water % for women was slightly lower, due to a natural gender difference in body fat amount. Intriguingly, both men's and women's body water compositions dance closely around the Golden Ratio within the Golden Prime Zone years of ages 19-31 (*see the Golden Prime Zone sections in Ch 10 & accompanying Rx*). Even though bioelectrical impedance testing is a modern technique of measuring body composition, there have been visionary artists that have masterfully captured different levels of body composition in their work. A prime example of Golden Ratio body composition is elegantly demonstrated in Leonardo da Vinci's *Vitruvian Man,*

2

Dehydration: Death By A Thousand Breaths

Many modern diseases are known as *silent killers*; two prominent examples are high blood pressure (hypertension) and chronic, low-grade inflammation. To this we must add chronic dehydration. While its symptoms are easily ignored, its effects are insidious—even deadly. One of the most overlooked sources of dehydration comes from the simple act of breathing, which accounts for about 0.5 liters of water loss daily. The exhaled water vapor from the entire human population adds up to around 3-4 billion liters of water per day. Just breathing, humankind has the ability to form clouds and make rain. If we don't replenish our water losses daily, we're a doomed and dehydrated species. Exercise, so highly touted, also causes rapid breathing and even greater dehydration. Breathing is clearly vital, *yet we must also recognize that replenishing the water lost in each breath is also critical.* It might seem impossible that the micro-droplets of water you exhale could add up to such a significant daily water loss. However, if you consider how a colony of ants builds an ant hill one grain of sand at a time, you'll get an idea of how your 23,000 breaths per day contribute to significant dehydration, micro-droplet by micro-droplet. This is another prime reason to upgrade both the quality and quantity of your daily water intake and stop the silent killer of dehydration in its arid tracks, one drink of water at a time.

in which we can clearly see the sleek, muscular build of a prototypical human male in his prime. Da Vinci demonstrated what ideal humans would look like with Golden Ratio proportions in both anatomical structure and body composition. We can surmise that these *Homo Vitruvians* would have approximately 62% total body water content, as shown in the optimal body water composition graphic on p. 74, where total body fat is relatively low (likely in the 8-10% range). Da Vinci's masterpiece holds many secrets, ideal Golden Ratio body composition included. **Muscle is composed of significantly more water than fat, so by increasing muscle your percentage of total body water naturally increases.** As an added bonus, every pound of muscle burns 50 calories per day whereas every pound of fat burns only 3 calories per day—yet another reason to build more muscle and reduce fat.

Macro & Micro Golden Water Ratios

Knowing that the Golden Ratio appears across all levels of scale, we can predict that in addition to water being about 62% of ideal total body weight, Golden Water Ratios might well be evident at the next lower scale of your water containing compartments.

In the diagram on p. 74, we see the Golden Ratio's universal design constant of the body's intracellular/extracellular fluid compartment ratios. These ratios have been scientifically measured to be within 1% of the 62%:38% Golden Ratio (*these ratios are given for a healthy young adult and are used to illustrate the general concepts pertaining to Golden Ratio water balance*). We can surmise that there is an incredible physiologic advantage in maintaining Golden Ratios in our dynamic internal aqueous environment. Water comprises 62% of body weight in an optimal human, and on a smaller fractal level our intracellular/extracellular water ratio falls into 62/38 Golden Ratio. Why else would a human being in the prime of life—a Homo-Vitruvian—exhibit these uncanny Golden Ratio values? Since we're basically water beings with an ocean inside us, we must avoid dehydration at all costs. Drought management becomes ever more important with age, as the tendency is for dehydration to silently manifest and build insidiously over time. With the NSN Hydration Rx's, you can help restore the fluid vitality of the ocean within, for smoother sailing on the seas of a high quality and increased quantity of life.

Dehydration, Decreased Performance & Aging

On the day we're born, we're at high tide. After that, very quietly,
the sea within us ebbs and ebbs, and as it goes... so do we.

Loren Eiseley, philosopher, literary naturalist

Studies of top athletes show that exercise performance deteriorates progressively as dehydration increases. With as little as a 2% loss in water weight, performance is significantly impaired and dehydration greater than 5% can decrease performance by as much as 30%. We know that a Golden Ratio percentage of body water weight is 62% in healthy males in their prime (5-8% less in females, due to naturally higher body fat), so *any* amount of dehydration will upset your Golden Ratio water balance in both intracellular and extracellular compartments. The end result is always compromised performance. *However, it's not just prime athletes who are susceptible to the double-edged-sword of dehydration and compromised performance; anyone who is aging is also vulnerable.* With advancing years, the dehydration of aging lowers body water percentage well below the 62% Golden Ratio amount and we see a concomitant decrease in both form and function. As spinal discs lose their water, we see a loss in height as well as in postural integrity. The typical stooped posture of aging is one of the hallmarks of a dehydrated body. Dehydrated cells aren't able to keep up with the demands of youthful performance and we see a slowing in all systems, from a generalized loss of energy to decreased cardiac output to slowed mental functions. A vicious cycle of spiraling dehydration and decreased functionality takes over as we age. Our sense of thirst becomes blunted with

2

The Miracle Molecules: Hydrogen & Oxygen

Hydrogen comprises 62% of the total atoms in your body, while oxygen comprises about 62% of your total body weight. Each element in its own unique way expresses the human body's ideal Golden Ratio composition. Bound together as water (H_2O💧) a magical universal solvent is created, the sacred liquid upon which all life depends. *This is a great reason to practice daily Golden Ratio gratitude for water, as it nourishes and purifies you from within—and cleanses and inspires you from without.*

each advancing decade, leading to a progressive and insidious process of accelerating dehydration. As we become increasingly dehydrated, different bodily systems begin to fail with our destiny being the ultimate state of dehydration—ashes and dust. While we may not be able to evade this destiny, we can slow it down by being mindful that Hydration is NSN driver #2, just behind #1 Air. A dramatic example of how devastating dehydration can be on physical performance is the death in January 2016 of extreme explorer Henry Worsley. On his attempt to be the first unassisted person to ski across 900 miles of Antarctic terrain to the South Pole, Henry succumbed to dehydration and malnutrition, just 30 miles short of his goal. It wasn't as if there was a shortage of water, as all of Worsley's water came from an endless source of melted snow. Yet due to the enormous physical strain of the journey, his sensation of thirst had become blunted to such an extent that he just didn't drink enough water. As survival psychologist John Leach reminds us, *Humans are notoriously bad at monitoring our own condition… If you're on your own, you're your only reference point. If your reference point starts to drift, you drift with it.*

Apparently Worsley wasn't able to *adequately sense* his progressive dehydration—a fatal factor in his untimely demise. Although it's unlikely that any of us will ever encounter the extreme Antarctic conditions that Worsley dealt with, it's still possible—and all too common—for anyone to develop a blunted sensation of thirst with resultant dehydration and decreased health and performance. *The simple work-around is to establish multiple hydration reference points in order to proactively intervene on your own behalf.* All you need to do is begin daily hydration charting in the 21-Day Priority Coach System at the end of this book. This sets the reference points and crucial daily reminders you need to establish a new habit of healthy water intake. With this simple behavior modification, you'll avoid chronic dehydration and improve your health, performance and longevity as you trek through life and any extreme conditions you may encounter along the way.

The Vitruvian Internal Fountain of Youth

*The Fountain of Youth...it's exercise, healthy diet, **lots of water**, lots of laughter, lots of sex...it's healthy, it's natural, it's what we're here to do!*

Cameron Diaz, actress

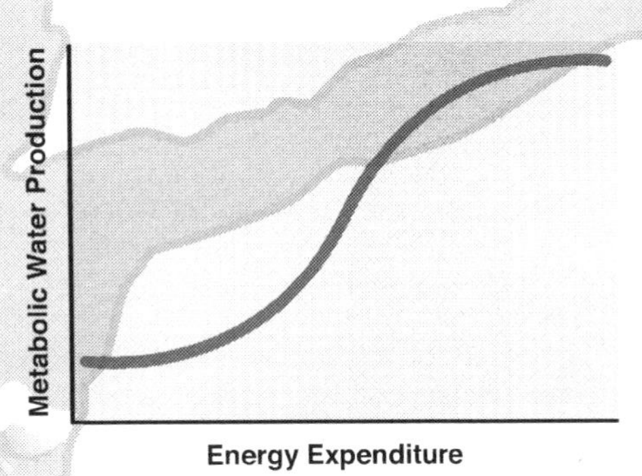

Cellular hydration increases proportionally with activity and exercise.

The Vitruvian Internal Fountain of Youth *internally* hydrates your cells, increasing your total percentage body water towards the 62% Golden Ratio level, that of a vibrantly healthy Vitruvian Man or Woman (p. 74). In order to increase your body water percentage towards the Vitruvian level, you must do three things. First, drink 1-2 liters/quarts of water per day. Second, consume foods high in natural water like fruits/vegetables; Third, release *intracellular metabolic* water from food, which can range anywhere from 250ml–800ml/day, depending on activity level. Water content of food that's directly absorbed in the intestines is additional to *metabolically produced intracellular water* (inside your cells). Metabolic water can be increased by burning more food through increased activity. Fat and carbs contain potential water, but it has to be released through intracellular oxidation. As exercise increases, so does the amount of metabolic water produced. This is a key reason the long-lived people in the world's Blue Zones (p. 284). routinely live 100+ years. With their naturally active lifestyle, they're continually burning carbs and fat and priming their Internal Fountain of Youth. Constant internal hydration keeps their cellular machinery running clean and at peak efficiency, contributing to longevity by protecting DNA telomeres (p. 291). An added benefit is that metabolically produced intracellular water is 100% pure—*no filtering needed*. By using the secret of increased intracellular hydration, you'll keep your body fat and water percentages in **Vitruvian Golden Ratio Range** and optimize your health and performance.

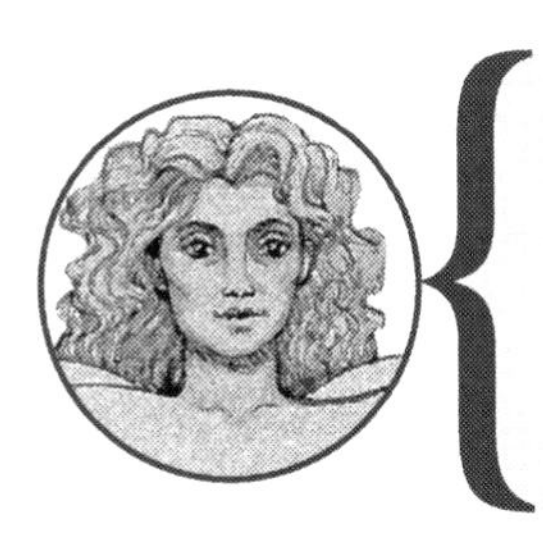

Remember, you're only as ***HYDRATED*** *as your last drink of pure* **Water**. So pay regular attention to what doctors and nurses call your I's & O's: Inputs & Outputs. Drink before you're thirsty and monitor the color of your urine to keep it in the clear-to-light Chardonnay range.

Sleep~Night & Wake~Sunlight: #3 dual drivers for full spectrum health

What's vital for sound sleep? **Total darkness**—essential for the release of melatonin.

Sleep deprivation impairs physical, mental & emotional health & causes obesity, heart & hormonal problems. **Don't cheat** on sleep!

What's the **Golden Sleep/Wake Ratio?** 9 hours sleep to 15 hours awake.

The **Quality** of your sleep is just as important as the **Quantity**. Upgrade both to enhance your total health.

Light & Dark are both essential in Golden Ratio amounts to insure vitality, peak performance & longevity.

The **Solar Collectors** on your **skin** surface make Vitamin D & the ones in your **eyes** regulate hormones, circadian rhythms & DC electric charging.

The happiness & well-being hormone **Serotonin** is initially generated via sunlight activation in the **retinas.**

Sun exposure can be either **medicine or poison** depending on dose; get regular **moderate** doses in Golden RAYtio amounts.

Sleep is just as important as diet and exercise.

Grant Hill, NBA basketball star

Here comes the Sun... it's all right.

George Harrison, The Beatles

3

Sleep~Night & Wake~Sunlight

Early to bed and early to rise,
makes a man healthy, wealthy and wise.

Benjamin Franklin

Sleep at Night & Wake to the Sunlight

The Cosmic Dance of Duality plays itself out beautifully in the constant flow between the dual NSN priority drivers Sleep~Night & Wake~Sunlight. Both darkness and light are vital MegaNutrients that all living things require in complementary doses daily. How well our circadian rhythms (internal body clocks) function is determined by the degree that we're synchronized with Nature's rhythms. Vitality, happiness, performance and longevity are all reflective of our alignment with these two basic evolutionary requirements—adequate quantity *and* quality of Darkness and Light. Viewed through the Golden Ratio lens, there are optimal amounts of Darkness and Light that ensure wellbeing. If we fall *out-of-ratio* with one of these MegaNutrients, by definition we're out-of-ratio with the other. The most common imbalance in our time is decreased sleeping to waking time. Since the hours of night and day are constantly changing over the year, our challenge as healthy humans is to dance with the seasons and maintain an approximate Golden

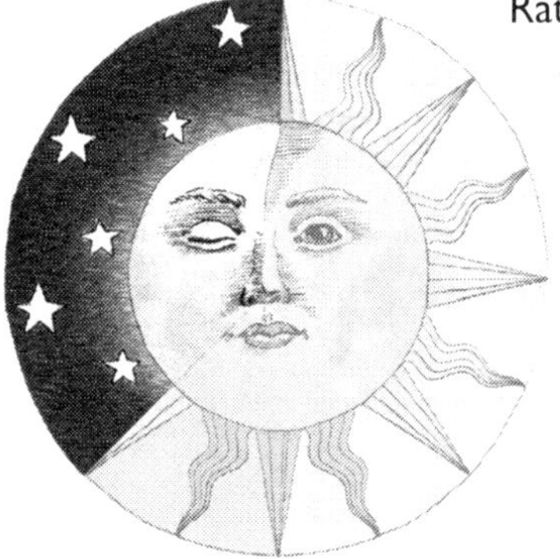

The eternal dance of Sleep~Night, Wake~Sunlight is Divinely Proportioned with a 1.6 Golden Ratio of approximately 9 hrs. sleep/rest to 15 hrs. awake every 24 hrs:

15÷9=1.6 Φ

Ratio of 9 to 15 hours of sleeping to waking on at least 3-4 days out of 7. If we stray too far to either side of this 9/15 Golden Sleep Ratio we can make ourselves susceptible to a wide range of modern diseases—and poor health and performance. By attuning our circadian rhythms to the Golden Ratio, we can extract maximum NSN from these health priority drivers, avoiding insomnia, injury and disease while supporting maximum life quality *and* quantity. In this section, we'll focus on key Golden Ratio aspects of Sleep~Night, where we spend the vital restorative hours of each 24-hour day. Starting on p. 98, we'll elucidate the Golden Ratio aspects of Wake~Sunlight, where we spend the waking, active hours of each 24-hour day.

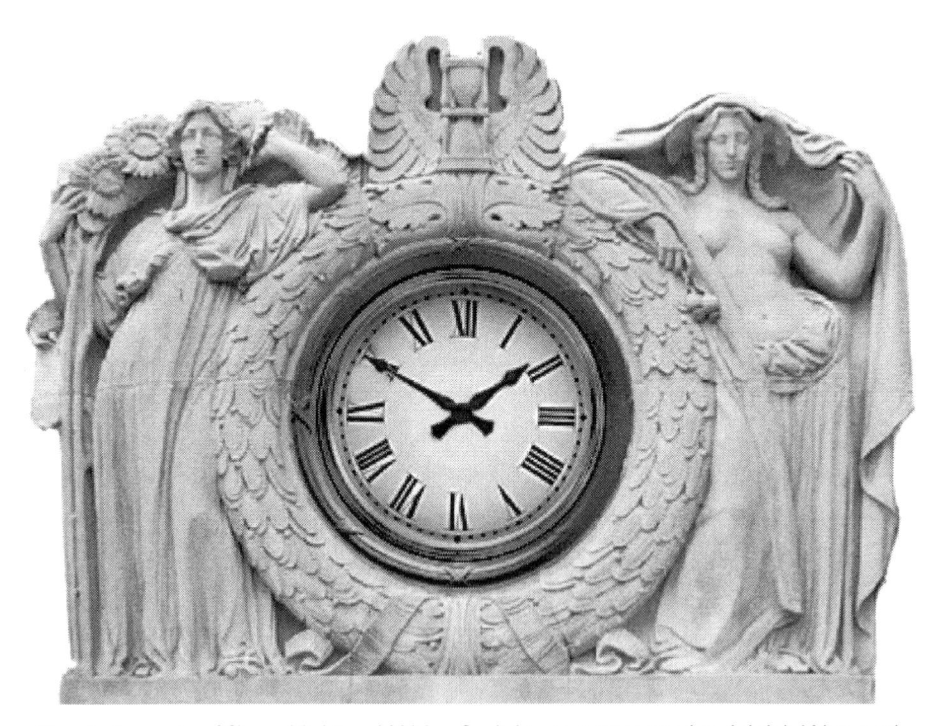

The dual aspects of Sleep~Night and Wake~Sunlight are represented in Adolph Weinman's *Day and Night* sculpture from New York City's magnificent, original Penn Station (1910-1963). With a winged hourglass & clock between them, Day (*L*) holds wide-awake sunflowers, while Night (*R*) holds drooping/sleeping poppy's. Note that clocks in advertisements often display 10:10 or 1:50, which neatly divides clockfaces into Golden Ratio angles (137.5/223.5).

SECTION 1: Sleep~Night

Sleep Deprivation

In the head of the interrogated prisoner, a haze begins to form. His spirit is wearied to death, his legs are unsteady, and he has one sole desire—to sleep... Anyone who has experienced this desire knows that not even hunger and thirst are comparable with it.

Menachem Begin, former Israeli Prime Minister, regarding his time as a KGB prisoner

3

As a result of extreme duress from sleep deprivation torture in a Russian prison, former Israeli Prime Minister Menachem Begin would likely have ranked his top-3 health drivers slightly differently than we did in this book's formulation. The contrast:

Menachem Begin's Probable Prioritization	The Authors' Prioritization
1. Air	1. Air
2. SLEEP	2. Water
3. Water	**3. SLEEP**

Although it would be extremely rare to die from sleep deprivation—like you certainly could from air or water deprivation—Menachem felt the extreme discomfort from not being able to sleep. Such is the power of sleep on our physiology. Nicole Bieske, of Amnesty International Australia, corroborated Begin's thoughts on sleep by stating, *At the very least, sleep deprivation is cruel, inhumane and degrading. If used for prolonged periods of time it is torture.* If top authorities recognize the destructive effects of sleep deprivation, why would we want to subject ourselves to such easily preventable self-abuse? The speed of life has clearly accelerated to the point where most people are undergoing a societally induced sleep deprivation—*in other words, torture.* A pernicious side effect of this slow, low-grade sleep torture is the disruption of our biorhythms. This leaves us vulnerable to many physiologic stresses including obesity, cardiovascular disease, hormonal problems and poor mental and emotional responsiveness, with attendant increased accident and poor performance risks. Normal circadian biorhythms are critical for maintaining healthy life quality and sleep is one biorhythm that we're all very familiar with. A century ago most Americans got around 9 hours of sleep a night—well before the modern era of 24/7 electromagnetic (EMF) bombardment, including television, computers, cell phones, PDA's, etc. Today the average amount of sleep per night is around 6.8 hours, while a third of the population struggles to get by on less.

People are getting between one and two hours less sleep a night than 60 years ago. We are the supremely arrogant species; we feel we can abandon four billion years of evolution and ignore the fact that we have evolved under a light-dark cycle. What we do as a species, perhaps uniquely, is override the clock. And long-term acting against the clock can lead to serious health problems.

Russell Foster, professor of circadian neuroscience, University of Oxford

Golden Ratio Sleep—And How To Get It

Sleep, the gentle tyrant—it can be delayed but not defeated.

Wilse Webb, Ph.D., sleep researcher

Sleep requirements vary throughout life, yet as children move into adulthood, sleep tends to decrease and gravitate around the Golden Ratio of 9 hours per night (15 hrs. awake / 9 hrs. sleep = 1.6, the Golden Ratio in two digits). After a landmark 2-year study, the U.S. National Sleep Foundation in 2015 released their healthy sleep recommendations by age group—which unsurprisingly confirmed the prevalence of Golden Ratio Sleep:

Life Stage/Age		*Healthy Sleep Range*	
Newborns	0-3 mos.	14-17 hrs.	
Infants	4-11 mos.	12-15 hrs.	
Toddlers	1-2 yrs.	11-14 hrs.	
Preschoolers	3-4 yrs.	10-13 hrs.	
School-aged	**5-12 yrs.**	**9-11 hrs.**	Φ *Golden Ratio Range*
Teenagers	**13-17 yrs.**	**8-10 hrs.**	
Young adults	**18-25 yrs.**	**7-9 hrs.**	
Adults	**26-64 yrs.**	**7-9 hrs.**	
Older adults	65+ yrs.	7-8 hrs.	

The Golden Ratio of 9 hours sleep per night is the *Just Right* amount that's advantageous for both the prevention of daytime fatigue and poor performance, and also as a window where a level of enhanced vitality, peak performance and longevity can be accessed and supported. A very small percentage of the population can get by on less than 7-9 hours sleep per night, e.g., the 1–3% of people with the "Thatcher Gene," a genetic variant named after British Prime Minister Margaret Thatcher, who needed only 4 hours of sleep nightly. Such outliers are envied for their gift of extra waking time that most don't have; just think of how much more *you* could accomplish with an

3 Different Sleep Patterns for Accessing Nature's Secret Nutrient/NSN

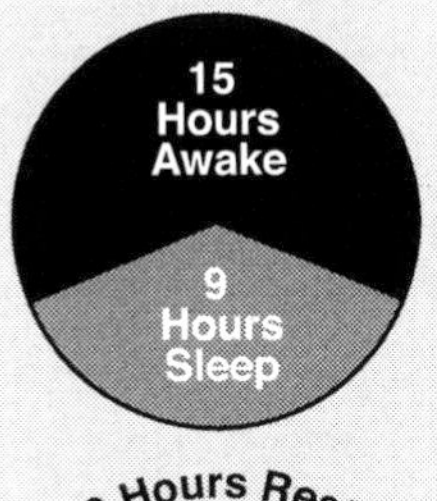

MONOPHASIC (one uninterrupted phase) sleep pattern: Although often challenging to do in modern times, 9 hours of uninterrupted sleep and 15 hours awake is the combination needed to obtain a 15/9 Golden Sleep Ratio. ***Great news:*** Achieving this ratio range on at least 4 nights a week lifts you into the Golden Ratio range for the week as a whole.

2 Hours Rest
7 Hours AM Awake
8 Hours PM Awake
7 Hours Night Sleep

SIESTA sleep pattern: Many cultures add in an afternoon nap or siesta to bring the total amount of sleep/rest closer to 9 hours in a 24-hour period, resulting in a 15/9 Golden Sleep Ratio.

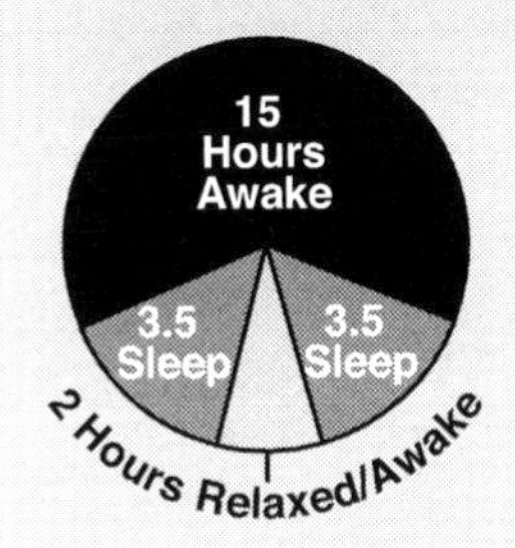

BIPHASIC (2-phase) sleep pattern: This is actually our deeply rooted ancestral pattern, composed of two 3.5 hour sleep segments, separated by a 1–2 hr. relaxed/awake phase for a total 9 hour sleep phase. This also gives a 15/9 Golden Sleep Ratio.

extra 2-5 hours every day. Yet the seeming gift of extra hours in the nocturnal realms may be a double-edged sword. Over time, those who sleep outside normal bounds may be covering up serious health problems that may one day present themselves as uninvited visitors. **An easy biohack to avert the tendency to undersleep is to negotiate a deal with yourself: aim to get 9 hours sleep on at least 3–4 nights per week, as 3–4 out of 7 nights is a rough approximation of the Golden Ratio. This unique biohack enables you to get a double dose of NSN—one nightly dose for when you do sleep 9 hours in one night and a second weekly dose for hitting that goal of 3–4 out of 7 nights in a week.** In addition to upgrading the *quantity* of your sleep, many of the other Rx's in the back of this book will upgrade the *quality* of your sleep as well. The ultimate aim? ***To help you awaken fully recharged to meet and surmount the challenges of the day with a strong wind—and enough winks—at your back.***

> *I have never actually met a true short sleeper. Most people who say they don't need a lot of sleep don't have that gene and they are just fooling themselves.*
> **Dr. Charles Bae, sleep specialist, Cleveland Clinic**

The Forgotten Healthy Biphasic Sleep Pattern

A fascinating historical and biological fact that isn't commonly known by modern health professionals and society at large is that prior to the 17th century (pre-industrial revolution), humanity followed a biphasic sleep pattern defined as an initial "first sleep" of around 3-4 hours, followed by a 1-2 hour period of awakening, followed by another 3-4 hour "second sleep." In Stephanie Hegarty's *The Myth of the Eight-Hour Sleep* (BBC News; 2.22.12) she highlights two books on the history of biphasic sleep during the transition from pre-industrial age to the present. Both Craig Koslofsky's *Evening's Empire* and Roger Ekirch's *At Day's Close: Night in Times Past* reveal that during the 1-2 hour sleep intermission, people would take advantage of this time by praying, meditating, reading, writing, smoking, lovemaking, etc. This middle-of-the-night waking time period wasn't resisted; it was instead accepted as a special time for contemplating life. Contrast that view to the anxiety that arises when a modern human awakens, worrying about life's problems and can't immediately go back to sleep, fearing that a day of fatigue and poor performance are ahead without a quick return to sleep. This innate biphasic sleep pattern is deeply ingrained in our physiology, but has become distorted with the emergence of a 24/7, light-based, electromagnetic-polluted civilization. Due to the pressures of our do-more society, we have overridden our genetic, biologic sleep imprint to the point that scientists and doctors now accept a new overlay—a monophasic (uninterrupted) sleep pattern of 7-8 hours per night—as being the norm. Virtually all books and research papers on sleep science use and portray a monophasic sleep pattern as the norm. A variation of the biphasic sleep pattern incorporates an afternoon nap or siesta in order to compensate for any nocturnal sleep deficit.

Alphabet Sleep

Nature structured our brainwaves in categories corresponding to approximate Fibonacci Sequence numerical divisions. Via an EEG (electroencephalogram), the divisions are measured in hertz (Hz) or *cycles per second*. From our alert Beta wave (13-34 Hz) waking state, we drift down through lighter stages of sleep (stages 1 & 2) where Alpha waves (8-13 Hz) and Theta waves (5-8 Hz) predominate. From there we descend into sleep's deepest stages (stages 3 & 4) where Delta waves (0.1-5 Hz) manifest.

- Φ Beta (13-34 Hz/above), when your mind is alert and active, i.e., daily waking activity.
- Φ Alpha (8–13 Hz) is the state where you are quiet and deeply relaxed, as in pre-sleep or meditation. It appears in Stage 1 and is also known as the "twilight sleep" zone you pass through just before falling asleep and just as you're waking up. Alpha is the magical "window state" for accessing latent intuition and also a most powerful

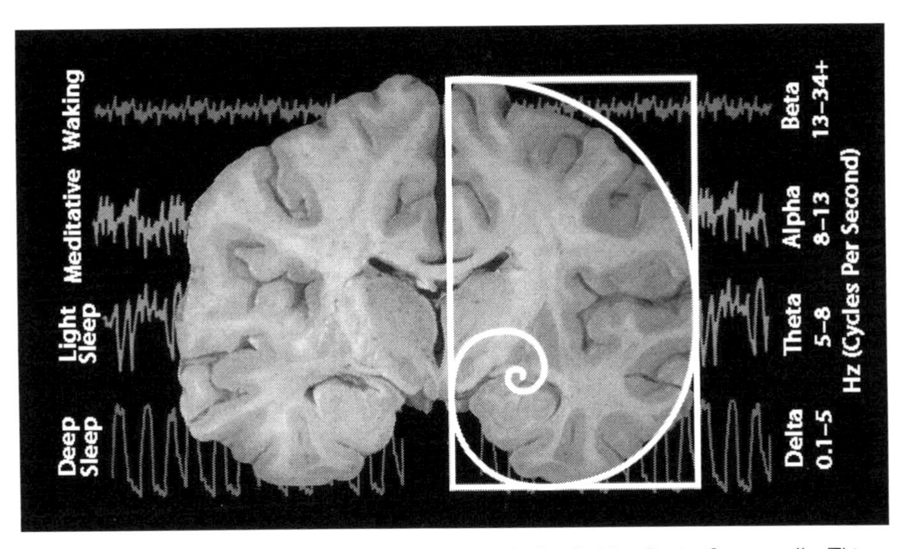

The human brain is designed structurally & functionally with the Golden Ratio. Structurally: This anatomical brain section fits perfectly in a Golden Rectangle, with contours following a Golden Spiral. Functionally: Brainwave frequencies (Hz) naturally mirror the Fibonacci Sequence. EEG signatures (electrical brain tracings) increase in amplitude & decrease in frequency (Hz) as they transition from beta > alpha > theta > delta.

state for creative visualization. Simply closing your eyes and then deepening and slowing your breathing with Fibonacci breaths can quickly induce the Alpha state.

Φ Theta (5–8 Hz) occurs in Stage 2 and is the level of superficial sleep or very deep meditation, in which many creative ideas originate. Theta also offers an expanded window into intuition and deep memory.

Φ Delta (0.1–5 Hz) is most prominent during Stages 3 & 4 deep sleep (slowest wave sleep); also associated with growth hormone secretion, healing and regeneration.

REM & Non-REM Sleep

In addition to viewing the spectrum of waking through sleep in terms of brain frequencies (beta, alpha, theta, delta), it can also be viewed in terms of two broad categories—REM and non-REM sleep. REM (Rapid Eye Movement) sleep periodically occurs at the transition zone between stages 1 & 2 and is where dreaming and mental/emotional processing occurs. Non-REM sleep occurs in stages 1-4, and ranges from light sleep to deep sleep. A night's sleep cycles between REM and non-REM throughout the night as many as 5 times. As the night progresses, we tend to spend longer and longer periods of time in REM. Our deepest sleep periods are in the early part of the night and this is where HGH (Human Growth Hormone) is secreted. Whenever you shortcut your total night's sleep quality or quantity, you reduce both REM and non-REM sleep. Your creativity and mental-emotional processing along with the HGH secretion responsible for regeneration and rejuvenation are all compromised. That is why it's so crucial to maintain a healthy base of sleep in the Golden Ratio range of 8–9 hours a night—whether uninterrupted or biphasic—making up any deficit through naps or siesta periods during the day. Due to our historical ignorance and modern bias, monophasic sleep is incorrectly thought to be the only healthy norm for a modern human being.

No scientist or doctor dares ask the question that perhaps there's a substantial benefit to a biphasic sleep cycle compared to a monophasic cycle. However, the monophasic sleep pattern is a very recent modern adaptation that rewrites our biologic history. There are consequences of superimposing an artificially accelerated evolution of sleep behavior on a species whose sleep patterns evolved over millennia. When people naturally awaken in the night between their first and second sleeps, it's likely diagnosed as a sleep disturbance and a prescription for a sleeping pill is commonly given, thereby overriding whatever the original function of the split-sleep cycle was. In a biphasic sleep pattern, the 2nd sleep phase potentially allows access to deep sleep stages 3 and 4 for a second time, thereby getting a second dose of the life elixir HGH in the same night's sleep. Biphasic patterns aren't seen only in sleep behavior, but have been beneficially used

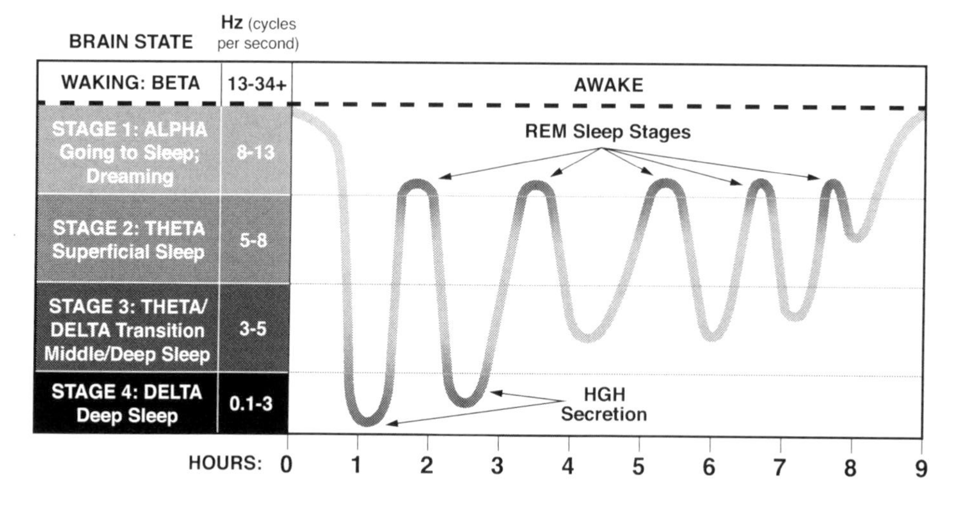

This graph is a generalized example of a sleep pattern tracing known as a hypnogram. A hypnogram charts electrical brain activity from the waking state in and out of the various stages of sleep (stages 1-4). On average, each sleep cycle lasts from between 90-120 minutes with our deepest sleep occurring in stage 4. REM sleep is associated with dreaming and psychological processing and is located at the transition zone between light sleep stages 1 and 2. Secretion of Human Growth Hormone (HGH) occurs in the first 2.5 hours of deep sleep, so it's important to access stage 4 for maximal cellular regeneration and rejuvenation.

by athletes for more efficient workouts. By splitting a longer exercise session into two shorter, separate sessions with several hours of rest in between, a net gain of up to 50% in exercise benefits is possible when compared to a single longer uninterrupted exercise session. No matter which sleep cycle you are accustomed to (biphasic, monophasic or siesta), you can still extract NSN by adjusting your total waking and sleep times to the Golden Sleep Ratio. Here are a few simple suggestions to help you gracefully walk the tightrope of sleep—making sure that your waking-to-sleeping time keeps you balanced on the narrow, healthy path of the 15/9 Golden Sleep Ratio.

3

- Φ If you awaken in the middle of the night, remember that it's just your body's deeply ingrained ancestral sleep imprint asserting itself. Try and accommodate the awakening, just like our ancestors did by taking advantage of the time to contemplate, meditate, pray, write or even make love. Acceptance of this natural biorhythm will likely become a satisfying and anticipated part of your night's sleep.
- Φ Take an afternoon nap or siesta to augment any sleep deficit that you might have incurred during the night. Even naps as short as 20 minutes can be highly refreshing and beneficial, recharging you for the rest of the day.
- Φ Remember that sleep is your #3 foundational driver for health, performance and longevity. Sleep doesn't cost anything other than a little energy and awareness in reprioritizing your activities, such that adequate sleep moves up the ladder of importance to its proper cornerstone position.
- Φ We've seen how Golden Ratio relationships permeate and elevate all aspects of human health and life. With this higher perspective, whenever we feel ourselves being pulled back into the prevailing modern paradigm that less sleep is both inevitable *and* a badge of honor, it's worth reflecting on Krishnamurti's sage wisdom:

  It is no measure of health to be well adjusted to a profoundly sick society.

We can conclude that in a truly healthy civilization that honored natural sleep requirements, most humans would thrive on a Golden Sleep Ratio. While through the lens of a sick society 9 hours of sleep/rest per 24 hours may seem excessive, 9 hours sleep to 15 hours awake is on the wise path to living a long, healthy and productive life. Individual variances will always trump blanket recommendations, so the final word is for each person to experiment on themselves in a neutral/non-alarm clock environment to

> *Sleep changes with aging, but it doesn't just change with aging;*
> *it can also start to explain aging itself.*
> **Matthew Walker, Ph.D., Sleep & Neuroimaging Lab, UC, Berkeley**

discover their own *just right* amount of healthy sleep to live and perform at their best. **Good sleep is like loading a catapult: the better you load it, the better it performs.**

Our Electromagnetic World: Outpacing Evolution

3

With the widespread increase in Internet and cellphone use, which really began to take off in the mid to late 1990's, similar increases in obesity and diabetes began to occur. At the root of these aberrations is the fact that over 40% of Americans don't get as much sleep as they would like or need. What we really need is not just an adequate quantity of sleep, but also a *high quality* of nighttime sleep, undisturbed by light, sound and EMF interference. Evolutionarily speaking, our high-tech, 24/7 society has outpaced our biological capacity to adapt. In the accompanying graph, we can see that the spike in Internet use began in the mid-1990's. Computers and cellphones became the norm, but the convenience and efficiency of the information and communication revolution has turned out to be a double-edged sword. We're still genetically programmed to rise with the sun and go to sleep shortly after sunset. Our circadian rhythms (24-hour biologic clock) are easily disrupted by artificial light and EMF exposure. The worst offenders for light and EMF disruption are evening TV, cell phone and web use that throw off normal biorhythms and the release of melatonin (sleep hormone), leptin (satiation hormone) and other neurotransmitters. This interferes with our biological clock's efficient operation. Once the timing of neurotransmitter and hormonal sequencing is disrupted, a critical downstream metabolic system is affected, i.e., regulation of adipose (fat) tissue. The normal communication between fat cells and the hypothalamus in our brain is disrupted, leading to aberrant hunger signals and abnormal fat metabolism. The end result is the explosion in rates of obesity, diabetes and many other chronic diseases we see today.

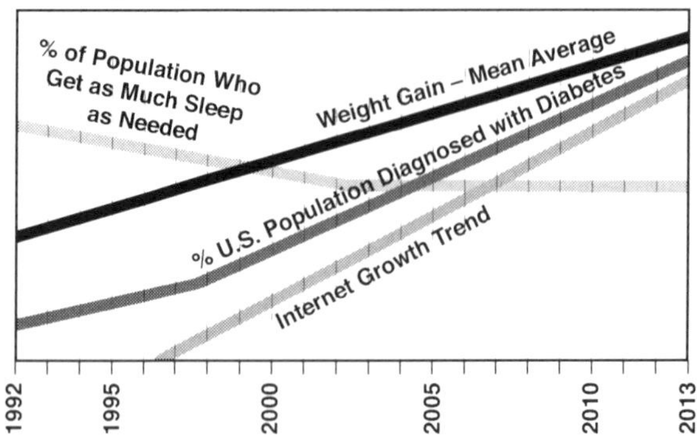

This composite graph illustrates the simultaneous upsurge in internet use with sleep deprivation, weight gain and diabetes. Increased EMF exposure and biorhythm disturbance may be factors in the recent health decline of our high-tech civilization.

Obesity & Sleep Deprivation

Research shows that adequate sleep is crucial for maintaining healthy weight, especially over time. Dr. Sanjay Patel, Professor of Medicine at Case Western Reserve University, conducted a study of nearly 70,000 women, which followed the effects of sleep on weight over a sixteen-year period (1986-2002). The study's major findings include:

Φ Compared with sound sleepers, women who slept 5 or less hours per night were 32% more likely to experience major weight gain (increases of 33 lbs.+).

Φ These same women were also 15% more likely to become obese, compared with women who got at least 7 hours sleep per night.

Φ The findings were unrelated to light sleepers who over-ate or under-exercised.

Φ The study results are said to apply equally to men and women.

Some of the mechanisms of how sleep deprivation may lead to weight gain include:

Φ Altered hormone secretion leading to increased hunger, via altered leptin and ghrelin secretion.

Φ Increased fatigue, leading to diminished/poor quality or no exercise the next day.

Φ Changes in basal metabolic rate (BMR; number of calories burned at rest).

Φ Sub-optimal digestion and diminished nutrient absorption, leading to increased food intake. As a result of this research, new, innovative weight loss systems include therapies that synchronize sleep/wake ratios with the Golden Ratio.

Depression & Weight Gain Can Result From Dim Light During Sleep

Sleeping with the light on could leave you feeling low the next day, researchers from Ohio State University have warned. They say that a night-light—however dim—may affect the structure of the brain, raising the odds of depression. The eerie glow emitted by a TV or the seemingly reassuring presence of a night-light could be enough to impact mental health, weight gain and have serious implications on overall health and happiness.

Key Point: Secure total darkness for your sleeping environment, to maintain optimal melatonin secretion to support and protect your health. If you need a night light, use a red frequency bulb which lessens impact on nighttime brain function.

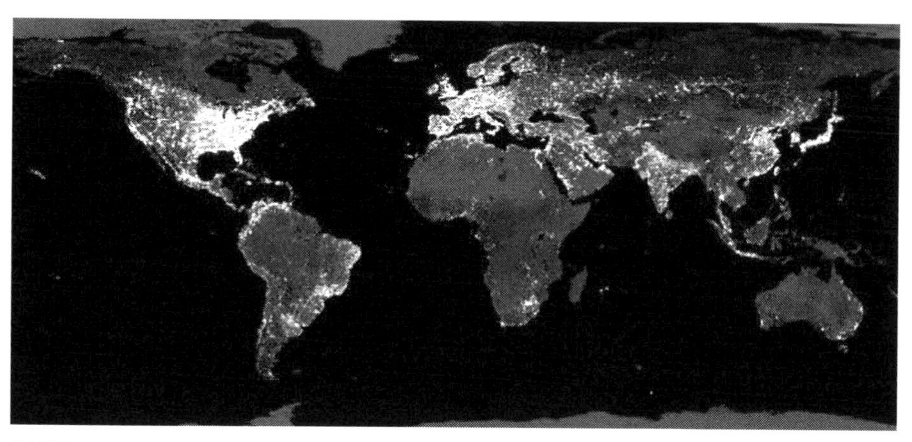

NASA composite night satellite photo of Earth, showing man's remarkably strong footprint of light. In large cities it can take extra diligence to insure a dark sleeping environment.

3

Naps Cut Heart Attacks by 37%

Siesta in Healthy Adults and Coronary Mortality in the General Population, a 6-year study of 23,681 Greek adults, showed that those who napped at least 3 times a week for about a half hour had a 37% lower risk of dying from heart attacks than those who didn't nap (37% is virtually the smaller part of the 38/62 Golden Ratio). The study's senior author and researcher Dimitrios Trichopoulos, M.D. remarked, *My advice is if you can nap, do it. If you have a sofa in your office, if you can relax, do it.*

Darkness & Silence: Two Essential Yet Underappreciated Sleep Nutrients

What hath night to do with sleep?

John Milton

In kind answer to John Milton we'd reply: *Night sets the stage for Darkness and Silence to appear, preparing the way for Sleep to make its grand entrance.*

Sleep has two key prerequisites, often overlooked. Darkness and Silence are the unappreciated necessities for healthy sleep to be established in the proper amounts and ratios. These include total hours of sleep as well as quality REM (Rapid Eye Movement) and non-REM sleep. What actually makes deep, restorative sleep possible is the fact that less auditory and visual stimuli are being registered in the brain. Darkness and Silence remove two key sensory inputs, which allows the brain to go fully offline in order for maximum restoration to occur. That's why it's critical to avoid as much light and sound as possible during the night, to access the key Sleep Nutrients Darkness and Silence.

(*L*) Noticing the number 6:18 on your clock AM/PM is a Golden Ratio wake-up. But faint light from clock radios and electronics disrupts nightly melatonin secretion, interfering with sound sleep. (*R*) Moon/stargazing has beneficial PM circadian synchronization impact—only moon/stargaze **before** retiring, for maximum sleep/health benefits. Even soft moonlight through your window can disrupt sound sleep.

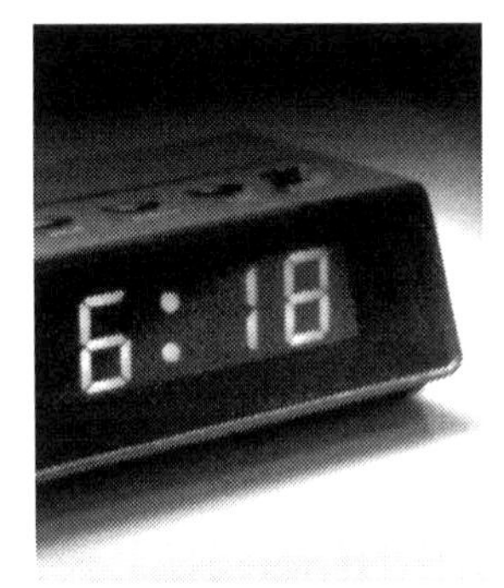

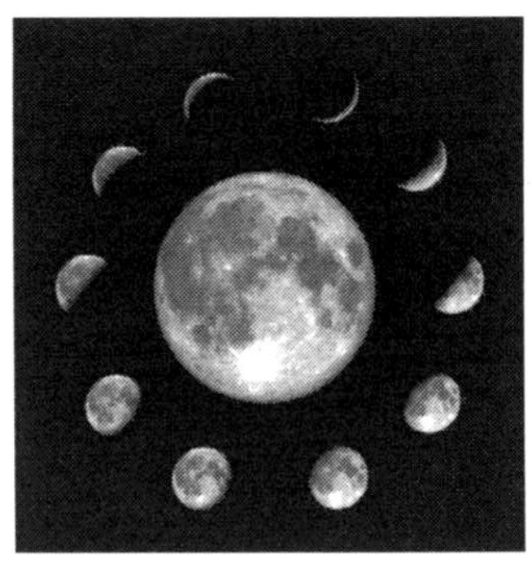

3

Sleep: The Keystone Habit

In the literature of habits, they talk about the keystone habit that you change, and then it becomes easier to change other habits. In my life, the keystone habit was sleep. I went from 4–5 hours to 7–8 hours. That was transformational. [Sleep] truly is a miracle drug.

Arianna Huffington, founder of *The Huffington Post*; author of *Thrive*

Hibernate Like a Bear: Nightly Sleep as Micro-Hibernation

A simple example of how exposure to light and darkness affects fat metabolism is a glimpse into the processes occurring in a bear during winter hibernation. After a summer of gorging on abundant food, the fat bear enters his cave at the onset of winter and goes into hibernation. His body temperature decreases, his metabolic rate slows and shifts to fat burning to stay warm. In the spring, a skinny bear exits the cave, having burnt off a large proportion of his adipose (fat) tissue in the process of staying warm. Exposure to darkness and cold stimulated his fat burning metabolism so he could survive the winter. For humans, each night's sleep is a tiny fractal of a bear's winter-long hibernation. Nighttime is when our neurohormonal system burns off a lot of fat—if operating correctly. Let's avoid as much nighttime light exposure as possible and commit to healthy, light free mini-hibernations every night. Your TV, web and cellphone usage need a good rest during those critical evening and nighttime hours. That's the only way you can reestablish a Golden Sleep Ratio of light/dark and arousal/sleep. Once balanced, Nature's Secret Nutrient miraculously appears and you wake up feeling energized, like a fully recharged yet skinnier bear, ready to roar and rule.

Darkness is as essential to our biological welfare,
to our internal clockwork, as light itself.

Verlyn Klinkenborg, *Our Vanishing Night, National Geographic* magazine

Keep Cooler, Sleep Better

The temperature of your sleeping room is critical for healthy sleep; optimal sleeping range is 60-68° F (15.5-20°C). Many people experience restlessness if the sleeping area temperature goes below or above this range. The 60-68° F range helps to moderately decrease core body temperature, supporting sound, healthy sleep.

Even the Ironman Needs the Golden Sleep Ratio

Mark Allen, "*The World's Fittest Man*" (from *Outside* magazine), won the grueling Hawaiian Ironman Triathlon a record-tying 6 times. A key factor in Mark's training regime was his dedication to getting 9 hours of sleep nightly, to sustain peak performance and optimize his recovery periods—and 9 hours of sleep/rest every 24 hours is the Golden Sleep Ratio. Allen also benefited from strategic longer rest/recharge periods in the time leading up to his races, a protocol aligned with Nature's Energy Wave / N•E•W (see p. 197). Mark was keenly aware of the importance of the right ratio *and* timing of rest/recovery phases to the active phases of training, telling co-author Matthew Cross that ***95% of athletes go into races overtrained [under-rested].*** In the *Business Insider* article *Professional Athletes Like To Spend As Much Time In Bed As Possible,* **Steve Fabregas & Cheri Mah** reported that the average amount of sleep of champions across a wide range of sports approximated the Golden Sleep Ratio range of 9 hours out of 24. Mah is a professional sleep coach working with top athletes whose research applies just as strongly to the rest of us, whatever our fitness regimen. Her findings include:

- Φ A 20-30 minute power nap improves alertness by 42%
- Φ Chronic sleep loss can lead to a 30-40% reduction in glucose metabolism
- Φ 2 days inadequate sleep can lead to a 3x increase in attention lapses & reactivity
- Φ Well-rested tennis players got a 42% boost in hitting accuracy
- Φ Sleep loss means an 11% reduction in time to exhaustion
- Φ A good night's sleep before the game = a winning game;
  a season of good sleep every night = a season of wins.

Tennis legend **Roger Federer** is a great example of the power of ample rest and recovery in support of peak performance. After a nagging knee injury in 2016 forced him to take 6 months off to heal, Federer roared back to win a then-record 18th Grand Slam title at the 2017 Australian Open (beating nemesis Rafael Nadal in a classic 5-set final). Evident to all was Roger's renewed endurance and focus, clearly tied to his unplanned 6-month catapult-loading rest and recovery break.

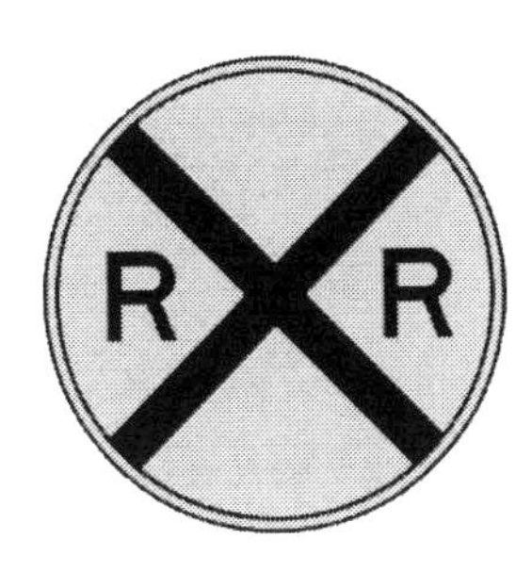

As at all Railroad (RR) Crossings, it's best to *stop* and be sure you have enough R&R (Rest & Recovery) before proceeding to the next health & longevity drivers. For example, it's better *not* to exercise—or engage in any activity requiring full presence and alertness—if you're sleep-deprived, to avoid the risk and dangers of injury, accident, heart attack, immune system stress, poor digestion and poor performance.

Sleep & Performance Insights from World-Class Athletes

Sleep is extremely important to me—I need to rest and recover in order for the training I do to be absorbed by my body.

Usain Bolt, sprinter; 9-time Olympic gold medalist & world record holder

Sleep is just as important as diet and exercise.

Grant Hill, NBA basketball player, Phoenix Suns

A hard work ethic needs to be balanced with a disciplined sleep ethic. Many athletes think they are overtrained, when in fact they are under-rested.

Deena Kastor, Olympic runner; 2:19:36 marathon

I sleep 8 to 9 hours a night, plus a 60-90 minute nap. Sleep is when my body grows stronger. I protect my sleep like a pot of gold.

Ryan Hall, Olympic runner; 2:04:58 marathon

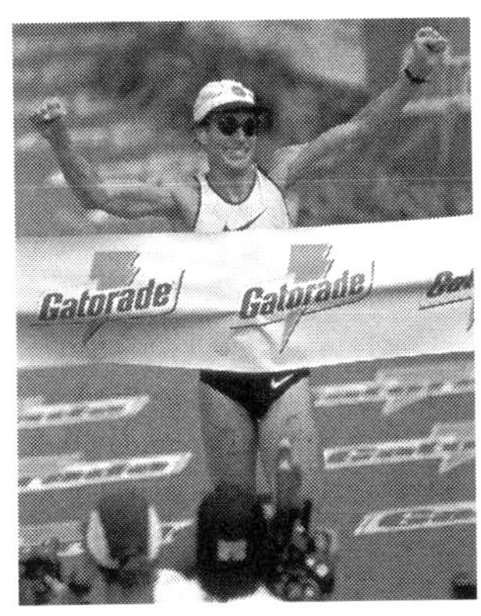

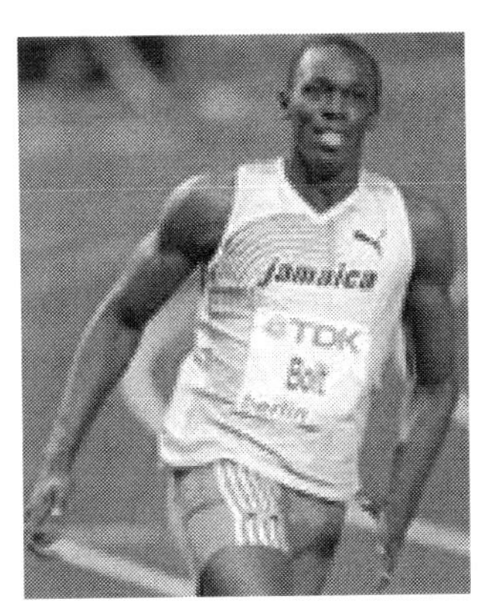

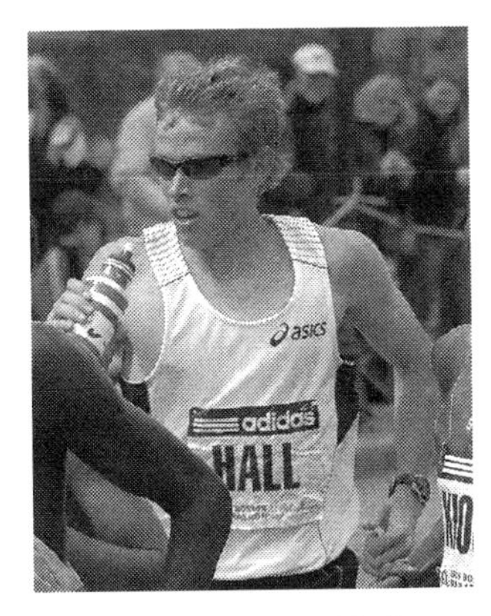

(*L*) A cornerstone in the training regime of 6-time World Ironman Triathlon Champion **Mark "The Grip" Allen** was his dedication to sleeping 9 hours a night to sustain peak performance and optimize recovery. (*Center*) **Usain Bolt** of Jamaica, legendary World and Olympic sprinting champion. Bolt's sound sleeping practice is a vital component to his world record shattering performances. (*R*) American running champion **Ryan Hall** protects his 8-9 hour nightly sleeping regimen "like a pot of gold."

A well-rested body is a healthier, more efficient, more capable one. This could be the hardest thing to accomplish on my to-do list, but it always makes a difference.
Kerri Walsh, Olympic beach volleyball champion

Napping every game day, whether you feel like it or not, has a positive effect on your performance and a cumulative effect on your body throughout the season.
Steve Nash, NBA basketball player, Phoenix Suns

3

To ↓ Risk of Cardiovascular Disease & Heart Attacks, Sleep B4 Exercise & Avoid the Toxic☠Brew of Sleep Deficit & Biorhythm Disturbance

A groundbreaking article in the journal *Hypertension*, 7/2016, by Grimaldi, et.al., showed that people who burn the candle at both ends or just don't get enough sleep have an elevated nighttime heart rate, along with elevated norepinephrine (stress hormone) levels. Healthy Heart Rate Variability (HRV) was also decreased, indicating increased stress on the autonomic nervous system. When sleep's normal restorative function on the heart and cardiovascular system doesn't occur, it leaves the unrested individual at higher risk of catastrophic cardiovascular events like heart attacks. **In short, adequate regular sleep is your vital nightly cardiovascular regenerator—a critical (and free!) life insurance policy for your heart.** Priority Coach takeaway: **Always be sure you're well rested before exercising.** If you stay up late often, are jet lagged or do shift work, *get some sleep before you do any exercise or vigorous activity.* This study affirms the wisdom of honoring the sequence of the NSN health priority drivers—remember that Sleep, co-#3 driver, comes before Exercise, driver #6. Poor sleep is often a clear symptom of excess stress/tension in your life and excessive stress/tension in life are often symptoms of poor sleep. It works both ways. Either way, such symptoms indicate the need for a *total* lifestyle upgrade vs. *just focusing on better sleep alone.* Working *both* sides of the equation supports peak health and performance in all life areas. All NSN health priority drivers must be properly supported, as they cross reinforce one another ongoingly.

Neil Patel: Master Entrepreneur & Golden Ratio Sleep Champion

Entrepreneur Neil Patel is another shining example of the power of dwelling in the Golden Ratio sleep zone. In the 12/2016 *Entrepreneur* article *How I Run 3 Multi-Million-Dollar Companies While Getting 9.25 Hours of Sleep a Night,* Patel reports that the upgrades he's enjoyed in his life and performance since he made sleep a key priority include dramatic increases in energy, focus, collaboration and productivity: *The more sleep I get, the more I'm able to achieve in less time. This is opposite from what most people think. We tend to think*

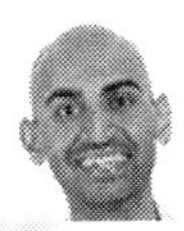

BEFORE	*AFTER*
Around 4 hrs. Sleep/Night	**9.25 hrs. Sleep/Night**
Depleted Energy • Lowered Focus	*Fully Energized • Laser Focus*
Poor Decision Making Ability	*Quality Decisions Faster*
Suboptimal Performance & Productivity	*Vastly Increased Performance & Productivity*

I Love Sleep! Multi-millionaire entrepreneur Neil Patel (in his custom pajamas) gets a Golden Ratio of just over 9 hrs. sleep nightly. He treats healthy sleep like a great business investment to be optimized.

3

that if we sleep less, we'll be able to accomplish more things… but what are you actually doing in your half-dazed, sleep-deprived, brain-numb condition? You're working slowly, inefficiently and miserably. Patel, a top web influencer who helps Google, Amazon, Viacom and businesses worldwide grow revenue, has been widely recognized in the media as well as by the United Nations and President Obama. His story adds to the growing research on the value of allowing your sleep to dwell in the Golden Ratio zone of 9+ hours sleep/rest per 24 hours. Visit NeilPatel.com to learn more about this Golden Ratio Sleep Champion & his work.

In the next chapter, we'll explore the crucial role regular healthy sunlight exposure plays in support of sound sleep and maximum vitality, performance and longevity.

Good sleep is like loading a catapult: *the better you load it, the better it performs.* Every catapult generates its power by going back *first.* Similarly, Golden Ratio-tuned sleep/rest is the vital *catapult loading phase* for optimal health, performance and longevity.

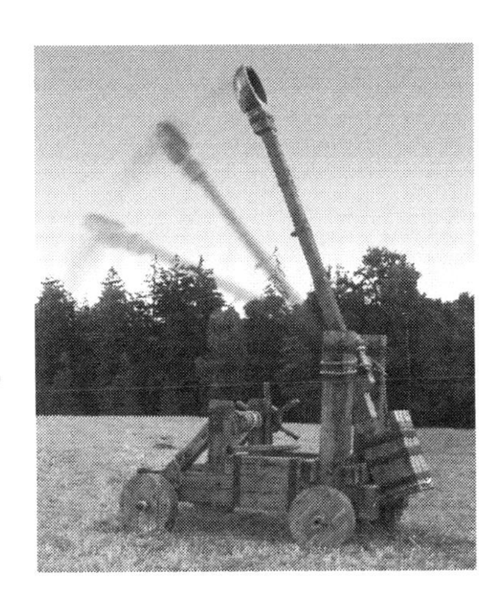

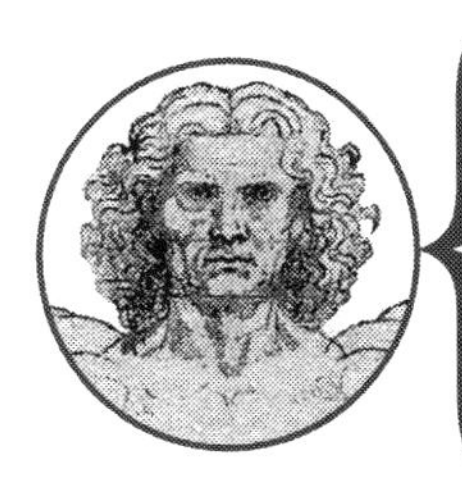

Remember, you're only as **Rested** *and recharged as last night's* ***SLEEP***. So load your sleep catapult by honoring the quality and quantity of your sleep by aiming to get a Golden Ratio of 8–9 hours of sleep/rest on at least 3 to 4 nights per week. Sleep in a dark, cool, relaxing and cozy space with no EMF's.

3

SECTION II: Wake~Sunlight

Solar Nutrition: The Bright Golden Key to Health, Energy & Happiness

Here comes the Sun King... Everybody's laughing... Everybody's happy...

The Beatles

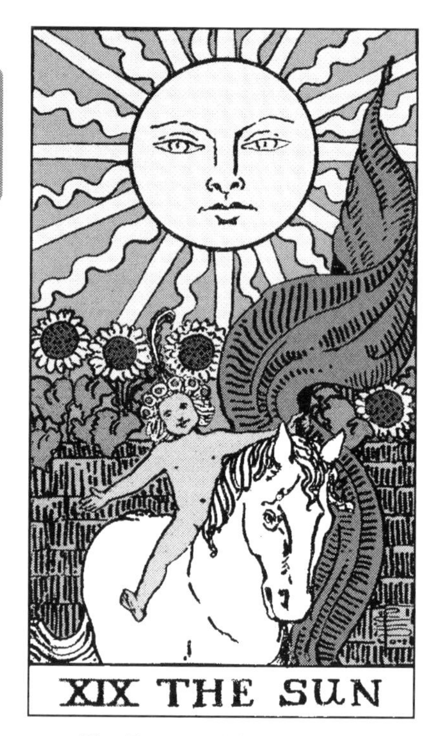

The Tarot card for the Sun is represented by the Roman Numeral XIX (19). Nineteen is the start of the Golden Prime Zone, that time in life between ages 19-31 when human vitality is at its peak (see Ch 9 for more on the Golden Prime Zone). The Sun brings health, happiness, vitality, enthusiasm and recharges body, mind and spirit.

Sunlight is the indispensable energy source necessary to ignite and sustain all life processes on earth. Sunlight energizes oceanic phytoplankton and terrestrial green plants to generate the oxygen that fills our atmosphere. Around 400 million years ago, enough oxygen had filled the atmosphere to support air-breathing terrestrial creatures. Over time, terrestrial creatures, including humans, evolved their own direct methods of harnessing various aspects of sunlight. The abundance of food on our planet is evidence of the photosynthetic processes that are continually going on in plants. Yet most people are unaware that we humans are also able to use sunlight directly, not for photosynthesis, but to regulate circadian rhythms and produce vitamin D, neurotransmitters and hormones. Without regular sun exposure we risk deficiency diseases of sunlight malnutrition, much like the vitamin deficiency diseases discovered over the last 150 years.

One of the most well known vitamin deficiency diseases is scurvy, a vitamin C deficiency that was remedied by British sailors who discovered that by simply consuming lemons or limes on their ocean journeys, they could avoid bleeding sores, infections and fatigue. They realized that humans weren't able to make their own vitamin C, but had to get it from various food sources. As is the case with vitamin C, we're not able to synthesize sunlight, so we have to get it from our environment, namely the sun. On our journey through the sea of life, many in this modern age are suffering from sunlight malnutrition that disconnects us from normal circadian rhythmicity, as well

The Timelessly Illuminated Message of the Sun Gods

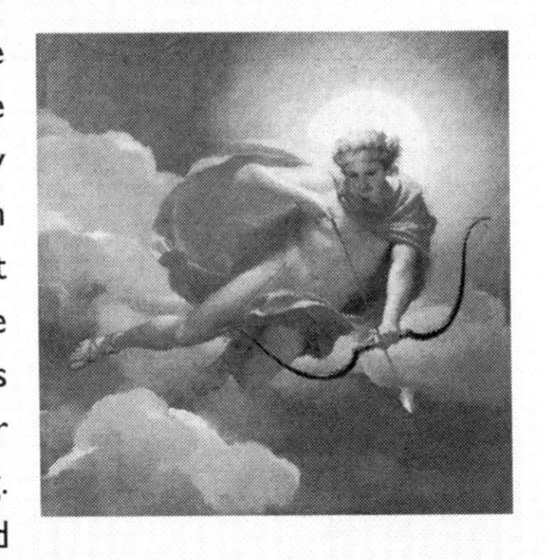

From the Greek Helios (pictured here) to the Roman Sol to the Egyptian Ra, sun gods have always bestowed the vitalizing power necessary for humanity to survive and flourish. Although earlier cultures that worshiped the sun didn't have our current scientific understanding of the physiological mechanisms behind sunlight, it was clear to them that sunlight was necessary for their physical, mental, emotional and spiritual well-being. Unfortunately, our current culture has dethroned the ancient sun gods and in their place has deified SSRI pharmaceuticals as the new wonder emancipators of depression. Yet we can easily restore the sun gods to their rightful place as the rejuvenators of mankind, by simply using Nature's **SSRI's**—**S**olar **S**kin & **R**etina **I**nvigorators—as more natural and effective remedies.

as vitamin D, neurotransmitter and hormonal production. One of the most common effects of solar malnutrition is a low energy state of the brain known as depression. This common affliction is usually not treated with the simple and free remedy of sun exposure, but has a medical and societal default to pharmaceutical antidepressants.

Antidepressant use in the United States among all ages increased nearly 400% from 1988–1994 compared to 2005–2008 (CDC data), with women having double the rate of antidepressant use compared to men. The most commonly prescribed antidepressants are the **SSRI's** (Selective Serotonin Reuptake Inhibitors) Prozac, Zoloft and Paxil. They keep what little serotonin has been released from being reabsorbed, thereby prolonging its action. This artificial, pharmaceutical mechanism does nothing to support naturally induced synthesis and release of new serotonin. Serotonin is one of many in a cascade of natural brain and body hormones closely associated with happiness and a healthy state of mind. Due to the usurpation of natural alternatives by the Medical Industrial Complex (MedIC), a critical, timeless panacea for health—the sun—has been unfairly demonized and thrown into the dust bin of carcinogens and beauty-destroying toxins. Yet we can easily turn the tables by simply using a remedy that's hidden in plain sight:

Nature's SSRI's: **S**olar **S**kin & **R**etina **I**nvigorators

Research has shown that serotonin production and uptake pathways exist in both the skin and the retina, yet need to be activated by the sun. The natural human proclivity for sunbathing is clear evidence that humans naturally feel better with sun exposure. On a practical level, our retina's and skin are the most amazing biosolar panels, which can charge and regulate all of our body systems. The right dose of Sun is a powerful healer, igniting our cells with the power to regenerate. Sunlight is both a physiological and a psychological nutrient, with the same requirements as other nutrients to dwell within the *Just Right* dosage zone for optimal vitality. We also know that when deprived of adequate sunlight—or at least regular doses of full-spectrum light—we can become depressed and unhealthy, a condition known as SAD—Seasonal Affective Disorder.

Healthy sun exposure can raise serotonin to clinically significant amounts necessary to negate the need for pharmaceuticals. With sun exposure as with all of the NSN health priority drivers, *the dose makes the medicine or the poison*. Each individual needs to determine proper timing, intensity and duration for themselves. Skin type as well as location, time of day and year are critical variables to get the *Just Right* amount of sunlight, without overdosing. Insufficient sunlight prevents serotonin, melatonin and vitamin-D synthesis and also increases the tendency for depression and possibly suicide. Alternatively, too much sun exposure (especially sunburn) increases photoaging of the skin, skin cancers and possible cataract formation and macular degeneration. There is essentially no risk of producing too much serotonin, melatonin or vitamin-D from sunbathing, as the body's natural intelligence has negative feedback loops that stop production when adequate levels are restored. In the end, personal responsibility is important when using sunlight as your personal health panacea. In this chapter you'll discover how to find the ideal, Golden Ratio amount of healthy sun exposure that also generates maximal NSN. This optimal sun exposure range aligns elegantly—like all NSN health priority drivers—with the timeless wisdom of the Ancient Greeks:

Meden Agan—Nothing in Excess

Photosynthesis Makes Sugar

People have known sunlight's life-giving effects for millennia. One magic aspect of sunlight's power is the process of photosynthesis in plants, whereby CO_2 and H_2O are catalyzed in by sunlight to make sugar, with oxygen as a by-product. The sun's energy is stored in sugar molecules like the charge in a battery. As sugars/carbohydrates are eaten and metabolized by humans and other creatures, energy is released in a slow manner via ATP and is used to power cellular processes. **Essentially, food is stored**

sunlight. Photosynthesis is an example of the interconversion of energy and mass as demonstrated in Albert Einstein's famous equation, $E=mc^2$. Plants make energy in the form of sugar molecules and humans reverse the process—releasing the stored energy by eating and metabolizing the food.

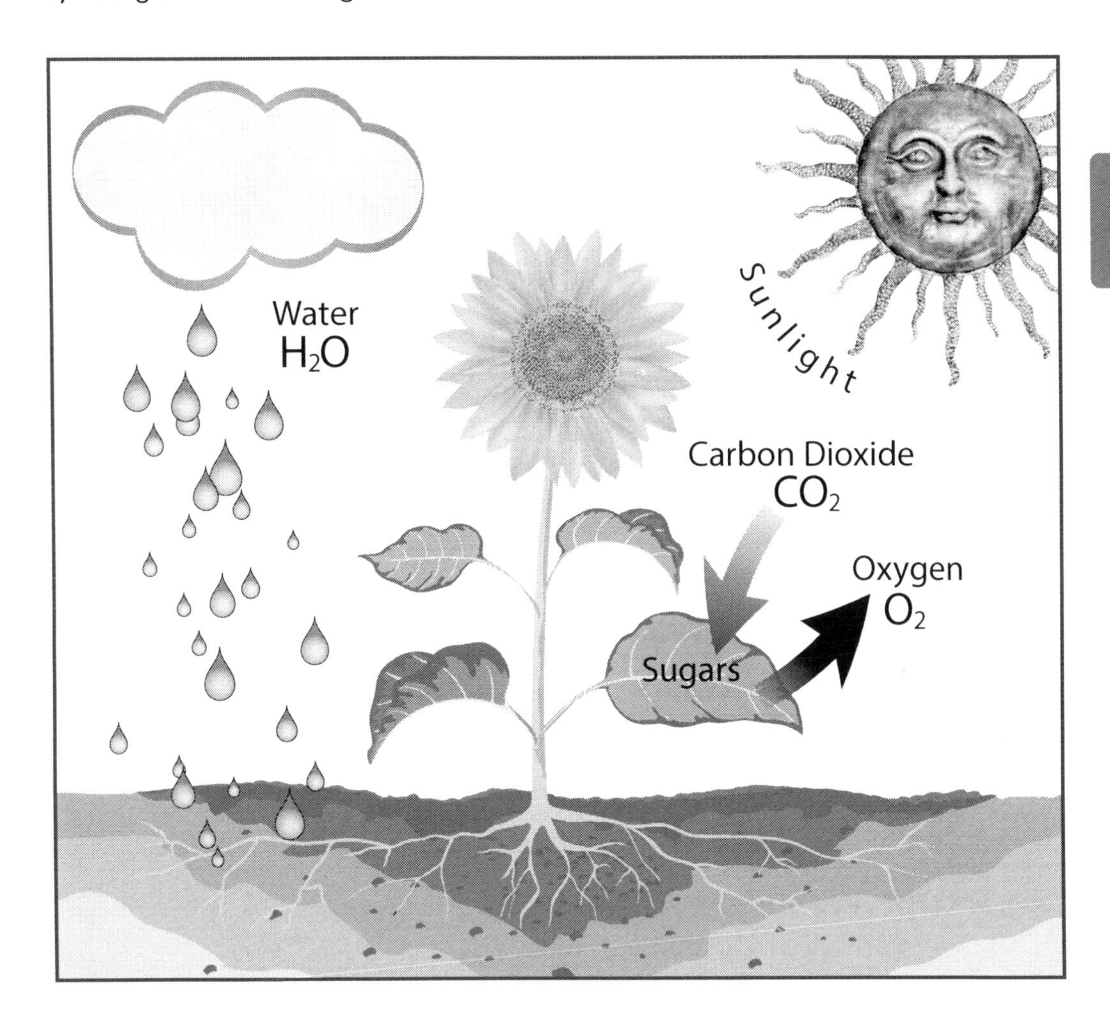

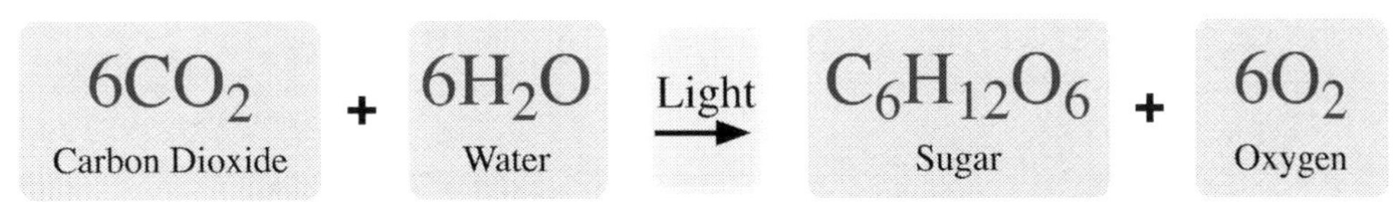

Photosynthesis: Macro & Micro Perspective

Top: How sunlight, air, water, plants and earth combine to make photosynthesis possible.

Bottom: The chemical process whereby sunlight catalyzes the formation of sugar from CO_2 and H_2O, with Oxygen (O_2) as a key by-product.

3

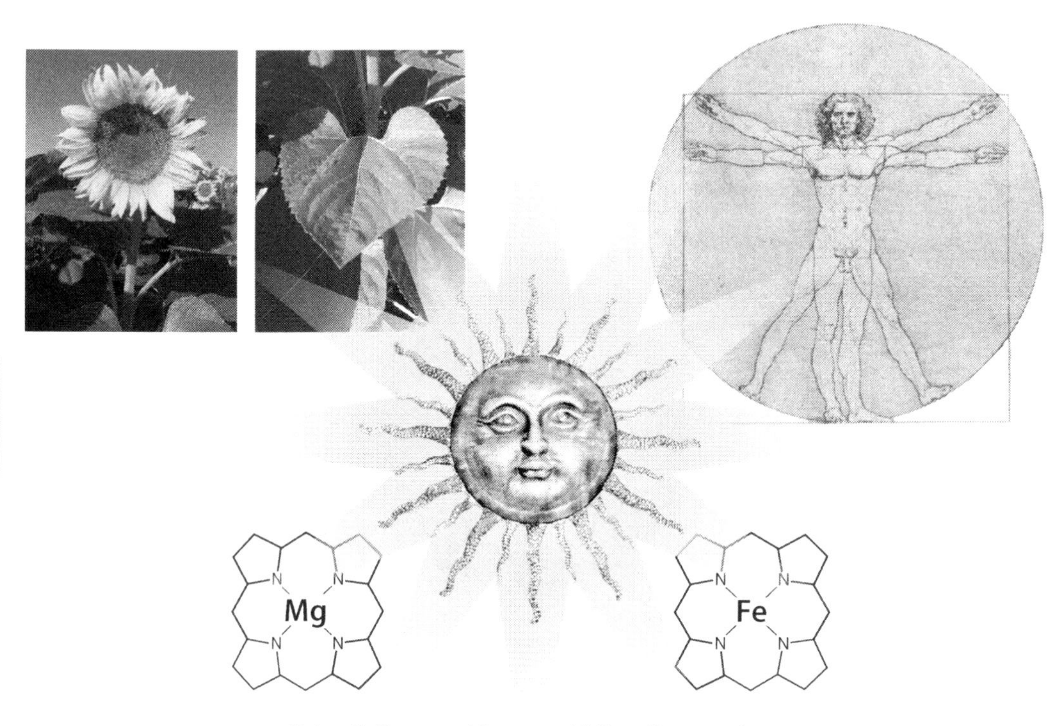

Solar Collectors: Macro and Micro Perspective

Top: Both sunflowers and human beings are Golden Ratio designed intermediaries between heaven and earth. To harness sunlight, each have their own specialized type of solar collectors—leaves & flowers on plants and skin and retinas on humans. Sunflowers track the sun's path to maximize sun exposure and take advantage of their Fibonacci structured (Golden Spiral) leaf and petal distribution for optimal sun, air and moisture exposure. Humans can learn from plants by making sunbathing a regular healthy habit.

Bottom: Sunlight is captured by chlorophyll in plant leaves and hemoglobin in blood as it flows through capillaries in human skin. (*L*) chlorophyll is green, having a magnesium molecule (Mg) at its center, while (*R*) hemoglobin is red, having an iron molecule (Fe) at its center. Both chlorophyll and hemoglobin can also transmute sunlight to structure and energetically charge intracellular and extracellular water (*EZ water*).

Golden Ratio Synthesis Makes NSN

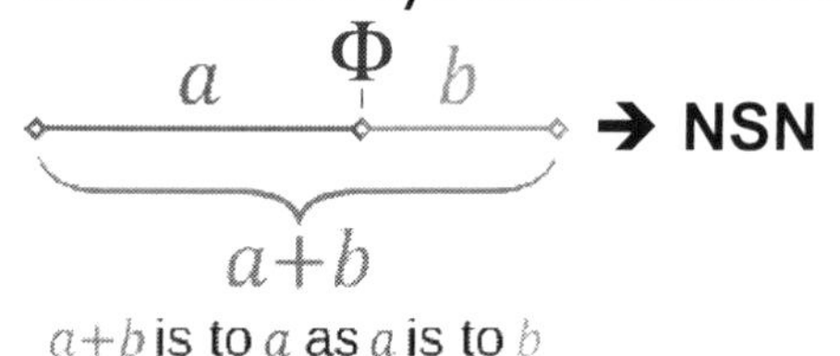

The simple yet powerful formula for Golden Ratio Synthesis. By combining the elements of each health priority driver in Golden Ratio proportions, a powerful synergy factor emerges that optimizes all human physical, mental, emotional and spiritual functions. **That synergy factor is known as NSN.**

Just as CO_2, H_2O and sunlight produce sugar, so is Nature's Secret Nutrient/NSN produced when the elements composing the health priority drivers are utilized in Golden Ratio. The general principle of Golden Ratio Synthesis can be described as follows. When two lines of specific lengths (**a & b**) are combined such that **a + b is to a, as a is to b**, NSN emerges as the MetaNutrient that super-energizes *all* MegaNutrient health priority drivers.

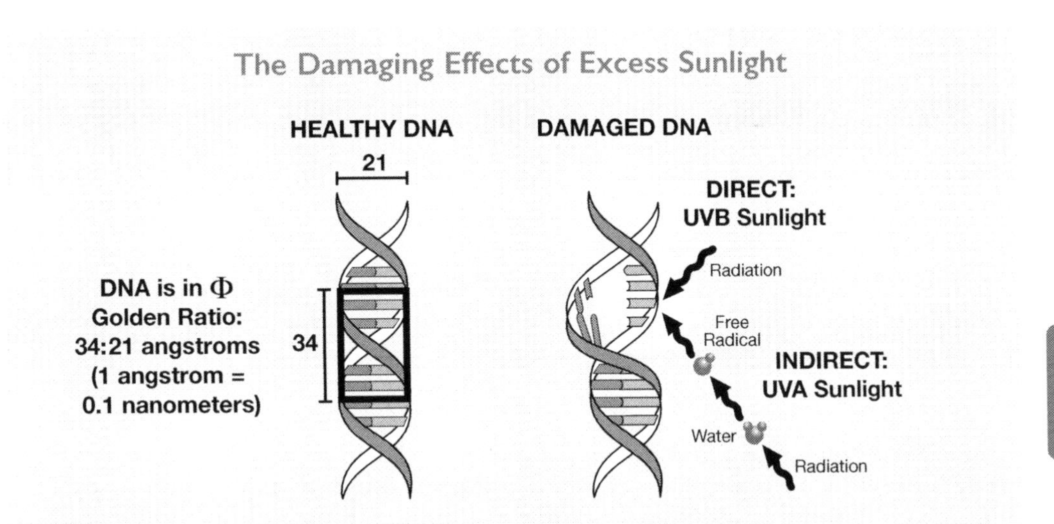

Excess UVB from sunlight can damage DNA, through *directly* disrupting DNA molecules, while UVA from sunlight *indirectly* damages DNA by creating free radicals, which then damage DNA. The result of excess exposure of either UVA/UVB is photoaging of the skin, damage to collagen, elastin and formation of spider veins, age spots and increased risk of skin cancers. Sunlight exposure's many benefits must be weighed against the risks; finding a Golden Ratio balance between the two is the aim.

The Sunlight Dose Makes the Medicine ℞ — Or the Poison ☠

The Goldilocks principle of finding the dose of *Just Right* applies to just about everything, including finding the correct dose of UV Sunlight, vitamin D and DHA. Too small a dose and there's no beneficial effect; too large a dose produces undesirable side effects. Essentially, as we see with all NSN health priority drivers, *The Dose Makes the Medicine or the Poison*. In addition to UVA and UVB, all visible wavelengths of light are necessary for our health—nutritionally, cosmetically and psychologically. The challenge is to absorb the sun's rays into our bodies in the most healthful way, getting not too little yet not too much. The tanning effect of the sun is due to the immediate effects of UVA on melanin pigment release in the skin, whereas UVB's tanning effects can take up to several days. Each person needs to determine their own ideal amount of sunlight to get, while avoiding the negative effects of over-sunning. UVB has been found to directly damage DNA, but at the same time is the critical wavelength of light that produces vitamin D. UVA gives us a healthy looking tan, yet prolonged exposure can result in the formation of damaging free radicals that can also damage DNA and collagen, causing skin aging and skin cancer. DNA structure is based on Golden Ratio proportions with a length/width ratio of 34:21 angstroms and these precise proportions can be disrupted from excessive UV exposure. **Once the Golden Ratio *form* of DNA is disrupted its *function* is altered as well.** Although DNA has self-repair mechanisms, they are occasionally inefficient, which can result in photoaging and skin cancers.

Jack Kruse, M.D.: The Renaissance Doctor Who Saw & Spreads The Light

One day light will be seen as important as diet and exercise.

Jack Kruse, M.D.

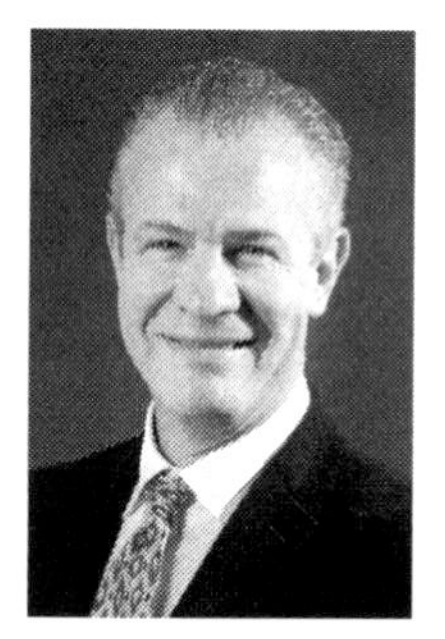

Jack Kruse, M.D., neurosurgeon, biophysicist, modern-day Renaissance man.

Jack Kruse, M.D. is a New Orleans-based neurosurgeon, biophysicist, author, modern-day Renaissance man and Biohacker (or in Dr. Jack's case, ***Bayou*Hacker**). While viewing Michelangelo's classic *David* statue in Florence, Italy in 2006, Jack had a profound epiphany regarding the workings of his own *inner David*. At the time Jack was a very obese 350 pounds, while *David* was a sleek, Golden Ratio-proportioned icon. Jack realized that his own 21st century environment was radically different compared to David's 16th century world. *David* reflected a man who's biology was finely-tuned to the circadian rhythms of natural sunlight, an unpolluted electromagnetic field and pure, energetically charged air and water. Jack's environment on the other hand was distorted by a radically altered artificial light spectrum, severe air and electromagnetic pollution and chemically treated, dead water. 500 years had made a huge difference in the environmental terrain and the ensuing epigenetic changes that presumably accounted for Jack's obesity. He surmised that by revising his relationship with these 21st century aberrations he could perhaps release his *inner David* and thus resolve his personal health challenge. After much research **it became clear that the *seemingly minuscule* effects of Sunlight, Magnetism and Water were really the *primary drivers* underlying biochemistry, physiology, nutrition and medicine.**

These ***Quantum ElectroDynamic* (QED)** effects are a great example of the butterfly effect—where small initial changes in one state of a nonlinear system can result in large changes downstream. When environmental conditions—sunlight, magnetism and water—are properly supported in the short run, they can lead to optimal health, performance and longevity in the long run. Prior to Jack's epiphany, the ***Quantum ElectroDynamic***/QED effects of physics were relegated to a separate arena, thought to be more or less independent from the more tangible medical sciences. Jack's solid research combined with his intuitive sense told him that *all* of the sciences needed to be reprioritized and integrated before his obesity could be effectively addressed and resolved.

He took action and designed a personal biohack that activated his evolutionarily programmed QED pathways, boosting energy production and fat burning in his body. This involved daily direct morning sunlight exposure to reset his circadian rhythms and fully activate his neurohormones, along with taking care to avoid the disruptive effects of artificial blue light in the evenings. His other activation key was bathing in ice-cold water, otherwise known as cold thermogenesis (see Ch 10 Longevity). *Through these combined effects he lost an astounding 137 pounds in just 9 months.* Jack became his own Michelangelo, sculpting his *inner David* by designing a reprioritized health pyramid, one with the QED effects of sunlight, water and magnetism at its base. His food choices were also supportive and geared towards getting optimal amounts of DHA, through high consumption of seafood/shellfish (DHA is necessary to prime the photon/electron pumps in the eye's retinas; see ***The Catcher in the Eye***, next section). A pyramid without a stable base is one that's likely to topple over; the shift of the QED effects of light, water and magnetism to the base of his health pyramid was the stabilization needed to kick his metabolism into high gear and resolve his obesity. Since that time, he's used these techniques to help countless patients break free of the diseases imposed by an out-of-control technological civilization. Bridging the gap between physics and the healing sciences is a paradigm shift in medicine and science and is Dr. Jack Kruse's outstanding gift to humanity.

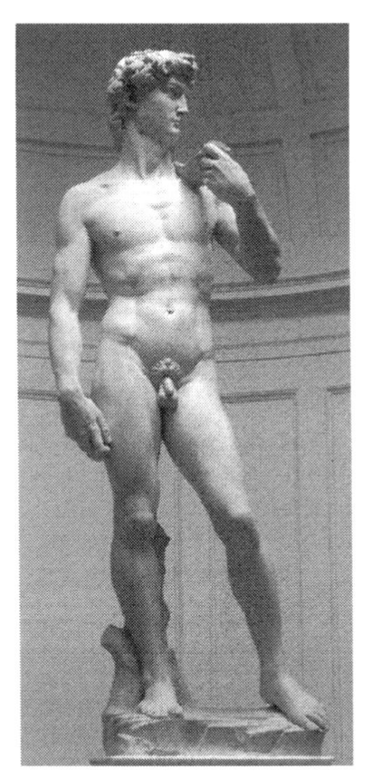

Michelangelo's Golden-Proportioned *David* was the catalyst for Dr. Jack Kruse's epiphany into how Quantum ElectroDynamic laws of physics interface with human biology.

On a related note, Kruse also received a healthy Golden Ratio imprint as he stood at the base of *David*, which Michelangelo had elegantly embedded in his timeless masterpiece. As we see in this book, the Golden Ratio is the universal blueprint integrating all NSN health priority drivers into a coherent, fractal method of rejuvenation and restoration. Dr. Kruse underscores this point in his insight regarding the ***As Above, So Below*** principle of Fibonacci math, i.e., the Golden Ratio:

> ***Fibonacci math*** *is tied directly to the fractal patterning of all living things found on this planet. This math shows us that everything that is used in our microcosm is patterned after*

the great design of our macrocosm. All one needs to do is look for the pattern and you will find it everywhere.

The Catcher in the Eye: DHA Omega-3 Fatty Acid Snares Sunlight

The more DHA you eat, the more gets into your tissues.

Jack Kruse, M.D., neurosurgeon, biophysicist

In a healthy human, DHA comprises 60% percent of the PolyUnsaturated Fatty Acids (PUFA) in the eyes' retinas and 40% in the brain, both approximate Golden Ratio distributions (62/38 being the next finer level of alignment). DHA is one of the omega-3 fatty acids derived from algae, fish and shellfish that catalyzed the massive increase in brain size that enabled our species to develop our uniquely human ingenuity and adaptability. Over the course of evolution, we evolved high concentrations of DHA (fish oil molecules) in our retinas (back of the eye) that facilitate the production of electrons (DC electric current) when photons from UV sunlight hit the DHA molecule. **This process is none other than a fascinating biological adaptation of Einstein's Photoelectric Effect, for which he was awarded the Nobel Prize in 1921.** This DC electrical current in turn moves through the optic nerve into the brain, where it activates the hypothalamus, pituitary, pineal and other brain structures to produce neurotransmitters and hormones. Just as with regular batteries, if the charge is low, the device (our brain cells) won't function effectively—if at all. Only by getting healthy

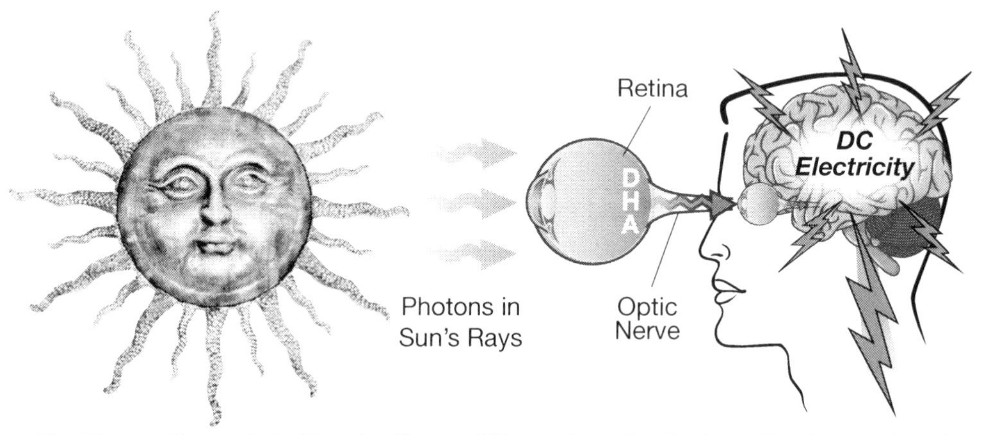

The Human Photovoltaic Charging System. We are charged and animated by the sun when the following sequence is activated: 1. Unfiltered sunlight exposure provides raw photons that enter the eye. 2. DHA molecules in the retina act as targets for photons (DHA is one of the omega-3 fatty acids derived from algae, fish and shellfish). 3. Photons generate DC electricity by knocking electrons off DHA molecules. 4. The DC electricity travels from the retina into the brain via the optic nerve. This sequence *supercharges* your brain and body—a prime example of **Quantum ElectroDynamics (QED)** in action—as well as energizing all NSN health priority drivers/MegaNutrients.

UV sunlight exposure and having an adequate supply of DHA in our retinae can we ensure that our neurohormonal circadian system will be activated and healthy on a daily basis and that we'll receive the full benefits the DC electric charging effect. When DHA decreases, so does the Sunlight-activated production of DC electric current. Viewed from our Golden Ratio perspective, once DHA levels in the retina fall below 60%, energy-dependent cellular processes in the brain will become inefficient. Initially, vague symptoms like lethargy, fatigue, depression, poor digestion and decreased libido inevitably arise. If the combined deficit of sunlight, DHA and low cellular charge continues, the vague symptoms can progress into actual disease states. Virtually all modern diseases can be accelerated through this low cellular charge state—obesity, diabetes, hypertension, heart disease, autoimmune diseases, as well as the recent increase in neurological and ophthalmologic diseases like Alzheimer's, Parkinson's and macular degeneration. What we're really looking at is a *Golden Ratio Threshold of Sunlight and DHA*, below which disease states begin to manifest. With that information in mind, the cure is both free and relatively simple: ***Increase Sunlight exposure in controlled doses throughout the day, along with consistent, adequate doses of DHA from seafood and/or supplements.*** A critical factor to remember: avoid the damaging blue light in the evenings from computers, cell phones, TV's as well as improper indoor lighting that can degrade DHA in the retina faster than it can be regenerated. As an overall measurement of DHA in your body, order the DHA finger-stick blood test from Life Extension Foundation; see Rx 2 in chapter 3/Sun; Rx section of this book.

3

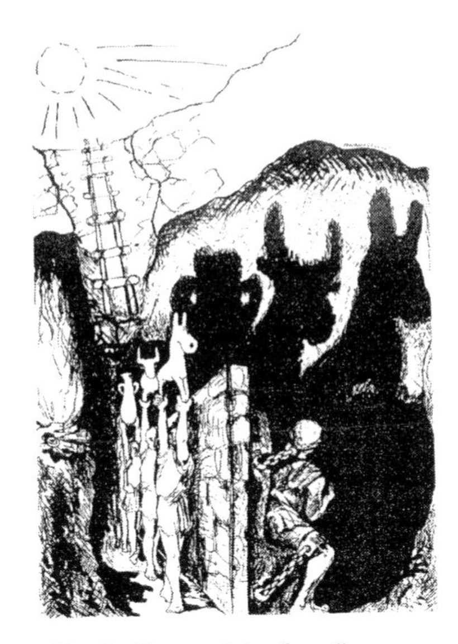

Plato's *Allegory of the Cave* illustrates the illusion of a false reality and the resulting freedom from it once illuminated by real Sunlight (illustration by Markus Maurer). Like a modern-day Plato, Dr. John Ott guided millions of modern-day cave dwellers from light malnutrition into full-spectrum light.

Dr. John Ott: Full Spectrum Light Genius

The world of our sight is like the habitation in prison, the firelight there to the sunlight here, the ascent and the view of the upper world is the rising of the soul into the world of mind.

Plato

In Plato's *Allegory of the Cave*, he describes a group of people who have been prisoners in a cave, only being able to see shadows cast on the cave wall by a fire behind them and believing the shadows to be reality. Once the prisoners are released from their limited perspective

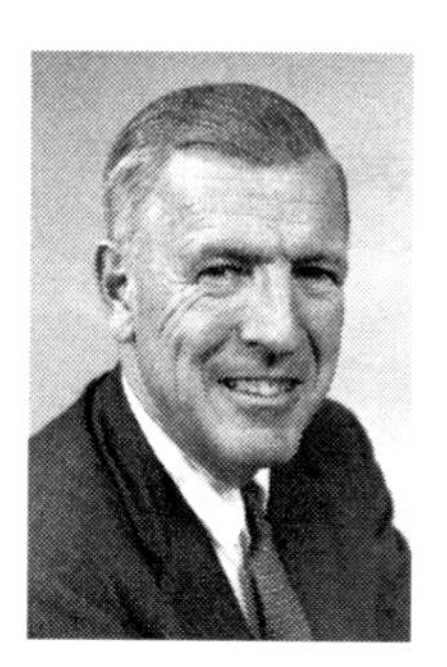
Dr. John Ott, pioneering cinematographer and photobiologist.

3

and exit the cave, they're able to see that the firelight and the shadows cast were mere illusion. The bright Sunlight outside of the cave at first hurts their eyes, but they eventually realize that the true Sun illumines the real world, forever destroying the false reality experienced in the cave. Like a modern-day Plato, Dr. John Ott had the insight and vision to guide generations of contemporary cave dwellers out of their culturally imposed light malnutrition and back into the awareness of full-spectrum light. Ott was a self-directed photographer and scientist who distinguished himself not only with his advances in time-lapse plant cinematography (leading to his recruitment by Walt Disney to collaborate on the groundbreaking film *Secrets of Life*), but also with his discoveries on the benefits of full-spectrum lighting in photobiology. Ott discovered that he could change various characteristics and behaviors of plants simply by modifying the color-temperature of the light they were exposed to. Certain light changes could influence the tendency to flower, bear fruit and could even change the gender of plants. His experiments expanded into the animal realm, where he demonstrated that light malnutrition could cause either health or disease in rodents.

The next logical step was to expand his theory of light malnutrition into the human realm. Ott performed experiments with school children using different groups who were exposed to full-spectrum natural lighting or standard fluorescent lighting. Dramatic differences were observed, where the children exposed to fluorescent lighting became hyperactive and disruptive, while the children exposed to natural lighting were more attentive, learned better and were better behaved. **Ott's breakthrough insight was that modern society is malnourished with respect to the natural light spectrum. Living behind light-filtering glass windows in houses, offices, cars—and even sunglasses—deprives people of the full spectrum of light frequencies necessary for health and vitality.** His discovery of light malnutrition in the 1960's was similar not only to Plato's Cave Allegory, but also analogous to the discovery of vitamin deficiencies over the last few centuries. Dr. Ott's hidden-in-plain-sight observation of light malnutrition had to be one of those *eureka!* moments, where a literal full-spectrum light bulb went off in his mind. Ott's genius included both identifying the problem and coming up with practical, easy solutions that continue to be used to this day, e.g., he developed full spectrum lights that mimic the natural light frequencies found in sunlight. The OttLite provides a precise balance of contrast and brightness that improves the ability to see colors and contrasts clearly.

The Conspiracy Against Sun/Natural Light

Dr. Ott's full spectrum indoor lighting is a major advance for humanity that has been replicated by other researchers since his death in 2000. Ott's insights into the natural human requirement for full-spectrum light gives contrast to what can only be called an insidious ***natural light conspiracy***, as revealed in the following enlightening points:

- Many doctors' ignorance of the essential benefits of regular, direct sun exposure.
- Many doctors' recommendations to avoid the sun at all costs, for fear of skin cancer.
- The media's parallel sensationalist propaganda on the dangers of sun exposure.
- The global multi-billion dollar sunscreen industry's promotion of UV-blocking and potentially carcinogenic products that also *prevent* vitamin-D synthesis.
- Creation of laws against incandescent bulbs, while simultaneously promoting energy efficient bulbs which have an increased toxic☠blue spectrum.
- The elevation of sun-blocking sunglasses as the ultimate "cool" fashion accessory.
- Proliferation of toxic☠mercury-containing Compact Fluorescent Light/CFL bulbs.
- The modern proliferation of Chemtrails that prevent sunlight from reaching earth, while discharging enormous amounts of toxic☠chemicals into the atmosphere.
- A subsection of Obamacare mandates a 10% excise tax on indoor tanning services. As a result of enaction of this law, within 5 years half of the tanning salons in the U.S. closed and thousands of jobs were lost. By keeping vitamin-D levels low in the population, this insidious law thwarted an easy preventive solution for numerous diseases along with a key factor in optimal health.

The Visible Light Spectrum

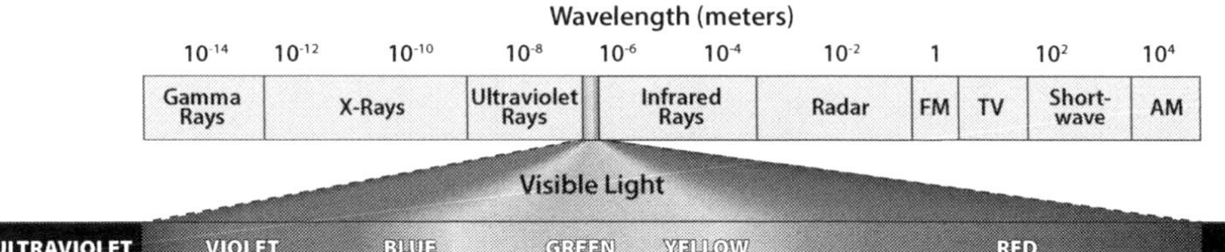

Visible sunlight is a small band in the electromagnetic spectrum ranging from around 380nm-750nm. Ultraviolet rays (UVA, UVB, UVC) have shorter wavelengths (100-400 nm), just overlapping into violet light and are mostly invisible to the human eye. Infrared rays are the warming rays of the sun with longer wavelengths (700 nm-1mm), just overlapping into visible red light. Visible blue light is from 450-495 nm. Excessive blue light has the undesirable properties of destroying DHA in the retina faster than it can be regenerated, as well as upsetting circadian signaling; hence the reason for avoiding blue light in the evenings from computers, cell phones, TV's, etc. Use blue blocker lenses or apps for more retinal protection from blue frequencies when using digital at night.

The antidotes to the conspiracy against sun/natural light are bright and clear:

Φ Educate yourself on the truths and vital benefits of heathy sun exposure.

Φ Get regular, safe sun exposure in healthy doses by following the recommendations in this chapter and its linked Rx section.

Φ When shopping for sunscreens choose only non-toxic, organic formulas.

Φ Use full-spectrum, mercury-free lights in your home and workplace.

Φ Share your newfound solar nutrition wisdom with family, friends and colleagues.

3

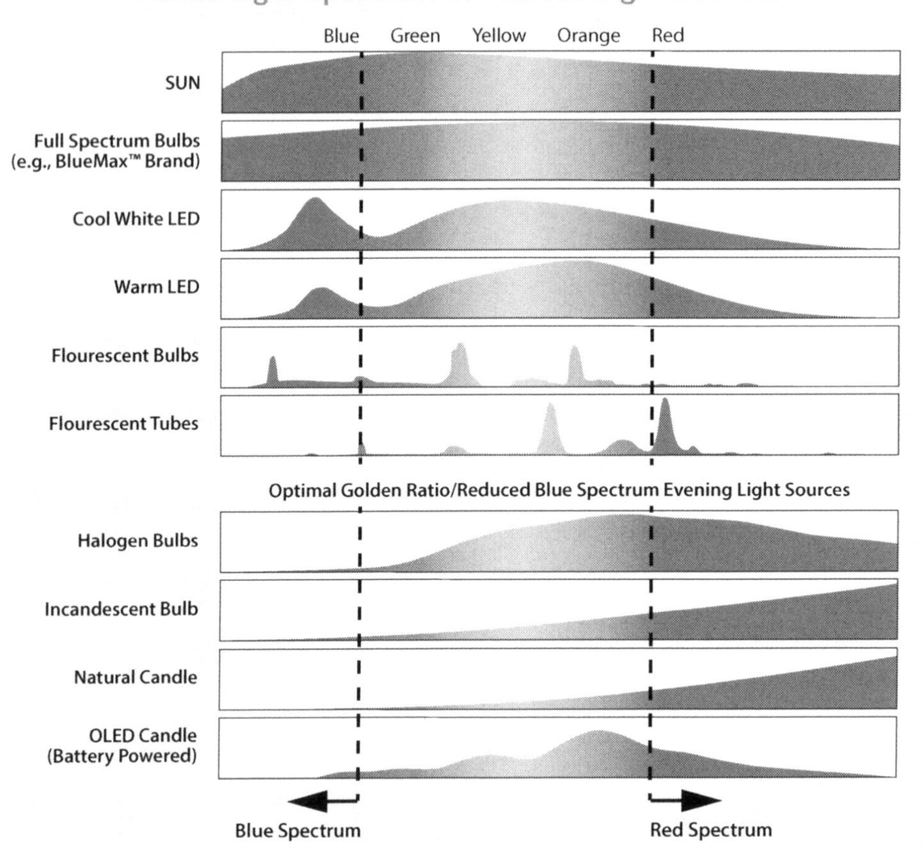

Different types of light bulbs emit different light frequencies, including various amounts of blue light. Although Sunlight has the highest amount of blue light, it of course only shines during daylight hours. **It's the artificial evening blue light that desynchronizes us from our natural circadian rhythms and wreaks havoc with normal hormonal secretions including melatonin, which induces sleep.** Of the common light bulbs compared, incandescent bulbs have the lowest amount of blue frequency emission; their spectral frequencies are shifted towards yellow, orange and red, while CFL and LED bulbs retain a fair amount of blue light emission.

The Golden Ratio Evening Light bulb

A theoretical ideal light bulb for evening use would emit light frequencies that are only in the 62% of the spectrum that encompasses *green/yellow/orange/red*. These frequencies avoid the toxic blue light that can disrupt our circadian rhythms if we're exposed to them after sunset. Candle light, candle light-style OLED's, traditional incandescent and halogen bulbs eliminate most of the blue light and thus fit into the Golden Ratio safe zone. The Golden Ratio division point is at 521nm, in the green part of the spectrum. As the evening progresses, so should your light bulbs move further to the right, towards the red frequencies. Light bulbs in the red range are also advisable for night lights.

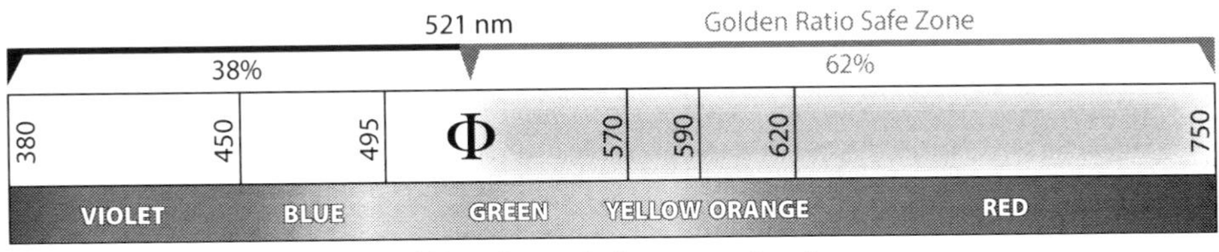

The Golden Ratio Φ division point is at 521nm, in the green part of the spectrum. As the evening progresses, so should your light bulbs move further to the right, towards the red frequencies. Light bulbs in the red range are also advisable for night lights.

Maui Snares the Sun

An ancient myth about the Hawaiian chief and cultural hero Maui is one that we modern humans can surely relate to. According to legend, Maui's mother was distraught because her clothes wouldn't dry in the Sun, due to the short days. Maui had an ingenious idea. At sunrise he climbed to the top of Haleakala volcano (*House of the Sun*) and snared the Sun's rays with a rope. After negotiating with the Sun for the terms of its release, it was agreed that summer days would be longer and winter days would be shorter. Although not chronicled in ancient Hawaiian lore, there was probably a hidden clause in Maui's bargain with the Sun that included a persistent lengthening of the days for future humans in the 20th and 21st centuries—that's us. The clause may have said something to the effect that daylight could be extended even longer by the invention of

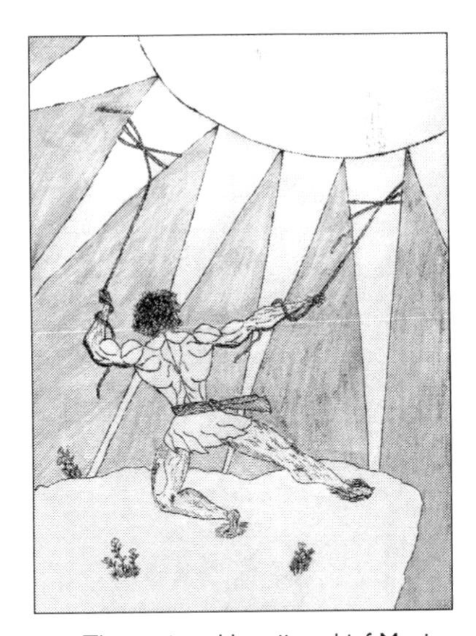

The ancient Hawaiian chief Maui snares the sun's rays. With the advent of modern indoor evening lighting, we have essentially "snared the sun's rays" and artificially elongated our days.

artificial Sunlight, i.e., indoor lighting. It seems that in our busy world of ever-unfinished business, we need Maui's blessing of longer days that artificial lighting bestows upon us. As in many myths, blessings often comes with a hidden curse. Such is the case with the circadian desynchronizing effects of artificial evening light, especially the toxic effects that come with our blue light-rich light bulbs and electronic screens. In order to regain our compromised health from over-exposure to excessive artificial evening light, we may need to petition Maui to release us from the blessing/curse of long days imposed by artificial lighting and allow us to return to the Sun's naturally allotted amount of daylight.

UV Distribution, Vitamin D & the Golden Ratio

We suspect the benefits to heart health of sunlight will outweigh the risk of skin cancer.
Dr. Richard Weller, senior lecturer in dermatology, Edinburgh University

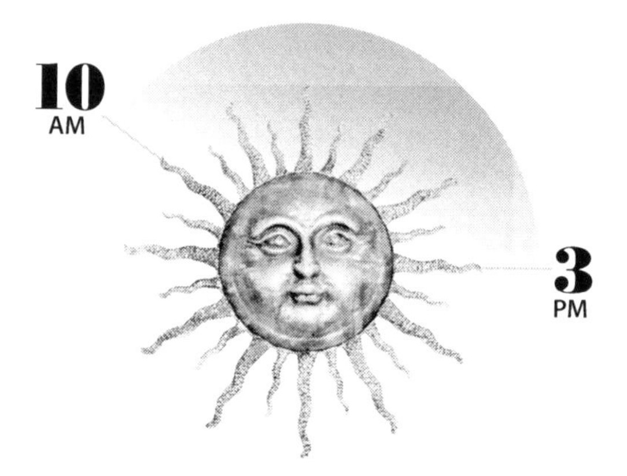

10am-3pm is the best time for maximum UVB exposure & vitamin D production. As summer sun is extremely strong, get your UV exposure at the edges of the 10am-3pm window during this season

The tropics of Cancer and Capricorn—at 23.5° North and South latitudes—are two key latitude lines determined by the annual movements of the sun that demarcate the Earth's northern and southern tropical climate zones. These tropical zones happen to be located within 2° of Golden Ratio harmonic points of the earth's latitude lines. As they say, *location is everything*. Such is the case with where you live and sunbathe in relation to the sun. As can be seen in the featured world map, UVB distribution falls in line with the tropics of Cancer and Capricorn. Depending on the time of year and angle of the sun towards the earth, UV levels can vary widely. Sunbathing in the summer months can provide enough UVB to maintain adequate vitamin D conversion in the skin to raise levels to the healthy range.

Since vitamin D is fat-soluble, your body can store it for months at a time. However, usually by January or February in the northern hemisphere and by June or July in the southern hemisphere, your Vitamin D stores are becoming depleted. This leaves your body more vulnerable to colds and various metabolic and immunologic problems, not to mention depressed psychological conditions such as SAD (Seasonal Affective Disorder). Only the southern part of the United States has any significant UVB during the winter, so

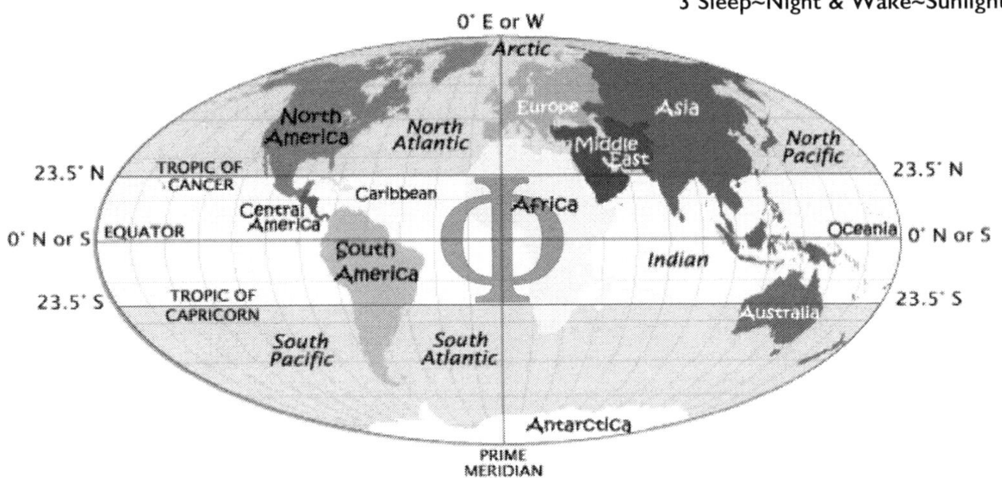

The Earth's mid-range between the latitude lines demarcating the Tropics of Cancer & Capricorn gets abundant ultraviolet (UV) sunlight throughout the year. With the tilt of the Earth through the seasons, northern latitudes receive abundant UV in June-July-August, while southern latitudes receive abundant UV in December-January-February. The surface area between the Tropics of Cancer and Capricorn comprises a little less than 40% of earth's total surface area, an approximate Golden Ratio division. Interestingly, the Golden Ratio symbol Φ (phi) is also commonly used to designate geographic latitude.

most people living in more northern latitudes become deficient during winter months. UVB is necessary for the conversion of a cholesterol-like compound in the skin into vitamin D_3. If you live above the latitude of Atlanta, about 33.7° N, you can't make any vitamin-D in your skin from November through March. Vitamin D_3 is actually a steroid-like molecule with numerous functions in the body including the regulation of calcium levels and prevention of bone diseases ranging from rickets to osteoporosis. A connection between insufficient vitamin D levels and various forms of cancer, autoimmune diseases including MS, diabetes and hypertension has also been found. In addition to latitude, season, altitude, weather and length of exposure, the effects of both UVA and UVB are also dependent on age, skin color/amount of pigment, amount of skin exposed and application of sunscreens. Older people and dark skinned individuals tend to make less vitamin D per amount of time in the sun. Since we don't get tropical or subtropical sunshine in the U.S. mainland (with the exception of the southern U.S.) and in Europe, we need to bring the benefits of those climates to us in the form of adequate vitamin D through food or supplements to make up the difference. Even the best food sources like salmon, mackerel, sardines and tuna may not give you enough vitamin D. The most concentrated food source of vitamin D_3 is cod liver oil, but due to variable vitamin A levels within different brands, it's not advised to take too much. The best ways to increase your vitamin D_3 levels are through a combination of sunlight, vitamin D_3 rich foods and targeted supplementation. Over-the-counter vitamin D_3 supplements come in various strengths, usually ranging from 100 IU's to 10,000 IU's. The best and only way to know if you're getting enough vitamin D_3—yet not too much—is to monitor your

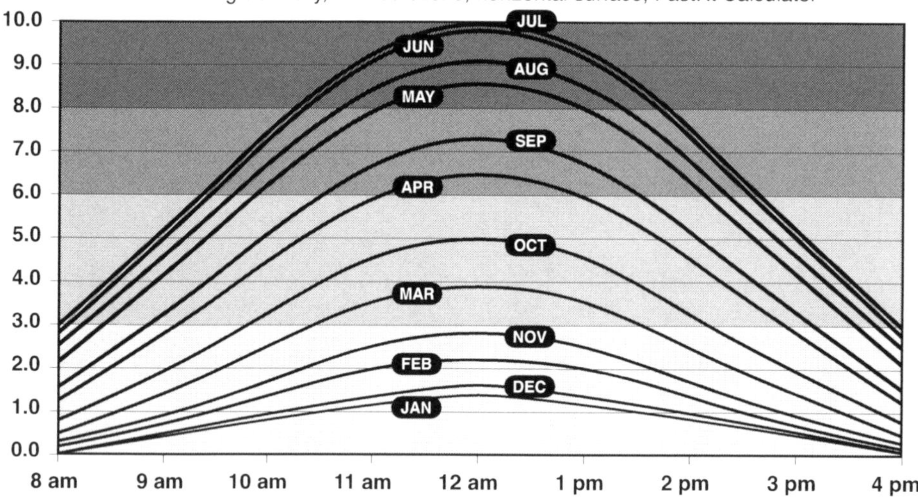

Variation of UV Index by time of day and month in New York City. Most of America has a low UV index during winter months, necessitating Vitamin-D supplementation—and ideally frequent trips to sunnier climates—for optimal year-round health.

blood level. On the top of the opposite page is a chart for recommended vitamin D, 25-Hydroxy levels adapted to Golden Ratio parameters. These levels fit closely to those recommended by **Michael Holick, Ph.D., M.D.**, a leading-edge endocrinologist and world authority on vitamin D. How do you get your vitamin D_3 levels into a therapeutic range without toxicity becoming a problem? By utilizing a combination of sun, vitamin D_3 rich foods and vitamin D_3 supplements in the proper amounts. In summer months you may need less from your diet due to increased UVB exposure, yet in winter, the reverse may be true. When using sun exposure to get vitamin D_3, remember that the sun is a double-edged sword with respect to UV rays: get just enough, yet not too much: *just right.* Remember that even sun bathing can't produce enough vitamin-D if there's a cholesterol deficiency in the skin. Note: Your vitamin D intake and levels should be monitored by your physician if you have malabsorption syndrome, AIDS, seizures, obesity, sarcoidosis or take prednisone or corticosteroids.

> *Up to 85% of people have insufficient levels of vitamin D & are unaware of their deficient state. While conventional media & medicine promote sun avoidance, doing so can actually put your health in grave danger & cause vitamin D deficiency.*
> **Dr. Joseph Mercola, Mercola.com; World's #1 natural health website**

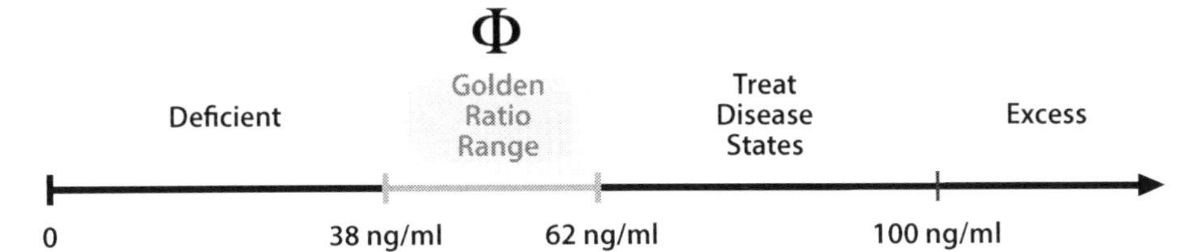

This chart shows ideal Golden Ratio 25-OH-Vitamin-D range of 38-62 ng/ml—very close to that recommended by Vitamin-D guru Michael Holick, Ph.D., M.D. (between 40–60 ng/ml). As vitamin-D synthesis is dependent on UVB light, this test can also be used as an indirect measure of UVB exposure. If your 25-OH Vitamin-D level is low, you know that you need to increase sun exposure or begin supplementing with oral or intramuscular Vitamin-D_3. The DMinder app tells you in real time how much UVB is available via sunlight according to season, location and duration of exposure. Vitamin-D test kits and DMinder app links are featured in this book's Ch 3 Rx section.

3

The Fibonacci Sunbathing Timer

Humans have a lot of beneficial biological processes that occur as a direct result of sun exposure. You might see a few of those with vitamin D supplementation, but not to the degree that you do with simply being out in the sun.

Michael Holick, Ph.D, M.D., director of Heliotherapy, Light & Skin Research, Boston University Medical Center

The Fibonacci Sunbathing Timer is an easy general guide for determining the duration of safe sun exposure. It uses Fibonacci Sequence Numbers as a progressive guide for how much time to stay in the sun without burning, tied to a person's skin type and sun sensitivity. Each person needs to find their own Golden RAYtio amount of sun exposure, where the dose becomes the medicine, but not the poison. The ideal way to get solar benefits while preventing over exposure is to *first sunbathe without sunscreen according to the Fibonacci Sunbathing Timer*. Then, after you've had a chance to absorb adequate sunlight, you can.

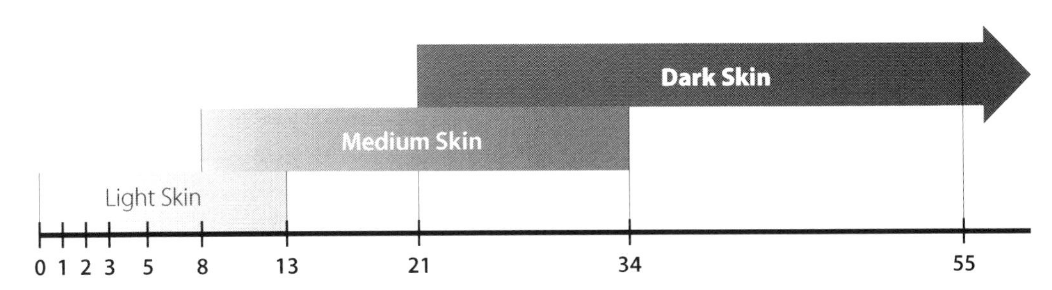

The Fibonacci Sunbathing Timer is a general guide for healthy sun exposure duration according to skin type. Each skin type has a range of minutes within which you can safely sunbathe. Depending on the season, sunbathing time can be adjusted up or down to accommodate stronger or weaker sunlight. See Rx section for this chapter for more details.

Even as little as 1 to 3 minutes may be the limit for those with light or extremely sensitive skin. Even if you're very sensitive to the sun, it's still possible to increase time in the sun as your skin develops more tolerance. These individuals can begin at the 1 minute mark and progress up to 3, 5 or even 8 minutes as their tolerance develops over time. Light-skinned people have less melanin pigment in their skin as an evolutionary adaptation to northern latitudes, where it was advantageous to maximize sun absorption in a low sun environment. Paradoxically, light-skinned people have an advantage over people with more pigmentation in that they don't need as much time in the sun to absorb an adequate amount of UV light. People with medium skin pigmentation have moderate sun tolerance and have a wider range of sun exposure on Fibonacci's Sunbathing Timer. These individuals can begin at the 13 minute mark and progress up to 21 or even 34 minutes as tolerance develops over time.

If any over-exposure occurs, you need to drop down to the next lower Fibonacci Number after your skin recovers and you're ready to begin again. Darker skinned people have the most resilient skin with more melanin protection and can easily tolerate intense sun exposure from 34 to 55 minutes or more. They need longer sun exposure to generate an equivalent amount of vitamin-D as the lighter skinned person. However, they benefit in not having to be as concerned with over exposure and burning as people with light and medium skin pigmentation. Sunlight has the potential to deliver life-giving medicine without side effects—if we monitor ourselves with respect to *duration, intensity and frequency*. As with all the NSN health priority drivers, remember the following:

- Start low & go slow.
- Moderation is the Key
- As sun intensity ↑, sunbathing time ↓
- As sun intensity ↓, sunbathing time ↑

Reset Your Circadian Rhythms Like the Sphinx

The Great Sphinx of Giza sits on the Giza Plateau and faces East, a perfect vantage point to see the rising Sun. Biophysicist and neurosurgeon Jack Kruse, M.D. points out that the Egyptians were clearly aware of the benefits of morning Sun gazing and purposely situated the Sphinx facing East as **a reminder to all humanity that the Sun's rays hold the secrets of health, spirituality and transformation** (interestingly, *Sphinx* contains the word **phi**, the Greek word for the Golden Ratio). The embedded word **phi** is a reminder for us to partake of the blessings of the Sun wisely and in measured doses—*nothing in excess.* The early morning rays of the Sun reset our circadian rhythms for the day and signal our brain to begin releasing the necessary hormonal and neurotransmitter cascades that enliven and focus us for the day ahead.

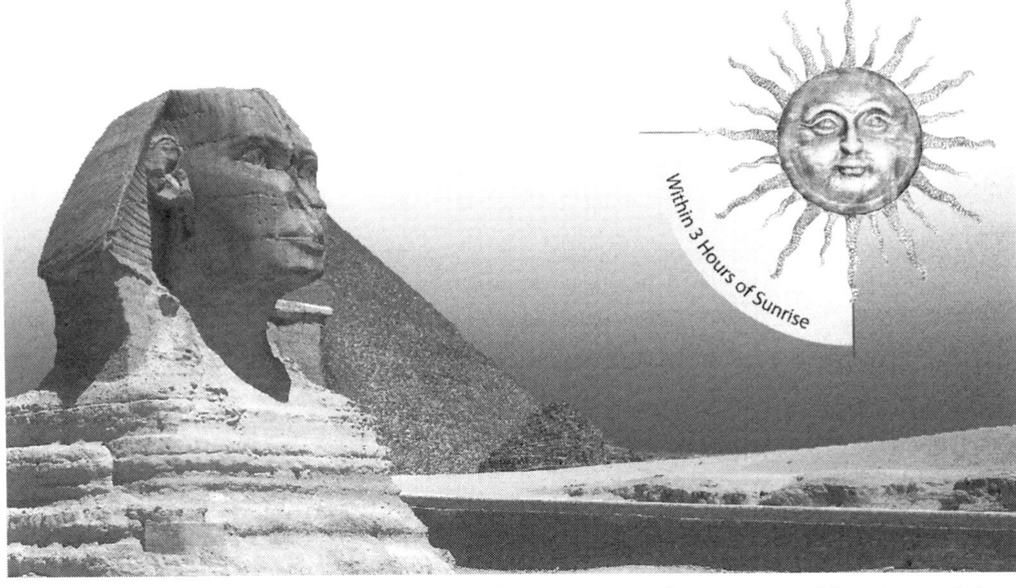

The Egyptian SPHInx and Dr. Jack Kruse remind us to get out early, turn east and face the sun daily for 3-5 minutes; however, don't look directly into the sun. This daily practice is a great morning ritual for the optimal circadian reset as well as for hormonal and neurotransmitter balancing.

Circadian Rhythms du Soleil: Morning Sun Supports Optimal Weight

The less energy you get from the sun, the more food you have to eat—
you get hungry to make up the deficit.
Jack Kruse, M.D., neurosurgeon & biophysicist

In modern times, keeping our circadian biorhythms aligned is an ongoing and often difficult task. Many people are indoors most of the day, subjected to a decrease in natural light, while receiving an increase in unnatural EMF's (Electro-Magnetic Frequencies) from computers, WiFi, cellphones and artificial lighting. This predisposes your body clock and hormonal systems to lose healthy synchronization, with various states of unwellness a result. As is usually the case, restoring your connection to Nature is the answer. This was recently highlighted in a study at Northwestern University Feinberg School of Medicine, where researchers Kathryn J. Reid, Giovanni Santostasi, et al., determined that **sunlight exposure of specific timing, intensity and duration was associated with a decreased BMI**. BMI (Body Mass Index) is a ratio of weight to height reflecting varying degrees of obesity or leanness. The researchers determined that there are 3 necessary elements (timing, intensity and duration) that when blended together elicit a decreased BMI, i.e., more leanness. Variations or absence in any of the 3 critical factors wouldn't decrease BMI. The specific requirements of the

3 elements of healthy sunlight exposure are:

Timing: Morning sun exposure between 8 am & 12 noon

Intensity: Natural outdoor sunlight—no windows or sunglasses

Duration: Up to 20 minutes of direct morning exposure daily.

This solar triangulation of fire practice is a simple, 3-faceted approach to activate and reset your biorhythms and support optimal weight reduction. By realigning with one of Nature's premier essential nutrients—the sun—you can lose weight, lower your BMI and experience improved health and vitality.

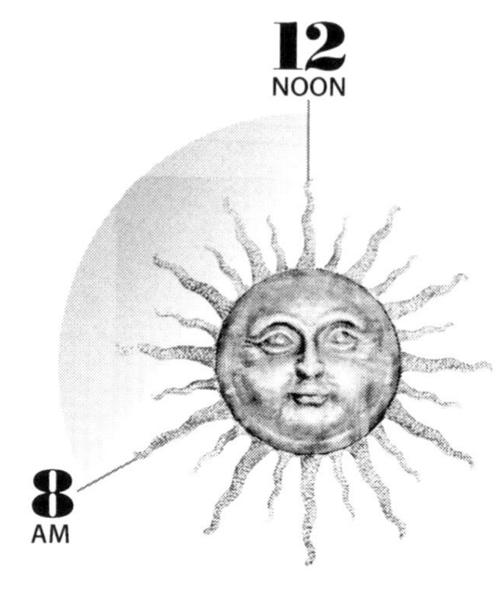

The best hours for sunning to activate weight reduction are between 8 am and 12 noon.

The Human Eye: A Two-Way Door for Sunlight & Spirit

Whereas once I was blind now I can see.

John 9:25, ***the Bible***

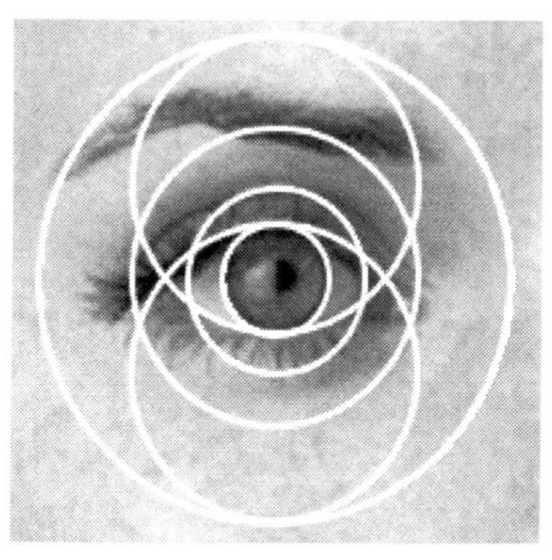

The human eye is a two-way door, allowing Sunlight to pass into the brain while simultaneously opening the way for outward Spiritual expression. Being remarkable in design, both structurally and functionally, it's only fitting that a Golden Ratio design of the eye would accompany it's amazing functionality. In this image, the superimposed circles delineate Golden Ratio relationships of the various eye structures.

The human eyes are truly Golden Ratio Windows of the Soul, through which our Spirit outwardly shines. It's only fitting that Sunlight—the prime animating and enlightening force on earth—should be ushered into our bodies in beautiful Golden Ratio style as well. By superimposing successively larger circles in Golden Ratio to one another over the eye, we see how the eye's structural landmarks correspond with this universal design blueprint. So much light, communication and feeling pass in and out of the eyes it's no surprise that Nature created beautiful, Golden Ratio–proportioned gateways for these full-spectrum energies.

In order to maximize the absorption of light in our bodies, Nature also designed the visual fields of the eyes with Golden Ratios in mind. Since Sunlight is our principle energetic nutrient, it's critical that we have good access to Sunlight in the most efficient way possible. Evolutionarily speaking, humans needed to protect themselves from predators mainly from the front or sides and less often from above or below. The most efficient way to balance these requirements as well as satisfy the nutritional need for good access to Sunlight was to design the visual fields according to the Golden Ratio, in both the vertical and horizontal planes, as the diagrams below illustrate.

We have two eyes, yet we see one seamless image due to the overlap in the center of the visual fields. Taken together, the combined visual fields of both eyes fit nicely inside a

Our Natural Golden Ratio Visual Field

Constructal Law originator and author of *The Physics of Life: The Evolution of Everything* Professor Adrian Bejan discovered that the horizontal orientation of the eye-eye axis approximates a Golden Ratio Rectangle, which facilitates the optimal flow of visual information to the brain. This highlights the fact that as humans we are oriented towards the world according to Golden Ratio structure and function.

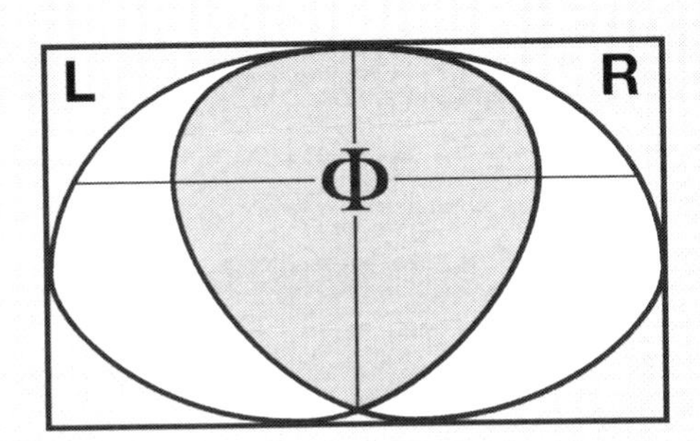

***Binocular* Visual Field**
We have two eyes, yet we see one seamless image due to the fact that our binocular vision receives overlapping images in the center of the visual fields. The visual cortex at the back of the brain processes the dual images from both eyes and fills in the blind spots where the optic nerves penetrate the retinas. When combined, the visual fields fit nicely inside a Golden Rectangle.

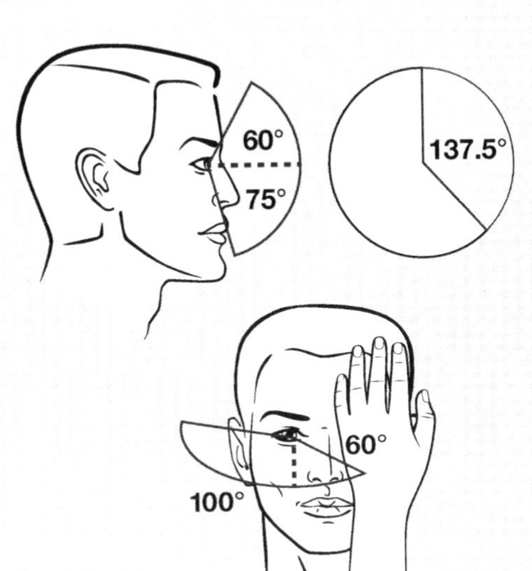

***Vertical* Human Visual Field**
Spans 60° above the direct line of sight and 75° below the direct line of sight. Added together, the total vertical human visual field spans a range of 135°, a close approximation of the small Golden Angle of a circle, 137.5°.

***Horizontal* Human Visual Field**
Spans 100° lateral to the direct line of sight and 60° medial. A 100° to 60° ratio (100:60) is also a very close approximation of the Golden Ratio.

Golden Rectangle. The Golden Ratio structure of the eyes enables them to functionally access Sunlight with Golden Ratio efficiency, maximizing intake of one of our most vital MegaNutrient priority health drivers—Sunlight.

The Golden Ratio Wide-screen & Binocular Vision

Wide-screen TV and computer monitors have varied in aspect ratio over the decades, fluctuating back and forth from 16:10, 16:9 and other ratios. Many reasons for the different designs have been given, with manufacturing costs being most prominent. Curiously absent from design considerations is the fact that the human visual field is designed with clear Golden Ratio parameters—**our vertical, horizontal and binocular fields are all resonant with the Golden Ratio**.

A design defect in the human eye known as the *blind* spot is where the optic nerve penetrates the retina, leaving a small central area of blindness. Everyone has this in each eye yet these blind spots aren't noticed, since brain processing of overlapping binocular images is able to compensate for the visual deficiency. Likewise, Wide-screen manufacturers have their own design and manufacturing blind spots in that they can't see how important it is to make Wide-screen monitors resonant with the human eye's innate blueprint, i.e., the Golden Ratio.

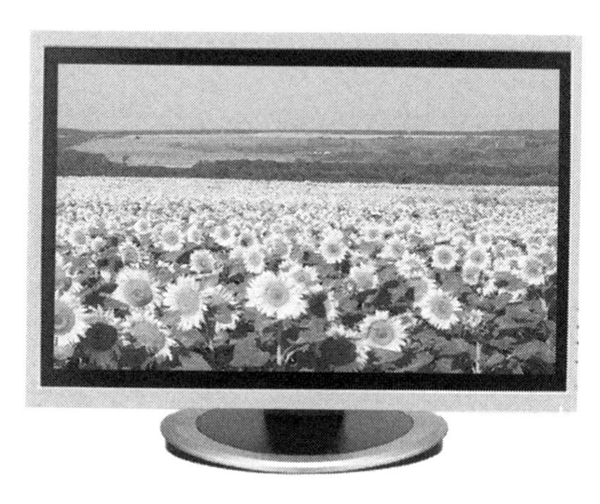

The human binocular visual field is structured according to Golden Ratio parameters. Although the current default dimensions of wide-screen monitors and TV's is a 16:9 aspect ratio, the ideal aspect ratio consistent with the human Golden Ratio structured binocular visual field would be the 16:10 dimension.

Wide-screen manufactures somehow stumbled upon the 16:10 Golden Ratio design, yet have jettisoned it for the 16:9 design by not considering how important it is to make Wide-screen monitor dimensions proportional to the human eye's optimal visual fields. The 16:9 aspect ratio shortens the vertical viewing field, creating a subtle tunnel vision effect which sub-optimizes visual-cognitive processing. A 16:10 Golden aspect Ratio harmonizes screen, eye and brain, thereby reducing eyestrain and enhancing our overall viewing experience. And of course when anything is done with the Golden Ratio in mind, a valuable opportunity to access NSN is at hand. Just viewing a 16:10 Wide-screen TV or computer monitor could be giving millions of viewers a consistent subtle dose of NSN.

Coffee: Sunlight's Liquid Circadian Surrogate

Daily morning exposure to sunlight is critical for the circadian reset that shuts off the sleep hormone melatonin and turns on and stimulates release of many essential daytime hormones and neurotransmitters. For optimal health and performance, the simple circadian reset of 3 to 5 minutes of direct sunlight on your face (eyelids closed) needs to happen every morning, the earlier the better. Since most people don't get these vital few minutes of direct morning sun, they can become disconnected from its powerful biorhythmic synchronizing effects. Absent this natural AM solar wake-up, coffee has become the sun's circadian surrogate; up to 80% of Americans use coffee or tea as part of their daily wake-up regimen. Along with the sense of well-being, heightened mental acuity and wakefulness, coffee consumption also stimulates autonomic nervous system reflexes that initiate a morning bowel

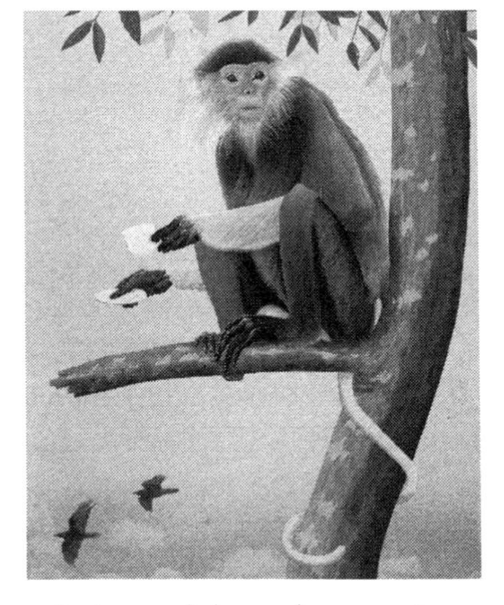

Perhaps early humans' consumption of the coffee bean was the impetus that got them out of the trees, walking, talking and socializing; in modern café culture, we're not that different from our hominid ancestors.

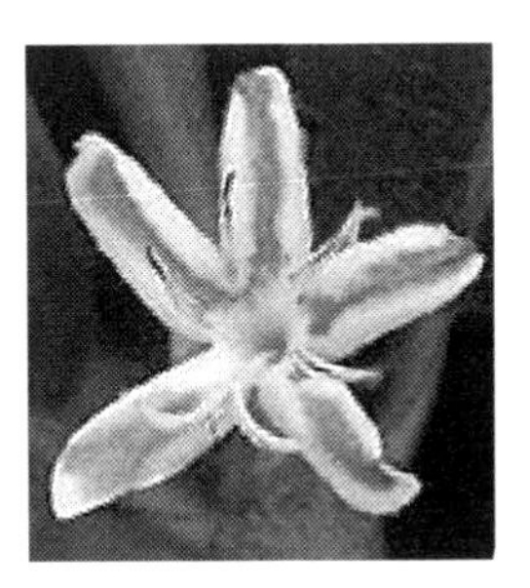

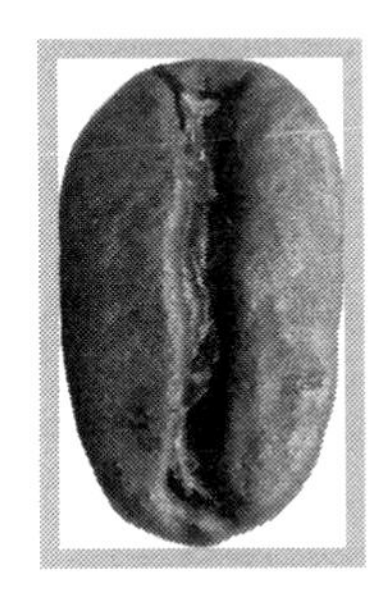

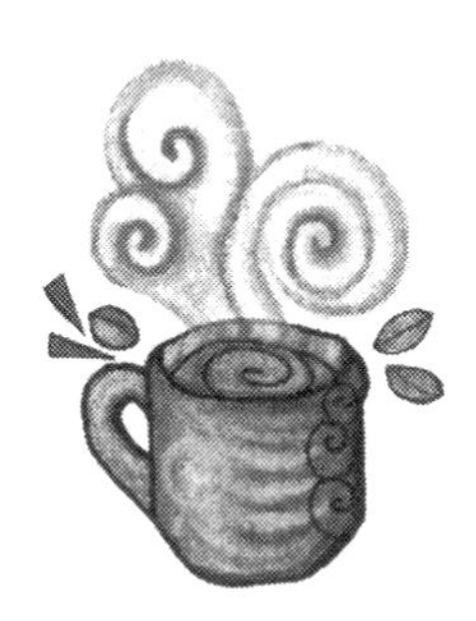

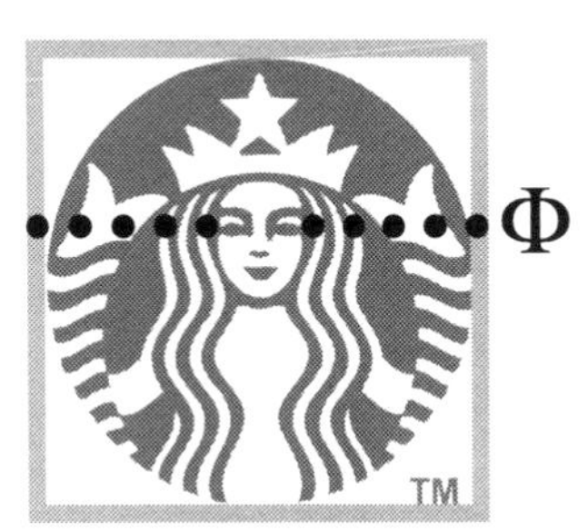

1. **Coffee Flower:** Coffee beans have their start as a majestic Golden Star flower. *2.* **Coffee Bean:** Roasted coffee beans tend to fit neatly inside a Golden Rectangle. *3.* **Coffee Cup:** Millions of people get a regular imprint of the Golden Ratio via the swirling Golden Spirals in the cream or milk in their morning coffee. *4.* **Starbucks Logo:** The (Starbucks) eyes have it: the familiar siren's eyes in the logo of the world's largest coffee company look out from the vertical Golden Ratio point of the design.

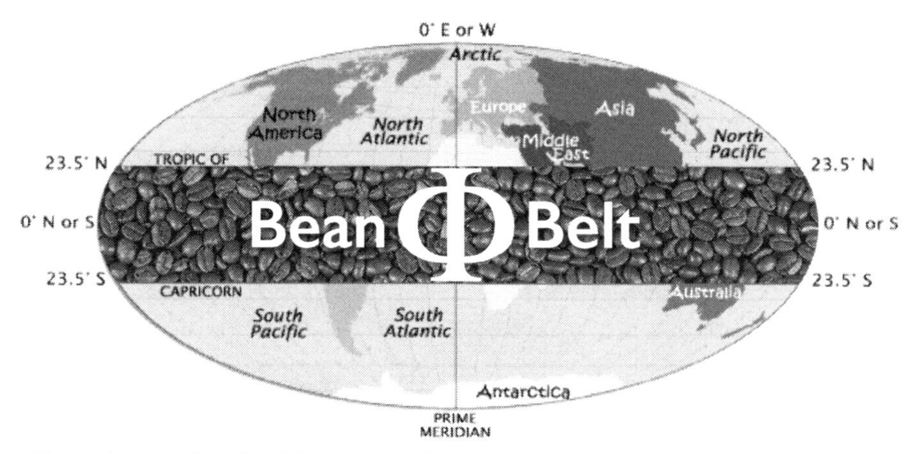

The mid-range of the Earth between the latitude lines demarcating the Tropics of Cancer & Capricorn gets abundant ultraviolet (UV) sunlight throughout the year. This tropical zone is also known as the **Bean Belt** (for coffee bean) and is the region on earth where coffee is predominantly grown. The surface area between the Tropics of Cancer and Capricorn comprises a little less than 40% of earth's total surface area, an approximate Golden Ratio division. Interestingly, the Golden Ratio symbol Φ (phi) is also commonly used to designate geographic latitude.

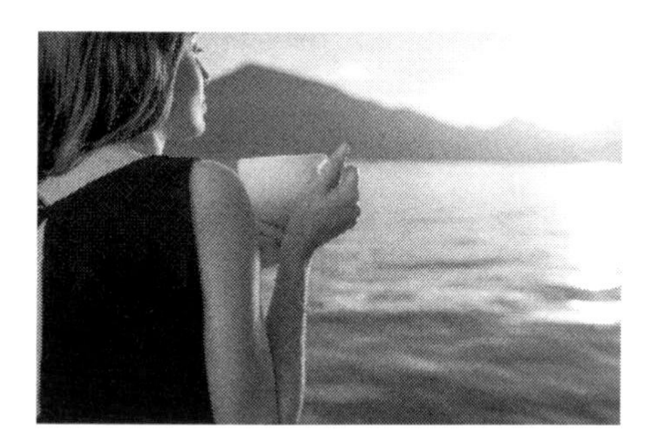

To assure an optimally bright start to every day, compliment your surrogate sunshine (morning coffee or tea) with a few minutes of the real thing—3 to 5 minutes of direct sun on your face and eyelids. You'll then get your circadian reset with a double shot of sunshine—in your cup *and* on your face.

movement, aka the AM-BM. If we greeted the morning sun with the same enthusiasm with which we greet our coffee cups, we would be more tuned into Nature's rhythms and healthier for it. Coffee's origins are in the tropical regions of the earth, between the tropics of Cancer and Capricorn—also known as the *Bean Belt.* The intense concentration of sunlight along with the perfect mix of climate and soil fostered the origin and proliferation of the Golden Ratio-imprinted coffee plant. With its 5-petaled flowers and roasted beans which tend to fit inside a Golden Rectangle, the coffee plant along with early modern humans emerged in Africa's Rift Valley from Ethiopia eastward. With the spread of coffee from its African origins to modern-day consumers worldwide, coffee is ushering in an era of hidden evolutionary adaptation to deficient morning solar nutrition. We're witnessing the emergence of a new species—*Homo coffeans*—who with the aid of percolators and espresso machines have figured out how to extract the concentrated energy and sunlight embedded in coffee beans, sidestepping millions of years of evolution underlying Nature's use of pure sunshine to wake us each day.

Purine: The Secret Ingredient in Coffee, Tea & Chocolate

The fascinating Purine family of molecules has a wide array of familiar derivatives including caffeine, theobromine, ATP and DNA (with its nucleobases adenine & guanine). The purine molecule is easily recognized as a combination of two Golden Ratio-based geometrical figures: the hexagon ⬢ and pentagon ⬟.

Your body has an amazing ability to transmute various purine-containing molecules, wherever and whenever needed. For example, have you ever considered that the caffeine and theobromine in your coffee, tea and chocolate are being used as building blocks for energy molecules (ATP) and genetic information (DNA) in your body? In that light, these little caffeinated and brominated pleasures of life can also be envisioned as great sources of NSN.

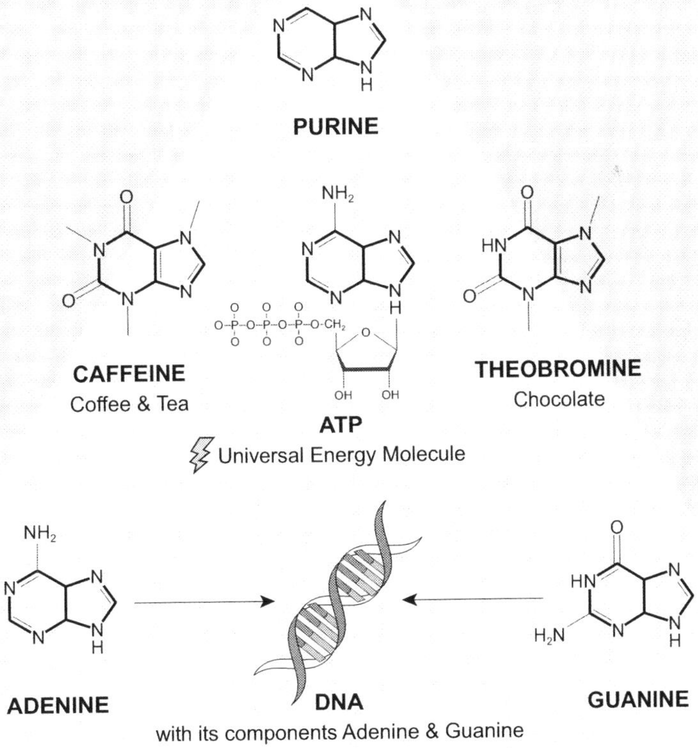

PURINE

CAFFEINE
Coffee & Tea

ATP
Universal Energy Molecule

THEOBROMINE
Chocolate

ADENINE

DNA
with its components Adenine & Guanine

GUANINE

The Purine Pyramid with the more familiar purine derivatives.

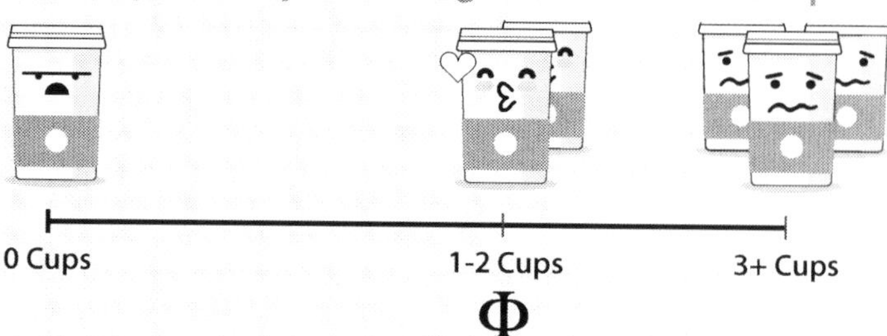

Φ

Coffee is the world's most popular beverage and principal source of antioxidants for many people, yet coffee consumption is no exception to the axiom of *All Things In Moderation*. Respect that limit or you'll likely suffer the consequences of anxiety, queasiness or even elevated blood pressure. Find your daily Golden Ratio of coffee with respect to the following considerations:

Quality: Go organic, as coffee is one of the heaviest toxic pesticide-sprayed crops on earth. While the weakness and jitters many feel after drinking coffee may be a result of too much caffeine, it can also just as well be due to the toxic pesticides or mycotoxins (mold toxins) present in non-organic coffee.

Quantity: Find your Golden Ratio quantity of coffee consumption to get the optimal dose of NSN. Long-term benefits from coffee include a lower risk of liver and colon cancer, decreased risk of type 2 diabetes, lowered risk of macular degeneration, improved memory, dementia prevention and delayed onset of Alzheimer's disease.

Timing: AM coffee is best, as it resets circadian rhythms for the day. Avoid coffee after 2pm; caffeine has a half-life of 5-6 hours & can disrupt sleep in the night ahead.

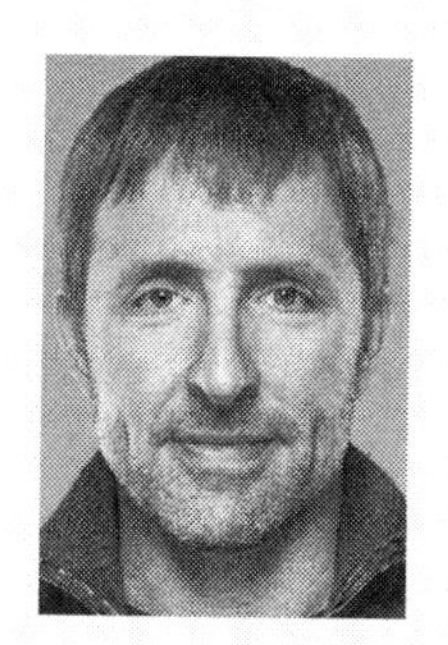
Dave Asprey, biohacking pioneer, Bulletproof entrepreneur and author of *Head Strong*.

Bulletproof® Coffee Biohack Enhances Quality, Quantity & Timing. Bulletproof Coffee (BPC) is a coffee innovation created by pioneer biohacker and entrepreneur **Dave Asprey**, inspired by an old Tibetan recipe that uses tea & yak butter. BPC is Dave's proprietary brand of single-sourced organic and lab-certified, mycotoxin-free coffee that leaves coffee connoisseurs free of toxin-induced crashes and side effects. Dave's unique recipe for BPC combines coffee spiked with grass-fed butter and Brain Octane (caprylic acid from coconut oil) that facilitates ketone generation, supporting steady energy and focus for 4-6 hours. It's a perfect circadian AM reset and also helps reduce cravings for that 2nd or 3rd cup. For added BPC detox benefits, see Ch 7/Detox. www.BulletProof.com

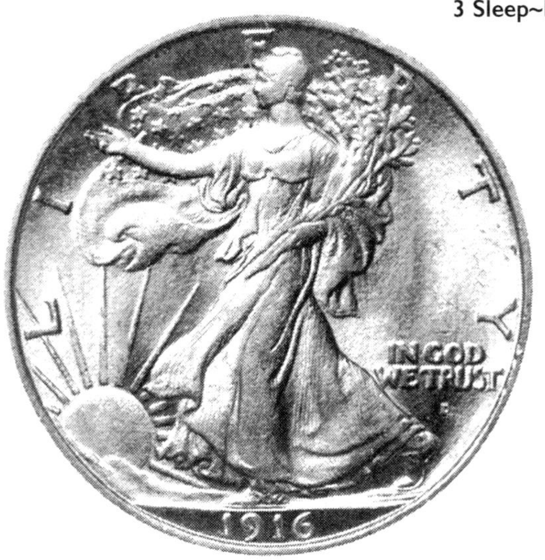

The beautiful *Walking Lady Liberty* emblazoned on 1916-1947 U.S. half dollars reminds us to face the morning Sun for Vibrant Health, Performance & Longevity. In our modern era it seems that we need to be reawakened to the ancient knowledge that the Sun can only bestow its salubrious effects *if we are out in it.* In addition to this vintage half dollar, master sculptor Aldolph Weinman also designed the sublime contrasting *Day and Night* sculpture at New York City's original Penn Station (see p. 82).

> *Learn to work with the light of the sun, for this light contains all riches.*
> **Omraam Mikhael Aivanhov, philosopher & mystic, referring to Surya (Sun) yoga**

The art and science of light in general and sunlight in particular, and their roles in human health and life, is as vast as it is fascinating. The same can be said of coffee. Like sunlight, coffee is one of Nature's under-recognized superfoods (in coffee's case, a *superliquid*). Coffee also spans at least 4 NSN health priority drivers—**Hydration** (water), **Sunlight** (circadian surrogate), **Nutrition** (top antioxidant source for many people) and of course **Happiness** (source of comfort and social magnet). For these reasons and more, coffee—and of course the sunlight MegaNutrient it represents—is a bright bridge to the next NSN MegaNutrient health priority driver, Nutrition.

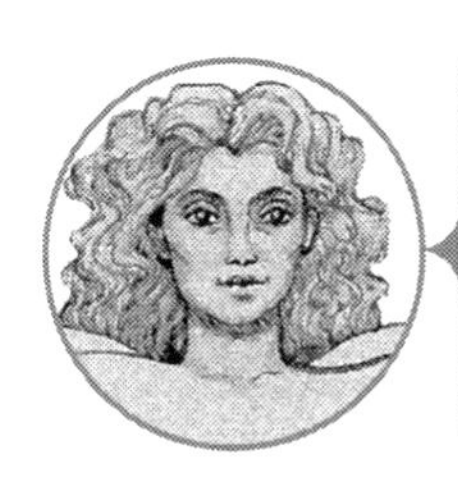

*Remember, you're only as **Charged Up** as your last healthy **SUN** exposure.* So be sure to get your morning sun circadian reset as well as a regular dose of UVB solar nutrition between 10am–3pm; this activates your vitamin D, neurotransmitter & hormone production, while supercharging your entire system.

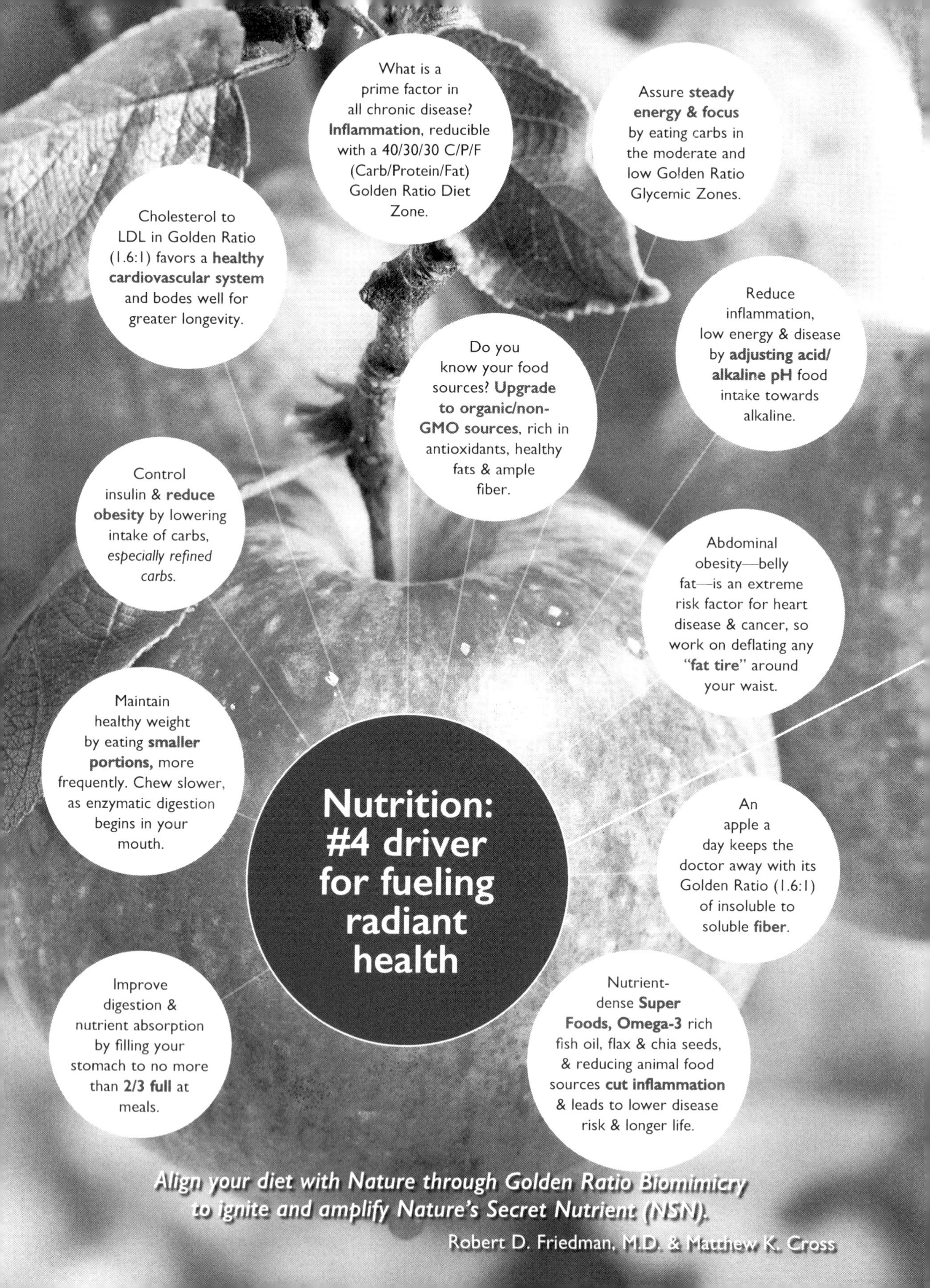

What is a prime factor in all chronic disease? **Inflammation**, reducible with a 40/30/30 C/P/F (Carb/Protein/Fat) Golden Ratio Diet Zone.

Assure **steady energy & focus** by eating carbs in the moderate and low Golden Ratio Glycemic Zones.

Cholesterol to LDL in Golden Ratio (1.6:1) favors a **healthy cardiovascular system** and bodes well for greater longevity.

Reduce inflammation, low energy & disease by **adjusting acid/alkaline pH** food intake towards alkaline.

Do you know your food sources? **Upgrade to organic/non-GMO sources**, rich in antioxidants, healthy fats & ample fiber.

Control insulin & **reduce obesity** by lowering intake of carbs, *especially refined carbs.*

Abdominal obesity—belly fat—is an extreme risk factor for heart disease & cancer, so work on deflating any **"fat tire"** around your waist.

Maintain healthy weight by eating **smaller portions,** more frequently. Chew slower, as enzymatic digestion begins in your mouth.

Nutrition: #4 driver for fueling radiant health

An apple a day keeps the doctor away with its Golden Ratio (1.6:1) of insoluble to soluble **fiber**.

Improve digestion & nutrient absorption by filling your stomach to no more than **2/3 full** at meals.

Nutrient-dense **Super Foods, Omega-3** rich fish oil, flax & chia seeds, & reducing animal food sources **cut inflammation** & leads to lower disease risk & longer life.

Align your diet with Nature through Golden Ratio Biomimicry to ignite and amplify Nature's Secret Nutrient (NSN).

Robert D. Friedman, M.D. & Matthew K. Cross

Nutrition

4

Your body has a BLUEPRINT, a SCHEMATIC of what perfect health is and it is constantly trying to achieve this perfect health for you. All that goes wrong is that you get in the way of this natural process.
Dr. Richard Schulze, N.D., natural healing authority

Have you ever wondered what the *true* goal of Nutrition is? If we answer the question by viewing it through the lens of the Golden Ratio, we could say that it is obtaining and maintaining that fine point of optimal sustenance—the point between being undernourished and over-nourished. In other words, we want to aim for the metabolic excellence of Da Vinci's evolved human—*Homo Vitruvius*—the place of ideal body composition and optimal physiologic function. We're searching for that diet that supports consistent health and efficient performance on all levels. **A quick look at numerous fleeting fad diets reveals that the majority are far from Golden Ratio balance by being extreme in either carbs, fat or protein.** Although some are beneficial for short-term therapeutic effect, few have hit the Golden Ratio mark for long-term practical use. By looking back to our paleolithic ancestors for insight, we see that their diet was one of *macronutrient moderation* consistent with Golden Ratio parameters. We'll be looking at various approaches to health and Nutrition that are able to provide support by reaching all the way down to the genetic level. These approaches also appear to be able to control one of the final common pathways to most disease processes—*inflammation.* Naturally, the dietary protocols we advocate closely conform to the Golden Ratio.

The Zone Golden Pro*Portion*: Activating Nature's Secret Nutrient/NSN

You're only as good as your last meal.

Barry Sears, Ph.D.

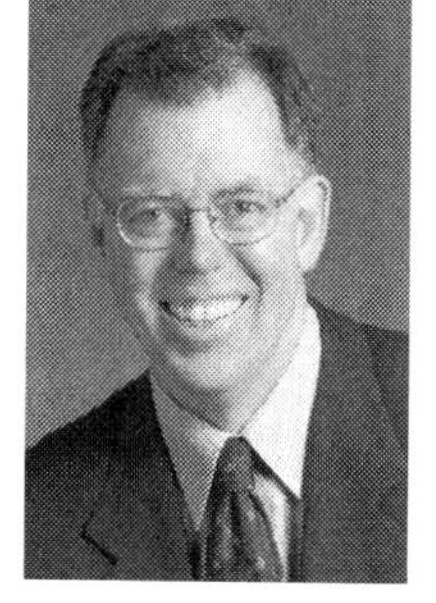

Dr. Barry Sears, world-renowned pioneer of *The Zone.*

Phenomenon is a fitting description for the 40/30/30 Zone lifestyle nutrition program pioneered by **Barry Sears, Ph.D.** This paleo-like diet, extraordinarily popular among world-class athletes and celebrities, is the epitome of moderation in the dietary world. The Zone emphasizes a 40/30/30 Carbohydrate/Protein/Fat (C/P/F) caloric intake ratio and has stood the test of time, while countless fad diets come and go. The Zone is a phenomenon because after years of extreme diets it's a scientifically researched, medically validated and finely-tuned daily eating plan for weight loss, peak vitality, performance and longevity. **Eating in the Zone normalizes blood pressure, balances insulin, cholesterol and triglycerides and decreases the leading cause of all disease: chronic inflammation.** With the Zone approach you simply aim for a ratio of 40% of your calories coming from Carbohydrates, 30% from Protein and 30% from healthy Fats and oils. What's especially important about this 40/30/30 food ratio is the degree to which it regulates insulin release. Insulin release is strongly activated by Carbohydrates, while Protein and Fat cause only moderate to minimal insulin release. Protein (30%) and Fat (30%) together equal 60%, thus the 40/30/30 C/P/F ratio becomes a simpler 40/60 ratio:

40% (Carbohydrates) to 60% (30% Protein + 30% Fat) 40/60 ~Φ

This 40/60 ratio approximates the Golden Ratio Φ. Upon approaching Golden Ratio balance, the NSN super-charging nutritional upgrade appears—no doubt a key reason the Zone approach is so effective in regulating metabolism, decreasing inflammation and promoting supreme health. Dr. Sears points out that the Zone's 40/30/30 ratio literally becomes ***a Potent Health and Longevity Drug—which you can take via every meal in your life*** (in true biomimicry fashion, the word *Drug* comes from *Droog*—Dutch for *Dried Plant*). Sears' scientifically validated Zone breakthrough powerfully resonates with the famous quote of the Greek father of medicine, **Hippocrates**:

Let food be thy medicine and medicine be thy food.

Stone Age = The Zone Age

In *The Omega Rx Zone*, Dr. Sears shares added Zone Diet insight, which mirrors macronutrient *ranges* of Paleolithic diets of East African, preagricultural, hunter-gatherers: *When broken down into percentages of Carbohydrates, Protein and Fat, it [the Paleolithic diet] comes to approximately 40% Carbohydrates, 30% Protein, and 30% total Fat.* Before the development of agriculture and industrialization, humans naturally ate a diet that essentially conformed to the Golden Ratio. A Zone/Paleolithic type of diet reflects the body's maximum metabolic efficiency ratio for utilizing macronutrients. It's similar to achieving the optimal fuel/air mixture in a finely tuned engine, thereby maximizing efficiency while minimizing waste and wear. Why is a Golden Ratio Pro*Portion* of nutrients so crucial in weight loss and health? A diet excessively high in carbohydrates—bread, pasta, grains, potatoes, fruit juices, sweets, etc.,—over-stimulates your pancreas to secrete insulin, resulting in what is known as **insulin resistance**. Since your body uses insulin to transport sugar molecules into the cells, the cells will become progressively less sensitive to insulin's actions as the amount of carbohydrates in your diet increases. To compensate for the insensitivity, your pancreas begins to secrete more and more insulin. Your metabolism switches from fat burning to fat storage. This can go on for years, resulting in Syndrome X, aka **The Metabolic Syndrome**, which consists of:

- Φ Obesity (excessive fat, especially around the mid-section)
- Φ High triglycerides and low HDL (good) cholesterol
- Φ Insulin resistance with glucose intolerance (elevated insulin & blood sugar levels)
- Φ Pro-thrombotic state (elevated blood clotting risk)
- Φ Elevated blood pressure (130/85 mmHg or higher)
- Φ Inflammation (elevated C-reactive protein)

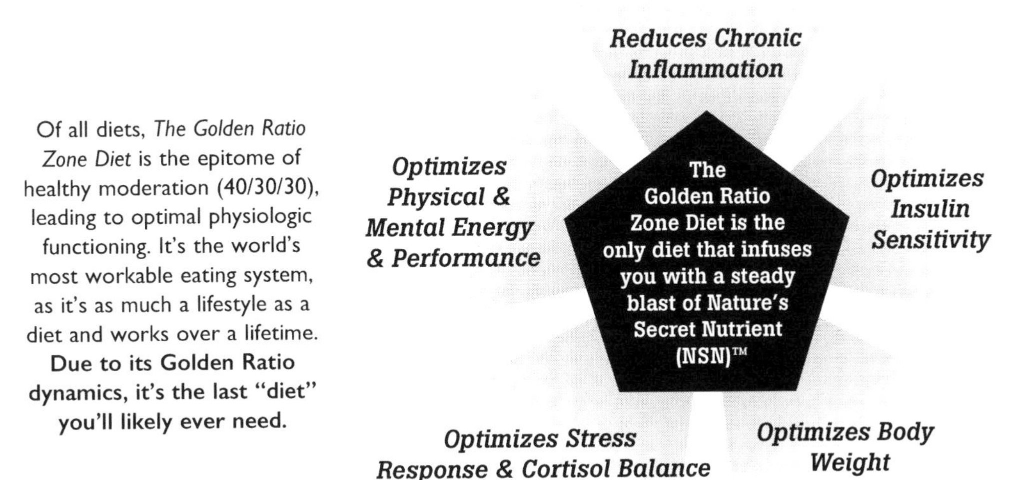
Reduces Chronic Inflammation
Optimizes Physical & Mental Energy & Performance
The Golden Ratio Zone Diet is the only diet that infuses you with a steady blast of Nature's Secret Nutrient (NSN)™
Optimizes Insulin Sensitivity
Optimizes Stress Response & Cortisol Balance
Optimizes Body Weight

Of all diets, *The Golden Ratio Zone Diet* is the epitome of healthy moderation (40/30/30), leading to optimal physiologic functioning. It's the world's most workable eating system, as it's as much a lifestyle as a diet and works over a lifetime. **Due to its Golden Ratio dynamics, it's the last "diet" you'll likely ever need.**

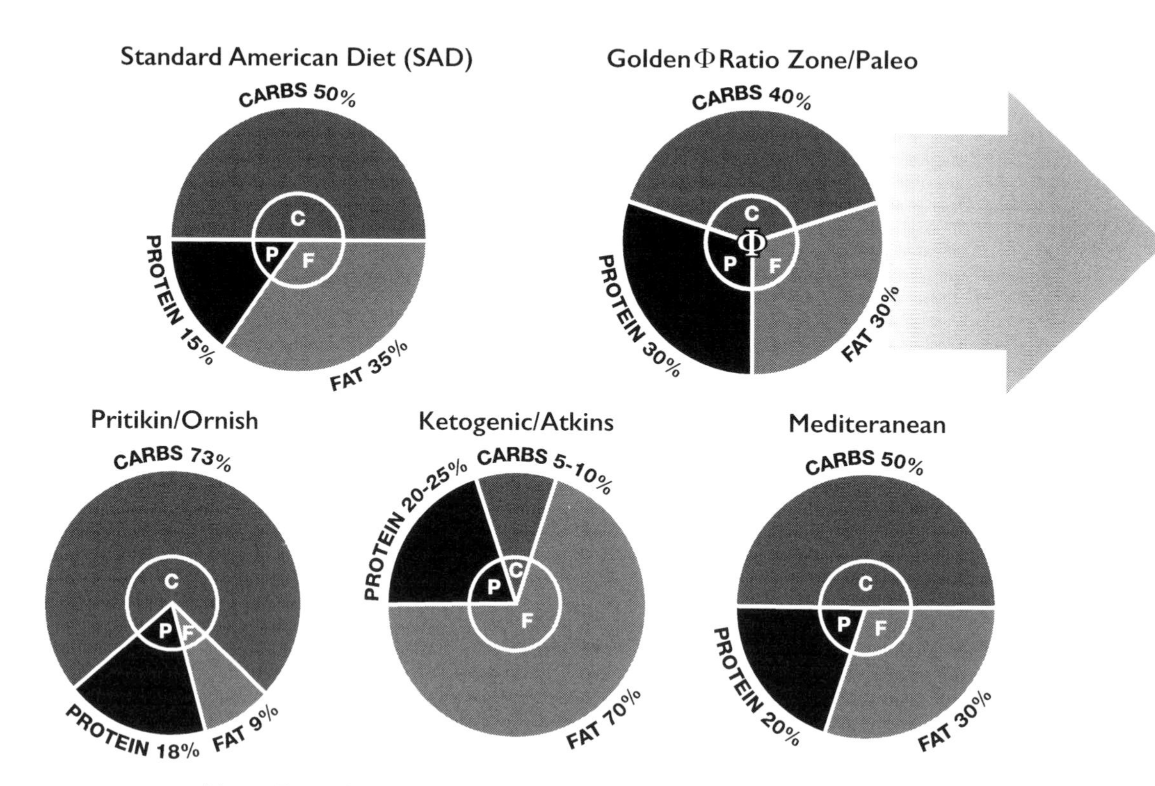

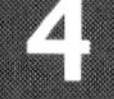

How Popular Diets Slice the Macronutrient Pie

The Golden Ratio Zone/Paleo is the only diet with a moderate, healthy balance of Carbohydrate/Protein/Fat (C/P/F). Other diets are extreme (≥50%) in either Carbs (C) or Fat (F); they may have therapeutic value yet are not well-suited for long-term adherence for most people. For example, the popular Ketogenic diet has proven medical benefits, yet may be difficult and impractical to maintain. An ideal scenario would be to integrate intermittent fasting with the Golden Ratio Zone/Paleo diet to get the best of both worlds (see Pac-Man/intermittent fasting, p. 133). The Golden Ratio Zone diet and other copycat diets ↓ inflammation, ↑ insulin sensitivity, optimize body weight, balance cortisol response & ↑ physical & mental energy & performance. *Note that C/P/F MacroNutrient balance doesn't address food* ***quality****; that's why the Standard American Diet (SAD) looks similar to the Mediterranean Diet, even though the Mediterranean Diet is vastly superior.* So be sure to eat *healthy* carbs: fresh, organic fruits & vegetables instead of SAD-predominant bread, pasta & potatoes.

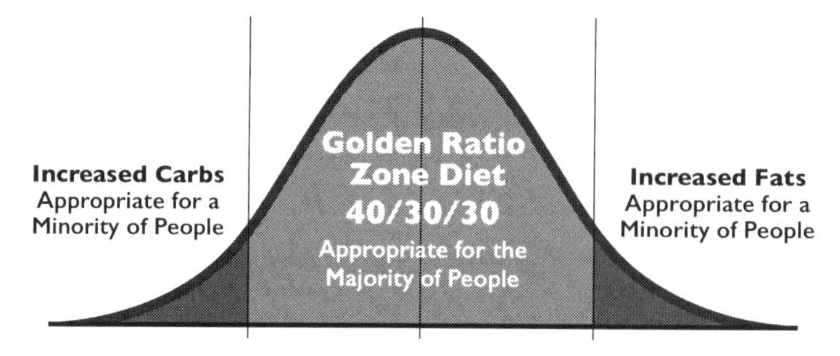

The Golden Ratio Zone Diet is appropriate for the majority of people (roughly 2 standard deviations of the Bell Curve). Since there's unique variability among humans, some outliers may benefit from more fat or more carbs, depending on constitution, season, medical conditions, therapeutic needs, performance requirements, age, economic constraints, etc. In contrast to carbs & fat, protein is moderate through most diets. As a life-long diet however, The Golden Ratio Zone Diet is a healthy lifestyle homing beacon that gives the *most* to the *most*.

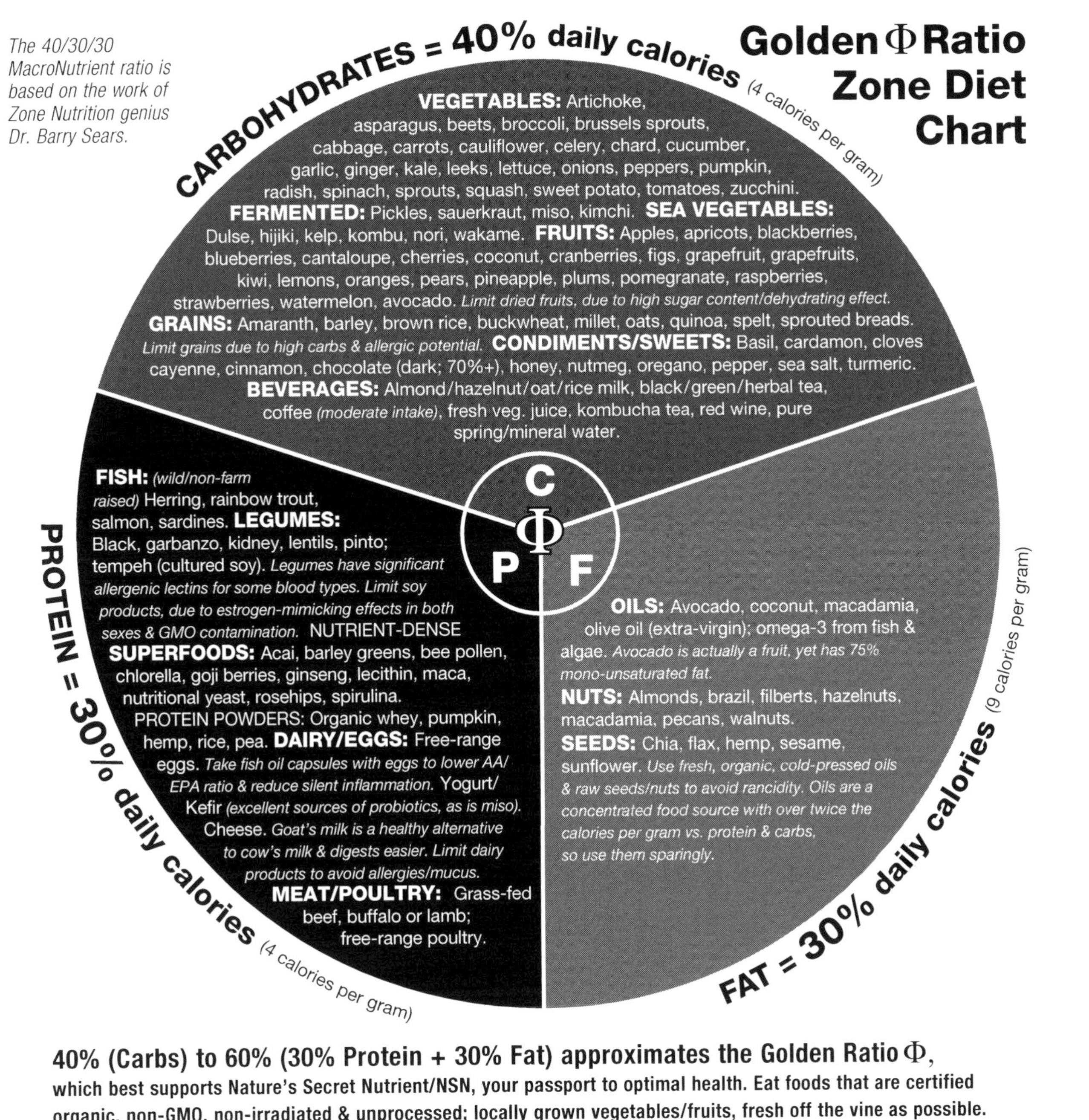

The 40/30/30 MacroNutrient ratio is based on the work of Zone Nutrition genius Dr. Barry Sears.
Golden Φ Ratio Zone Diet Chart
CARBOHYDRATES = 40% daily calories (4 calories per gram)
VEGETABLES: Artichoke, asparagus, beets, broccoli, brussels sprouts, cabbage, carrots, cauliflower, celery, chard, cucumber, garlic, ginger, kale, leeks, lettuce, onions, peppers, pumpkin, radish, spinach, sprouts, squash, sweet potato, tomatoes, zucchini.
FERMENTED: Pickles, sauerkraut, miso, kimchi.
SEA VEGETABLES: Dulse, hijiki, kelp, kombu, nori, wakame.
FRUITS: Apples, apricots, blackberries, blueberries, cantaloupe, cherries, coconut, cranberries, figs, grapefruit, grapefruits, kiwi, lemons, oranges, pears, pineapple, plums, pomegranate, raspberries, strawberries, watermelon, avocado. Limit dried fruits, due to high sugar content/dehydrating effect.
GRAINS: Amaranth, barley, brown rice, buckwheat, millet, oats, quinoa, spelt, sprouted breads. Limit grains due to high carbs & allergic potential.
CONDIMENTS/SWEETS: Basil, cardamon, cloves cayenne, cinnamon, chocolate (dark; 70%+), honey, nutmeg, oregano, pepper, sea salt, turmeric.
BEVERAGES: Almond/hazelnut/oat/rice milk, black/green/herbal tea, coffee (moderate intake), fresh veg. juice, kombucha tea, red wine, pure spring/mineral water.
C
Φ
P
F
PROTEIN = 30% daily calories (4 calories per gram)
FISH: (wild/non-farm raised) Herring, rainbow trout, salmon, sardines.
LEGUMES: Black, garbanzo, kidney, lentils, pinto; tempeh (cultured soy). Legumes have significant allergenic lectins for some blood types. Limit soy products, due to estrogen-mimicking effects in both sexes & GMO contamination.
NUTRIENT-DENSE SUPERFOODS: Acai, barley greens, bee pollen, chlorella, goji berries, ginseng, lecithin, maca, nutritional yeast, rosehips, spirulina.
PROTEIN POWDERS: Organic whey, pumpkin, hemp, rice, pea.
DAIRY/EGGS: Free-range eggs. Take fish oil capsules with eggs to lower AA/EPA ratio & reduce silent inflammation. Yogurt/Kefir (excellent sources of probiotics, as is miso). Cheese. Goat's milk is a healthy alternative to cow's milk & digests easier. Limit dairy products to avoid allergies/mucus.
MEAT/POULTRY: Grass-fed beef, buffalo or lamb; free-range poultry.
FAT = 30% daily calories (9 calories per gram)
OILS: Avocado, coconut, macadamia, olive oil (extra-virgin); omega-3 from fish & algae. Avocado is actually a fruit, yet has 75% mono-unsaturated fat.
NUTS: Almonds, brazil, filberts, hazelnuts, macadamia, pecans, walnuts.
SEEDS: Chia, flax, hemp, sesame, sunflower. Use fresh, organic, cold-pressed oils & raw seeds/nuts to avoid rancidity. Oils are a concentrated food source with over twice the calories per gram vs. protein & carbs, so use them sparingly.

40% (Carbs) to 60% (30% Protein + 30% Fat) approximates the Golden Ratio Φ,

which best supports Nature's Secret Nutrient/NSN, your passport to optimal health. Eat foods that are certified organic, non-GMO, non-irradiated & unprocessed; locally grown vegetables/fruits, fresh off the vine as possible.

- Reduces silent inflammation, a key underlying cause of heart disease, cancer, Alzheimer's & most chronic diseases.
- Normalizes insulin levels, assuring steady energy & protection from diabetes.
- Supports optimal weight, loss of toxic belly fat, better use of stored body fat & decreases food cravings.
- Assures maximal physical & mental performance while supporting an enhanced sense of well-being.
- Many foods in this chart fit in multiple categories & are placed here in their dominant category, e.g., many nuts & seeds are good sources of both protein *and* fat.
- Fill your plate about 1/3 with protein & 2/3 with colorful, non-starchy vegetables. Restrict grains, breads & pastas (infrequently & in small amounts). Add small amounts of oil, seeds, nuts or condiments.
- For optimal digestion & absorption, eat consciously, in a relaxed manner. • Chew well, eating only to about 2/3 full (about what would 2/3 fill both hands cupped together). • Eat proteins first & then pause a few minutes.
- Rotate foods—only eat same food every 3rd to 4th day, to avoid allergies. • You'll get ample fiber eating from this list.
- Reduce consumption of meat/animal products, as the slimmest, longest-lived people eat small amounts, infrequently.
- Due to increasing seafood toxicity (heavy metals, PCB's, radioactivity, etc.), taking chelating compounds with fish gives extra protection. Good oral chelators are vitamin-C, garlic, chlorella, EDTA, zeolite.
- Your metabolism is unique; customize above recommendations to support individual requirements & satisfaction.

Insulin resistance is often accompanied by reactive hypoglycemia. After eating unopposed carbohydrates or sugary foods, insulin is rapidly released into the blood, causing blood sugar levels to plummet. This results in dizziness, sweating, weakness, irritability and foggy thinking. Typically, people respond by consuming more carbohydrates, which only leads to a roller coaster ride of blood sugar peaks and valleys. This puts an enormous strain on your nervous and endocrine systems, which are trying to compensate for the metabolic stress. Over months and years of out-of-proportion carbohydrate consumption, insulin resistance may worsen and blood sugar levels may rise, leading to diabetes. Yet diabetics are usually advised to follow standard dietary recommendations with abundant carbohydrates at the base; insulin resistance only worsens as does its associated problems. *By keeping your carb/protein/fat in the 40/30/30 range will you improve insulin sensitivity, normalize blood pressure, triglycerides & cholesterol, restore ideal weight—and keep deadly inflammation at bay.*

The Golden Ratio Glycemic Zone: Upgrading Your Carbohydrate Quality

Building on our knowledge that the healthiest *quantity* of carbohydrates is defined by the 40% carbohydrate, 30% protein and 30% fat Golden Ratio Zone, we now offer critical new insight for improving the *quality* of your carbohydrate consumption. This data focuses on the selection of the healthiest types of carbohydrates and compliments the 40/30/30 *quantity* adjustment. Once you've zeroed-in on the right *amount* (ratio) of carbs to eat, you might ask: *are all carbs created equal?* The surprising answer is a resounding NO; ***All Carbs Are NOT Created Equal.*** Each carbohydrate type has a different rate at which the component sugar molecules are broken down and absorbed into your blood stream. Absorption rates of hundreds of foods have been tabulated into the **Glycemic Index (GI)** on a 0–100 scale, with pure glucose having the fastest absorption rate of 100. Other foods like breads, cereals, fruit and beans have differing absorption rates. This ground-breaking research was published by Jennie Brand-Miller, Ph.D., et al., in *Diabetes Care*, vol.31, no.12, Dec. 2008. We've reformatted the standard Glycemic Index with the Golden Ratio to further enhance your body's natural functioning and physiology. A 0-100 scale is ideal for superimposing Golden Ratio divisions, as 38 and 62 on any 100-pt. scale divides it into Golden Ratios. Our physiology so often mirrors a Golden Ratio distribution when we look for it, remembering that it's Nature's universal design blueprint. We call this new measure of carbohydrate absorption rate the *Golden Ratio Glycemic Zone*. It offers an easy and powerful way to fine-tune your system by optimizing blood sugar levels. Foods from 100-62 fall into the **High** *(not best)* Golden Ratio Glycemic Zone, with fast absorption rates. Foods from 62-38 have **Moderate** rates, while foods

Golden Ratio Pac-Man Weight Loss & Health Secret: Timing is Key

In a study with profound implications, **Dr. S. Panda's** (Salk Institute, San Diego) time-optimized eating discovery showed that mice whose feeding window was tuned to around 9 hrs. in a 24-hour day had *dramatic improvements in health—everything from weight loss, reversal of type 2 diabetes and lower cholesterol.* This means that the remaining 15 hrs. of no-meals time was like a daily mini-fast, which gave the mice a chance to effectively clean out cellular waste products (*autophagy*) and optimize cellular metabolism. These animal studies are now being extrapolated to humans for similar benefits, including metabolic improvements as well as cancer prevention and anti-aging benefits. It's likely that the generation of ketones via intermittent fasting are responsible for many of these beneficial effects. Not surprisingly, this (intermittent fasting) 9:15 hour feeding/fasting ratio closely approximates the Golden Ratio. This is an easy and very effective way to add another Golden Ratio biohack to your NSN health, peak performance and longevity regimen. *Simply eat only during a 9-hour window during your day.* This means you'd do a 15-hour mini-fast for the remainder of your day/night. For example, you'd eat from **7am–5pm • 9am–6pm • 11am–8pm,** or select your own 9 hour eating window. What you eat is up to you—however, superimposing the Golden Ratio Diet on top of this 9:15 meal timing schedule will give you a double dose of the amazing plus factor that supercharges all NSN protocols. The 9:15 schedule may be challenging in the beginning, so work your way up to the Golden Ratio 9:15 eating window; try narrowing your eating window by as little as 15-30 mins. weekly. This is especially true for people with medical conditions or hypoglycemic tendencies. Don't worry if you skip a day or two here or there; the original mice research protocols were still successful whenever the mice took weekends off and fed freely.

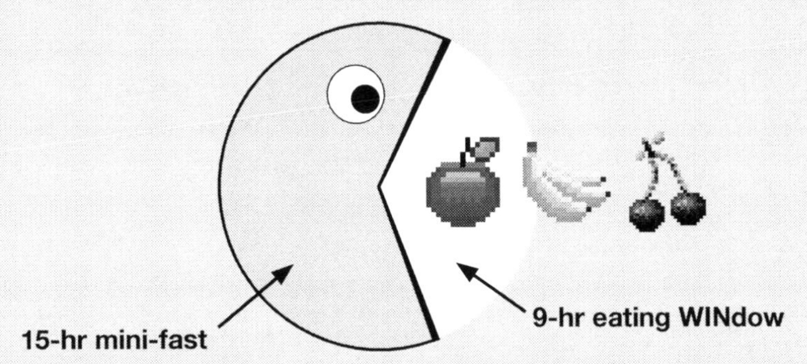

Navigate your Golden Ratio Pac-Man through the maze of always available food to achieve optimal weight loss and health. By simply keeping your meals within a 9-hour window out of 24, you tap a powerful NSN principle for sustainable weight loss—and win the game of long-term health.

less than 38 have **sLow** rates. **Ideally, we want to eat foods in the Moderate-to-Low Golden Ratio Glycemic Zones to prevent insulin spikes common with high glycemic foods.** Typically, more complex carbohydrate foods absorb slower and fall into the low/moderate zones. Surprisingly, some simple carbohydrates like sucrose have a lower than expected **Glycemic Index (GI)**. Many heavily sugar-laden foods like ice cream also naturally contain protein and fat, slowing their sugar/carb absorption and thereby lowering their GI. Remember that glucose is the standard for the highest glycemic zone carbohydrate at 100. Sucrose (white sugar) and high-fructose corn syrup (HFCS) are both strongly associated with obesity, diabetes and many other diseases. Sucrose is made up of one molecule each of glucose & fructose bonded together, whereas HFCS has one molecule each of glucose & fructose, but the two molecules aren't bonded together. Crystalline fructose is at 25 on the GI, while pure glucose is 100; that's why HFCS & sucrose (both a mix of glucose & sucrose) are 55-65 on the GI.

Refined sugars including white sugar and high-fructose corn syrup pack an added pernicious punch, as both are strongly associated with obesity, diabetes and a host of disease conditions. Sucrose—ordinary white table sugar—is made up of one molecule each of glucose & fructose. Even though refined sugars have a high carbohydrate *macronutrient density* (calories), they have a zero *micronutrient density* (vitamins, minerals and phytonutrients). In order to be metabolized at the cellular level, critical micronutrients need to be borrowed or leached from existing micronutrient stores in your body when you consume high carb, low/no nutrition foods. Over time various nutritional deficiencies and health challenges can develop as critical micronutrients in your body are depleted. On the other hand, *unrefined* carbohydrates have variable macronutrient density, while also having high micronutrient density. Nature in her genius designed whole, natural foods with "batteries included," i.e., micronutrients. The micronutrient profile of 100 grams of broccoli compared to 100 grams of cotton candy is vastly different. This is a critical reason to limit refined sugar, high-fructose corn syrup and other highly processed carbohydrates and eat predominantly whole, unrefined and slower-burning micronutrient-dense carbohydrates. The Golden Ratio Glycemic Zone Thermometer Infographic at right offers key insight and an easy way to upgrade your carbohydrate intake towards healthier, unrefined carbs.

Some key notes on the Golden Ratio Glycemic Zone Thermometer at right:

- Φ Fructose—in its natural, whole-fruit form—is complexed with fiber and varying amounts of glucose and is highly beneficial. For example, apples contain pectin and fructose (with a smaller amount of glucose) and are found in the low Golden Ratio Glycemic Zone, with a GI of only 36.

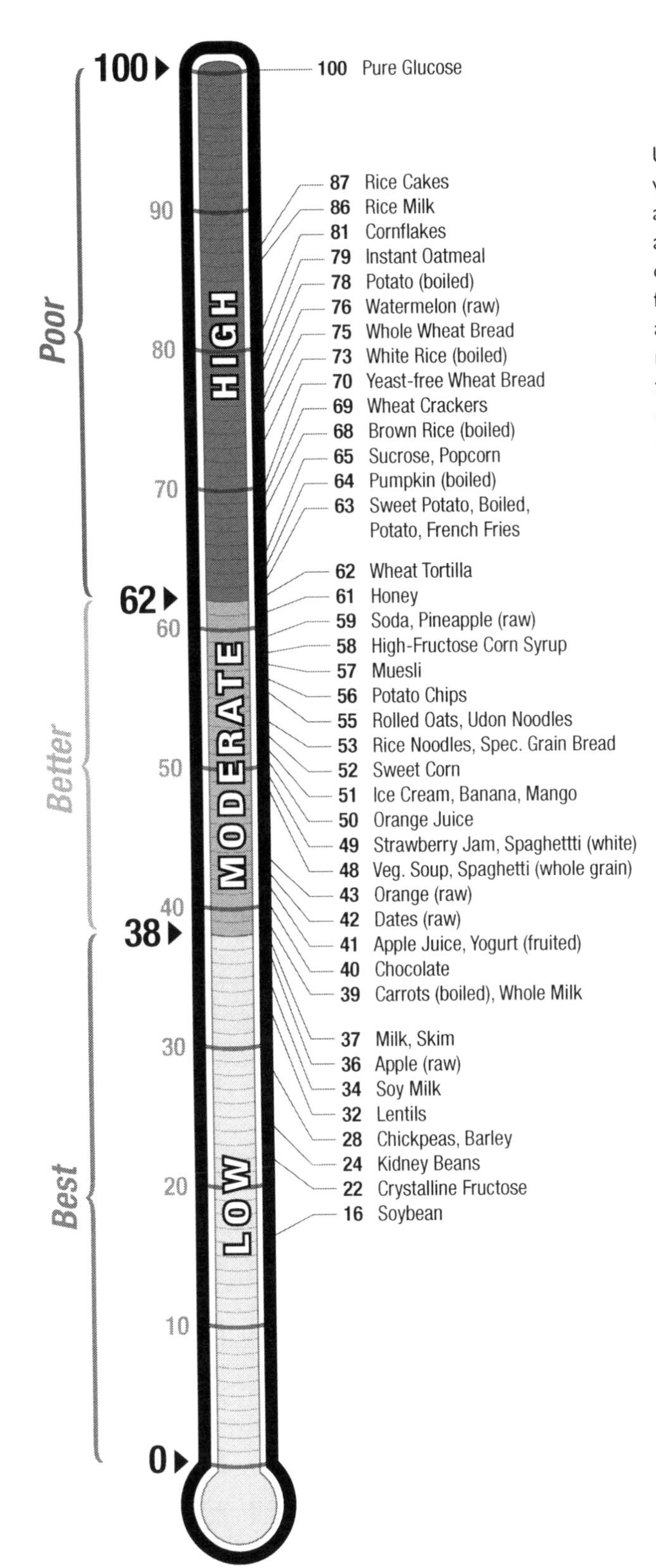

Golden Ratio Glycemic Zone Thermometer Infographic

Use of Golden Ratio divisions as a tool with which to categorize glycemic values is an easy and powerful way to understand this concept and thereby make better carbohydrate food choices. The glycemic index measures how fast blood sugar rises after ingesting specific amounts of different carbohydrates. Original research organized the carbohydrate into 9 food groups, e.g., high-carb foods, breakfast cereals, fruit and fruit products, vegetables, dairy products and alternatives, legumes, snack products, and sugars. With this perspective, the foods in each group are seen to have glycemic indices with wide-ranging values. We re-organized the carbohydrates into just 3 groups (instead of 9) according to Golden Ratio divisions, resulting in the user-friendly infographic at left. Using the Golden Ratio, Nature's prime design blueprint, we can now clearly see the various carbohydrate foods not only according to their absorption rates (low, moderate, high), but also by their potential for health (poor, better and best).

The upper section from 62-100 includes carbs with rapid absorption. These carbs are fast burners and cause large insulin spikes, with resultant hypoglycemia and endocrine stress. In the long run, glycemic stress is at the root of inflammation, hormonal aberrations and a multitude of degenerative diseases.

The middle section from 38-62 borders both the upper and lower divisions. It includes carbs with both moderately rapid absorption (at the upper end) and moderately slow absorption (at the lower end). Eating carbs from this range is moving you in the right direction by decreasing absorption rate and dampening the insulin response.

The lower section from 0-38 includes carbs with the slowest absorption rates. These carbs are slow burners and are highly beneficial and help to establish a balanced insulin response. Eating carbs from this list can prevent and possibly reverse many of the degenerative diseases prevalent today.

How Different Carbohydrates Affect Blood Sugar Levels

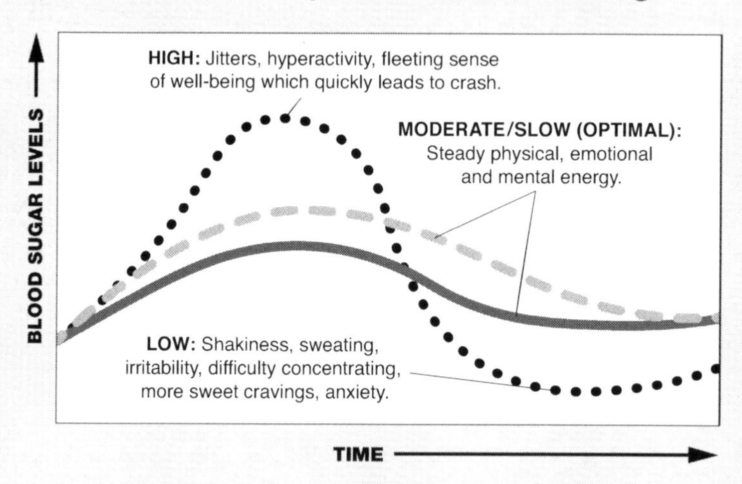

Glucose tolerance curves show blood sugar ups & downs over time after ingestion of 3 different classes of carbohydrates. Negative side effects result from eating fast-absorbing carbs (dotted line), while positive effects are associated with moderate and slow absorbing carbs (dashed and solid lines). Data below correlates with the Golden Ratio Glycemic Zone infographic, p.135.

•••• Fast absorbing carbs > 62, like cornflakes, white rice, boiled potatoes.

▬ ▬ Moderate absorbing carbs 38 to 62, like oats, bananas, vegetable soup, and ice cream.

▬▬ Slow absorbing carbs < 38, like barley, chickpeas and lentils.

An apt analogy to better understand differing carbohydrate absorption rates is obtained by looking at the varying burn rates of different kinds of fuel. For example, using gasoline for a fire gives a quick flash, yet no lasting flames. This is similar to what happens when you eat sugary, high carbohydrate sweets without any accompanying fat, protein or fiber to slow the absorption rate. A rapid burst of energy followed by hypoglycemia—low blood sugar—is a predictable result. Other kinds of fuel tend to release their energy slower, yet last longer, e.g., hardwoods like oak will burn with steady heat for hours. Likewise, complex carbohydrates take longer to digest and absorb, providing a steady release of energy and preventing large insulin swings.

- Φ Proteins and fats don't contain carbohydrates and therefore have no effect on blood sugar; hence, they don't appear on the Golden Ratio Glycemic Zone Thermometer. However, different proteins and fats have variable insulin responses and can have indirect effects on blood sugar.
- Φ The absorption rates of carbohydrates on the thermometer can be slowed by any accompanying proteins and fats in a given meal. **In a typical meal, many different foods are combined with a mix of all three macronutrients—Carb, Protein and Fat.** The resulting carbohydrate absorption rates are inevitably slowed compared with individual carbohydrates eaten separately as listed on this infographic.

Nevertheless, it behooves anyone interested in improving their glycemic response and both short and long-term health to select foods from within the lower two categories—**Moderate, Low**—on the Golden Ratio Glycemic Zone Thermometer.

The Golden Ratio Glycemic Zone guides us to eat more foods from the moderate and low carbohydrate categories. This simple yet powerful practice decreases insulin and leptin resistance and avoids the devastating sequelae of inflammation, obesity, diabetes, heart disease, cancer and innumerable other chronic diseases. Here's the magic formula for both fine-tuning the *quantity* and *quality* of your carbohydrate consumption, as well as extracting the maximum possible dose of Nature's Secret Nutrient from your diet:

Golden Ratio Zone Diet + Golden Ratio Glycemic Zone = Optimal Health & Energy

Abdominal Obesity Is Far Worse than Overall Body Obesity

In the April 2008 issue of *Circulation,* **Dr. C. Zhang** et al., reported that the health risks of abdominal obesity (belly fat) are even greater than those incurred by overall body obesity. Women with a waist circumference greater than 35 inches or waist/hip ratio greater than 0.84 had a 60%–70% greater risk of all-cause mortality, compared to women with a waist circumference less than 28 inches or with a waist/hip ratio less than 0.73. The authors emphasized that, *Although maintaining a healthy weight should continue to be a cornerstone in the prevention of chronic diseases and premature death, it is equally important to maintain a healthy waist size and prevent abdominal obesity.* **Essentially, keeping weight off your waist is even more important than keeping your overall body weight down.** With every excess inch of belly fat, the odds of disease and premature death increase proportionally. By decreasing the width of your midsection you can increase the length—and quality—of your life.

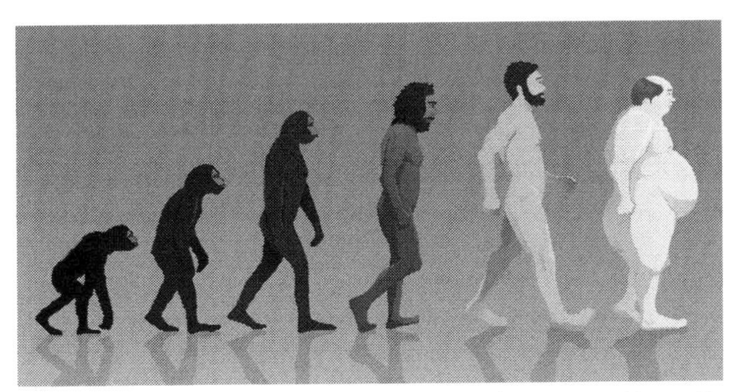

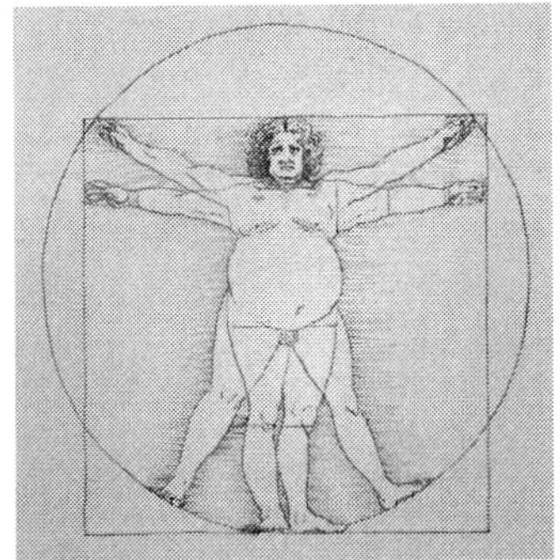

Human *devolution*, culminating in Homo-Fatruvius' high waist/hip ratio, i.e., extreme abdominal obesity (belly fat).

Abdominal Obesity Distorts Spinal Balance

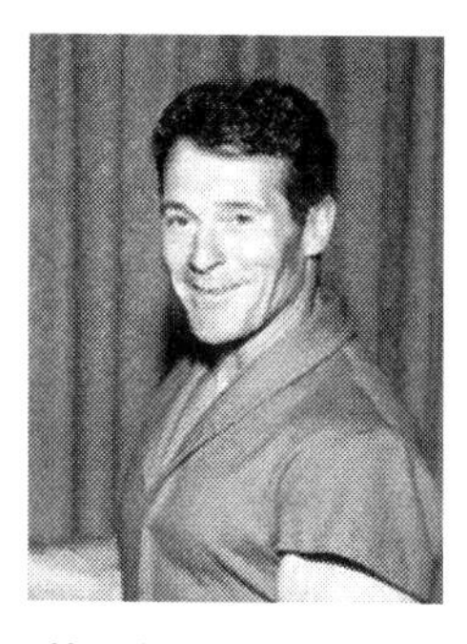

Your Waistline is Your Lifeline. Jack LaLanne, fitness pioneer.

Extra abdominal fat can also throw off spinal health and biomechanics by pulling your lumbar spine forward, causing an accentuated lumbar curvature (lordosis). This stresses your lower back and disrupts the alignment of your whole spine, predisposing you to back pain, slipped vertebrae and ruptured discs. Abdominal organs, including the organs of digestion, are also pulled out of alignment, compromising their function. The lumbar back area is also opposite the navel—the main vertical Golden Ratio dividing point of the body. Abnormal spinal alignment distorts normal Golden Ratio balance between the upper and lower segments of the body and negatively affects overall body function and energetics.

A Body Shape Index (ABSI): Body Mass Index (BMI) + Waist Circumference (WC)

Even before modern times, artists and scientists were fascinated with the proportions of the human body. Leonardo da Vinci's iconic drawing of the **Vitruvian Man**, the Golden Ratio archetype of humanity, illustrates that even in the year 1490 there was a consensus that slim and sleek body types, at least for males, were considered ideal. Other than visually illustrating the relationship between a person's height, weight and body shape, there was no scientific way to describe these relationships until the years 1830-1850 when Belgian polymath **Adolphe Quetelet** devised a formula we know today by the acronym **BMI** (**B**ody **M**ass **I**ndex). BMI is obtained by simply dividing a person's weight in kilograms by their height in meters squared. The number obtained reflects the degree of leanness or obesity that can then be used to predict mortality rates. Yet the accuracy of BMI is unreliable in many cases because there's such a wide range of variability within the so-called normal range. In addition, certain body types like athletes have an increased muscle mass and will appear to have elevated **BMI's**, when clearly their increased body mass is due to muscle and not fat. Another major limitation of the BMI measurement is that it doesn't specify where a person carries their excess weight. Contrast the BMI to the simple **WC** (**W**aist **C**ircumference) measurement that also has its own mortality prediction charts. As we've seen, increased abdominal obesity or "belly fat" has been clearly shown to be its own independent risk factor for increased mortality. WC charts show that it's more risky to carry excess weight as an "apple" shape rather than a "pear" shape. To clarify and resolve the discrepancies and limitations inherent with both BMI and WC, researchers **Nir Y. Krakauer** and **Jesse C. Krakauer, M.D.**, from City College of New York came up with an ingenious way of integrating complementary information from both systems. They developed their own unique method that was significantly more accurate than either the BMI or WC for predicting mortality rates. The acronym for their system is **ABSI—A B**ody **S**hape **I**ndex. **The main message from their research is that independent use of either WC or the outdated 19th-century BMI method can give misleading predictions regarding your mortality risk.** Instead, use the online ABSI calculator, which integrates both BMI and WC. The calculator can be found online at: www.absi-calculator.com

Losing Weight & Gaining Health

Here's great news for those wanting to lose weight: Lowered insulin levels mean that your body won't store as much fat. This allows you to better access stored body fat for energy, as well as for warding off hunger. A Golden Pro*portion* intake of carbohydrates to protein and fat keeps your blood sugar and insulin levels on an even keel. You use stored fats for their intended purpose—expending physical and mental energy. In the sage words of of *Zone* Master Dr. Barry Sears:

> *It is excessive levels of the hormone insulin that make you fat and keeps you fat. How do you increase insulin levels? By eating too many fat-free carbohydrates or too many calories at any one meal. Americans do both. People tend to forget that the best way to fatten cattle is to raise their insulin levels by feeding them excessive amounts of low-fat grain. The best way to fatten humans is to raise their insulin levels by feeding them excessive amounts of low-fat grain, but now in the form of pasta and bagels.*

Eating Divine Pro*portions* (40% carbohydrates to 60% fat + protein) is meant to become a consistent healthy eating pattern. If you decide to test it, use the 21-Day Priority Coach System at the back of this book to embed it into your daily behavior. Celebrate your progress on the Fibonacci days (1, 2, 3, 5, 8, 13, 21...) and remember to build up some escape velocity to get beyond the usual bog-down around day 13. Always remain sensitive to which foods and how much you eat. Become attuned to the pro*portions* of the food you take into your body during a meal.

Inflammation: The Silent, Deadly Threat to Your Health & Longevity

In Dr. Sears' book *Omega Rx Zone* he upgrades *The Zone* approach by the addition of high doses of pharmaceutical grade fish oil to the diet, to control the ratios of hormonally

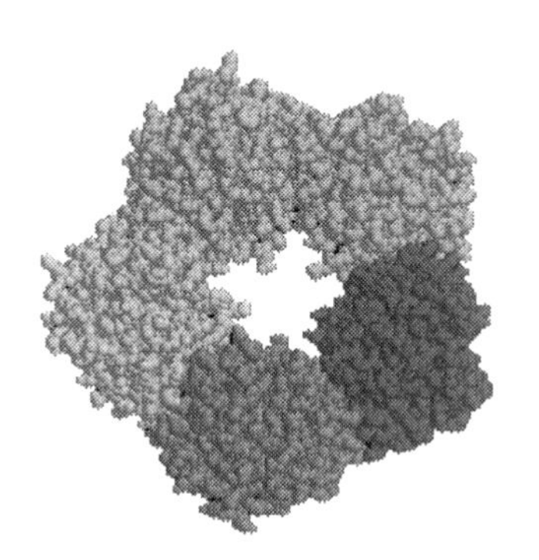

C-Reactive Protein (CRP) has a distinct pentagonal Golden Ratio shape and is a sensitive blood marker for inflammation and heart disease.

important fats called **eicosenoids**. These eicosenoids profoundly influence inflammation in your body. This eicosenoid balance completes the one-two punch along with the Zone Diet for controlling insulin. This combination is a superior way to achieve high-level health and performance and treat chronic diseases. Interestingly, the best way to measure eicosenoid balance is with a blood test. The ideal ratio of bad to good eicosenoids (Arachadonic Acid/EPA) is around 1.5. This matches the ratio of numbers early in the Fibonacci Sequence—3:2—moving towards the Golden Ratio of 1.618. Again, the genius of Dr. Sears:

In the final analysis, it's all about your genes, especially how an anti-inflammatory diet, like the Zone Diet, can turn off inflammatory genes and simultaneously turn on anti-inflammatory genes that promote cellular rejuvenation, repair and healing. ***Your ability to control inflammation becomes the molecular definition of wellness.***

The Golden Ratio of Evolution: Omega-6 to Omega-3 Balance

Living in the Rift Valley of East Africa 100-200 thousand years ago, our Homo Sapiens ancestors' diet was composed of up to 12% lake fish and shellfish that had a polyunsaturated fatty acid—omega-6 and omega-3—content very close to that of the human brain. Those dietary conditions favored the evolutionary spurt of the human brain's neocortex that gave our ancestors the survival advantage needed to flourish. The quantum jump in brain evolution correlated with a diet consisting of an omega-6 to omega-3 ratio that ranged from between 1:1 to 2:1, a range that **Artemis P. Simopoulos, M.D.** termed the "Ratio of Evolution." **With our Golden Ratio lens, we can see that Dr. Simopoulos' fatty acid Ratio of Evolution encompasses the Golden Ratio of 1.618:1.** Knowing that Nature always works with Golden Pro*portions* first in mind, we can refine the terminology, calling it the *Golden Ratio of Evolution*. This ratio was the most efficient physiologic path for evolutionary progress to occur.

Over the millennia, our species evolution has gone through fits and starts that have had a high correlation to dietary conditions. Much of the world, including Western civilization, may currently be going through a period of *devolution* as a result of mass dietary ignorance and resulting poor dietary habits. In Western diets, the omega–6 to omega–3 ratio is around 16.7:1. This ratio is about 10 times greater than the ideal *Golden Ratio of Evolution*: 1.618:1.

In some countries, such as India, the ratio is as high as 38:1. Not surprisingly, India has extremely high rates of cardiovascular disease and diabetes. Researchers **Veronique Chajès** and **Philippe Bougnoux** have discovered that an omega–6 to omega–3 ratio from between 1:1 to 2:1 has a protective effect against the development and growth of breast and colon cancers. Studies have also determined that a ratio of omega–6 to omega–3 of about 2.5:1 may protect against colorectal cancer.

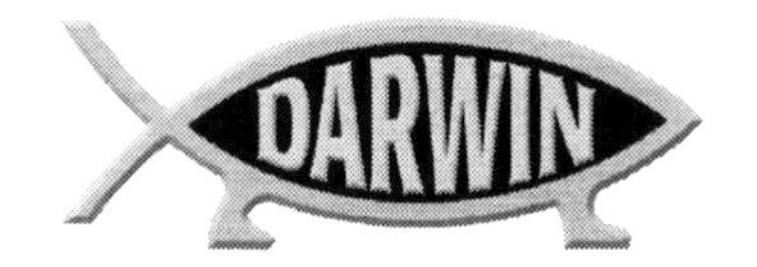

Darwin's evolutionary fish glyph takes on an entirely new meaning when one considers the impact of fish oils on human brain development and evolution.

Japanese researchers **Tomohito Hamazaki** and **Harumi Okuyama** have produced more evidence of a Golden Ratio connection regarding omega-6 to omega-3 ratios. Even though Japanese diets have a relatively favorable omega-6 to omega-3 ratio of 4:1, these researchers are recommending even lower omega–6 to omega–3 ratios in the range of 2.7–3.6:1. Again, these ratios are in line with Golden Ratio harmonics of 2.618:1 and 3.618:1 and are consistent with the master efficiency principle of the Golden Ratio. Over-consumption of omega-6 fats in relation to omega-3 fats leads to an increase in inflammation and an increased tendency for blood clot associated heart attacks and strokes. Chronic inflammation also has negative effects on cellular membranes and is also associated with many chronic diseases including arthritis, diabetes, cancer and dementia. The cellular health membrane diagram above illustrates how shifting your essential fatty acid intake towards the Golden Ratio of Evolution's omega-3 to omega-6 balance helps make cellular membranes softer and more permeable.

DHA: the Golden Ratio Omega-3 Fatty Acid

DHA (DocosaHexaenoic Acid) is found in fish and micro-algae and makes up around 40% of the brain's polyunsaturated fatty acids as well as about 60% of the retina's polyunsaturated fatty acids. As you recall, 40% and 60% are close approximations of Golden Ratio percentages, i.e., 38% and 62%. DHA is recognized as being so important for infant brain and eye development that it's found in most infant formulas. In adults, a high concentration of DHA has preventive properties against Alzheimer's and Parkinson's diseases as well as protective properties against cardiovascular disease and stroke. Anti-aging properties of DHA have also been discovered, with the mechanism being a slower rate of telomere shortening. See Ch 10 Longevity for more on telomeres.

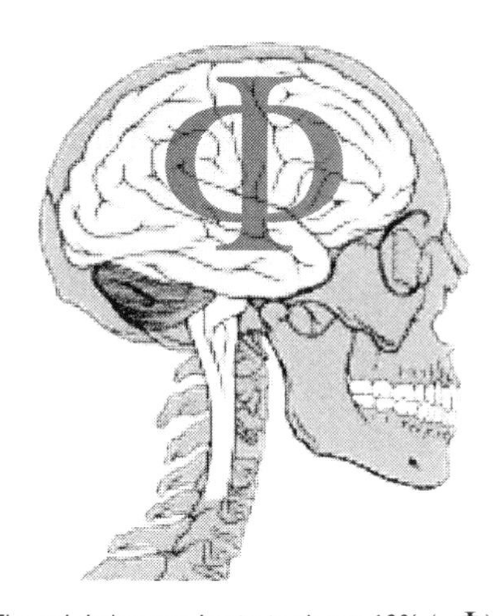

The adult human brain is about 60% (~Φ) lipid (fat), another amazing correlation with the Golden Ratio, and a strong added reason to make sure your diet contains ample levels of DHA & EPA omega-3 oils.

This improves intra and extracellular signaling, enhancing nutrient absorption and toxin elimination. **Vibrant health and performance is a result of the healthy interaction between our** *external* **electromagnetic environment and our** *internal* **cellular environment—with a healthy cellular membrane being the prime interface between these macro and micro levels.** Thus it's imperative to achieve and maintain an optimal ratio of omega-3 to omega-6 fats in your system. Simply including omega-3-rich fish oil along with chia and flax seeds in your diet—while reducing omega-6-rich food intake—insures the health and integrity of your 30 trillion+ total cells. As our daily cellular turnover averages about 50 billion cells, everyone has a golden opportunity to elevate their total health by restoring healthy omega-3 and 6 fat ratios. Most fish (especially salmon, mackerel and sardines), krill and plankton have high omega-3 levels and are recommended. Avoid toxic farm-raised fish, which are ironically also fed high omega-6 grains. Limit/avoid large fish like tuna, shark and swordfish due to their increased mercury content; avoid shellfish due to increased heavy metals/toxicity from bottom feeding. Avoid Pacific seafood due to probable radiation contamination from the ongoing 2011 Fukishima, Japan nuclear disaster. With canned fish, get water-packed vs.

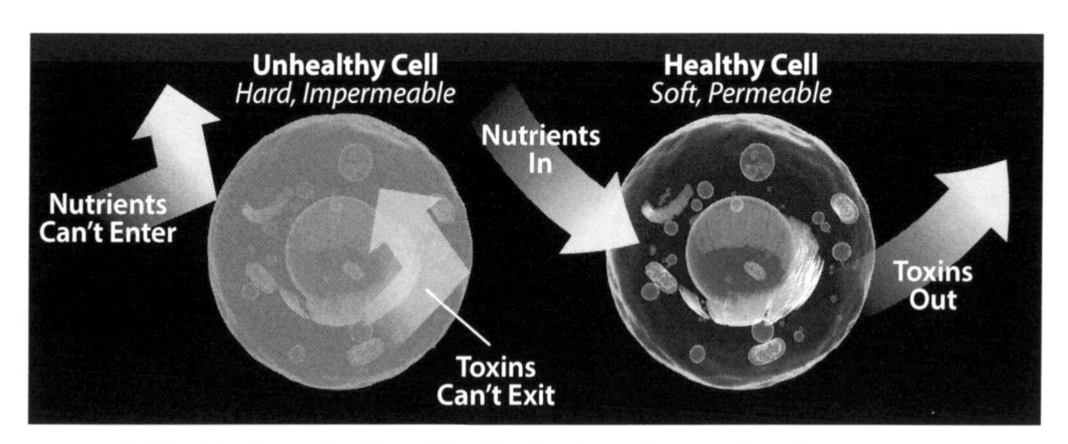

Cellular Membrane Health and Healthy Fat. By avoiding trans-fat and optimizing your intake of healthy fat, including a good ratio of omega-3 to omega-6 fat, your cell membranes become softer and more permeable, improving nutrient absorption, toxin elimination, cellular vitality and overall health *(after diagram by Chris Johnson, OnTargetLiving.com).*

omega-6 oil packed, e.g., sunflower, soy or sesame. Taking fish or krill oil supplements is another option, as is non-fish omega-3 oil derived from algae grown aquaponically. This vegetarian omega-3 source avoids all contamination present in ocean-sourced omega-3. While green vegetables like spinach and kale have good omega-3 to omega-6 ratios, their total omega-3 content is quite low and can't match that from fish or algae. Most nuts and seeds have high omega-6's, a big exception being **chia and flax seeds, which are very high in omega-3's** (though not in the same metabolically active form as in fish, krill or plankton). Grains are high in omega-6 and are thus not your best choice for omega-3's; they should also be kept to a minimum as they are less favorable carbohydrates, due to their increased contribution to inflammation and often being allergenic. Fruits are negligible fat sources; best to minimize fruit sugar intake due to their excessive carbohydrate load and adverse insulin level impact.

Bread: The Golden Ratio Staff of Life

Stick to the 5:3 Ratio and you're Golden.

Michael Ruhlman, author of *Ratio: The Simple Codes Behind the Craft of Everyday Cooking*

Bread became the Staff of Life as the transition from the Paleolithic to Neolithic era began around 10,000 years ago. The Paleolithic nomadic diet that had high omega-3's from seafood and wild game slowly gave way to a high omega-6 grain-containing diet. Through trial, error and the magic of serendipity, humans learned how to transform grains into bread. Just as amazing, from our perspective, is that this simple combination of flour, water, baking yeast and salt has Golden Ratio proportions. It is known as a baker's percentage and utilizes weight instead of volume to measure ingredients. The classic ratio of flour to water is 100:60, which closely approaches the Golden Ratio (100:62). The addition of yeast and salt brings the ratio very close to a perfect Golden Ratio and a perfect loaf every time. By simply remembering the Golden Ratio, you will never have to look up the recipe for bread again. If you want an even simpler formula, use the Fibonacci numbers 5 and 3. Five parts flour (ideally organic, non-GMO whole-grain flour) to three parts water (by weight) will give you essentially the same proportions. This universal constant is essential for you to "rise to the occasion" of life on planet Earth. For other interesting recipe ratios see the great book *Ratio: The Simple Codes Behind the Craft of Everyday Cooking*, by Michael Ruhlman. For those who are bread aficionados, try and keep your bread intake on the low end so that you'll have room for healthy vegetables in your Golden Ratio carb allotment.

Bon Golden Appetite!

Nature's Secret Nutrient/*NSN App:* Why An Apple a Day Keeps the Doctor Away

The apple is Nature's prototypical Golden Ratio fruit, with a pentagonal seed array, five-petaled blossoms and a perfect 1.6:1 Golden Ratio of insoluble to soluble fiber (See Ch 7 Detox). Apples also have an unidentified, mysterious "X-Factor" that lifts them above all other fruits in the prevention of lung cancer and asthma.

Researchers are aware that antioxidant and anti-inflammatory effects of apple phytonutrients are involved, yet this doesn't fully explain why apples shine above every other fruit in this area. Since apples are one of Nature's prime examples of Golden Ratio balance, they also logically contain high levels of Nature's Secret Nutrient/NSN, endowing them with their phenomenal health-giving benefits.

The Amazing Health Benefits of Apples—*Live Happley and Prosper!*

- Regular apple consumption is associated with a decreased risk of cancer, heart disease, asthma, diabetes and obesity.
- The phytonutrients in one apple have the equivalent antioxidant activity of 1,500 mg of vitamin C.
- The antioxidant protection from eating an apple lasts only about 24 hours; hence, eating "An Apple a Day" keeps your antioxidant levels replenished and lowers your risk of the above-mentioned diseases.
- Apple peels have significantly higher antioxidant activity than the fruit flesh, so eat the whole apple, raw and unprocessed; chew well to maximize nutrient uptake and make sure your apple is organic so it's pesticide-free.
- Cholesterol and triglyceride levels can be lowered simply by eating apples, as apple pectin binds cholesterol-derived bile acids in the gut.
- Antioxidant potency varies greatly between types of apples; darker red apples contain more beneficial anthocyanin antioxidants.
- Apples favorably alter intestinal bacteria. Apple extracts have even been shown to inhibit cholera bacteria.
- Eating an apple 15 min. before meals can significantly lower your appetite.
- Apple consumption reduces C-Reactive Protein (CRP), a key blood marker of inflammation, a leading cause of many diseases including heart disease.

Raw, Green & Lean

Nothing could be better than consuming greens and nothing could be faster than consuming blended greens.

Victoria Boutenko, author of *Green for Life*

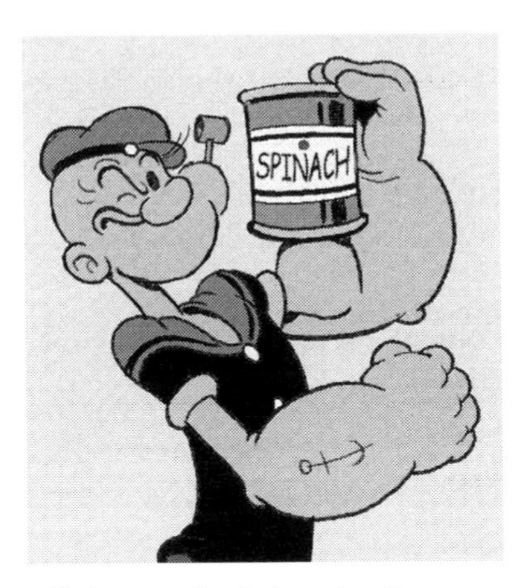

Early green food champion Popeye.

As we saw in the previous section, The Golden Ratio of Evolution, the evolution of the human brain was driven by an increased dietary intake of omega-3 essential fats like EPA and DHA, resulting in a lower ratio of omega-6's to omega-3's that approached the Golden Ratio. Yet, since humans can't live on omega-3's alone, what else are we supposed to eat? One researcher, raw food proponent Victoria Boutenko, has theorized that since humans and chimpanzee's have around 99% of their DNA in common, humans might benefit from eating a diet similar to what chimps, who along with gorillas are known for their great strength, naturally eat in the wild. Interestingly, a chimp's diet has a natural Golden Ratio balance, with around 60% fruits and 40% green leafy plants, nuts, seeds, insects and occasionally a small amount of meat. This primitive, elemental diet supplies them with high amounts of enzymes, chlorophyll, vitamins and minerals.

Boutenko noticed that a favorite chimp delicacy was a simple banana wrapped in a green leaf. Yet short of eating banana wraps, how could this chimp entrée be adapted to finicky humans? Her intuitive flash was to combine the ingredients into a blended green smoothie. By putting the ingredients into a blender, the combination would be much more palatable—as well as making it easier to predigest the fibrous greens. The total surface area of the food would also be vastly increased for more thorough and rapid absorption. One of the most potent and easily available greens for the recipe is kale, which has one of the highest antioxidant profiles of any vegetable. This brassica/ cruciferous family representative also has one of the highest nutritional values for the fewest calories of any vegetable. In addition, kale normalizes bowel functioning, increases liver detoxification and reduces the incidence of many cancers. The smoothie recipe is almost too good to be true in that it also satisfies Golden Ratio health driver #2 for water/hydration. By consuming up to 32 oz. of water (or more) with the blended ingredients, chronic dehydration can easily be overcome in a short time. The large increase in fluid intake flushes the kidneys, relieves constipation and also improves skin

Iron Man's Secret: Tapping the Power of Green

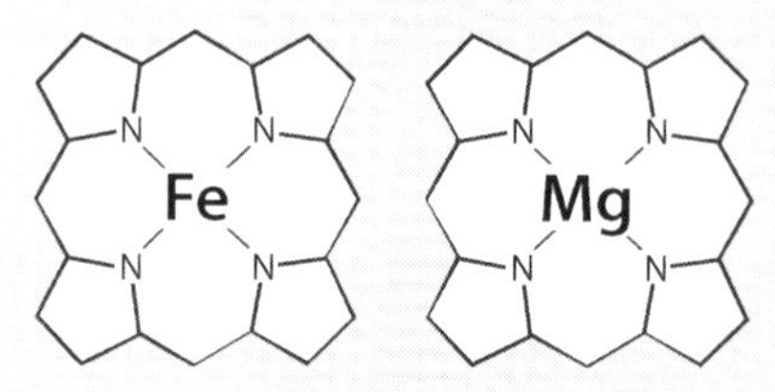

Both hemoglobin (*blood's red pigment, left*) and chlorophyll (*plant's green pigment, right*) are the O_2/CO_2 carrying molecules in humans and plants. Both are composed of 4 Golden Ratio-shaped pentagons (*porphyrin ring*). The key difference between the two is that hemoglobin has an iron molecule (Fe) at its center, while chlorophyll has a magnesium molecule (Mg) at its center. *Although not experimentally proven, many nutritionists theorize that by eating green leafy plants, our bodies transmute chlorophyll into hemoglobin, thereby boosting our blood's oxygen carrying capacity.* Whether it's Popeye and his can of spinach or the color of the Incredible Hulk, green is associated with super strength and vitality. The Golden Ratio Iron Ape Green Smoothie (see Rx section) is like getting a super energy-boosting natural blood transfusion. Is this why Iron Man's alter-ego Tony Stark (Robert Downey, Jr.) drinks a green smoothie in the hit film *Iron Man*?

Green superfood Spirulina, from an illustration in the Florentine Codex (c. 1585), showing how the Aztecs harvested Spirulina off lakes by skimming the surface with ropes; then drying the algae into square cakes to make a nourishing condiment. Spirulina, chlorella, wheat and barley grasses, as well as kale and romaine lettuce are power-packed green sources of chlorophyll-rich nutrition.

4

tone and texture. Last but not least, the smoothie is incredibly quick to make. You can take the extra leftover smoothie with you to work or a workout. In her book, *Green for Life*, Boutenko documents some of her family's amazing healing stories as a result of adopting this simple smoothie into their daily diet (she personally lost over 180 pounds). **In the Ch 4 Nutrition Rx section of this book there's a supercharged version of Boutenko's original smoothie: The Golden Ratio Iron Man Green Smoothie.** This version unleashes the combined energy of King Kong, Iron Man, The Incredible Hulk and Popeye by lifting the original ingredients a few notches up the evolutionary scale: more towards the carb/protein/fat ratios and antioxidant levels that our Zone/Paleolithic ancestors would have thrived on. Remember that the evolution of our physiology was tuned and refined over millions of years, and that agriculture was introduced only about 10,000 years ago in current history. The modern era of processed-for-profit, denatured, nutritionally deficient and chemically/genetically violated foods has only occurred over the last 150 years or so. It's illogical, if not insane, to think that we can disregard millions of years of our natural evolution on whole, unadulterated healthy foods and still be optimally healthy and enjoy maximum longevity. Nature is our eternally bright North Star guiding us to great health, happiness and longevity and NSN elegantly aligns us with Nature's North Star.

Fast-Track to Health: The Fasting Mimicking Diet & Fibonacci Connection

Everyone has heard of WMD, but now there's a new diet called FMD—and it doesn't stand for Fat Mass Destruction. **Dr. Valter Longo** of the USC School of Gerontology dubbed his new system **FMD**, which stands for **F**asting **M**imicking **D**iet. **The FMD rejuvenates the body through a metabolic and immune system reprogramming induced by a modified fasting protocol which only requires 5 days a month.** The diet purportedly reduces risk factors for a wide range of conditions including premature aging, diabetes and cardiovascular disease. Dr. Longo incorporated his remarkable immune system restoration discovery into a simple 5-day fasting protocol that works by decreasing the number of daily calories consumed to between 34% and 54% of the calories that a person would normally eat in a given day. The Fasting Mimicking Diet is done for 5 days in a row, moving from 54% of daily caloric intake for the 1st day down to 34% for the next 4 days. In addition, it only needs to be done monthly or even quarterly. Amazingly, Dr. Longo and his team have mirrored two sequential Fibonacci numbers—34 and 55—as recommended percentages of caloric consumption. This is one of countless, clear examples of how Golden Ratio Biomimicry unexpectedly appears in scientific research—even when the researchers may have unknowingly used Golden Ratio parameters in the design of the experiment. But that's not all, as there's even more Fibonacci/biomimicry resonance in the diet.

On Day 1 of the diet, the recommended fat to carbohydrate ratio also uses Fibonacci numbers—56% fat to 34% carbohydrate. This double-layered Fibonacci embedding assures the dieter of a hefty dose of NSN that can modulate and soften the impact of caloric deficit. Interestingly, the Fibonacci-based Fasting Mimicking Diet (FMD) with its 34% to 54% caloric reduction range is very similar to the NSN/Golden Ratio caloric reduction method featured in Ch 4's Rx section. Instead of using Fibonacci numbers to delineate the caloric range, the NSN Rx defaults to two easier-to-use Golden Ratio protocols: **1**: Either eat 62% (slightly less than 2/3) of your normal daily caloric intake, or **2**: Further reduce it to 38% (slightly more than 1/3) if more accelerated weight loss is desired. The NSN approach may promote greater adherence, due to the fact that the NSN Rx is less calorically restrictive than the FMD protocol. A main attraction of the FMD is the fact that it only needs to be done monthly or quarterly, whereas the NSN Rx can be

4

Zer0 Nutriti0n for Regenerati0n & Rejuvenati0n

To lengthen thy life, lessen thy meals.

Benjamin Franklin

Throughout history, virtually every ancient culture and religion on earth has recommended the practice of *Zero Nutrition*, otherwise known as fasting, for spiritual and physical renewal. We normally consider nutrition as the ingestion of something solid, something that we can smell, taste and swallow as the food that nourishes us. Yet science has recently confirmed that the *absence* of food—*Zero Nutrition*/fasting—has the unique ability to powerfully regenerate and rejuvenate our bodies. What's new regarding the *Zero Nutrition* approach is that clinical research has caught up with timeless ancestral wisdom, finally explaining how the beneficial effects of fasting actually occur. Dramatic results from a study published in the 6/5/14 edition of *Cell Stem Cell* revealed that mice and men with damaged immune systems, some from aging and others from chemotherapy, fasted anywhere from 2-4 days. In the initial stages of the fast, old or otherwise damaged white blood cells underwent a process of self-digestion and recycling known as autophagy. The proteins of the defective white blood cells could then be recycled and used to regenerate new cells. At the same time, molecular signaling activated a new crop of stem cells that were programmed to regenerate and replace the damaged white blood cells. Lead researcher **Dr. Valter D. Longo** noted,

> *The good news is that the body got rid of the parts of the system that might be damaged or old, the inefficient parts, during the fasting. Now, if you start with a system heavily damaged by chemotherapy or aging,* ***fasting cycles can generate, literally, a new immune system.***

This echoes the wry wisdom of **Mark Twain**, who said: *A little starvation can really do more for the average sick man than can the best medicines and the best doctors.* By expanding the range of what we consider a nutrient, in this case a *Zero Nutrient*, we open ourselves to the probability of even greater health and vitality. The short and long-term benefits of *Zero Nutrition*/fasting can almost magically manifest rejuvenation and regeneration. If you decide to integrate periodic *Zero Nutrition*/fasting into your health and longevity regimen, consult with your doctor, as there are important details that need to be customized to your particular needs.

done once or twice a week. Both approaches offer unique methods for regeneration and rejuvenation in that they take advantage of NSN's Golden Ratio Biomimicry technology.

Golden Ratio Longevity Code & Caloric Reduction

Research from the Washington University School of Medicine in St. Louis indicates that caloric reduction can significantly lengthen life expectancy, reduce incidence of disease, increase overall health and lead to sustained optimal weight. As reported by Rob Stein in the *Washington Post* on April 20, 2004:

> *Small groups of people who are drastically restricting how much they eat in the hope of slowing the aging process have produced the strongest support yet for the tantalizing theory that very low-calorie diets can extend the human life span. The first study of people who voluntarily imposed draconian diets on themselves found that their cholesterol levels, blood pressure and other major risk factors for heart disease—the biggest killer—plummeted, along with risk factors for diabetes and possibly other leading causes of death such as cancer and Alzheimer's. While it's long been known that eating well and staying trim helps people live healthier lives and avoid premature death, evidence has been accumulating that following extremely low-calorie diets for many years may do something more—significantly extend longevity beyond current norms. 'It is a very important paper,' said Roy L. Walford M.D., Biospherian and professor emeritus at the UCLA School of Medicine. 'You may well be able to choose between [caloric restriction] and that double-bypass cardiac surgery you are not looking forward to.'*

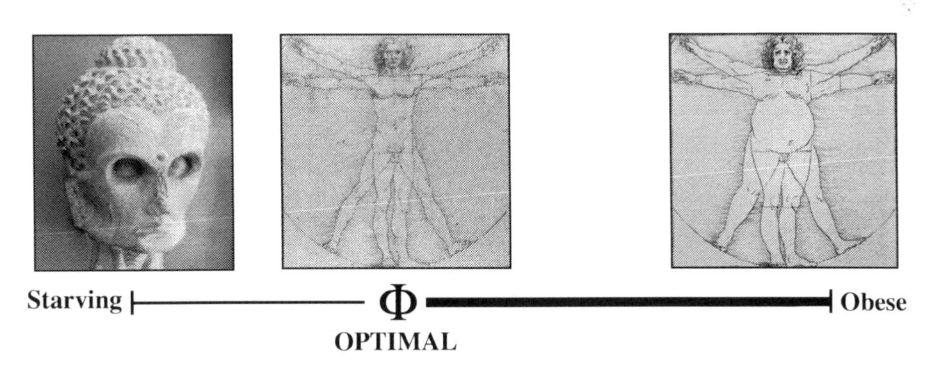

This bust of a calorically challenged and pre-enlightened Buddha (*left,* 2nd century, C.E.) demonstrates the result of an ascetic approach towards life and diet. Extremely restrictive diets or eating disorders result in neither good health nor do they put an end to human suffering. The ***Vitruvian Man*** (***center***), the ideal human prototype, shows the possibility of what can result from following a supremely balanced lifestyle and diet. Nature's Secret Nutrient is not extreme in restriction nor indulgence and results in optimal health and an ideal muscle/fat ratio. The ***Fatruvian*** Man (***right***) is the epitome of an indulgent lifestyle and diet, similar to the condition of a large percentage of the population in most western countries. **The extreme of obesity—especially abdominal obesity—is just as unhealthy as being too thin.**

One member of the Caloric Restriction Society who inspired the above study, **Dean Pomerleau**, decreased his intake of calories from around 3,000 to 1,900 daily. In other words, he allowed himself approximately 63%—very close to the 62% Golden Ratio—of his normal daily calories. To reap the benefits of caloric reduction without going to extremes, one could mirror the formulae of these life-enhancement pioneers. To calculate your daily Golden Ratio-adjusted target intake of calories, simply multiply your current total daily calories by 0.618, e.g. 3000 x 0.618 = 1854. Remember: Nature's Secret Nutrient is about *bringing one's dietary habits into balance and harmony.* It has absolutely nothing to do with the draconian, extreme measures typical of many weight loss diets or extreme caloric restriction. In the following section we will see how an innovative doctor unknowingly used the Golden Ratio to integrate sensible caloric reduction into his weight loss program in an ingenious, manageable and low-stress way.

The Alternate-Day Diet: Sensible Caloric Reduction Boosted with NSN

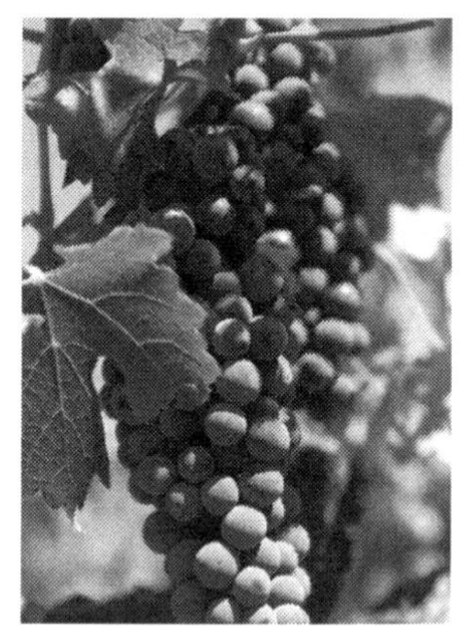

Grapes contain the nutrient Resveratrol, which slows the aging process by the same genetic mechanism as caloric reduction (activation of the SIRT-1 "skinny" gene).

As we have seen, Dr. Roy Walford's innovative discoveries in the area of caloric reduction have opened the door to a new era of health and longevity. However, not many people are able to put themselves through the rigors of daily caloric reduction without feeling deprived, tired or unable to function well. Taking Dr. Walford's premise to a more practical level, **James Johnson, M.D.** discovered some fascinating research and devised a more realistic approach to caloric reduction. He discovered an ingenious way to take caloric reduction from the deprivation level and make it tolerable—even fun—while maintaining its effectiveness. Earlier animal studies had shown that, by fasting the animals only on alternate days, they still experienced weight loss, increased health and longevity. Perhaps there was some way that he could apply these animal experiments to humans. Johnson noted,

> *I knew I wouldn't be able to fast on alternate days, but I thought I might be able to restrict my calorie intake enough every other day to reap the same health benefits as those mice. I decided to become my own lab mouse and began to restrict my calories to 20 percent of what I normally ate on alternate days. On nonrestrictive days I ate whatever and as much as I wanted.*

Reducing Calories May Protect Your Brain From Alzheimer's Disease

Research in non-human primates at the Mt. Sinai School of Medicine in New York City has shown that a lower calorie diet triggers the production of an anti-aging protein, SIRT-1 (the "Skinny Gene") that protects the brain from Alzheimer's-like disease. This protein has been shown to curtail and reverse the production of plaque in the brain, a common attribute of the disease. The message is clear: *eat less/live more—more years with more quality.*

This was the birth of what Johnson calls the Alternate-Day Diet. He found that **by alternating eating normally one day, and then calorie reducing the next, he avoided the compulsions and cravings induced by other diets.** After a while on most diets, one's metabolic rate and weight loss plummet while food cravings increase. Not so with the Alternate-Day Diet. Johnson lost 35 pounds by week 11 of his alternate-day regime and reports that he's been able to keep it off since that time (2003).

The secret to the tolerable and steady weight loss is activation of the SIRT-1 or "skinny gene" (SIR stands for Silent Information Regulator), which once activated has the ability to prevent oxidative damage, inhibit fat storage and decrease inflammation at the cellular level. What this means on a practical level is that in addition to keeping your metabolic rate elevated and losing weight, you are decreasing your chances of developing chronic degenerative conditions such as arthritis, allergies, asthma, cancer, infection, stroke, heart disease, etc. Johnson says that by instituting alternate-day caloric reduction, a built-in cellular stress response or *hormesis* is activated that in addition to facilitating weight loss, increases one's resistance to disease. He explains hormesis as follows:

> *The most widely accepted theory of why calorie restriction prevents disease and/or delays the onset of age-related diseases is called "hormesis," which means that a harmful stress—one that might be fatal in large quantities—is beneficial in small amounts. Thus, if an animal is starved, it dies, but if its daily calorie intake is reduced to 60 percent of normal, it lives longer in very good health.*

Of particular interest is how Johnson's Alternate-Day Diet adheres to principles of the Golden Ratio, in that reducing calories to 60% of normal (averaged over a two day period) approximates a Golden Ratio calorie reduction. Johnson's practical caloric reduction breakthrough has taken the inspiration of Roy Walford, M.D. to a new level.

This is a huge upgrade in our understanding of how to achieve and maintain vibrant health and maximum longevity. **Using scientifically proven genetic and metabolic discoveries, you can now comfortably reduce your calories according to Golden Ratio principles and reap the benefits of weight loss, weight maintenance, disease prevention and increased longevity—in an easy to practice manner.**

Dr. Johnson has unknowingly harnessed Nature's Secret Nutrient/NSN with his Alternate Day Diet and has taken advantage of one of its many important, paradoxical properties: *Nature's Secret Nutrient has zero calories—and massive nutritional value.*

A Profound New View of "Fullness"

As seen on the opposite page, the human stomach is shaped just like a Golden Spiral. Since the stomach structurally follows the pattern of the Golden Ratio, it stands to reason that it should functionally follow it as well. This would mean that the stomach is ideally meant to be no more than 62% full (and 38% empty) after a meal, for optimal digestive efficiency. Anything higher than 62% full will likely impede the healthy digestive process, in the same way an overloaded washing machine cannot properly wash clothes. The simplest way to assure you don't overeat at any meal is to use the finest meal portion measuring system ever invented: your hands. **It turns out that there is a close correlation between the size of your stomach and the volume of both of your hands when cupped together.**

So, regardless of your plate size, only fill your plate with about as much food as would fill about 2/3rds of your hands cupped together. The resulting portion will equal slightly less than 2/3 of the total volume of your stomach. If you eat in a relaxed manner, pause occasionally and chew well, you'll usually find this portion size amply satisfying. An all-too common challenge to healthy portion sizes and digestion is rushing our meals and eating amidst distraction or while multitasking, to the point where we've lost awareness of our body's natural satiety signaling system. Relaxed, mindful eating is a great way to reactivate this system and support healthy digestion. In her article *Eating in the Slow Lane* from the October 2004 issue of *Alternative Medicine Magazine*, **Judith S. Stern**, Vice President of the American Obesity Association, notes that it takes about 20 minutes for the mind to get the message that the stomach is full:

> *If you eat too fast you outpace your body's natural signaling system. Studies show that if you draw out the meal, build in pauses, and allow for satiety signals to come into play you will eat less.*

The Ancient Wisdom of Eating to Only About 2/3 Full

Caloric reduction—smaller, more modest meal portions—is naturally practiced by the Japanese people in Okinawa, who have a low amount of body fat (low body mass index or BMI) resulting from self-restraint in over-eating. Okinawans also have some of the lowest mortality rates in the world, presumably from their modest dietary portions along with a genetic predisposition for longevity. Their genetic predisposition may be inexorably interwoven with century-old lifestyle habits—especially the tendency to avoid overeating.

In his book *The Three Pillars of Zen*, author **Philip Kapleau** relates wisdom from 1300's Zen master Yasuntani, who recommended that Zen students eat only to about 2/3's full. We can upgrade the common 1/3 to 2/3 (rule of thirds) default to the more precise unifying ratio found in Nature, the Golden Ratio of 38% to 62%. The practice of caloric reduction, whether on laboratory rats or in everyday human life, appears to delay chronic diseases of aging and increase life expectancy.

So remember, **your stomach is about the size of both of your hands cupped together**—so only eat the amount of food that would fill them to about 2/3 full (Zen style), or about 62% full (Golden Ratio Zen style).

Φ

Golden Spiral-shaped stomach, at 62% or about 2/3rds full.

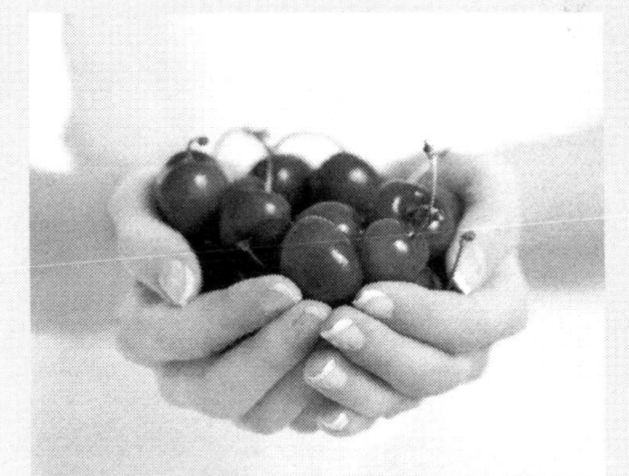

Cupping both hands together biomimics the natural, just under 2/3rds Golden Ratio meal capacity of your stomach. This easy guide supports optimal meal portions and healthy digestion.

Stern's point is well taken. However, the ideal objective is to sense our natural Golden Ratio satiety signal: not eating until you are 100% full, but eating no more than the Golden Pro*portion* of about 62% full. This profoundly redefines what "fullness" actually is. This profoundly redefines what "fullness" actually is. Biospherian Roy Walford, M.D. echoes the *doing more with less* principle when he said,

> *Optimal fullness equates to getting maximal nutrition with minimal calories.*

The message is simple: relax when eating. Enjoy your meals without distractions whenever possible. Don't drive, listen to the radio, watch television, surf the web or text/talk on your cellphone when eating. Learn to pay better attention to your body's natural signals to pause and put down the fork from time to time. Finally, always give yourself permission to stop eating—even if there's food left on your plate. This will rarely happen if you follow the twin Golden Ratio Portion Guidelines: 1. Only fill your plate to the Golden Pro*portion* (slightly less than 2/3 full) and, 2. Only eat at one meal as much as would fill both hands slightly less than 2/3 full when cupped together. You'll feel better and support your efforts to reach and maintain your optimal weight. At the same time you'll awaken your ability to eat—and live—within the optimal Golden Ratio Zone.

Cholesterol: It's ALL About the Ratio

Heart disease is the number one killer in modern times. To counter this trend, the American Heart Association recommends that you lower your LDL-C (LDL cholesterol) level to under 100 mg/dl. Yet by looking only at absolute, single values such as isolated LDL-C levels, the enormous predictive and therapeutic power of ratio is lost. These recommendations don't take into account whether a persons total cholesterol is 200 mg/dl or 300 mg/dl; the same sub-100 mg/dl LDL-C level is recommended. That being said, there are some ratios that are used by many physicians and labs, such as cholesterol/LDL-C, cholesterol/HDL-C, triglyceride/HDL-C and Apo B/Apo A-1. However, these ratios haven't been referenced to Nature's universal optimal design constant—the Golden Ratio. Nature has given us the gold standard by which to measure and optimize our physiology, so let's use it.

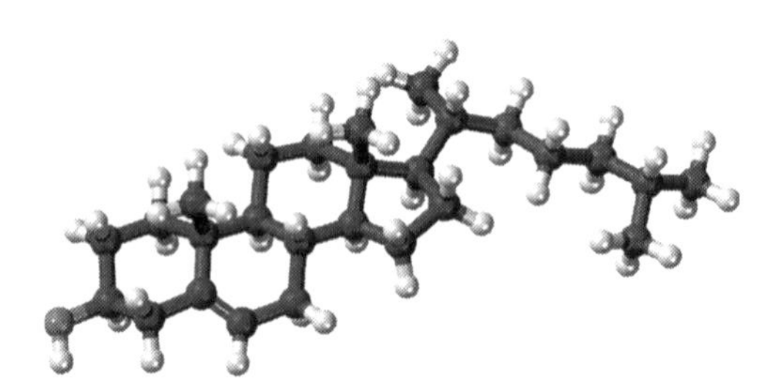

The much misunderstood cholesterol molecule. Cholesterol is a major and essential building block of our cell membranes as well as being the mother of all steroid hormones, including vitamin D, estrogen, testosterone, progesterone and cortisol.

The distribution of cholesterol throughout the body moves in two directions: from the liver to all cells and also in the reverse direction, from the cells back to the liver. The cholesterol pool in the liver is either formed into bile and released into the intestines, or repackaged and sent out to the body for another delivery. The water-insoluble cholesterol can't circulate by itself through the blood, so it's packaged into and transported inside of lipoproteins that are water-soluble, e.g., VLDL (very low density lipoprotein), IDL (intermediate density lipoprotein), LDL (low-density lipoprotein) and HDL (high-density lipoprotein). When these lipoprotein carriers are complexed with cholesterol, they're denoted as such by adding the letter C after the specific type, e.g., LDL-C, HDL-C. What we're looking for is the optimal ratio of the to-and-fro movement of cholesterol, such that cellular requirements are adequately supplied without too much cholesterol being distributed peripherally, congesting the arteries and fueling the atherosclerotic process. Using the Golden Ratio to evaluate basic cholesterol data gives you a yardstick to compare its subtypes. VLDL-C, IDL-C, LDL-C and HDL-C exist not only as independent entities, but as interactive particles embedded in a dynamic system. Philosopher **Stephen McIntosh's** description of the Golden Ratio and its dynamic unity function is applicable to the cholesterol family of lipoprotein subtypes:

The Golden Ratio relationship is an expression of unity—a unity pattern—because each part is defined completely by its relation to the whole.

Below are two line diagrams showing the essential Golden Ratio unity pattern. The first line diagram shows total cholesterol in relation to its largest subfraction, LDL-C. The second line diagram shows the largest cholesterol subfraction, LDL-C, in relation to the remaining smaller cholesterol subfractions. Only when the parts are in Golden Ratio divisions to one another does perfect integration with respect to the to-and-fro movement of cholesterol occur.

- Total Cholesterol is to LDL-C...the whole to the largest part as...
  LDL-C is to (VLDL-C + IDL-C + HDL-C)...the largest part to the smaller parts
- Φ denotes Golden Ratio division (optimal balance) between large & small part(s).

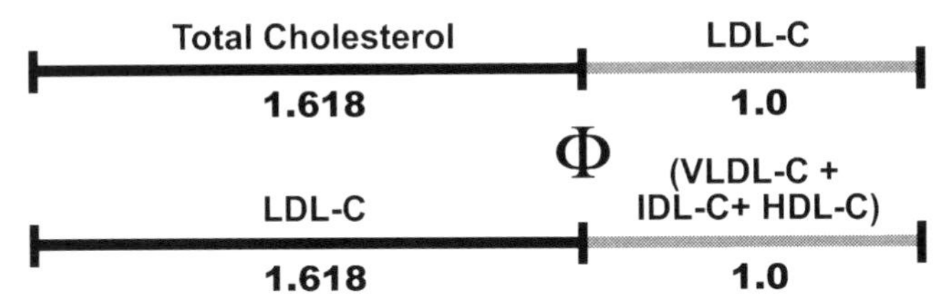

Optimal cholesterol ratio. Your body's cholesterol ratios ideally should be in the Golden Φ Ratio range of 1.618:1. The large section of the line is in ratio to the small section as the whole line is in ratio to the large section. When the ratio of total cholesterol to LDL ratio is in Golden Ratio, greater health is a natural result.

Through anecdotal clinical observation of numerous lab reports, it became evident to the authors that the total cholesterol/LDL-C ratio approximated 1.62:1 in an unusual number of healthy subjects. **The Golden Ratio is indicative of a system in optimal balance**, e.g., with just the right amount of cholesterol in the right parts of the body. This observation warrants serious study in the future, since it is a paradigm shift in viewing how the body's intelligence organizes organic processes in line with the optimal design constant that is the Golden Ratio. A cholesterol/LDL-C ratio in the Golden Ratio range of 1.62:1 may promote the ideal balance of cholesterol transport in *both* directions:

From the Liver ➔ Cells **From the Cells ➔ Liver**

In the state of Golden Ratio cholesterol balance, arteries remain clear and hormones and cell membranes have adequate cholesterol to satisfy the various cellular functions. Cholesterol dietary intake and bile/bowel excretion are additional modulating factors that can influence overall cholesterol balance towards Golden Ratio proportions. Although the Golden Ratio proposition of cholesterol balance is theoretical at this point, our aim is to have it thoroughly studied and evaluated in the near future.

Cholesterol: The Demonized Molecule That's *Essential* For Life

Sorely maligned by mainstream medicine for the last 50 years, cholesterol is in reality one of Nature's foundational requirements for life and health. The truth is, without cholesterol we'd be dead. With current abnormally low LDL-C recommendations (less than 100 mg/dl), cells lack one of their basic building blocks—cholesterol. In addition:

- Φ Cholesterol is vital for the synthesis of *all* steroid hormones, e.g., the sex and adrenal hormones—**testosterone, estrogen** and progesterone, cortisol and aldosterone, etc. Sexual dysfunction is a predictable result of inadequate cholesterol as well as adrenal related problems including hypoglycemia and decreased stress resistance.
- Φ The brain is especially dependent on cholesterol, as 25% of the body's cholesterol is located in the brain and spinal cord, where it's used for cell membrane and myelin sheath formation (myelin is a vital electrical insulator that speeds nerve conduction). Depression, memory loss, dementia and suicide are associated with low cholesterol levels in the central nervous system.
- Φ Vitamin D is also dependent on cholesterol for its synthesis and when a cholesterol deficiency exists, even sun bathing can't produce vitamin D.
- Φ Over time, a lack of cholesterol results in intestinal malabsorption and vitamin deficiency problems, since cholesterol dependent bile salts are needed to absorb fats and fat-soluble vitamins (A, D, E and K).

Low cholesterol-related conditions are commonly overlooked by practitioners who have an aggressive, misplaced obsession with extremely low LDL-C levels. **The beauty of referencing cholesterol levels to the Golden Ratio is that it's the perfect way of finding that optimal balance where just the right amount of cholesterol is available for cellular processes, yet not too much that would favor the atherosclerotic process.** When high total cholesterol levels occur, it's usually because the body is trying to produce more cholesterol dependent hormones/membranes/bile, etc. Of importance isn't the absolute level of total cholesterol or LDL-C, but whether or not the total cholesterol to LDL-C is in Golden Ratio.

Golden Ratio cholesterol balance is only one of many other factors involved in the atherosclerosis process that should also be addressed. These include particle size and number, apolipoprotein ratios as well as the many biochemical processes such as cholesterol oxidation, inflammation and glycation. Nevertheless, balancing basic cholesterol ratios according to the Golden Ratio is a wise first step on the journey to health and longevity. The grand overlying principle—the Golden Ratio—guides not only the formation of spiral galaxies in the heavens and DNA spirals at the molecular level, but everything in between—including healthy cholesterol lipoprotein distributions (See Ch 4 Nutrition Rx's to see if your cholesterol/LDL-C is in Golden Ratio).

Absorbing NSN From Your Five Senses

All human senses, including hearing, touch, taste, vision, smell
and pain receptors, have not only spiral physiology, but also response
curves that are logarithmic (having a Fibonacci structure).

Frederick A. Hottes, M.D., anatomic & clinical pathologist

As shown throughout this book, our bodies are designed in form and function according to the Golden Ratio; even our senses reflect this principle of peak efficiency and performance. However, we don't often consider that everything we see, hear, touch, smell and taste also has nutrient potential. Like air, water and sleep, each of our five senses can be classified as a MegaNutrient, that class of vital sustenance consumable in very large amounts, although sometimes difficult to quantify. For example, it's hard to say that we consumed a certain number of grams of beauty on a walk through a forest or ample units of healthy touch in a day. Nevertheless, **we're being continually nourished—or not—by the multisensory inputs from our**

environment. What is overlooked is that our multi-faceted sensory input should be considered absolutely essential nutrients, as explored in the provocative section ahead.

Touch: Our Primal Sensory Nutrient

Touch is a great example of vital sensory nutrition, being the first sense to develop in humans. Yet touch is not traditionally considered a "nutrient"—even though newborn babies can die when touch deprived—or survive, grow and thrive when touch is provided in adequate amounts. Touch malnutrition at *any* age is implicated in a wide array of physical, psychological and social health conditions. A 1997 *Life* magazine article, *The Magic of Touch*, by George Colt explored touch's vital role in human health:

> *...we instinctively know that touch is a primal need, as necessary for growth as food, clothing or shelter. Michelangelo knew this: when he painted God extending a hand toward Adam on the ceiling of the Sistine Chapel, he chose touch to depict the gift of life. From the nuzzles and caresses between mother and infant that form the foundation of the self, to the holding of hands between a son and his dying father that allows a final letting go, touch is our most intimate and powerful form of communication.*

Tactile & Visual Synergy: Michelangelo's 500 Year-old Secret

Michelangelo's painting *Creation of Adam* is stunning to anyone who's been to the Sistine Chapel in Rome. Even looking at pictures of the spectacular church ceiling boggles the mind. Our simple Golden Ratio analysis reveals an amazing find. The exact point where God's and Adam's fingers touch is the Golden Ratio point formed between "God's brain" and Adam's body. This simple measurement confirms the fact that Michelangelo used the Golden Ratio in his work. But that's just the surface of the secret. For 500 years, everyone took the section of God bestowing life to Adam at face biblical value—until 1990, when **Frank Meshberger, M.D.**, through his deeper sense of sight/insight, saw something even more incredible. The ellipsoid shape in which God rests actually bears an uncanny resemblance to a *human brain*, complete with amazingly accurate anatomic detail. Compare Michelangelo's painting overlaid with an anatomic drawing of a human brain below. You can clearly see the unmistakable resemblance of the brain's prominent lobes, complete with an emerging spinal cord—all artistically embedded in the masterpiece. Dr. Meshberger didn't just look at the artwork on the surface, he really saw with his depth of vision what Michelangelo had embedded in his painting in plain sight. Why was Michelangelo so secretive in his depictions? As it turns out, like his contemporary and rival Leonardo da Vinci, he had a clear ulterior motive. Since the Catholic Church

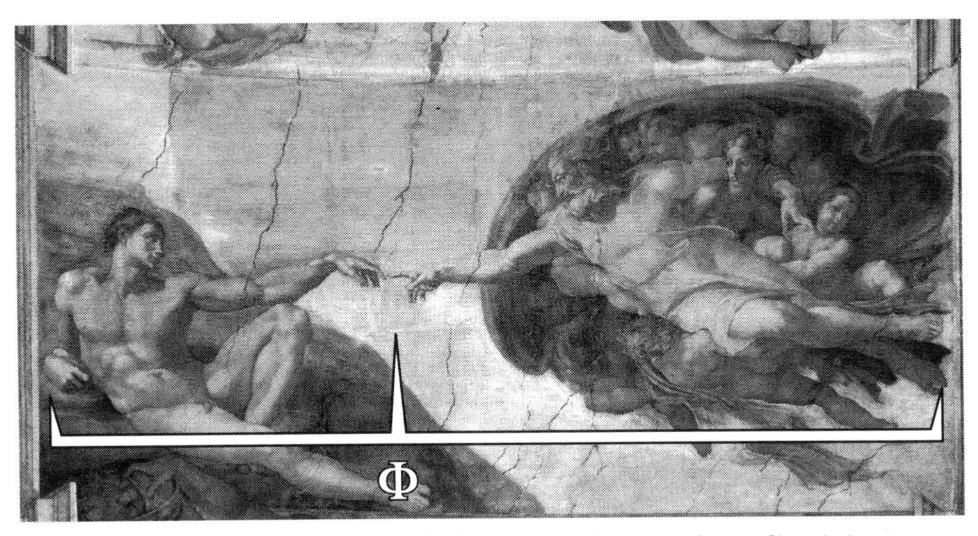

Michelangelo's *Creation of Adam* (1512), from the ceiling of the Sistine Chapel, showing God giving Adam the "Touch of Life" at the precise 38/62 Golden Ratio point between them.

forbade grave robbing and dissection of cadavers, Michelangelo had to hide his anatomical discoveries to avoid persecution or even death. The simplest and most ingenious way to document his discoveries was to secretly embed the information within his paintings. Luckily for him and for us, the Church never found out. Our sense of sight allows us to perceive Michelangelo's mastery, while we also appreciate the vital sense of touch that's highlighted by God touching Adam and bestowing the evolutionary power of conscious thought which elevated him to human level. This synergy only comes together in a once-in-a-millennial masterpiece. These secrets lay dormant for 500 years—until Dr. Meshberger had the depth of vision to see what had literally been right in front of everyone for centuries. Likewise, we can enliven all of our 5 Senses by simply *slowing down and committing to see, hear, smell, feel and taste with more presence in the moment.*

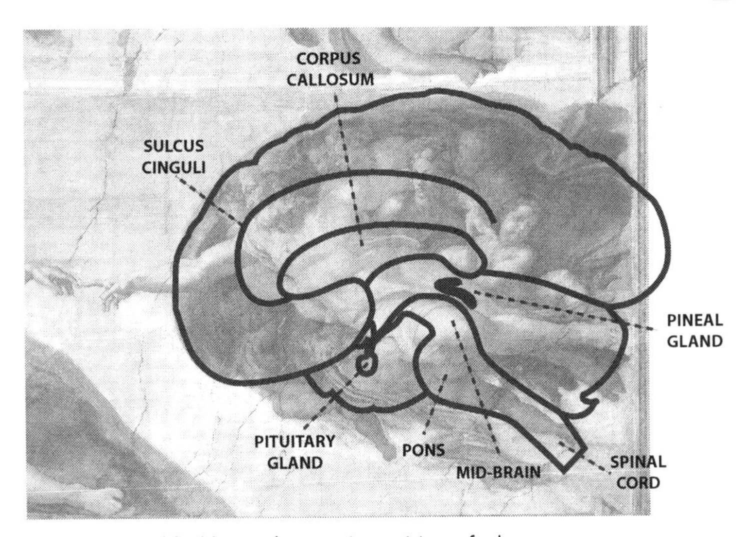

Dr. Meshberger's superimposition of a human brain over Michelangelo's *Creation of Adam.*

As **William Osler, M.D.** said:

> *Use your five senses. Learn to see, learn to hear, learn to feel, learn to smell, and know that by practice alone you can become expert.*

> *Feelings aroused by the touch of someone's hand, the sound of music, the smell of a flower, a beautiful sunset, a work of art, love, laughter, hope and faith—all work on both the unconscious and the conscious aspects of the self, and they have physiological consequences as well.*
> **Bernie Siegel, M.D., author of *Love, Medicine & Miracles***

4

The Sensory Synergy of Food

Whether your sensory input is nutritious or more of a toxic burden to your system, you can improve the quality of your sensory diet by shifting your sensory exposure to as many Nature-based frequencies and input sources as possible. By natural default, we would thus be consuming Golden Ratio-designed substances and frequencies and therefore more NSN. Spending time in Nature is the easiest way to absorb the panoply of life-enhancing sounds, sights, smells, textures and tastes. More often than not, sensory input isn't through a single sense, it's from a combination or symphony of sensations.

Your senses of taste, touch, smell, sight and sound blend together in a broad palette of choices available in your food and menu selections. We all know the pleasure that comes from a colorful, tasty, aromatic and nutritious meal prepared with an artist's touch. The sensory benefits are in addition to the multiple nutritional benefits received from consciously prepared, healthy organic food. Golden Ratio aficionado Dr. Mehmet Oz highlights the synergy of food's visual and nutritional aspects:

> *Foods with bright, rich colors are packed with flavonoids and carotenoids, powerful compounds that bind with damaging free radicals in your body, lowering inflammation. Eat nine fistfuls of colorful fruits and vegetables each day and you'll reap the benefits without having to give up other foods. Whenever I shop in the produce aisle, I'm reminded that these foods are often more powerful than the drugs sold in pharmacies.*

Sensing the Rose's Beauty & Aroma

Just as in the example of tasty, rainbow colored foods, it's common to have multiple senses blending together in a magical synergy of amplified delight, which nourishes the soul. One of the most spectacular blending of the senses of sight and smell is in

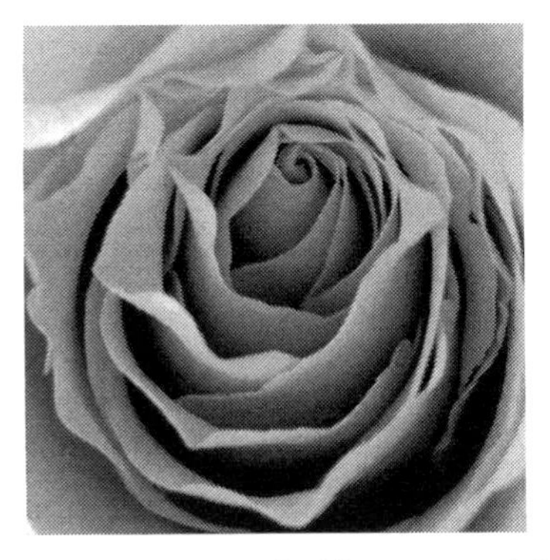
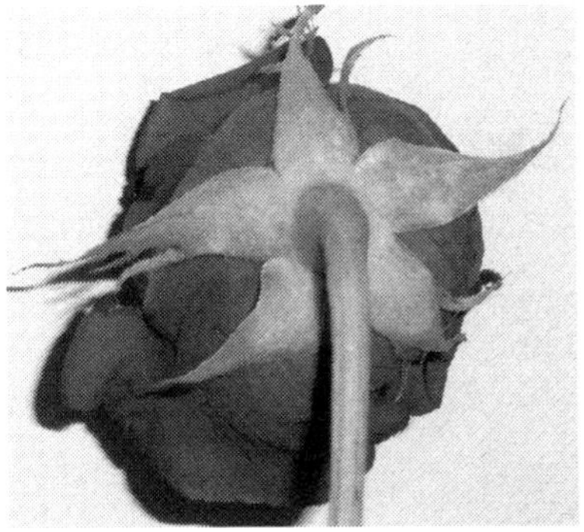

Every rose contains a double imprint of the Golden Ratio, hidden in plain sight: petals embedded in Golden Spirals on the front and a five-pointed Golden Star on the back.

the beautiful and aromatic rose. At first glance, most just see the basic shape, color, petals, stem, leaves and thorns. Yet if we look deeper, with a relaxed eye for patterns, we clearly see the universal imprint of the Golden Ratio. Multiple, elegant Golden Spirals are formed by the petals in the face of every rose. Turning the rose around, we can see the Golden Star pentagram, formed by the leaves on the backside of the rose. While the amazing scent of the rose is virtually impossible to quantify, many people would no doubt name the rose as the archetype of lovely aromas. If we were to measure a rose's key aromatic attributes with precision, it's reasonable to expect that they would reflect Golden Ratio proportions.

We can see that nutrition is a multifaceted, multidimensional source of NSN, free for the taking if the secret nourishment factor of the Golden Ratio is consumed like one's daily bread. As Hippocrates, the father of medicine might have said:

Let NSN be thy medicine and the Golden Ratio be thy food.

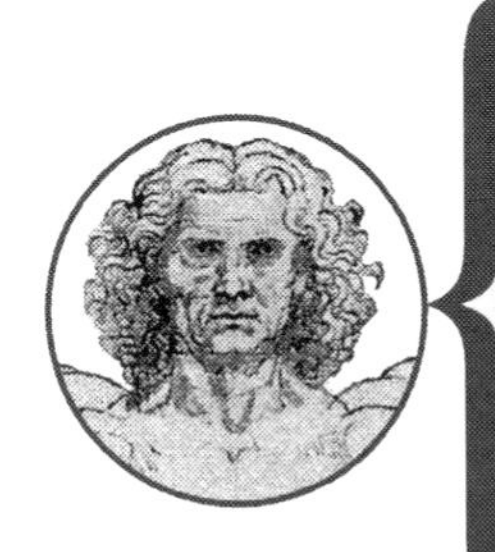

Remember, you're only as well ***NOURISHED*** *as your last healthy* ***Meal.*** So eat in the Golden Ratio Zone: 40% carbs, 30% protein and 30% fats. Use organic, fresh, unprocessed, non-GMO food and integrate nutrient-dense Superfoods into your diet to boost total nutrition. Eat only to a little less than 2/3 full: a Golden Ratio ProPORTION. Prepare and enjoy your food with presence, relaxation and gratitude.

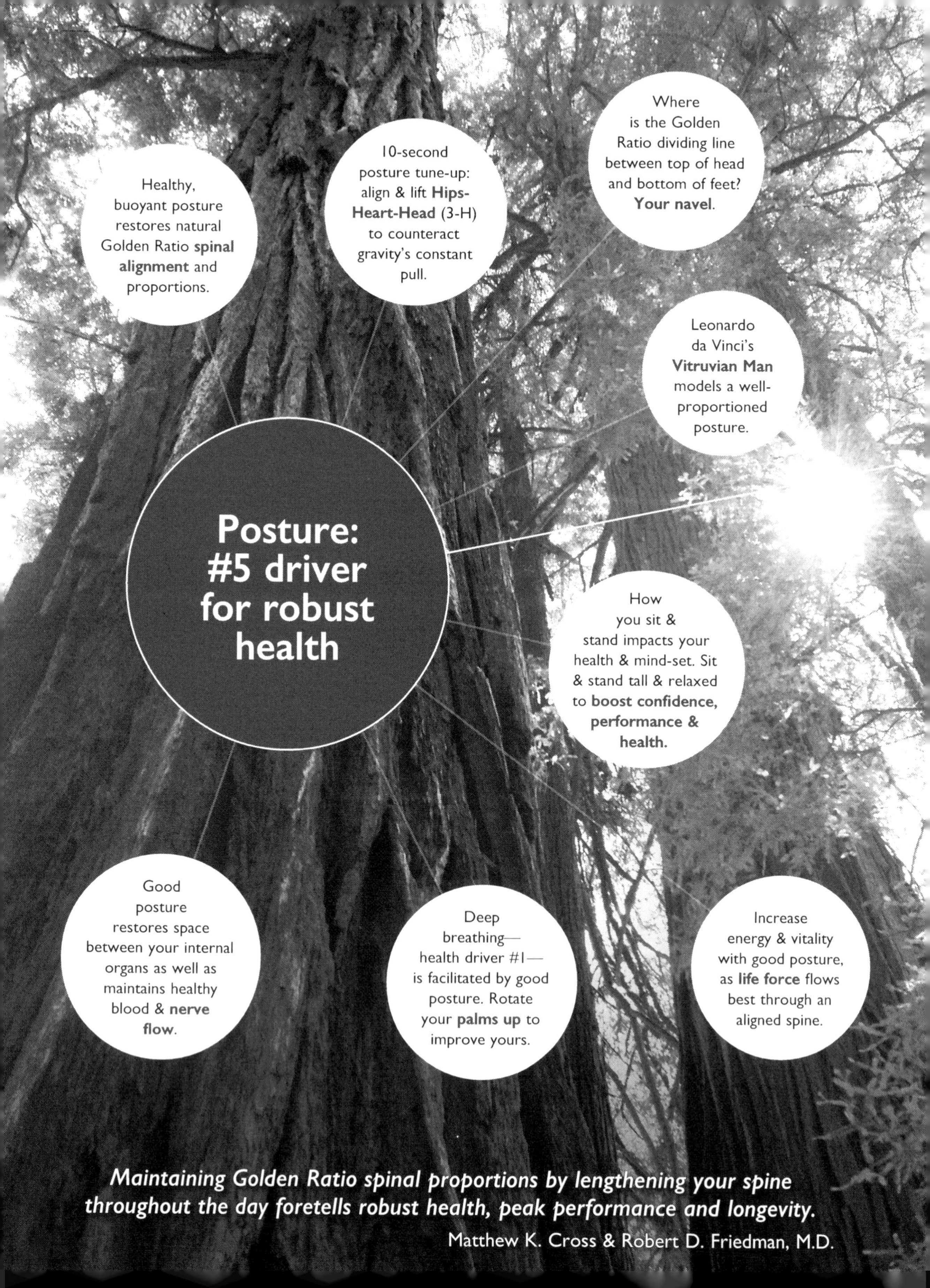

Posture: #5 driver for robust health

Healthy, buoyant posture restores natural Golden Ratio **spinal alignment** and proportions.

10-second posture tune-up: align & lift **Hips-Heart-Head** (3-H) to counteract gravity's constant pull.

Where is the Golden Ratio dividing line between top of head and bottom of feet? **Your navel**.

Leonardo da Vinci's **Vitruvian Man** models a well-proportioned posture.

How you sit & stand impacts your health & mind-set. Sit & stand tall & relaxed to **boost confidence, performance & health.**

Good posture restores space between your internal organs as well as maintains healthy blood & **nerve flow**.

Deep breathing—health driver #1—is facilitated by good posture. Rotate your **palms up** to improve yours.

Increase energy & vitality with good posture, as **life force** flows best through an aligned spine.

Maintaining Golden Ratio spinal proportions by lengthening your spine throughout the day foretells robust health, peak performance and longevity.

Matthew K. Cross & Robert D. Friedman, M.D.

5

Posture

A good stance and posture reflect a proper state of mind.

Morihei Ueishiba, founder of Aikido

Golden Ratio Spinal Dynamics

The beautiful and curvaceous human spine is an engineering marvel, in both form and function. The Golden Ratio-encoded gentle S-curve of the human spine is the result of evolution's continual improvement and adaptation, as our species gained upright posture. The awareness and maintenance of an optimal spinal S-curve allows us to efficiently harmonize with gravity, instead of working against it. Only through regaining awareness of what our ideal relationship is to gravity can we begin to restore and sustain good posture. It's unlikely that a fish ever considers the fact that it's wet. Similarly, we live and move under the influence of a gravitational field that has become so second nature we forget that it even exists. Yet the sense of gravity that has become mostly unconscious still exerts its constant downward force upon us, 24/7. This relentless force field eventually takes its toll on our posture if we're not aware of its constant presence. Posture is that counterbalancing force that allows us to stand upright within gravity's field. If we have healthy posture there's no problem, but for most people this isn't the case. The ideal Golden Ratio Spinal Curve is possible when the cervical, thoracic and lumbar regions

Head Over Heels for the Golden Ratio

The human skull and spine are engineering marvels, fusions of Golden Ratio design in form and function. This dynamic Golden Ratio synergy endows us with extraordinary postural alignment, optimal strength, protection, flexibility and endless variety in movement. In the spine the Ratio is seen between the 5 vertebral structural divisions when healthy posture is present. This ensures that the navel naturally rides at or near the body's vertical Golden Ratio division point from head to toe.

Golden Ratio spinal alignment also supports optimal breathing, circulation, nerve function and adequate space for healthy organ function in the chest and abdomen. Drs. R. J. Tamargo and J. A. Pindrik have discovered Golden Ratio relationships between the skull's cranial bones. This compliments our finding of the brain's enfolded Golden Spiral shape and corresponding delta/theta/beta/alpha brain waves in Golden Ratio. At all scales the brain's master form and function GR code is apparent and astonishing.

Bregma
Nasion
Inion
Cervical
Thoracic
Navel
Lumbar
Sacral
Coccygeal

5

Golden Ratio Skull Landmarks

Inion External occipital protuberance; bump at base of skull.
Bregma Φ Junction of sagittal & coronal sutures; top of skull.
Nasion Junction of frontal (forehead) & nasal bones.

Posture Check ✔: Your spine is naturally meant to form a gentle S-curve. Sit and stand tall, lifted and relaxed, with ankles, knees, hips, shoulders and ears aligned like the example at right.

have an ideal amount of curve—not too curved and not too straight—just right. Golden Ratio relationships between vertebrae enable optimal strength and flexibility as well as the ability to maintain effortless, upright posture within the gravitational field. Any out-of-ratio posture inevitably gives rise to disc and nerve compression, degenerative arthritis, restricted motion and accompanying back pain; physiologically, impeded breathing and compromised organ function result in decreased energy and poor performance. **You know when you have a Golden Ratio Spinal Curve because your head will be perfectly aligned over your hips, knees and ankles and you'll move more effortlessly through the gravitational field.** Adequate Hydration (chapter 2) also plays a hidden yet vital role in healthy posture, by maintaining the suppleness and integrity of the intervertebral discs; it's no accident that fallen leaves curl up in a reverse Golden Spiral as they dehydrate—the fate of far too many dehydrated, aging spines.

Your Natural Golden Φ Ratio Body Symmetry

Structurally and functionally all the bones in your body—arms, legs, fingers and toes—closely approximate the Golden Ratio in their relationships to one another. Your skull and pelvic bones reflect the Golden Ratio, as does the gentle wave curve of your

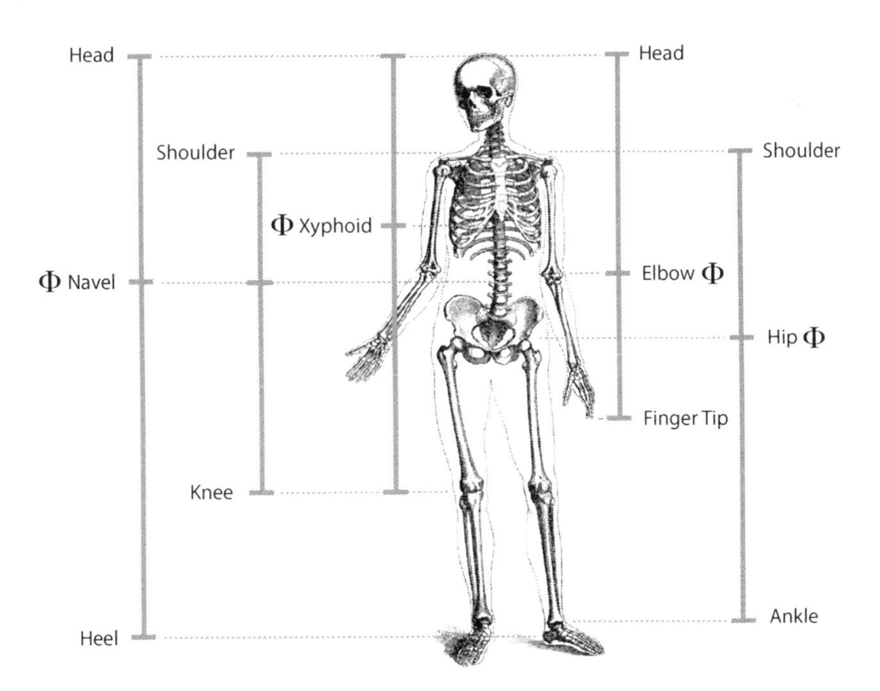

Some classic structural Golden Φ Ratios in the human body.
Individual variants dance around the ideal Golden Ratio.

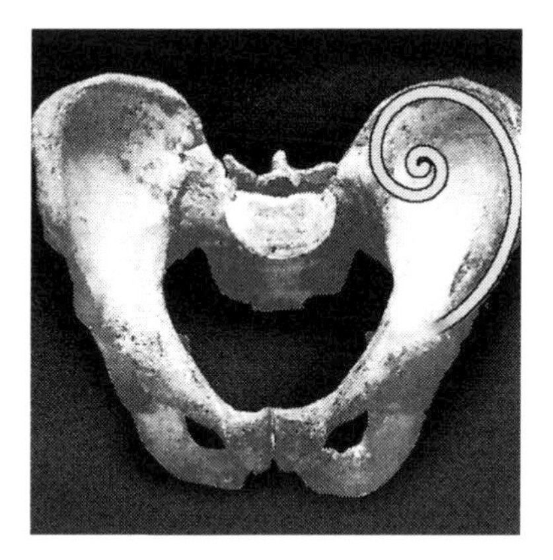
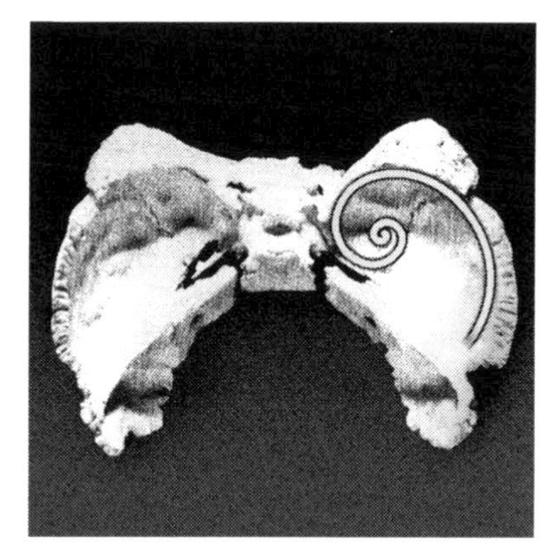

(*L*) Pelvis, (*R*) Temporal and sphenoid bones of the skull; all with Golden Spiral structure.

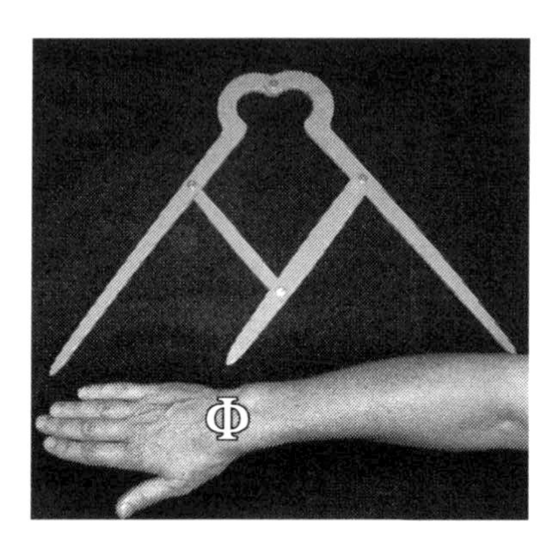

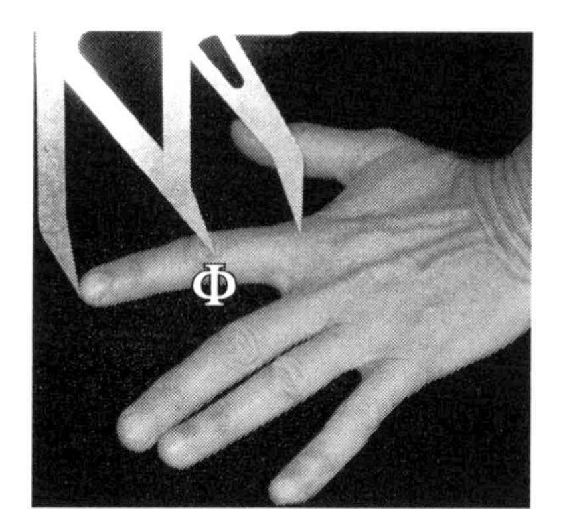

Man is the Measure of All Things – Protagoras. All parts of your body reflect the Golden Ratio at every scale, in endless variety.

spine. As a general tendency, the ratio of the distance from your navel to your feet compared to your navel to the top of your head approximates the Golden Ratio. All of the parts of your body, indeed your entire body—bones, muscles, tendons, ligaments and organs—exhibit the Golden Ratio, in endless manifestations of the universal design principle we all reflect.

> *Phidias, the Greek sculptor, revealed the Golden Ratio in his work—for example, in such proportions as the relation of the width of the head to the width of the throat, the width of the forearm to the wrist, the width of the calf to the ankle, and so on.*
>
> **James Wyckoff, author of *Pyramid Energy***

Whenever you discover an expression of the Golden Ratio in anything, you can be sure it's also embedded at both micro and macro levels. For example, each bone in your finger is in Golden Ratio to the adjacent bones in that finger. And the length of that finger is in Golden Ratio to the length of your hand. As the length of your hand is in Golden Ratio to the length of your forearm, it should come as no surprise that the length of your arm is in Golden Ratio to the length of your entire body... and so on. Another fascinating manifestation of the Golden Ratio in our bodies is in the actual shape of some of our bones. For example, you can clearly see the shape of the Golden Spiral in the pelvic, temporal and sphenoid bones. The cervical, thoracic and lumbar vertebrae exhibit a smooth transition in size that reflects the Golden Ratio. When you curl your hand into a fist, it naturally takes the shape of the Golden Spiral.

> *Man is all symmetry, full of proportions, one limb to another, and all to all the world besides. Each part may call the farthest brother, for head with foot hath private amity, and both with moons and tides.*
>
> **George Herbert, English priest & poet**

The anatomical Golden Ratio points of the body's length are in dynamic flux during human development, from our beginnings as a Golden Spiral-shaped embryo to full-grown adulthood. In infants, the Golden Ratio points are at the level of the heart or at the genitals, depending upon which direction (head or feet) one measures from.

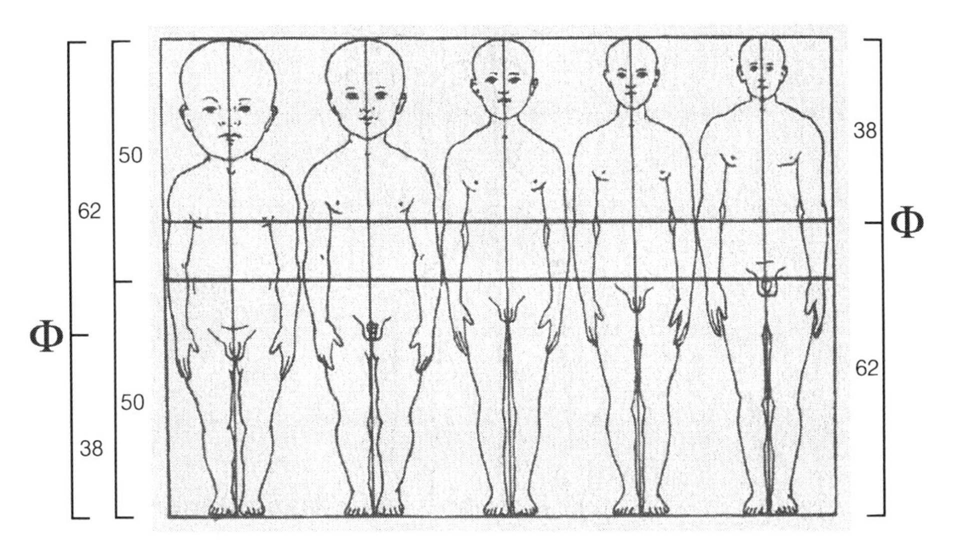

Dynamic flux of the Golden Ratio points of the human body, from infant to adult. The navel's position changes from the 50:50 point in the infant to the 38:62 Golden Ratio point in the adult, while the position of the genitals changes from 38:62 in the infant to 50:50 in the adult (not to mention that fact that the reproductive systems in both sexes, from testes to ovaries and beyond, exhibit Golden Spiral design).

As the body grows and develops, the Golden Ratio point is seen to shift to the level of the navel in the adult. Actual navel measurements are not always exactly at the 0.618 ratio point and can vary within individuals according to Fibonacci Sequence ratios. Since there are always variations in human proportions, some people's navels will be at the 0.618 cut point whereas others may be slightly off. For example, some people may have a 2/3 (0.66), a 3/5 (0.6) or a 5/8 (0.625) ratio. This variability is known as dancing around the Golden Ratio.

Golden Ratio Postural Alignment

The prime Golden Ratio division of your body in the vertical plane is at the level of the navel. This ideal upper body-to-lower body ratio is important to maintain throughout life. The most common cause of loss of Divine Proportion in our stature is due to poor postural habits. *Slumping posture and rounded shoulders result in a loss of vertical height in your spine.* Your spine's natural, gentle S-shaped curve can become deformed with an accentuation or loss of curvature in the cervical, thoracic or lumbar regions. Poor postural habits are commonly seen and become fixed in the way that many people sit at their desks or computers, or work on their smartphones or tablets when standing.

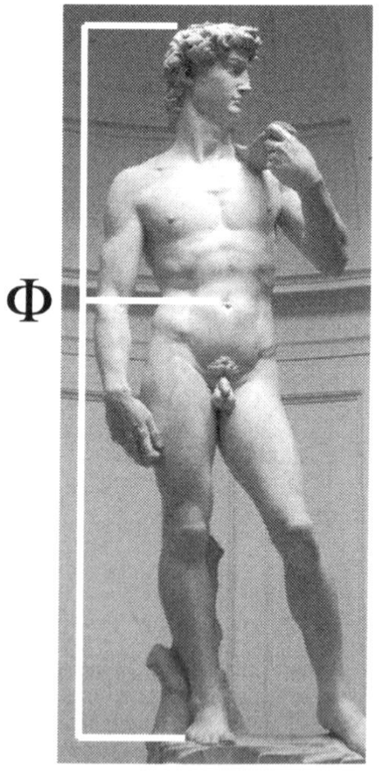

Michelangelo's *David*, the archetype of Golden Ratio body symmetry.

Over time, the slumping position becomes integrated into permanent posture with tight muscles pulling the spine, shoulders, arms, legs and pelvis out of natural alignment. This results in an avalanche of undesirable domino effects. In addition to harmful wear on your vertebral discs and spine as a whole, internal organs have less space in which to move and their healthy physiological function is inhibited. Blood flow is decreased in compromised areas and headaches, tight shoulders and sore back muscles are some of the more obvious symptoms. Poor digestion and elimination are also common symptoms when internal organs are cramped. When poor postural habits combine with the aging process and hormonal decline, osteoporosis may result. Osteoporosis further accentuates loss of height in the spine, due to vertebral collapse and increased curvature of the spine. This process only worsens the deviation from the Golden Proportion between the upper and lower body. The further from Golden Proportion your posture becomes, the less efficient is your mobility and physiological functioning. Loss of natural Golden

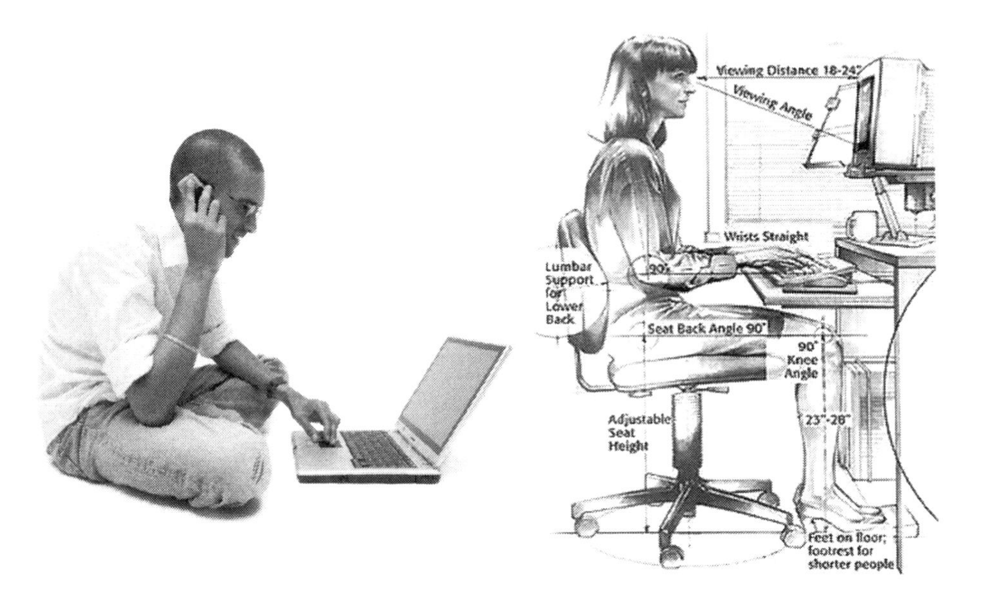

(*L*) This all-too-common hunched-over position pulls one out of healthy postural alignment.
(*R*) Ergonomically correct desk posture for sitting. While good sitting posture is important, a growing body of research reveals that sitting for too long poses serious additional dangers to health and longevity. See the Ch 5 Posture Rx section for targeted posture improvement suggestions.

Posture's Cascade Effect on Health & Longevity

Your posture initiates the following continuous causal chain:

Poor posture	**Good posture**
↓	↓
Rounded shoulders	Open shoulders
↓	↓
Lung compression	Lung expansion
↓	↓
Hypoventilation (restricted breathing)	Healthy ventilation (deep, full breathing)
↓	↓
Decreased Vital Lung Capacity	Increased Vital Lung Capacity
↓	↓
Decreased vitality, mental acuity & sexual potency	Increased vitality, mental acuity & sexual potency
↓	↓
Decreased life expectancy	Increased life expectancy

Golden Posture: Direct Link to Confidence & Performance

Good posture not only projects a favorable image to others, it also self-reflects, giving you more confidence in your own thoughts. In a study on the link between posture and attitude, people who were told to sit up straight were more likely to believe thoughts they wrote down about their qualifications for a job. Yet those who were slumped over their desks were less likely to accept these written-down feelings about their qualifications. According to **Richard Petty**, co-author of the study and professor of psychology at Ohio State University:

> *Most of us were taught that sitting up straight gives a good impression to other people... but it turns out that our posture can also affect how we think about ourselves. If you sit or stand up straight, you end up convincing yourself by the posture you're in... sitting up straight is something you can train yourself to do, and it has psychological benefits... people assume their confidence is coming from their own thoughts.* ***They don't realize their posture is affecting how much they believe in what they're thinking...***

This study reveals intriguing insight into the body-mind connection of healthy posture, and as we have seen, better posture is always more reflective of Golden Proportion in both form and function.

Proportions in how you carry yourself has a powerful butterfly effect on your entire state of health, and thus your *quality*—and *quantity*—of life. As with anything we wish to upgrade, restoring postural Golden Proportions first requires awareness of its vital importance. Greater health and longevity are directly connected to this simple awareness and practice. Some easy ways to do this are to get in the habit of regular ***posture check-ins*** regarding how you're sitting, standing or moving in any moment. Pay special attention to the position of your pelvis, which is the critical First 15% of healthy spinal alignment, along with the placement of your feet when sitting and standing.

For example, **how are you sitting as you read these words right now?** Is your spine upright and flexible, with your head gently "floating" on top of your neck? Are your breaths full and deep? If not, gently correct whatever feels *out of proportion* in your body right now. Therapies that reverse the daily stresses on the spine are an excellent daily practice. Any regular, balanced exercise regimen which invites you to expand

WARNING: Years of poor postural habits, osteoporosis and dehydrated discs result in back pain, loss of height and poor overall health and energy.

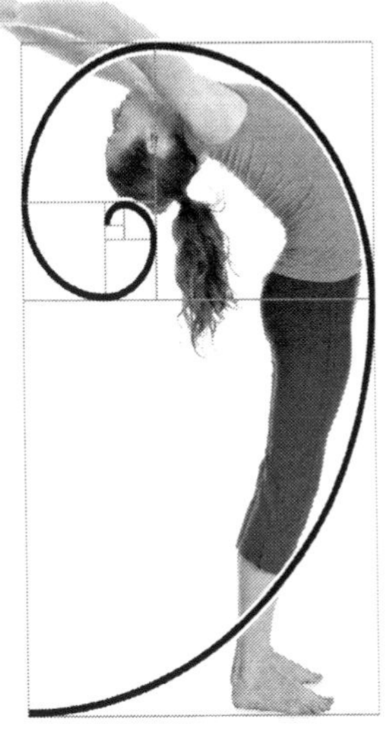
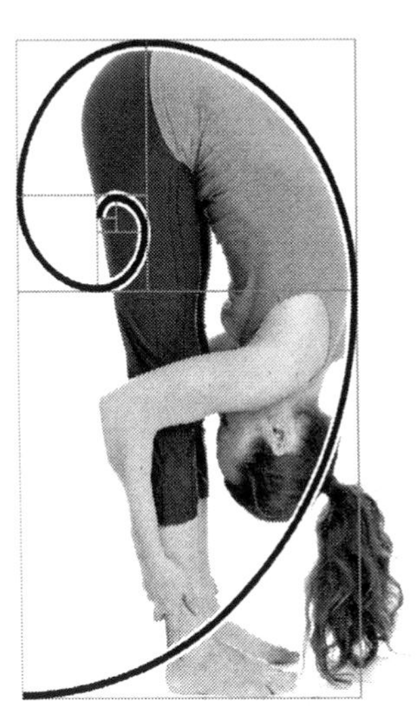

Gentle Golden Ratio Spiral flexion/extension poses can help reverse the effects of gravity and poor postural habits. When combined with ample hydration, exercise and the NSN health drivers, they help support maximum height and healthy, buoyant posture for a lifetime.

your body's range, e.g., yoga, Pilates, dance, Bob Cooley's Resistance Stretching®, etc., are essential to regaining and maintaining proper spinal dynamics and good posture. In addition, Core Strength Training builds a strong foundation for healthy posture, prevents osteoporosis and counters the effects of aging. Gravity inversion devices such as the DEX-II (See Ch 5 Posture Rx section) are also an effective way to gently traction your spine and relieve pressure on intervertebral discs. Make sure that your nutritional status is optimal, paying special attention to your hydration and mineral intake. Consult with your doctor to explore if bioidentical hormonal therapy may be of value for you in preventing/reversing osteoporosis, if this is an issue for you. As Thomas Edison said,

> *The doctor of the future will give no medicine, but will interest his patients in the care of the human frame, in diet and in the causes and prevention of disease.*

The Golden Ratio Power Pose

As Morihei Ueishiba, founder of the peaceful martial art of Aikido, observed: *a good stance and posture reflect a proper state of mind.* This sage insight reflects a *top down* approach—the state of mind being the *driver* which results in good stance and posture. This is a *Mind–Body* approach. Conversely, Harvard psychologist **Amy Cuddy, Ph.D.**,

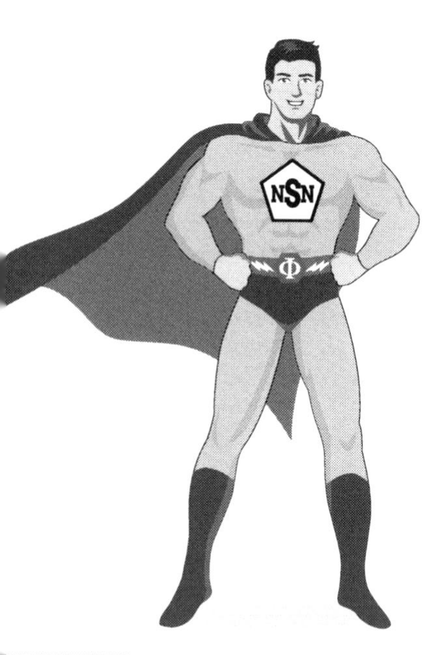

author of *Presence: Bringing Your Boldest Self to Your Biggest Challenges*, has demonstrated in her work that *a proper state of mind reflects a good stance and posture.* Dr. Cuddy's research reflects a *bottom up* approach—good stance and posture are the *drivers* that cause a proper state of mind. This is a *Body–Mind* approach.

Dr. Cuddy's research focuses on the science of *Power Posing*, where expansive, confident postures are held for 1-3 minutes, such as those typically modeled by superheroes like Wonder Woman, Batman, Superman, NSN Man and when your hands are thrust high over your head in the classic "V" for Victory pose. She found that there were powerful positive downstream effects of such poses in subject's cognitive, emotional and behavioral areas, especially in dramatically increased self-confidence. The physiological effects were also impressive, with power poses resulting in ***increased*** testosterone (power/confidence hormone) saliva levels of up to 20% and ***decreased*** cortisol (stress/anxiety hormone) levels up to 25%. With something as easy as changing physical posture, anyone can send immediate, strong subconscious signals to themselves that result in increased confidence/performance for any upcoming situations requiring enhanced self-assurance, performance and power, e.g., public speaking, job interviews—any situations where a Superhero-like mind-set andpresence would result in a favorable outcome.

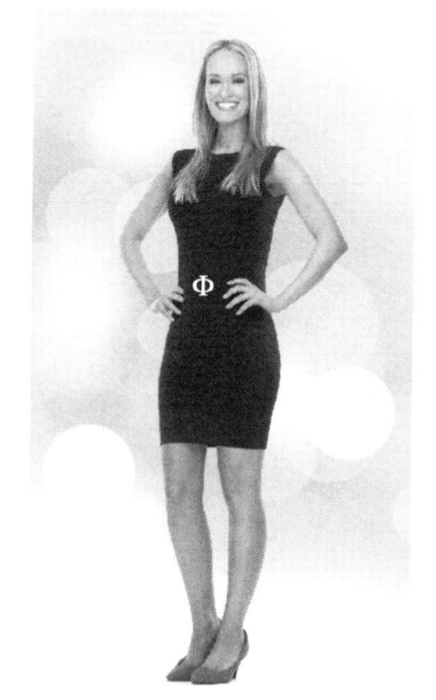

A Golden Ratio secret hidden-in-plain sight of standing in superhero Power Poses is that your hands are resting at and pointing directly to your navel region—which is the main Golden Ratio division or Power Point of your whole body. The Golden Ratio division point of your body—your navel region—is a most powerful first 15% starting point for building core strength, posture and balance. It's no coincidence that the martial arts place such a strong emphasis on this region known as the *hara*, which is slightly below the navel. In addition, the solar plexus, the 2nd largest nerve center in your body, known as the *second brain*, is slightly above the navel. This core postural/neural/

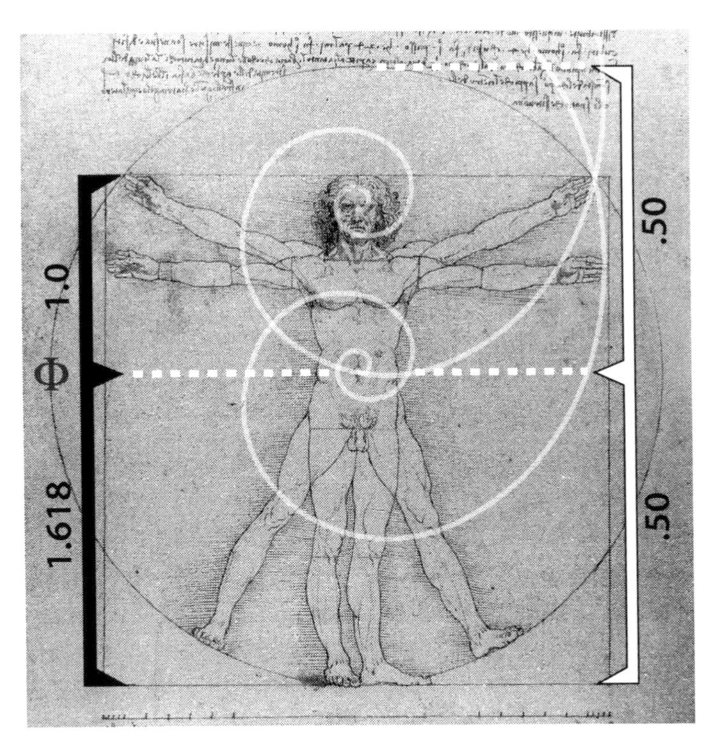

Da Vinci's *Vitruvian Man*, showing the Golden Ratio, 1.618:1, the height of *Vitruvian Man* (the square) as well as the 50:50 measurement of the encompassing circle. Both measurements meet at the navel—Da Vinci's way of showing how the human being contains the secret of the ages, depicted as the *Squaring of the Circle*. When posture is properly aligned, you more efficiently access and increase Nature's Secret Nutrient/NSN throughout your whole body.

gravitational matrix that surrounds your navel—above, below, sides and back—also strengthens your balance, poise and focus. This translates into strengthening the same qualities in your mind, emotions and spirit as well. An alternate Golden Ratio Power Pose is elegantly demonstrated by the *Vitruvian Man* (which Cuddy calls the "Starfish pose"). Leonardo da Vinci positioned V-Man in a most expansive, robust and inspiring pose which has captivated mankind for over 500 years.Vitruvian Man's variant Power Pose (above) encompasses both the *Mind–Body* and *Body Mind* approaches of **Morihei Ueishiba** and **Dr. Amy Cuddy**. Here we see an integration of the two complementary approaches where,

A good stance & posture reflect a proper state of mind—and—
a proper state of mind reflects a good stance and posture.

It elegantly works both ways:

Φ Calm your mind and align your body: ***As above, so below***.

Φ Align your body and calm your mind: ***As below, so above***.

> *The ideal posture we seek results from consistently optimizing our strength-to-flexibility ratio, to support coming ever closer to our own perfect body balance. This balance is always being challenged by gravity, which we must diligently learn to work with if we are to succeed. Lifting upward towards the sky, let us be like the young sapling* [Biomimicry]; *tall, straight, and flexible, able to bend with the strong wind yet not break.*
>
> **Robert Kaehler, master body balance coach**
> **& former Olympic rower (USA); KaehlerCore.com**

Dr. Cuddy points out that high-power yoga poses also show a direct correlation between the pose and a corresponding rise in testosterone and drop in cortisol. For example, after just 2 to 3 minutes in the classic cobra pose, testosterone levels *increased* by about 16%, while cortisol levels *decreased* by about 10%, with *"every single person in the study showing that pattern of changes."* Of course, this +16% to -10% ratio (1.6) reveals the dynamic Golden Ratio in action.

By practicing power poses, whether superhero, Vitruvian Man or yoga, you are amplifying and broadcasting your hidden-in-plain-sight Golden Ratio power to yourself

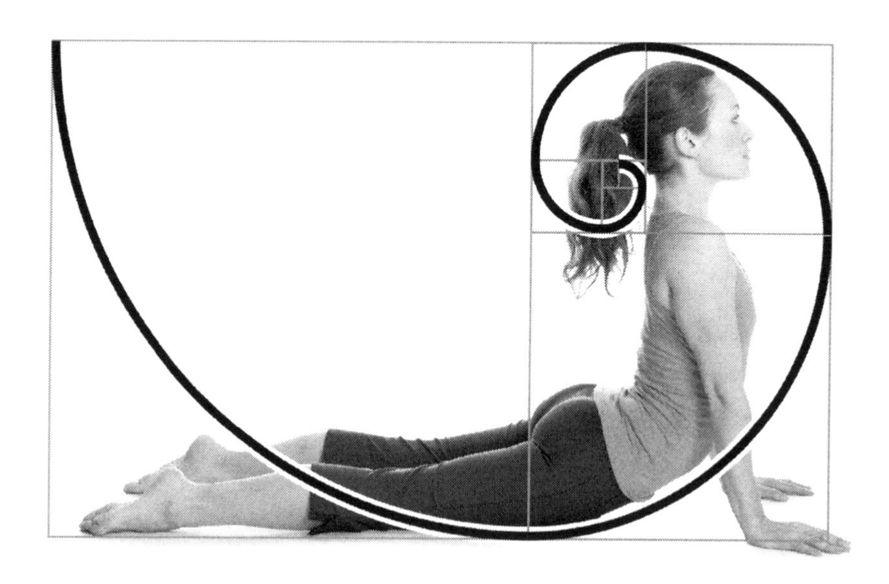

The human spine naturally tracks a Golden Ratio Spiral in both extension and flexion.
In addition to being a healthy posture reset, just 2-3 minutes in Cobra pose (above) simultaneously increases testosterone/power & confidence hormone by about 16% and reduces cortisol/stress/anxiety hormone by about 10%. This +16%, -10% ratio is the Golden Ratio in dynamic action.

and to the world. So what are you waiting for? Next time you need to amp-up your confidence, power and effectiveness before an important interview, meeting, presentation or competition: **1. Center your mind; 2. Imagine your favorite superhero (or make like a cobra); 3. For 1 to 3 minutes, go ahead and** ***strike a pose!***

Spirituality & the Spine

Sir John Woodroffe, aka **Arthur Avalon** wrote in his classic book *The Serpent Power: The Secrets of Tantric and Shaktic Yoga*, that the body's primal Kundalini/life energy, aka "serpent power," is coiled up 3 1/2 times at the base of the spine. When the Kundalini/life force is activated, it moves up the spine and is associated with varying degrees of psycho-spiritual development. As this subtle energy moves up the spine, it sequentially activates the body's seven subtle energy centers, known in Eastern traditions as the chakras (Sanskrit for "wheel," literally a "wheel of light"). The chakras have a correspondence with various endocrine glands (testes/ovaries, adrenals, pancreas, thymus, thyroid, pituitary, hypothalamus and pineal) and nerve plexi (sacral, lumbar, solar, cardiac, etc.). The ultimate result of the Kundalini rising up the spine and into the seventh chakra is variously known as spiritual enlightenment, nirvana, samadhi or bliss. The seat of this infinite power is always referenced as being at the base of the spine, which is composed of the coccyx and sacrum.

5

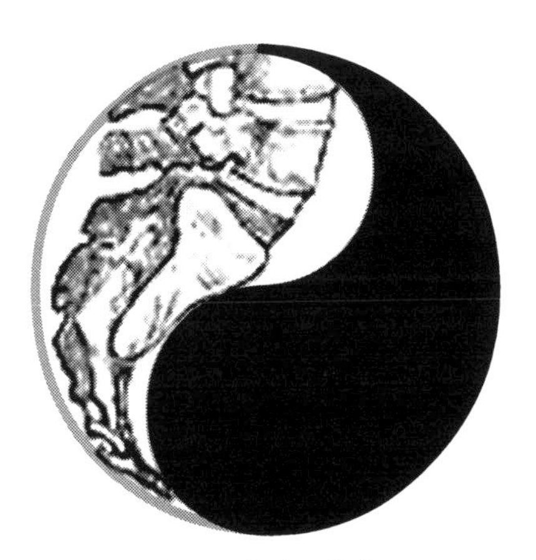

Origin of so-called ***coiled serpent*** Kundalini/Life Energy at the base of the spine mirrors bi-directional yin/yang-like ☯ Golden/Spirals, beginning at the 1st chakra level of the coccyx/sacrum.

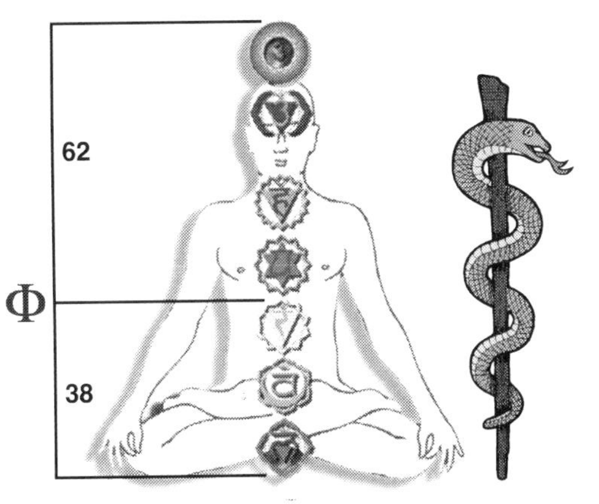

The crossing points of the winding serpent on the Rod of Asclepius occur at the levels of the Golden Ratio–spaced chakras (seven primary energy centers). The Golden Ratio dividing point between the upper and lower chakras is between the solar plexus and heart chakra. This signifies the bridge between the lower, more primal urges and the more humanistic and spiritual aspirations above.

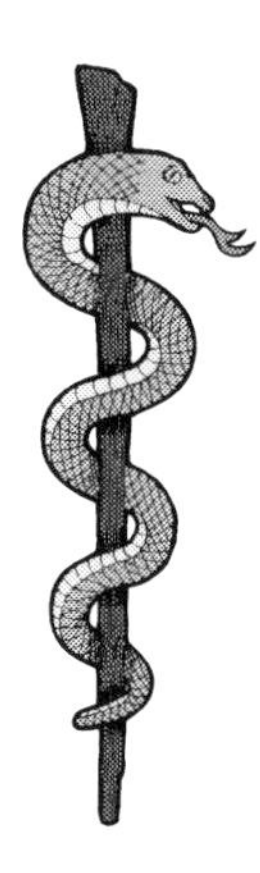

Both the Rod of Asclepius (*L*) and the Caduceus (*R*) are symbolic representations of the integration of form and function within the spinal system. The Rod represents the spine; the coiled serpent the movement of life force energy. The Caduceus' wings represent both the sphenoid bone at the base of the skull and the emerging higher consciousness, while the ball represents the sacred pineal gland—which up close resembles a pinecone with elegant Fibonacci spirals.

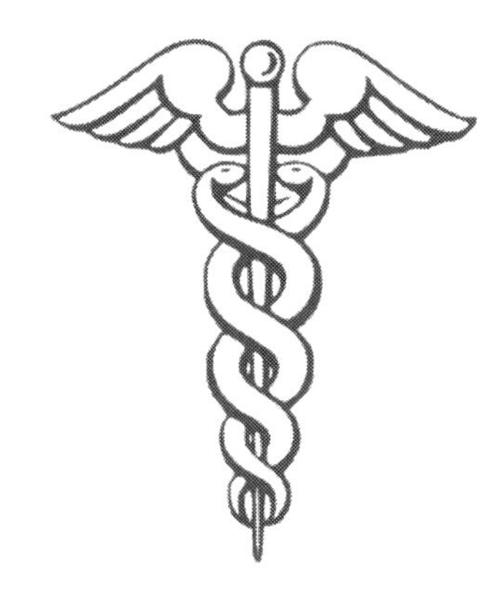

Traditional anthropologists view the coccyx, otherwise known as the tailbone, as a vestigial tail remnant with little or no value. Yet could the coccyx and sacrum have a powerful yet hidden function? Among other things, tailed animals use their tails to maintain balance in movement. Humans have adapted to being tail-less by developing large gluteal muscles, which act as torso stabilizers during movement. The coccyx is composed of 3 to 5 fused vertebrae attached to the sacrum by fibro-cartilaginous ligaments. The sacrum is a triangular-shaped bone composed of 5 fused vertebrae (note the Fibonacci numbers). When you view the sacro-coxygeal segment from the side, its distinct Golden Spiral shape is visible. It looks like a curled fetus, a shrimp or even a cuckoo's beak (coccyx translates as "cuckoo's beak" in Greek). It is also interesting that the translation of the word sacrum is "sacred bone." It would appear that the ancients knew that sleeping in the structure and function of the sacred sacral bone was potential Divinity. Could it be that the mysterious coiled serpent power revered by yogis throughout time is synonymous with the Golden Spiral? The Golden Spiral and Ratio don't limit themselves to the base of our spines of course, as they can be seen throughout the spine in the ratios of the cervical, thoracic, lumbar, sacral and coxygeal segments to one another.

The Rod of Asclepius, the Caduceus & the Spine

A symbol universally associated with medicine and healing is the serpent-entwined Rod of Asclepius. Bearing an uncanny resemblance to a single coiled strand of DNA, it rises in serpentine fashion around a staff that represents the spine. The ancients clearly understood the vital importance of the healing and enlightening power associated with energy moving freely along the spine. Good posture smooths the pathway for the unimpeded transmission of neural impulses—the Kundalini or life force—up and down the spine. When these neural impulses rise to their full potential, you can be sure that spiritual, scientific and/or artistic creative insights will emerge. The Rod of Asclepius is the true symbol of medicine yet it's often confused with a similar appearing symbol, the Caduceus. The Caduceus, ancient symbol of Hermes/Mercury, is also commonly associated with medicine and health care in modern times, yet more accurately symbolizes the arenas of commerce, negotiation, and as some would claim, the business side of medicine. As we've seen, proper posture, via the beautiful structural integrity of the human skeleton, is the critical Golden Ratio **Form** supporting healthy neurosignal transmission and life energy through the spine and thus the whole body. In Ch 6 Exercise, we'll explore how this optimal Form supports our fluid, unified **Function** through time and space. As legendary architect and Golden Ratio genius **Frank Lloyd Wright** said,

Form and function should be one, joined in a spiritual union.

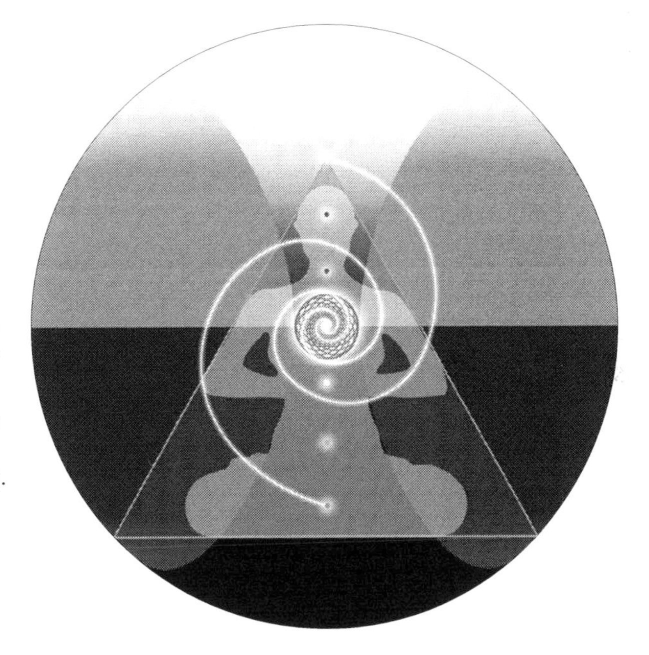

Healthy, buoyant posture showcasing the human chakra system, with double golden spirals emanating from the heart center. This classic artwork by author and architect **Scott Onstott** beautifully illustrates the Divine Proportion of the human form and the intrinsic matrix for the optimal transmission of life force energy throughout the body (www.SecretsInPlainSight.com).

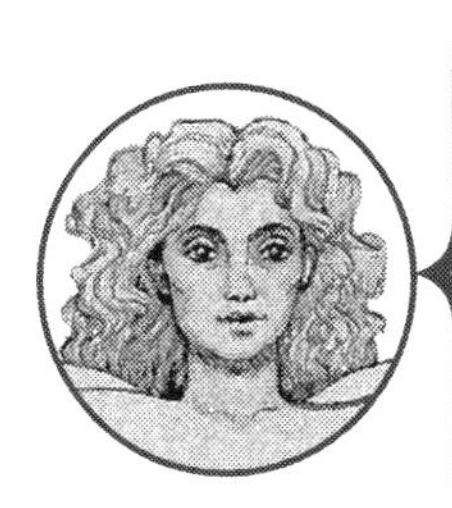

*Remember, you're only as well **Aligned** as your **POSTURE** is right now.* So sit and stand tall, relaxed and poised to support and maintain Golden Ratio skeletal alignment within the gravitational field. Strengthen your Golden Ratio Core Zone to enhance spinal health and posture. Practice yoga and use Power Poses to further boost total body alignment and confidence.

Exercise: #6 driver for dynamic health

The **human heart** is a Golden Ratio design marvel, both structurally & functionally.

Optimize performance, prevent injuries & burnout with the **Fibonacci Interval Training (FIT)** Workout Waves.™

Practice some form of **fun, dynamic** movement at least 4 days out 7 to keep your body strong & supple.

Ignite more energy for exercise by applying NSN in quality **small steps (*Kaizen*)** to upgrade breathing, hydration, sleep, nutrition, posture & detox.

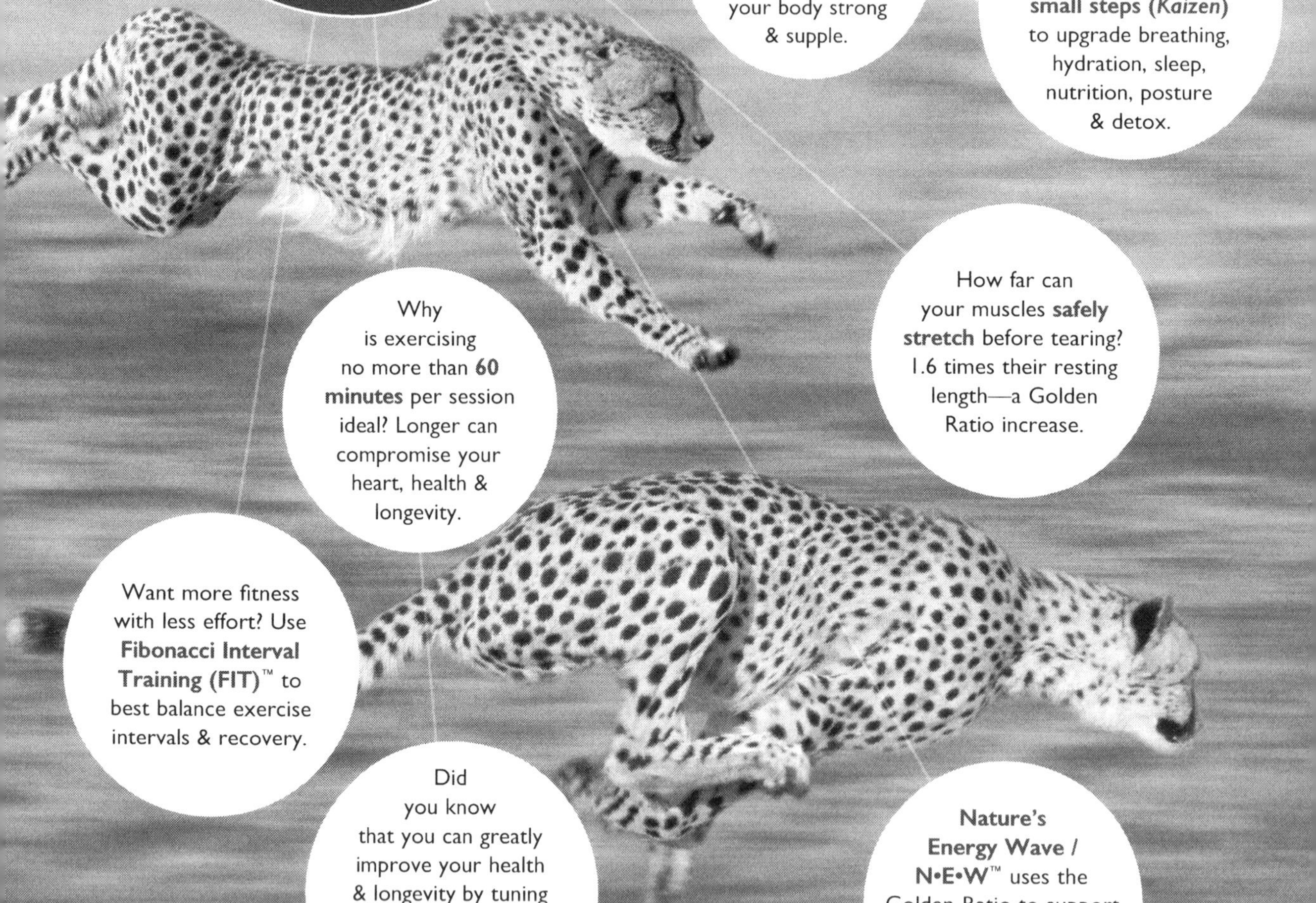

How far can your muscles **safely stretch** before tearing? 1.6 times their resting length—a Golden Ratio increase.

Why is exercising no more than **60 minutes** per session ideal? Longer can compromise your heart, health & longevity.

Want more fitness with less effort? Use **Fibonacci Interval Training (FIT)**™ to best balance exercise intervals & recovery.

Did you know that you can greatly improve your health & longevity by tuning your **blood pressure** (systolic/diastolic) to the Golden Ratio?

Nature's Energy Wave / N•E•W™ uses the Golden Ratio to support predictable peak performance and optimal fitness.

***The most perfect actions mirror the patterns found in Nature* [Biomimicry].**

Morihei Ueshiba, Founder of Aikido

6

Exercise

Nature's Path of Least Resistance, Maximum Efficiency and High Performance follows the Golden Ratio.
Dr. Ronald Sandler, Golden Ratio peak performance pioneer

6

A great hallmark of the Golden Ratio is the unification principle that arises when Golden Ratio relationships are established between the parts of any system, practice or regimen. A higher order functioning emerges when all the drivers of the NSN system are fine-tuned to the Ratio. This especially applies to NSN MegaNutrient #6, Exercise. Of all the writings on exercise, *very* little has focused on applying Golden/Fibonacci Ratios to working out. Research has shown that either too little *or* too much exercise is a risk factor for sudden cardiac death, yet the billion-dollar question is: *how much exercise is ideal for you?* Surely there's a way to customize exercise to each person's specific needs and requirements. As it turns out, that way is revealed to be the application of the Golden Ratio to your exercise—in particular, to the interval ratios within and between exercise sessions.

In SECTION I, ***Exploring the Extremes of Exercise,*** we'll get a higher perspective on what our optimal amount of exercise actually is. We'll look at extremes of exercise, ranging from HIT (High Intensity Training) to the low-intensity Blue Zone longevity exercise approach. This contrast gives anyone who works out at any level priceless insights about their own exercise regimen. We'll look first at the physical consequences of excess exercise in high aerobic sports like distance running and in anaerobic sports like body building. In contrast to Western exercise practices, we'll consider the benefits enjoyed by low-intensity exercisers from the worlds' longevity Blue Zones, where people often live healthy into their 90's+. Their exercise is built into their daily activities and lifestyles and as such tends to be generally of lower-intensity and lower stress.

SECTION 2, ***Fibonacci Interval Training (FIT) Waves,*** introduces a revolutionary new approach to exercise for both fitness exercisers and competitive athletes. The 3 FIT Waves—Short, Medium & Long—are exercise intervals lasting seconds, minutes or hours, while Nature's Energy Wave / N•E•W carries this principle into days, weeks and months. The system combines the wisdom of both low and high-intensity exercise approaches and tempers them with a dose of the Golden Ratio, expressed via Fibonacci Sequence numbers. The Waves generate NSN, the unique vitality factor that both maximizes overall health and fitness *and* gives the competitive athlete an unparalleled advantage. As an added benefit, athletes training over extended periods of time are at decreased risk of injury and burnout, due to the protective effect of Golden Ratio-structured exercise/rest cycles.

SECTION 3, ***NSN Fitness Innovations,*** explores physiology and practical methods, including the Benefits of Split Workouts, the Golden Olympic Training (GOT) Ratio, Dynamic Golden Ratio Movement, Active Isolated Stretching & Resistance Stretching, Golden Spiral Fitness, the Martial Arts and WrightBalance Sports System.

SECTION 4, ***Golden Ratio Cardiovascular Dynamics,*** reveals how the Golden Ratio can be easily used to measure and improve physiologic parameters of your cardiovascular system. We share some innovative methods for evaluating and synergizing blood pressure, breathing and heart function (ECG) that gives new insight on how to best synchronize with Nature's Path of Least Resistance and Maximum Performance.

SECTION 1: Exploring the Extremes of Exercise

Historical Insights on Pushing the Limits of Exercise

The right amount of nourishment and exercise,
not too little, not too much, is the safest way to health.

Hippocrates, The Father of Modern Medicine, 440 B.C.

Exercise holds a unique place in the Nature's Secret Nutrient system in that it integrates all of the other drivers into a strong cross-reinforcing system of health and

Phidippides: The Original Marathoner's Race... *to Premature Death*

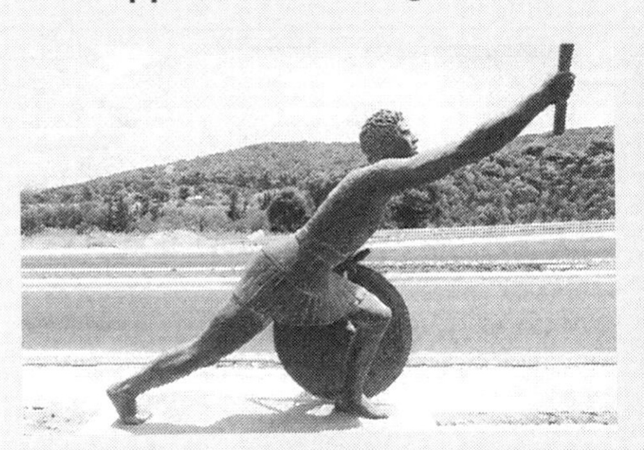

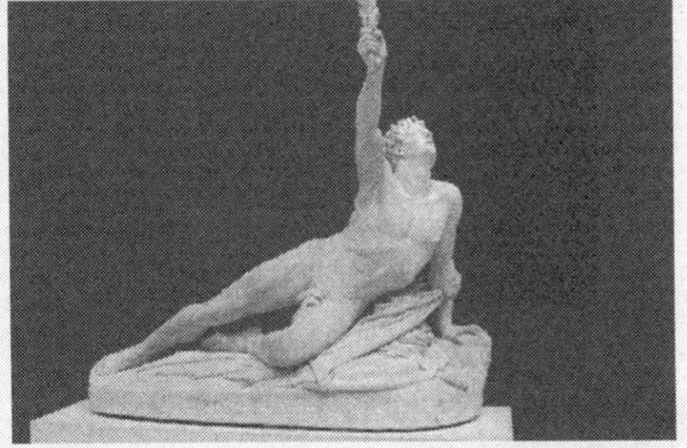

Two statues of Phidippides embody contrasting expressions of the human spirit. (*L*) The figure running the original marathon to Athens shows the dynamic yet extreme endurance and athletic prowess possible in a human being, while the collapsing figure (*R*) Phidippides' arrival in Athens reveals man's vulnerability when pushed to excess. Phidippides' death from physical overexertion can be extrapolated to our modern era, where going outside the bounds of the Golden Ratio "just right" zone in any aspect of life—including exercise—can lead to a sometimes heroic, yet often tragic outcome.

longevity. When exercising you of course must breathe, drink water, be well nourished and well rested, with good posture for a healthy workout. Ideally you'll also sweat a bit, get rid of some toxins and simultaneously release natural feel-good endorphins. Not only will your body, personal power and attractiveness improve, you'll likely also feel happier, with a greater sense of purpose and peace. If you continue this process over decades, you may well end up living vibrantly to/beyond a ripe old age. In line with Hippocrates' (the Greek Father of Modern Medicine) admonition of *not too little and not too much*, **modern medical research shows that the extremes of either too little or too much exercise are risk factors for sudden cardiac death.** Excess exercise is nothing new, as illustrated by another historical Greek, the famous runner Phidippides, who lived by and eventually died by the sword of long distance running. As the tale goes, after the Athenians defeated the Persians in the Battle of Marathon in 490 B.C., Phidippides, a military courier, ran the victory message from the battlefield at Marathon back to Athens (roughly 26 miles). Upon arriving in Athens he announced Victory, shouting the Greek word NeNIKÉkamen (Νενικήκαμεν, *Victory*)—the origin of the word NIKE. Phidippides proceeded to collapse from exhaustion, dying shortly thereafter. His legacy is the modern 26-mile, 385-yard (42.195 kilometer) marathon, initially run in the 1896 Olympics in his honor. The thrill of *Victory* has been

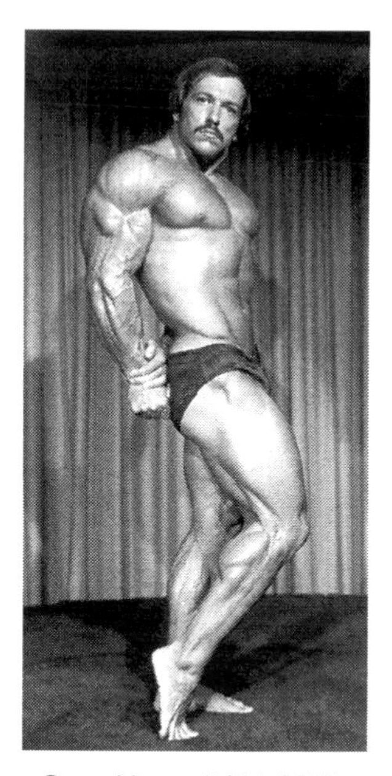

Casey Viator (1951–2013), Mr. America & Mr. Olympia.

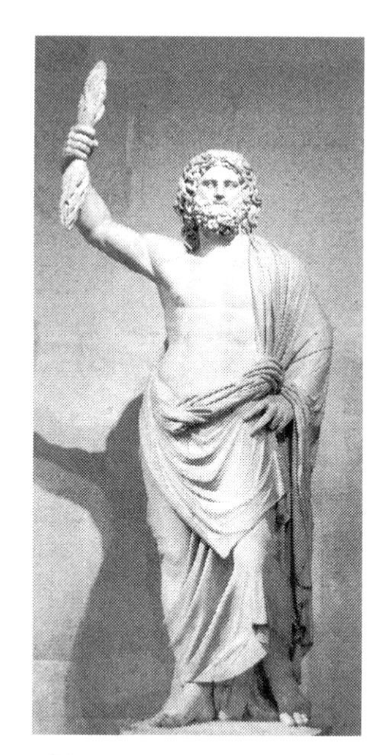

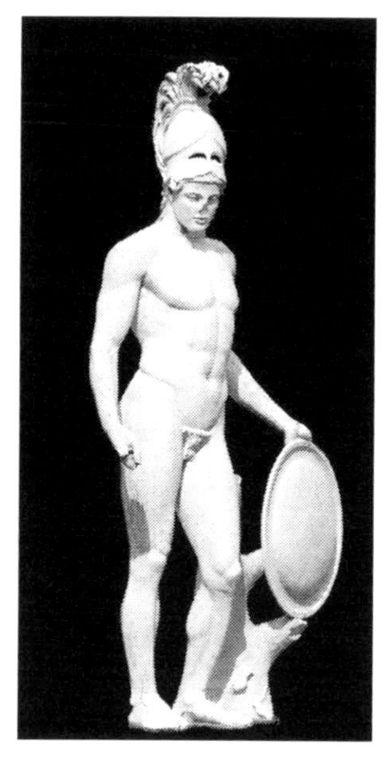

Zeus & Ares: Two of the ancient "Twelve Greek Olympians" that have become archetypes for modern-day bodybuilders.

the inspiration for generations of long-distance runners since Phidippides, with many suffering the consequences of overtraining and a few even succumbing to sudden death.

From Marathon to Muscle-Bound

In addition to the hordes of modern-day Phidippidian marathoners that emerged into the world of distance running over the last half-century, another group of athletes decided to also follow the Greek theme by resurrecting the ancient Greek archetypal image of strength and power through bodybuilding. Many bodybuilders turned to various extreme training regimens to emulate the powerful physical prowess of legendary Greek Gods. Through advances in exercise physiology and pharmaceutical science, bodybuilders seemingly hacked their way into a time warp, taking them back to the time of Zeus and Ares. Just like Michael Crichton and Steven Spielberg did by resurrecting extinct dinosaurs in *Jurassic Park*, leading exercise physiologists like **Arthur Jones** effectively brought these archetypal Greek Gods back to life for all to see. But unlike the *Tyrannosaurus Rex* in *Jurassic Park* which was created with harmless special effects, the flesh and blood human bodybuilders weren't immortal like Zeus and Ares and many suffered long-term consequences from overtraining. Although they developed impressive physiques on the outside, there were many unseen chinks in their internal armor that rendered them susceptible to cardiovascular disease and premature death. Following the original **H**igh **I**ntensity **T**raining (**HIT**) method developed by Arthur Jones (inventor of the Nautilus exercise equipment system), Casey Viator attained uncanny Golden Ratio measurements in his Greek God-like appearance and won titles in Mr. America and Mr. USA divisions. The essence of the HIT method is to use maximal exertion with minimal repetitions, followed by longer than usual recuperation periods. Muscle fibers can thus be super-stimulated into maximal hypertrophy (growth) in minimal time. The results obtained were phenomenal, as evidenced by the subsequent flurry of bodybuilding adherents to the HIT system. Yet the extreme short and long-term cardiovascular stresses were vastly under-appreciated in light of the spectacular gains achieved; also, most of the bodybuilders who achieved massive gains didn't use the HIT system alone. The other half of the equation was the addition of steroids and other Performance Enhancing Drugs (PED), which are known to damage the heart and vascular system. Viator died at age 62 from a massive heart attack. If his death was a singular occurrence, there would be no reason to associate it with the intensity of exercise and training protocols that preceded it. Yet Viator wasn't the only one who would succumb to the negative effects of HIT mixed with purported use of PED. This potent mix of HIT and PED could be typified as "short-term gain, long-term drain" syndrome. One has to seriously ask if the *end* (short-term gains in muscle mass and competitive wins) justifies the *means* (extreme HIT training and PED with associated risks).

6

Another one of Jones' protégés and trainees was the amazing **Mike Mentzer**, a Mr. America and Mr. Olympia winner who wrote one of the earliest High Intensity Training books, *High-Intensity Training the Mike Mentzer Way*. Mentzer consolidated the HIT principles and claimed that for optimal results in bodybuilding, workouts needed to be **brief, infrequent and intense**. Although the short-term effects of the High Intensity Training were profound, the extreme intensity of the workouts was apparently not healthy over the long run, as Mentzer died at age 49 due to heart complications—and was also known to combine HIT with PED. If Viator and Mentzer were isolated deaths from HIT and associated drug use, it would be a sad note in the annals of sport. Yet they weren't the only ones, as countless other bodybuilders have also died at young ages from the deadly mix of HIT combined with PED.

The Race to HIT Across Exercise Disciplines

One of the earliest applications of HIT-like workouts in the cardio/aerobic training arena was Fartlek or speed-play interval training, originated in 1937 by Swedish running coach **Gösta Holmér**. Fartlek training alternates periods of jogging interspersed with

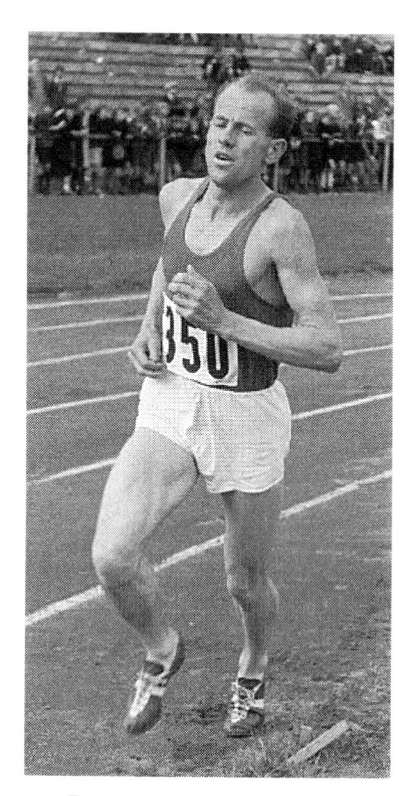

Emil Zátopek is known as the "Greatest Runner of All Time" (*Runner's World Magazine*, 2013), having won 3 Gold Medals in the 1952 Olympics (5K, 10K and marathon). Zátopek pioneered the use of Fartlek training (alternating periods of jogging and sprinting), the precursor to modern interval training.

6

sprinting bursts to increase a runner's dynamism, efficiency and endurance. Olympic triple gold medal running legend **Emil Zátopek** is one of many standout athletes who demonstrated the great power of the Fartlek or HIT approach. Zátopek won 3 gold medals in the 1952 Olympics: the 5K (3.1 miles), 10K (6.2 miles) and marathon 42.2K (26.2 miles). He's the only man to *ever* achieve this superhuman feat and was ranked by *Runner's World* magazine in 2013 as *The Greatest Runner of All Time*. As in bodybuilding, the HIT approach in endurance sports results in maximum short-term gains in a minimum amount of time. The endurance adaptations of HIT build lean body mass while simultaneously decreasing fat stores, resulting in a lean, cut look—ala Da Vinci's divinely-proportioned *Vitruvian Man*. These metabolic adaptations are mediated through increased release of hormones, including Human Growth Hormone (HGH) and testosterone. These insights inspire the question: *Who needs Performance Enhancing Drugs (PED) when you have HIT?*

Fartlek training has been shifted into overdrive via HIT methods, now becoming, as Mentzer would say, **brief, infrequent and intense**. A series of short, all-out sprints, each separated by a variable recovery period, constitutes the 1 to 2 times-a-week HIT workouts. The entire workout could be as short as 13 minutes or less, as opposed to traditionally tedious workouts of an hour or more. Recent research into HIT for cardio/aerobic training is corroborating what Jones, Viator and Mentzer proved decades ago in bodybuilding: the HIT method can be a super-efficient way to train in general—and can be done in a fraction of the time required for traditional workouts. Kinesiology professor **Martin Gibala** of McMaster University, a leading HIT scientist and author of *The One Minute Workout*, reports that **HIT training can provide big returns from small amounts of exercise time invested:** *Our study demonstrates that interval-based exercise is a very time-efficient training strategy. This type of training is very demanding and requires a high level of motivation. However, short bursts of intense exercise may be an effective option for individuals who cite 'lack of time' as a major* *impediment to fitness. Intensity is more important than duration... Relative to all sorts of health benefits, it is more time-efficient to exercise hard for a short amount of time than it is to exercise easy for a long amount of time...*

Vary Your Exercise Intensity for Increased Health & Longevity

It is now known that varying your training duration and intensity are the best ways to promote the health and efficiency of your cardiovascular system. In retrospect, you wouldn't want to use the traditional **L**ong-**S**low-**D**istance (**LSD**) cardio training method, as did **Jim Fixx**, author of *The Complete Book of Running*. With the steady, unchanging pace of the LSD method, Fixx likely *deconditioned* his heart and autonomic nervous system, thereby decreasing his **H**eart **R**ate **V**ariability (**HRV**), which refers to the beat-to-beat variation in heartbeats. The greater your HRV, the more dynamism—and health—your heart and autonomic nervous system have. Just as you gain more range and flexibility in your muscles from stretching, **your heart gets more dynamism from increasing the range within which it functions.** Fixx's LSD workouts had an overly monotonous, steady pace that likely *decreased* his HRV and contributed to the sudden-death heart attack he died from in his early 40's; poor diet and excess stress were also likely additional contributing factors. Monotonous, low-range LSD workouts keep your heart rate unchanged for long periods of time and can *decondition*—and ultimately damage—the responsiveness and overall health of your heart and autonomic nervous system. Although Fixx's cardio workouts were totally different in type, duration and intensity than the heavy strength training workouts of Viator and Mentzer, they all were clearly training in ways that were detrimental to their health and subsequent longevity. Their workouts are contrasted as follows:

6

Fixx's: *Long, Slow, Distance (LSD);* *Aerobic for Endurance.*	**Viator's & Mentzer's:** *Brief, Infrequent & Intense (BII)* *Anaerobic for Strength & Bulk*

Although Viator and Mentzer had variability built into their workouts, their intensity levels were overly excessive as were the duration and frequency of Fixx's workouts. We don't know what the HRV's of these 3 example athletes were, as HRV testing wasn't available at the time, yet the fact that they all died young from heart attacks suggests that they all also very likely had low HRV's. **An increased HRV (increased beat-to-beat variation in heart rate) reflects more dynamism and adaptability of the autonomic nervous system and has also been shown to improve hormonal functioning, emotional balance and slow the effects of aging.** It's far healthier to include frequent variability in the duration and intensity of your individual workouts, as well as between your workouts over days, weeks and months. Workouts that vary your heart rate result in a greater beat-to-beat variation—increased HRV—as well (see the Ch 6 Exercise Rx on measuring your HRV).

Exercise: The Dose Makes the Medicine ℞ — Or the Poison ☠

*Exercise, like any potent drug, follows the formula of **Too Little = No Benefit; Too Much = Harm*** [to which we'd add: ***the Golden Ratio amount = Just Right***].

James O'Keefe, M.D., author of *The Forever Young Diet & Lifestyle*

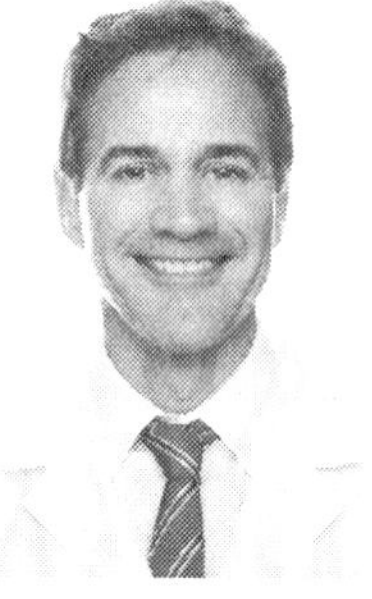

Dr. James O'Keefe, cutting-edge preventive cardiologist.

The current rush of enthusiasm for extreme HIT exercise protocols adapted to cardio/aerobic sports in light of its history in bodybuilding is especially concerning, when viewed from a long-term health and longevity perspective. We wonder whether the unwitting public is setting themselves up for a fate similar to that of bodybuilders Viator and Mentzer by subjecting themselves to overly intense exercise training protocols over years and decades. Although there is currently no data to conclusively answer the question of whether or not HIT protocols present any meaningful cardiac risks long term, there is emerging evidence indicating that excess endurance training over decades may be detrimental to cardiac health. **James O'Keefe, M.D.**, a leading cardiologist from the Mid-America Heart Institute in St. Louis has reported preliminary evidence that Excessive Endurance Training/EET over decades, as performed by endurance athletes such as marathon runners, ironman triathletes and long distance cyclists, may increase several key cardiac risk factors, including arrhythmias, accelerated atherosclerosis and myocardial fibrosis (scarring of the heart). After racing, marathon runners were found to have elevations in the same cardiac enzyme (troponin) found in patients who have had a heart attack. Troponin levels returned to normal after the runner's hearts repaired the damage—but repeated insults from excessive running result in repeated scarring in the heart muscle, heart valves and nerve conduction system. Dr. O'Keefe doesn't yet know how pervasive this pathology is in extreme endurance athletes, as his research is ongoing. Yet from what he *does* know thus far he's **strongly recommending that we practice predominantly moderate intensity and duration of exercise—anywhere from 30 to a maximum of 60 minutes per session**—correlating with Fibonacci Numbers 34 & 55. This range promotes excellent health and longevity benefits, *without the potential serious risks of overexertion.* Future research will further reveal the risk/benefit curves of extreme

Golden Spiral Exercise Benefit Curve™: Targeting *Just Right*

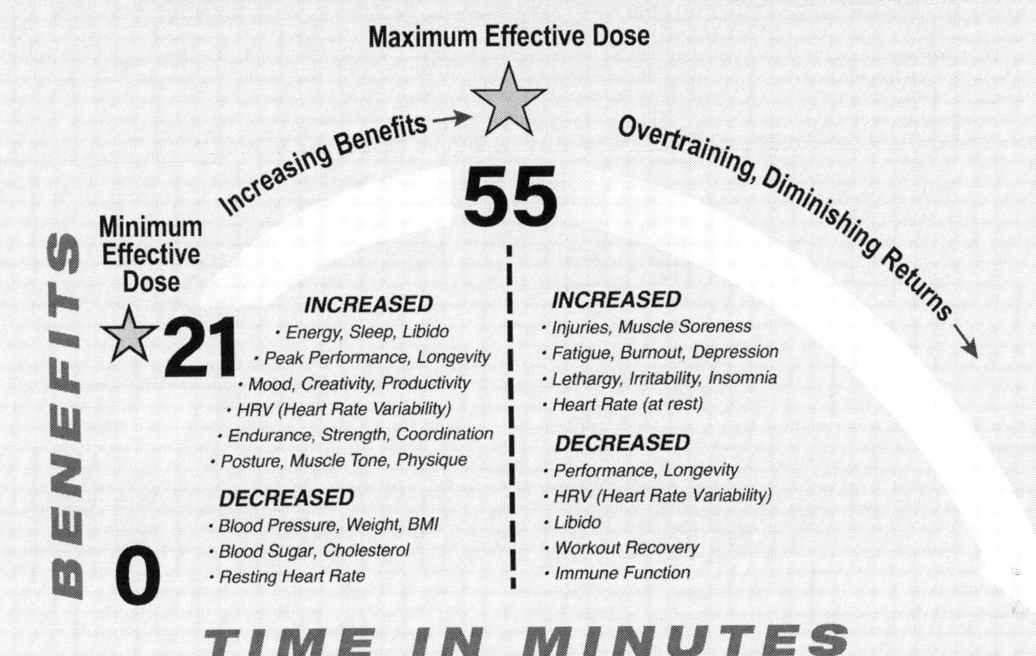

Exercise Time Per Workout Session: Minimum Effective Dose = 21 min. (could be combined total from 2 split sessions in same day); Maximum Effective Dose = 55 min. Over 55 min. = overtraining. The American Academy of Sports Medicine recommends 150 min./wk. total of moderate intensity exercise for adults, which is around 21 min./day.

This Exercise Curve is applicable to anyone, regardless of age or exercise goals. It doesn't matter if you're a fitness walker or an Olympic athlete, the principle of smart moderation holds true. **There is an ideal amount of exercise for each individual that promotes health, well-being and optimal performance, beyond which the benefits may be overshadowed by a continuum of diminishing returns, including overtraining syndrome and reduced life expectancy.** More is not better; the *just right* zone is our aim.

The benefits and risks of exercise are demonstrated in this Golden Spiral Exercise Benefit Curve. Most of the health-promoting benefits from exercise come early on, with the steep increase at the left section of the curve. This translates to as little as 21 minutes total/day. With a little more exercise, e.g., 34-55 minutes/day, you receive optimal benefits. **Past 60 minutes you become vulnerable to the risks of overtraining, with diminishing returns for your time and effort.** The exception is any exercise over longer periods which has frequent breaks, e.g., hiking, tennis, soccer, yoga, etc. Vigorous games/workouts can exceed 60 minutes, as long as they have rest breaks with enough recovery. In other words, keep to the left/middle range of the Exercise Curve to get the most from your exercise time and reduce the downside risks. Dr. James O'Keefe has shown that long-term—over a period of decades—Excessive Endurance Training/EET (over 60 minutes uninterrupted per session) may well increase the risk of cardiac atherosclerosis, fibrosis and arrhythmias. As Albert Einstein might have said,

Exercise as little as necessary, yet not less than that, or,
Exercise as much as necessary, yet not more than that.

vs. moderate endurance exercise, as well as optimal cardio aerobic HIT protocols. Extreme sustained activity (similar to a human running a marathon), is rare to non-existent in mammals. Therefore, we may want to take a hint from Nature through **Biomimicry** and avoid *extreme sustained* activity and the potential harm therein. We know from author **Dan Buettner's** research into the world's longevity "Blue Zones" with the oldest living people that these centenarians routinely exercise up to 5 hours per day. *Yet their exercise is crucially different from our commonly understood concept of exercise.* Blue Zone exercise is more a natural, harmonious part of one's daily lifestyle, moderate and undulating like gentle ocean waves. It includes farming, gardening, lifting, carrying, walking, climbing and bicycling. Intense exercise—*for the sake of exercise alone*, e.g., heavy weight lifting or strength training, extreme cardio/aerobic or long-distance running—are simply nonexistent in the daily lives of long-lived Blue Zone people. In fact, **Buettner found this gentle style of natural, Lifestyle Exercise to be the most significant single lifestyle factor shared by healthy centenarians in all Blue Zones worldwide.** Clearly a *moderate* exercise regimen helps win the longevity race, while the modern *more/harder is better* exercise obsession may well be a shortcut to the finish line of life.

Even though it may be decades too soon to have sufficient data to evaluate the risks and benefits from long-term studies of cardio/aerobic applications of HIT, Blue Zone centenarians are an easy study of what natural, low-to-moderate intensity interval training does for people. We can contrast the many reports of untimely deaths of professional bodybuilders who used HIT with the exceptional longevity of Blue Zone centenarians who get their exercise from the simple, less strenuous tasks of daily life. The question is whether cardio/aerobic use of HIT is worth the short-term gains in lieu of the possible long-term risks. Since the risk/benefit statistics won't be known for decades, it may be wiser to follow a more moderate exercise protocol when interval training. Perhaps there's a way to extract the benefits that both Blue Zone centenarians and HIT proponents enjoy, with minimal risks. Can we have the dynamic, robust health of a trained athlete while also living the full lifespan of a Blue Zone centenarian? Let's explore how to find the best of both worlds through the integration of the Golden Ratio into moderate, sensible interval training and exercise in general in the pages ahead.

> *If you look into Nature and our deep past, you can find the template* [Golden Ratio **Biomimicry**] *for ideal health, even in our modern world.*
>
> **James O'Keefe, M.D., cardiologist, from his TEDx talk**

Balancing the 3 Variables of Exercise: Intensity, Frequency & Duration

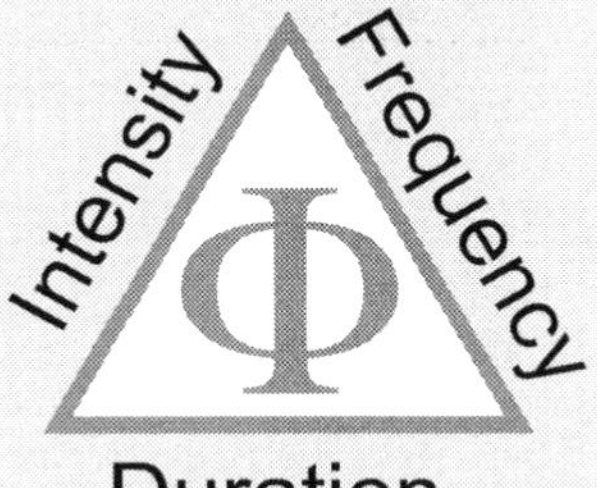

As much as you might want to max out your exercise sessions to improve as rapidly as possible, the reality of how our bodies regenerate in response to exercise stress must be considered. Successful athletes know from experience that they must vary the Intensity, Frequency & Duration of workouts to allow for sufficient recovery time.

As one variable goes up, the other two must come down to avoid overtraining. For example, as Intensity goes up, Frequency & Duration must come down. Of necessity, high-intensity sprints are of short duration and it's counterproductive to do them more frequently than two days a week. Likewise, when Frequency of training sessions goes up, both Intensity and Duration of workouts must come down to prevent poor performance and burnout. And of course we know that when Duration of workouts increases, both Intensity and Frequency of workouts must decrease in order to prevent overtraining and decreased Heart Rate Variability (HRV).

The secret lies in finding the particular relationships between these three variables so that they maximally support one another. A creative way to balance them is by using Fibonacci Numbers to designate the percentages of each allocated to Intensity, Frequency & Duration. The Fibonacci Numbers 5, 3 and 2 can be used as the basis for using the percentages 50%, 30% and 20% to make up 100% of your workout. These percentages automatically build in the Golden Ratio between Intensity, Frequency & Duration. **Key Point: for optimal training results, discover your ideal Golden Ratio balance of Intensity, Frequency and Duration.**

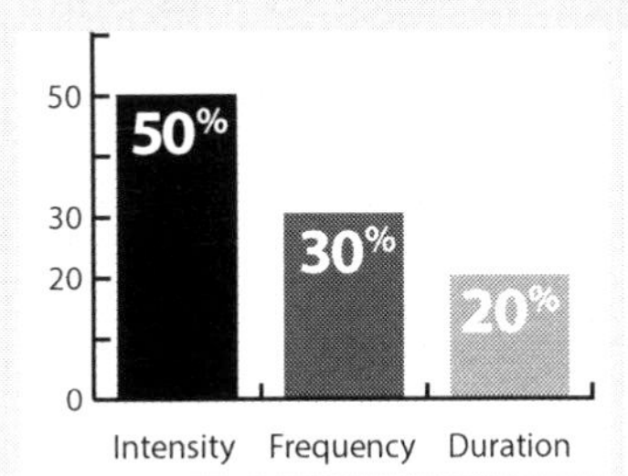

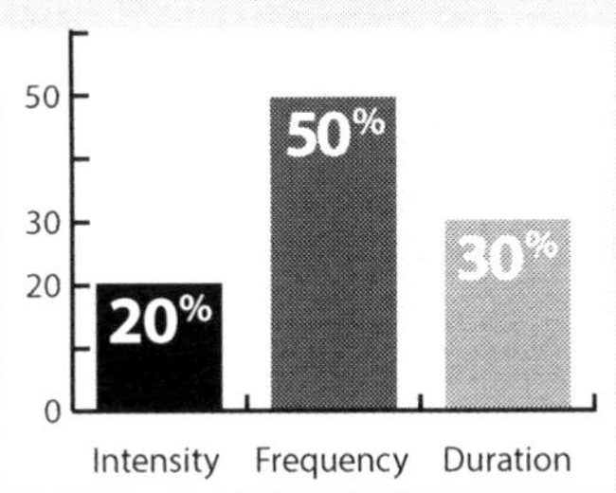

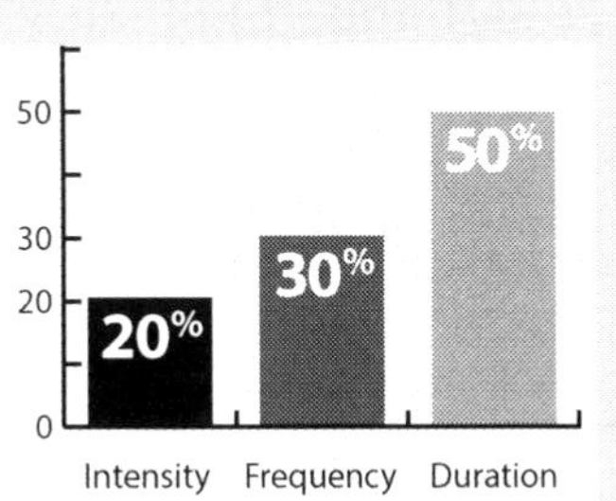

The three graphs above show how Intensity, Frequency and Duration are proportioned in Fibonacci Ratios: 50%: 30%: 20%. As one variable becomes dominant, the other two must go down to give your body the best chance to progressively build endurance, strength and flexibility—while simultaneously preventing injury and burnout. By finding a Golden Ratio balance between the three variables, you'll get more NSN out of your workouts with less effort.

SECTION 2: Fibonacci Interval Training (FIT) Workout Waves: World's 1st Golden Ratio Total Fitness & Performance System

The Super Synergy of FIT Waves

Fibonacci Interval Training (FIT) Workout Waves introduce a revolutionary new approach to exercise for both fitness exercisers and competitive athletes. All 3 FIT Waves—Short, Medium & Long—are exercise intervals that tap the power of the Golden Ratio via Fibonacci Sequence Numbers. Each FIT Wave is scaled to its own time frame: seconds, minutes or minutes/hours. Since all 3 FIT Waves are based on Fibonacci Sequence Numbers and the Golden Ratio, they're all fractals (self-similar on different scales) and can all be superimposed on one another to create a super-synergy effect. This allows any fitness exerciser or competitive athlete to create robust health and optimize peak performance, while simultaneously preventing injuries and burnout.

FIT SHORT Wave: Uses Fibonacci Numbers on a scale of *seconds*. High intensity sprints range from 8 to 55 *seconds*.

FIT MEDIUM Wave: Uses Fibonacci Numbers on a scale of *minutes*. Workout duration ranges from 13 to 34 *minutes*.

FIT LONG Wave: Uses Fibonacci Numbers on a scale of *minutes* & *hours* to schedule workouts & rest periods. Workout duration ranges from 55 to 144 *minutes* (~1 to ~2.5 *hours*).

Note: ALL FIT Workout Waves have built-in variable rest/recovery periods—*the downwaves*—dependent on recharge time needed.

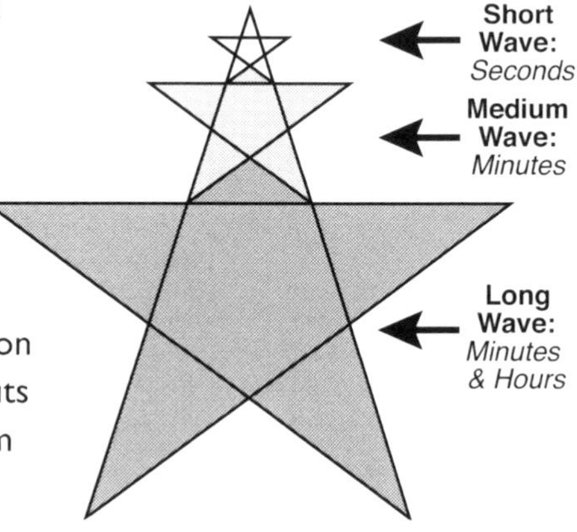

The FIT Wave Workout Stars: three self-similar (fractal) Waves embedded in one system.

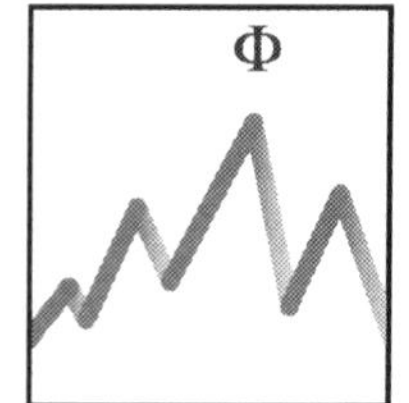

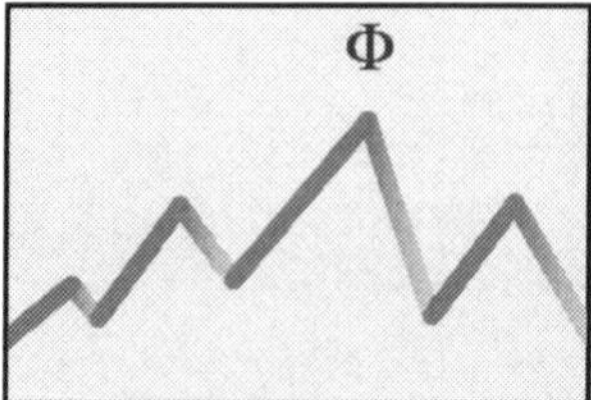

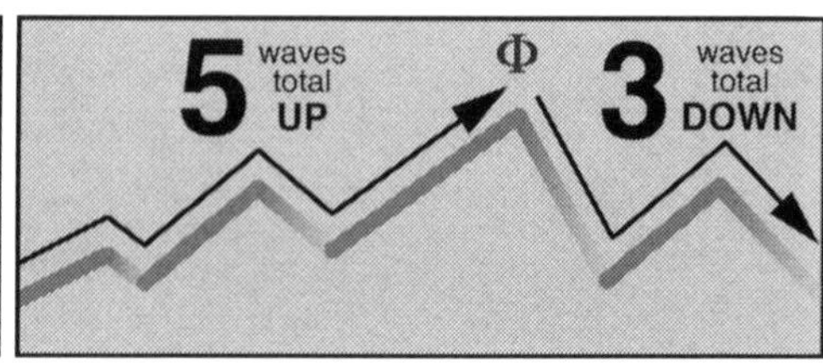

Short Wave: *Seconds* **Medium Wave:** *Minutes* **Long Wave:** *Minutes & Hours*

The 3 FIT Workout Waves: Short (seconds), Medium (minutes) and Long (minutes & hours). As the Golden Ratio-based star allows for fractal embeddings of self-similar, smaller stars, so do the 3 FIT Fibonacci-based training waves embed within one another for super-synergy fitness and performance. **NOTE HOW ALL FIT WAVES exhibit the classic Elliott Wave pattern of 5 total waves UP to 3 total waves DOWN.**

FIT Short Wave: Interval Training in *Seconds*

The FIT Short Waves are exercise sprints delineated by Fibonacci Numbers, ranging from 8 to 55 seconds. They have variable rest/recovery periods dependent on the time needed to catch your breath, clear lactic acid from muscles and regain a sense of well-being. The exercise sprint cycles cross-reinforce one another via Golden Ratios formed between the Fibonacci Numbers. The end result of this type of numerical-based exercise is that Golden Ratio harmonics are generated in all bodily systems, e.g., musculoskeletal, neurohormonal and cardiovascular. All 3 FIT Wave Workouts can be used by fitness exercisers and competitive athletes alike. Fitness exercisers can exert as much or as little intensity as desired, while competitive athletes can exert up to their full intensity according to their training goals. Everyone will get a powerful shot of Golden Ratio resonance in their system and generate a healthy dose of NSN. **No other exercise fitness system offers this Golden Ratio super-boost as an exercise optimizer.**

When you exercise with short, intense sprints, as in FIT Short Wave Workouts, you'll be burning fuel anaerobically. That's when your cellular machinery generates energy (ATP) without oxygen. This type of energy production can only be sustained for short periods of time; that's why the Short Wave sprints are only from 8–55 seconds long with variable recovery periods tuned to your personal needs. You want adequate time for your system to get rid of the lactic acid and generate more ATP, so that your cells are stimulated to build more strength and endurance. The Fibonacci-Numbered sprint intervals easily form Golden Ratios and are the keys to efficiency. These ratios are in strong alignment with Nature's Path of Least Resistance and Optimal Performance. They give your body just the right amount of stimulation from interval to interval—*not too little, not too much—just right*. As we'll see in the **Nature's Energy Wave / N•E•W** section ahead, Golden Ratio performance pioneer Dr. Ron Sandler has shown that the secret to injury-free exercise and peak performance lies within the application of the Golden Ratio to human performance. **Following the old adage of "no pain, no gain" actually increases your vulnerability to injury and burnout.** It sets you up to work against Nature's Path of Least Resistance, as opposed to having a strong, steady wind at your back. There is a better way—the FIT Workout Wave System.

All FIT Wave System exercise phases are stair-stepped up and down in Golden Ratio throughout the workout, corresponding to Nature's universal blueprint for optimal form and function. You'll increase and decrease in increments that aren't too steep on both the increasing and decreasing phases. These ratios are in the same proportion that you see in the ratios of clockwise to counterclockwise seed spirals and leaf distribution

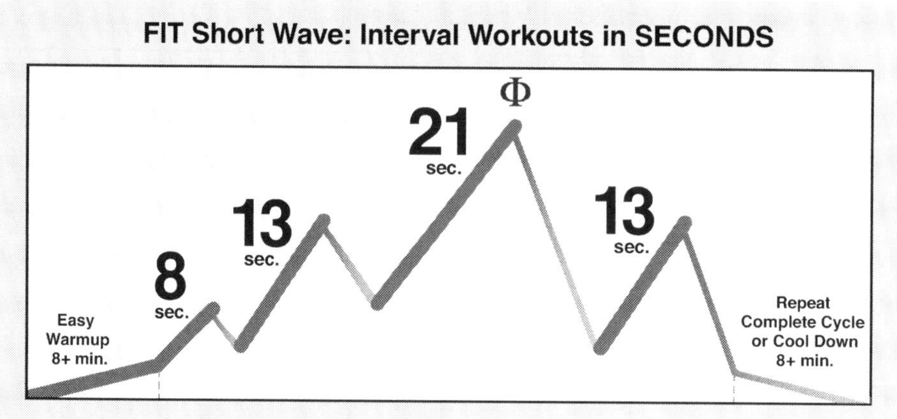

55 second FIT Short Wave workout example. The FIT Short Wave interval sprints are delineated by Fibonacci Sequence numbers, forming Golden Ratios between intervals. All *Downwaves* are recovery phases, loading the catapult for the next Upwave. You determine the length of each recovery phase, based on subjective & objective feedback of readiness/recovery for the next sprint. For shorter or longer workout options, see the FIT Short, Medium and Long Wave Workouts in the Ch 6 Rx section.

6

in a sunflower. The seeds and leaves are maximally packed and arranged like that for a reason; to enable the sunflower to carry out its functions—e.g., extracting maximum light and nourishment from the sun—with maximum efficiency and impact. All of its tasks are more easily performed when the plant is synchronized with Golden Ratios, just as Nature ingeniously designed. Maximum efficiency in growth, function and beauty are among the unique plus factors seen in the archetypal sunflower—so why not biomimic a sunflower (and *all* of Nature) and integrate these vast benefits into your exercise regime? When you align your exercise with these principles, the exponential plus factor/NSN you receive upgrades the efficiency of *all* your workouts and rewards you with rapid physical improvement in health and performance. To easily embed the Golden Ratio into your workouts, you simply use Fibonacci Sequence Numbers to delineate the number of seconds for each sprint. This applies whether your intervals are of easy, moderate or high intensity. Here's a quick review of the beginning numbers in the Fibonacci Sequence:

0, 1, 1, 2, 3, 5, 8, 13, 21, 34, 55, 89, 144...

(you can also try cycling between ***38 and 62,*** *the two key Golden Ratio marker numbers)*

The Fibonacci Sequence numbers used in the FIT Short Wave examples in the Exercise Rx section of this book are designed to optimally train your anaerobic zone. In the Short Wave *easy* example, your first sprint is 8 seconds followed by a 13-second one, followed by a 21-second one and then back down to a 13-second sprint to complete the cycle. Depending on your fitness level, you can repeat the FIT Wave interval sets

1, 2 or 3 times and then begin your final cool down. You'll have accessed the anaerobic zone in your peak sprints, balanced with adequate rest/recovery periods to facilitate your optimal recovery and recharge. You'll have given your entire system a Golden Ratio imprint that instantly rewards you with a healthy dose of NSN. By using Fibonacci numbers to orchestrate your workouts, you'll send repeated Golden Ratio homeostatic balancing signals to your cardiovascular, neuroendocrine and musculoskeletal systems. **This approach transforms the concept of *working smarter, not harder* into your secret exercise/training weapon and brings the Kaizen principle (continuous improvement in small steps) to life in your fitness regimen.**

FIT Medium Wave: Interval Training in *Minutes*

The FIT Medium Wave uses Fibonacci Numbers in workouts ranging from 13 to 34 minutes, with each interval being followed by flexible recovery period. The Golden Ratio is embedded into your workouts simply by using Fibonacci numbers to delineate the number of minutes you spend in each interval phase. These intervals are similar to the FIT Short Wave workouts, yet on a longer scale of minutes vs. seconds. In the Medium Wave workouts, depending on your chosen goals, you can vary your intensity such that you'll have the option of exercising in the aerobic zone for low to moderate intensity; or if you choose a more intense workout, you can also exercise in both aerobic and anaerobic zones. Exercising in both the aerobic and anaerobic zones allows you to

6

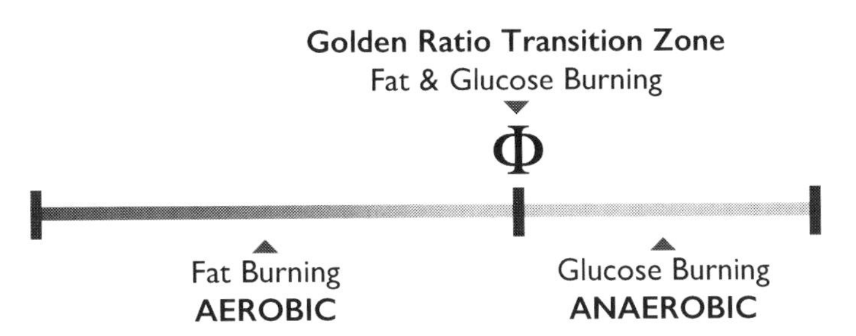

develop greater endurance in both glucose and fat energy production systems. In the aerobic phase, some glucose, yet mainly slow-burning fat is used to generate ATP, the universal energy molecule. As you speed up and transition to the anaerobic phase, your cells switch to quick-burning glucose to generate ATP. You'll know when you've gone too far into the anaerobic zone and depleted your ATP stores, because your breathing gets rapid and you begin to feel the burn of lactic acid in your muscles. This intensity of exercise can't be sustained for very long, so you need to back off the pace into a recovery zone until the lactic acid is cleared. During the recovery phase you drop back

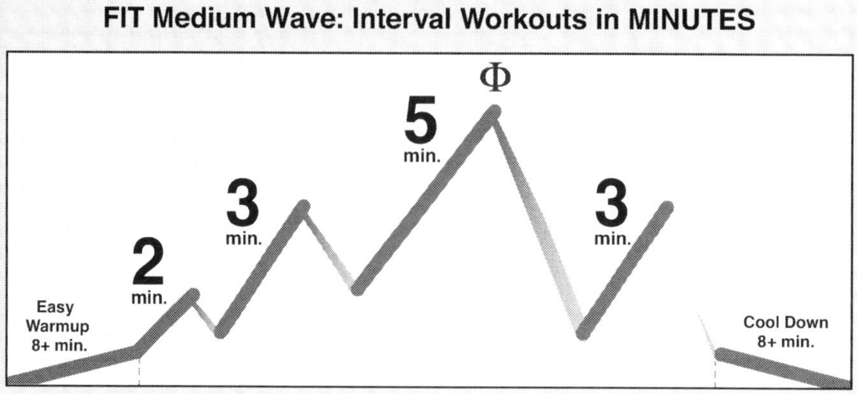

FIT Medium Wave: Interval Workouts in MINUTES

13 minute Medium Wave Workout example. The FIT Medium Wave intervals are delineated by Fibonacci Sequence numbers, forming Golden Ratios between intervals. All *Downwaves* are recovery phases, loading the catapult for the next Upwave. You determine the length of each Downwave recovery phase, based on subjective & objective feedback of readiness/recovery for the next sprint. For shorter or longer workout options, see the FIT Short, Medium and Long Wave Workouts in the Ch 6 Rx section.

into the fat-burning aerobic metabolism. **There's a transition zone where you're burning both fat and glucose—and that special zone neatly spans the Golden Ratio dividing point between aerobic and anaerobic metabolism.** In an interview with Bulletproof CEO Dave Asprey, Harvard researcher Dr. Richard Veech noted that when running mid to long distances, your liver begins producing ketones from fatty acids, which generate 38% more energy for the heart than glucose. The beauty of Fibonacci Interval Training (FIT) is that intensity, frequency and duration are customizable according to your particular needs on any given day, or even over weeks and months. In order to avoid complicated heart rate calculations and the use of bulky heart rate monitors, **all you need do is adjust your intervals according to varying Fibonacci Sequence numbers**, such that you're able to comfortably complete each workout. By establishing Golden Ratios between intervals, your autonomic nervous system (sympathetic/parasympathetic) quickly develops a dynamic response to the stress of exercise that improves all aspects of health. As your endurance, strength and flexibility improve over time, you can adjust the intensity, frequency and duration of your workouts accordingly. Another benefit of using the FIT Wave System is that no matter what your level of proficiency, whether fitness exerciser or competitive athlete, you don't need to go all-out to reap the benefits of FIT workouts. The unseen benefits result from application of Golden Ratios between interval cycles. By combining this training strategy with other NSN techniques such as Fibonacci breathing, you can extract even more NSN from your workouts. These Medium Wave workouts can be seamlessly integrated with the Short and Long Wave workouts for added impact. In weight lifting terminology this is known as *stacking*, where various performance-enhancing substances/techniques are combined or *Biostacked* for an amplified effect. The FIT Wave System does this naturally, allowing you to safely maximize the benefits of your exercise in whatever form or intensity it takes. A super-synergy emerges when you combine the 3 FIT Waves—Short, Medium and Long—via this unique approach. By establishing Golden Ratios between exercise intervals, it's possible to achieve and maintain rapid gains in endurance and health, with benefits accruing over time. In addition you won't be over-stressing your system and will greatly reduce the chances of injury, boredom and burnout. The FIT Wave System also delivers other priceless health benefits, including improved Heart Rate Variability (HRV), lower resting heart rate, lower blood pressure, increased metabolic rate, improved blood sugar regulation, more weight loss as well as improved hormonal secretion and more graceful and even reversed aging. **With FIT, you receive the combined benefits of high intensity exercise with Blue Zone moderation: the best of both worlds.**

FIT Long Wave: Interval Training in *Minutes & Hours*

The FIT Long Wave applies the same NSN generating principles as the FIT Short & Medium Waves, yet over longer periods—from 55 minutes (~1 hour) to 144 minutes (~2.5 hours) and above. We know from the research of cardiologist Dr. James O'Keefe that **nonstop exercise of around one hour is a safe limit, past which the risks of**

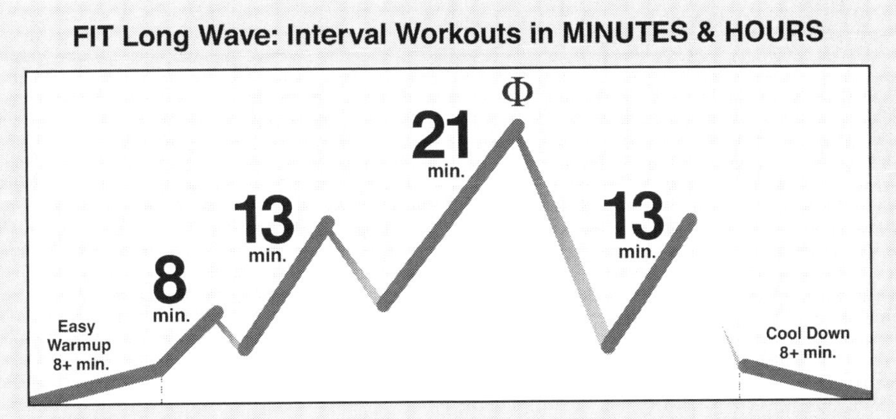

55 minute (~1 hour) Long Wave Workout example. Just as with the FIT Short and Medium Wave Workouts, the FIT Long Wave Workout intervals are delineated by Fibonacci Sequence numbers, forming Golden Ratios between intervals. All Downwaves are recovery phases, loading the catapult for the next Upwave. You determine the length of each Downwave, based on subjective & objective of readiness/recovery for the next sprint. For shorter or longer workout options, see the FIT Short, Medium and Long Wave Workouts in the Ch 6 Rx section.

overtraining begin to exceed the positive benefits of exercise. Many sports/games routinely exceed one hour in duration, yet due to the nature of the sport they have natural built-in breaks that give the heart time to recover. This avoids the nonstop stress on the heart that is seen for example in long-distance endurance athletes who routinely train with workouts of over an hour. Sports/games where frequent rest/recovery breaks can be used to natural advantage to safely exercise over an hour include hiking, cycling, swimming, tennis, basketball, soccer, skiing, etc. For the average recreational or fitness exerciser this isn't a consideration, as most people's workouts are usually around an hour or less. However, for competitive or professional athletes, longer exercise sessions can be done safely by simply incorporating the FIT Long Wave and its strategic rest breaks into their workouts. Three FIT Long Wave options for safe, extended workouts are featured in the Ch 6 FIT Rx section.

The Breakthrough Nature's Energy Wave / N•E•W: Optimizing Workouts & Rest/Recovery Periods Over Days, Weeks & Months

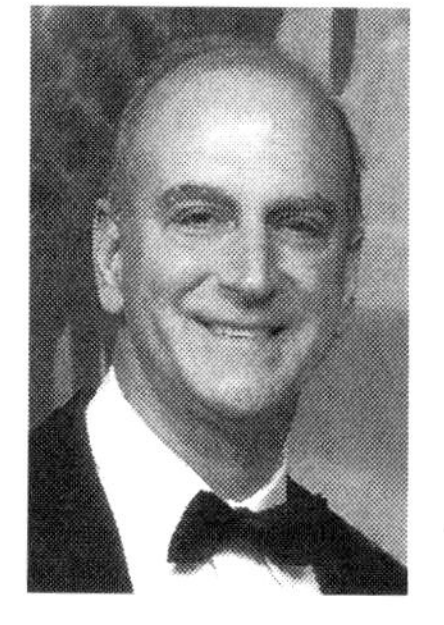

Dr. Ronald Sandler, Golden Ratio Peak Performance Pioneer

Nature's Path of Least Resistance, Maximum Efficiency and High Performance follows the Golden Ratio.

Dr. Ronald Sandler, peak performance pioneer

Peak performance pioneer **Dr. Ronald Sandler** is the man behind the Golden Ratio exercise training breakthrough—**a Copernican revolution in fitness and training.** He created what we describe today as Nature's Energy Wave / N•E•W, originally presented in his ground-breaking book *Consistent Winning*, which shows how anyone can optimize training periods of activity and rest by scheduling workouts according to Golden Ratios (Dr. Sandler's reengineered new book for the 21st century, *50 Pages to Peak Performance in Sports, Fitness & Life* will be released in 2022). By tuning exercise and rest/recovery periods to Fibonacci Sequence numbers spaced over days, weeks and months, a super-synergy emerges that bestows any athlete with a massively powerful yet totally natural performance advantage.

This dynamic metabolic catapult becomes a secret weapon strategy for scheduling workouts and rest periods in order to predictably peak on a selected future date. In 1982, Dr. Sandler discovered how to maximize the impact of any workout, regardless of intensity, without investing unnecessary effort and time—while simultaneously minimizing the chances of overtraining and injury. He had the flash of insight into how cycles of human activity, as reflected in Nature and the ups and downs of the stock

Nature's Energy Wave™ [N•E•W]: Peak Performance & Fitness on Demand

Nature's fundamental wave motion, mirrored by the Golden Ratio Spiral & Fibonacci Sequence, can be harnessed to schedule Peak Performances on exact days, weeks or months ahead. **N•E•W** puts the wind at your back to be your best when you need it most, while building in the vital rest/recovery catapult loading periods optimal performance requires. All athletes & fitness enthusiasts can use the Wave to safely maximize health & fitness, keep workouts fresh and optimize sports performance and enjoyment over a lifetime. Whether on the field or in the classroom, boardroom or stage, anyone wanting to perform their best in any arena can use Nature's Energy Wave as their secret success weapon.

- **NATURE'S ENERGY WAVE [N•E•W]** tapers you **up** for 2 days prior to your event vs. tapering **down** as in conventional systems. *A predictable peak occurs on the 3rd day back after a rest/recovery period.*
- **TO SET YOUR PEAK PERFORMANCE** count backwards from your event/race date, using the 1-wk (6-day), 3-wk (26-day), 5-wk (35-day) or 3-month (97-day) cycles. All 4 cycles can be superimposed for maximum synergy.
- **N•E•W REST & RECOVERY** down-waves are essential to load the Fibonacci catapult effect: 3 steps back/5 steps forward, or 5 steps back/8 steps forward.

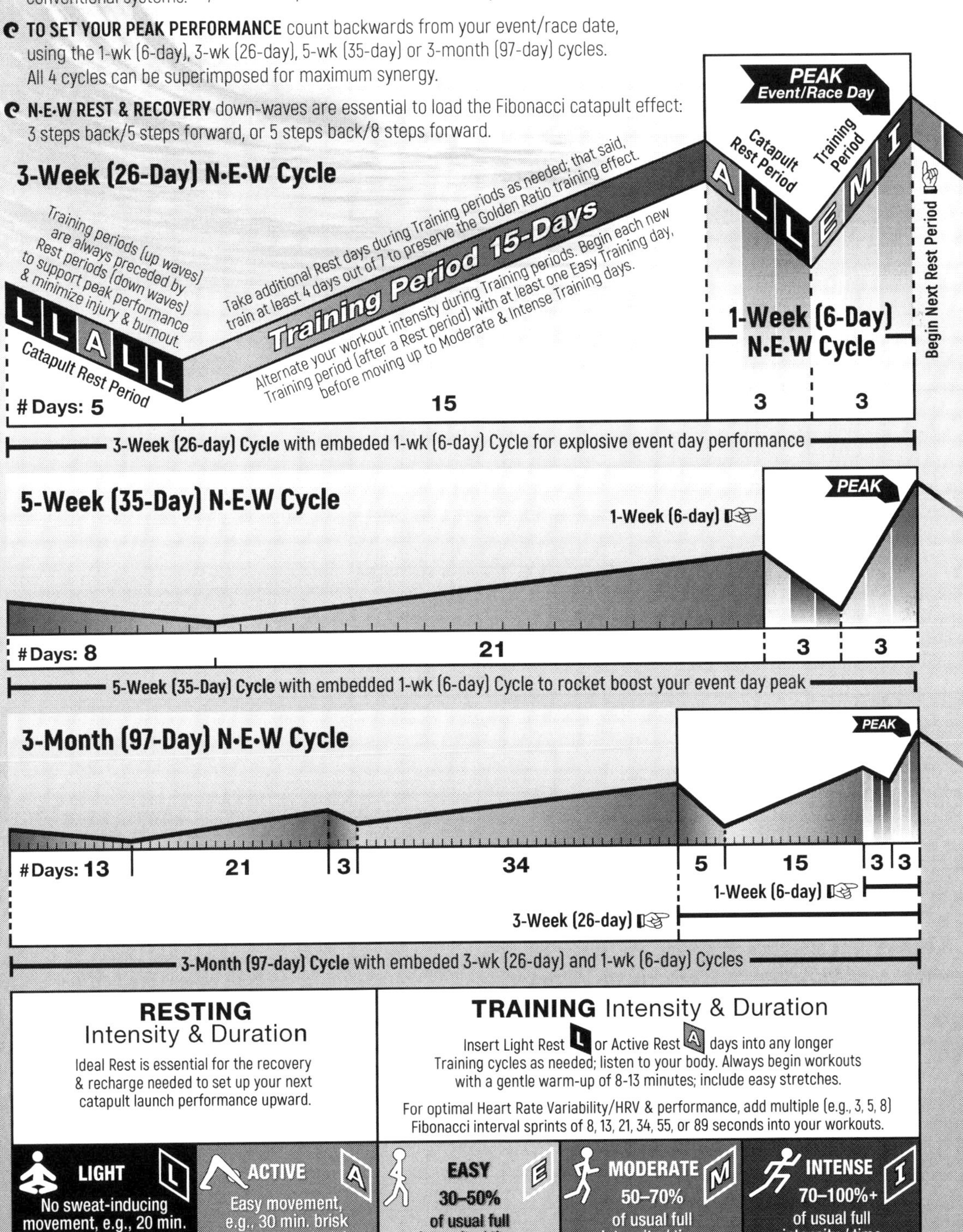

PEAK
Event/Race Day
3-Week (26-Day) N•E•W Cycle
Training periods (up waves) are always preceded by Rest periods (down waves) to support peak performance & minimize injury & burnout.
Take additional Rest days during Training periods as needed; that said, train at least 4 days out of 7 to preserve the Golden Ratio training effect.
Training Period 15-Days
Alternate your workout intensity during Training periods. Begin each new Training period (after a Rest period) with at least one Easy Training day, before moving up to Moderate & Intense Training days.
Catapult Rest Period
Training Period
L L A L L
A L L E M I
1-Week (6-Day) N•E•W Cycle
Begin Next Rest Period
Days: 5
15
3
3
3-Week (26-day) Cycle with embeded 1-wk (6-day) Cycle for explosive event day performance
5-Week (35-Day) N•E•W Cycle
PEAK
1-Week (6-day)
Days: 8
21
3
3
5-Week (35-Day) Cycle with embedded 1-wk (6-day) Cycle to rocket boost your event day peak
3-Month (97-Day) N•E•W Cycle
PEAK
Days: 13
21
3
34
5
15
3
3
1-Week (6-day)
3-Week (26-day)
3-Month (97-day) Cycle with embeded 3-wk (26-day) and 1-wk (6-day) Cycles
RESTING
Intensity & Duration
Ideal Rest is essential for the recovery & recharge needed to set up your next catapult launch performance upward.
TRAINING Intensity & Duration
Insert Light Rest L or Active Rest A days into any longer Training cycles as needed; listen to your body. Always begin workouts with a gentle warm-up of 8-13 minutes; include easy stretches.
For optimal Heart Rate Variability/HRV & performance, add multiple (e.g., 3, 5, 8) Fibonacci interval sprints of 8, 13, 21, 34, 55, or 89 seconds into your workouts.
LIGHT L
No sweat-inducing movement, e.g., 20 min. easy walk, yoga, stretch
ACTIVE A
Easy movement, e.g., 30 min. brisk walk, yoga, stretch
EASY E
30–50%
of usual full intensity / time
MODERATE M
50–70%
of usual full intensity / time
INTENSE I
70–100%+
of usual full intensity / time

Ironman Dave "The Man" Scott: The Vast Power of Rest & Recovery

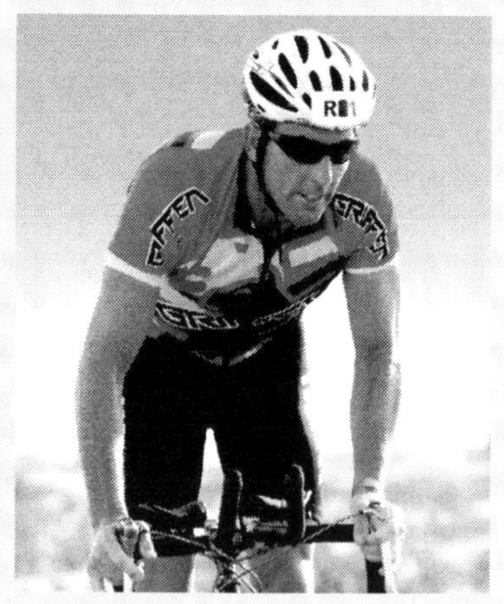

Dave "The Man" Scott, 6-time Ironman World Triathlon Champion.

Among his compelling research stories, **Dr. Ronald Sandler** describes how Dave Scott, six-time winner of the grueling Ironman Triathlon, unknowingly utilized the essential Fibonacci-based Golden Ratio training technique enroute to his 1986 and 1987 Ironman victories. The legendary Scott found himself forced to take many unintentional rest periods of three to five days due to speaking engagements and other commitments, before the 1986 and 1987 races. Initially, Scott was concerned that these unplanned rest periods would negatively affect his race performance. To his great surprise however, the opposite proved true:

The more time I missed the better I did. After about five days off I felt lethargic and stiff, but then I felt better in training than before.

6

In the 1986 Ironman Scott set a course record. In 1987 he won again, in what he considered to be his best race—even though his time was 5 minutes slower than in 1986 due to far tougher conditions, including severe headwinds. Scott's unintentional, Golden Ratio resting periods played a strategic role in his victories. Dave retired from competition in 1989 at 35, around the time Dr. Sandler introduced him to the Golden Ratio training system. 5 years later, at age 40, Scott made a stunning comeback at the Ironman, coming out of retirement to celebrate becoming the Ironman Hall of Fame's first inductee. His finishing time that year, 1994, won him 2nd place, *eclipsing all six of his previous first-place finish times* and missing winning his 7th title by just 4 minutes. In 1996, at 42, Scott returned, this time placing 5th and clocking his third-fastest finishing time—*which again beat all six of his previous first-place finish times at the Ironman.*

Dave Scott's Ironman Finish Times

Year	Age	Place	Time
1980	26	1	9:24:33
1982	28	1	9:08:23
1983	29	1	9:05:57
1984	30	1	8:54:20
1986	32	1	8:28:37
1987	33	1	8:34:13
1994	40	2	**8:24:32**
1996	42	5	**8:28:31**

market, could be applied to athletic performance. In the case of human athletic performance, it was the natural exercise and rest cycles that were related through the Golden Ratio and Fibonacci Sequence. Dr. Sandler realized that just as stock market fluctuations move up and down in Golden Ratio (via what are known in the finance world as **Elliott Waves**), so are optimal exercise and rest cycles similarly related. He subsequently amassed extensive data to support his theory through decades of observational study, personal experience and real-world application with patients and athletes from multiple sports, from weekend warriors to world-class competitors. With N•E•W you can successfully ***plan ahead*** for peak performance, while avoiding injury and burnout. Best of all it works for both competitive and noncompetitive athletes—and performers in any arena, on the field or off.

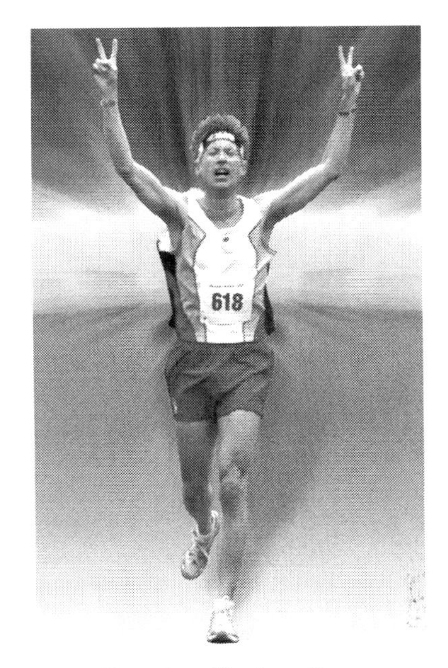

Co-author Matthew Cross utilizes Nature's Energy Wave to train for and win 5k races; he's seen here demonstrating a power pose variation, the classic arms-high "V for Victory."

Every athlete, competitive or those just wishing to stay fit, knows that some days you just don't have it, no matter how consistently or how hard you train. Yet on other days you feel an unexpected surge that enables you to turn in a great performance. How can you better understand those days of sustained energy and those of unexpected lethargy? The secret lies in honoring the ratios between exercise and rest periods required to balance and energize your whole body, mind and spirit. As we've learned in Ch 3/Sleep from World's Fittest Man and 6-time Ironman Triathlete champion **Mark Allen**, *95% of athletes are over-trained [under-rested]*. Nature's Energy Wave / N•E•W uses precise ratios of training and rest/recovery tuned to the Golden Ratio, assuring that you're *optimally* vs. *over* trained. These waves are a natural yet latent element of your physiologic cycles and biorhythms. Learning to ignite and manage these waves so you maintain high energy and drive—and peak when needed if you're competitive—is what Nature's Energy Wave / N•E•W delivers. To recap Nature's Energy Wave / N•E•W's benefits to guide your training:

- Φ You can predict, plan and schedule *in advance* when your peak day will be—with great accuracy—weeks and even months ahead of your event or race! **The predictive power of this universal principle applies to athletes at all levels, from fitness exercisers to competitive and world-class athletes.**
- Φ You can greatly reduce the potential for injury, while virtually eliminating burnout.

Just as we've seen how the FIT Short, Medium and Long Wave workouts make use of the Golden Ratio to structure exercise intervals over *seconds, minutes and hours,* the Nature's Energy Wave / N•E•W system likewise uses the Golden Ratio to plan exercise and rest/recovery cycles, **yet over extended time cycles—days, weeks and months.** N•E•W workouts are especially applicable for competitive athletes who want to plan a peak performance on a specific day in the future, such as for a race. The system also applies just as well to fitness exercisers who want to optimize their exercise regimen over time. Since N•E•W structures exercise in Fibonacci-numbered days, weeks and months cycles, they create a similar Golden Ratio catapult effect as do the FIT Short, Medium and Long Wave workouts, yet over longer cycles of time. The beauty of the N•E•W system is that it creates a large container within which the FIT Wave Workouts can be embedded. All FIT Waves can be easily superimposed upon one another, creating the conditions for NSN super-synergy and resulting predictable peak performance—the Holy Grail of competitive athletic training. In addition to turning in stellar performances, the most overlooked benefits of using FIT Waves concurrently are the prevention of injury and burnout. **These benefits alone are worth their weight in gold.** For competitive athletes interested in improving conditioning for athletic competition, the total FIT Wave approach (Short, Medium & Long Waves) combined with Nature's Energy Wave / N•E•W is a powerful secret weapon. *It loads your metabolic catapult, ensuring predictable peak performances in any chosen competition—days, weeks or even months away.* For non-competitive fitness exercisers, it also offers an enjoyable and efficient way to safely stair-step your way up to increasing levels of health and fitness.

SECTION 3: NSN Fitness Innovations

Split Workouts: *Increase* Exercise Benefits in *Less* Time

When NBA superstar **Baron Davis** was with the New Orleans Hornets basketball team, he demonstrated the little-known yet astonishing benefits of splitting workouts. At that time, due to overtraining and resulting poor performance, Davis' $80 million contract was in jeopardy. Instead of continuing his downward spiral by working out for six hours straight as was his usual practice, Davis' lead trainer **Dartgnan Stamps** split his off-season daily training regimen into two separate sessions—one in the morning, the other that afternoon. In so doing, they took advantage of a little-known leverage principle in fitness dynamics. **By splitting his workout in two—with rest and refueling in between—Davis was able to substantially increase the impact of his training.** He regained his superstar status and was able to perform at his full potential. For the average person, this means for example that two separate 20 minute sessions,

Maximizing Exercise Benefits: Smart Intensity, Frequency & Duration

Exercise in our time, like nutrition, has become a subject filled with countless interpretations, misunderstandings and in many cases, sheer dread. The entire concept of "scheduled regular exercise" in itself is a relatively recent phenomenon. **Throughout history exercise was simply *movement*—a natural part of daily lifestyle, not something that had to be jammed into a schedule.** In addition, exercise has become ruled by the *More/Intense is Better* mind-set. This has resulted in the unquestioned excesses of intensity, frequency & duration, coupled with unhealthy Heart Rate Variability (HRV) and insufficient rest/recovery. In addition, many people falsely believe that they can exercise healthfully even when they're under-slept. Be smart and safe: exercise when you're well-hydrated, well-rested and well-nourished. **Last yet not least, remember to keep it FUN. Enjoyable Movement = Sustainable Fitness.**

Key obvious POSITIVE Effects of Exercise, when in PROPER RATIO

- Regulates and optimizes all body processes, including digestion, sleep, hormones and sexual function.
- Tonifies, detoxifies and beautifies the body.
- Builds a sense of accomplishment and self-esteem.
- Clears the mind, enhances creativity and sharpens focus.
- Improves strength, endurance, flexibility and coordination.
- Reduces stress & releases endorphins, elevates mood, bestows a natural high.

Key not-so-obvious NEGATIVE Effects/Risks of Exercise, when OVERDONE

- Over-exercising causes inflammation, a leading cause of disease, dysfunction and premature aging.
- Over-exercising can result in muscle damage: micro tears—and if too long and/or intense, macro tears—in the form of strains and resultant scarring. This is especially concerning when you consider the impact of long-term repeated micro scarring on your **#1 life and longevity muscle: your HEART.**
- If overdone, can result in skeletal, ligament or tendon injuries, which can sideline you for weeks or even months—never fun.
- When exercise reaches into the zones of excess intensity, frequency, duration and/or monotony, e.g., extreme steady-state or Long Slow Distance/LSD, coupled with insufficient recovery, it can result in injuries, immune system suppression, burnout, compromised longevity and even premature death.

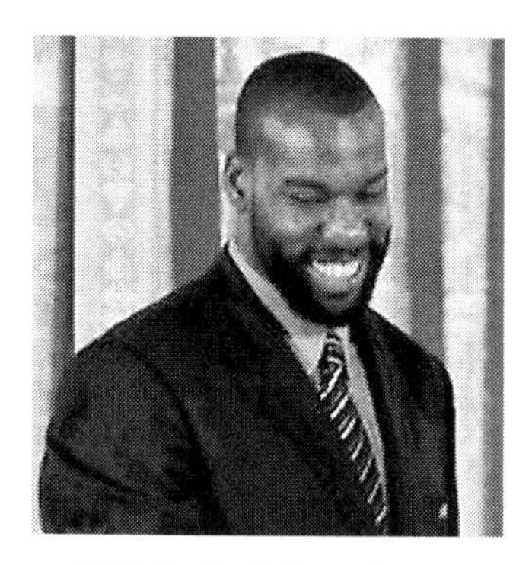

NBA basketball star Baron Davis demonstrated the great benefits of split workouts for peak performance and strong recovery.

with rest and refueling in between, could be as beneficial as one continuous 60-minute workout—a vast gain in exercise efficiency and impact. **This simple, powerful method of achieving more results with less effort was successful because of the increase of the *ratio* of rest to exercise.** Another great example of the benefits of increasing the rest-to-exercise ratio is research conducted at the Human Energy Research Laboratory at the University of Pittsburgh. This study revealed the hidden advantages of multiple, shorter daily workouts. It showed that women who did two or three separate daily 15–20 minute workouts—instead of the typical longer 30–60 minute single workout—burned more fat and lost up to 25% more weight. They were also far more likely to stick with their exercise regimen over time. This research exploded the popular myth that you have to exercise a minimum of 30 minutes or more to receive an aerobic or fat burning benefit. Multiple same-day exercise sessions, as short as 13 minutes each, can provide greater benefits than longer, single workout sessions. When combined with Fibonacci Interval Training (FIT), superior fitness in less time becomes a sustainable reality.

> *Iron rusts from disuse; water loses its purity from stagnation...*
> *even so does inaction sap the vigor of the mind.*
>
> **Leonardo da Vinci**

In these examples, the subjects were honoring the crucial rest phase in relation to the exercise period—and reaping the massive rewards. You can also strongly amplify the positive effects of your exercise by simply breaking it into two or more smaller sessions over the course of a day. This practice maximizes recovery and healing, while simultaneously minimizing the chances of burnout and injury. When you know that two daily workouts as short as 10 minutes each can actually be equivalent to 30 minutes of total exercise, you're far more likely to get in that 10 minute walk or run in the morning and then again that afternoon or evening. An easy way to generate NSN from a split workout is to do a FIT Medium Wave 13 minute AM workout, followed by a 21 minute PM workout. Depending on your goals and time, the duration of your AM/PM workouts can be changed to different Fibonacci Numbers—21/34, 34/21, 34/55 or 55/34.

GOT *Ratio*? The **G**olden **O**lympic **T**raining Ratio for Optimal Endurance, Strength & Flexibility/Balance/Coordination (FBC)

Dawn Saidur is a former world-class sprinter and the first person from Bangladesh to represent his country in the Olympics (1984, Los Angeles). Now based in Mamaroneck, NY, Dawn owns and operates the popular Mozart Café. As a sports performance psychologist, he also trains competitive athletes. Dawn notes that the optimal training ratio time spent on Endurance, Strength and Flexibility/Balance/Coordination (FBC) regardless of one's total weekly training hours, is *not* an even 3-way split. **Instead, this Golden Olympic Training Ratio turns out to be a 40/30/30 split, tailored to your specific sport or fitness aim.** Recall from Ch 4 Nutrition that a 40:30:30 ratio can be reconfigured as a 40:60 ratio and used as an approximation of the 38:62 Golden Ratio. This ratio supports a dynamic, cross-reinforcing balance of Endurance, Strength and FBC. The example pie graph below is weighted towards Endurance—40%. If you wanted to focus more on Strength for a specific sport, strength training would move into the 40% position. Accordingly if you wanted more Flexibility/Balance/Coordination (FBC), you'd increase FBC to 40%, and so on. Finding your personal Golden Olympic Training Ratio is a golden key to maximizing the efficiency and enjoyment of your chosen sport.

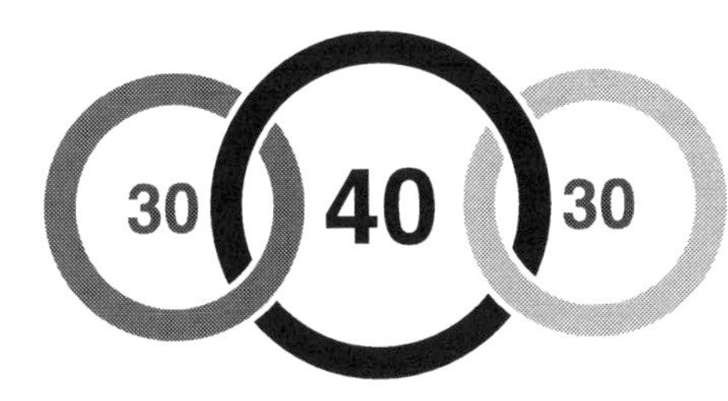

Example of endurance-weighted **G**olden **O**lympic **T**raining Ratio of Endurance, Strength and Flexibility/ Balance/Coordination (FBC). The larger/40% segment is always weighted towards your chosen sport's focus, to optimize your results in that arena. Maintaining a customized balance of these 3 training segments is a cornerstone of optimal fitness, performance and longevity.

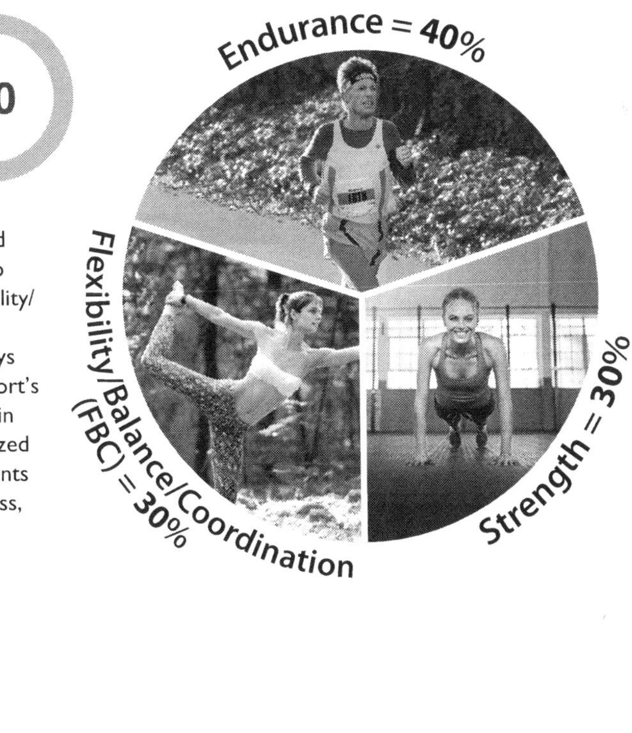

6

Active Isolated Stretching (AIS): Finding Your Golden Ratio Limit

Active Isolated Stretching (AIS) is a revolutionary physical therapy for restoring flexibility and range of motion to muscles, tendons and joints. Developed by Kinesiotherapy pioneer **Aaron Mattes**, Active Isolated Stretching (AIS) has helped rehabilitate many top athletes, e.g., football legend Johnny Unitas, Olympians Carl Lewis and Michael Johnson, tennis champions Pete Sampras and Andre Agassi, basketball greats Michael Jordan and Shaquille O'Neill and many other athletes. **Mattes discovered that muscles can stretch 1.6 times (the Golden Ratio) their resting length before tearing—yet another great example of the Golden Ratio's embeddedness in our physiology at all levels.** Mattes' method might be considered unorthodox, according to conventional wisdom, e.g., he's a proponent of short dynamic stretches vs. long static stretches, advising that the longest a full stretch be held is ***2 seconds.*** Six-time Ironman Champion triathlete & *Outside* magazine's *World's Fittest Man* **Mark Allen** told co-author Matthew Cross that ***full stretches should never exceed a half-second.*** According to *Stretching USA:*

> *Over the past decades many experts have advocated prolonged stretches up to 60 seconds. For years, this prolonged static stretch technique was the gold standard. Yet prolonged static stretching actually* ***decreases*** *the blood flow within the tissue, creating localized ischemia and lactic acid buildup.* ***This potentiates irritation or injury of local muscular, tendinous, lymphatic as well as neural tissues, similar to the effects and consequences of trauma and overuse syndromes*** [authors' emphasis].

6

The Active Isolated Stretching (AIS) System challenges long-standing principles popular in yoga and other traditional stretching systems. The age-old notion of holding stretches for long periods needs critical reevaluation. Mattes' research reveals that remaining in a pose for an extended amount of time may not be the optimal way to stretch. In addition to inhibiting your protective stretch reflex, holding postures and stretches too long can cause actual tissue suffocation, enabling lactic acid and other metabolites to build up to toxic levels. Long-held static stretches prevent the adequate blood circulation needed to oxygenate tissues and clear toxins. Muscular micro-tears are also far more likely under

Relaxed Muscle Length 1.0

Maximum Muscle Stretch Range 1.6

$1.6/1.0 = \Phi$

The Golden Ratio Muscle Stretch Range. Master Kinesiotherapist Aaron Mattes discovered that muscles will stretch 1.6 times (the Golden Ratio Φ) their resting length before tearing. He recommends not holding any stretch longer than 2 seconds; 6-time Ironman Triathlon Champion Mark Allen suggests just a half-second.

these hypoxic (low oxygen) conditions. Innovative stretching and movement approaches like Mattes' AIS system—with full stretches not exceeding 2 seconds—and other dynamic systems such as ***The Genius of Flexibility*** **Bob Cooley's Resistance Stretching®** (utilized by Olympic gold medal swimmer Dara Torres) are highly recommended. These breakthrough systems in stretching and movement therapy can replace other potentially damaging stretching methods. They support the healthy restoration and maintenance of your body's natural Golden Ratio proportions *and* performance.

Golden Ratio Movement: Maximum Efficiency, Minimum Effort

The impulse of all movement and all form is given by Phi Φ [the Golden Ratio].

Schwaller de Lubicz, *The Temple of Man*

Eastern mind-body exercise disciplines such as yoga, tai chi, karate and other martial arts are based on principles that integrate and unify the natural spiral anatomy of the spine, bones, muscles and organs. These disciplines teach you to be aware of your breathing, body and its responses as you perform specified movements. Since your body's structure and form are designed with the Golden Ratio, you'll find that your body naturally functions best when moving to the Golden Spiral—the path of least resistance and flow. A simple example:

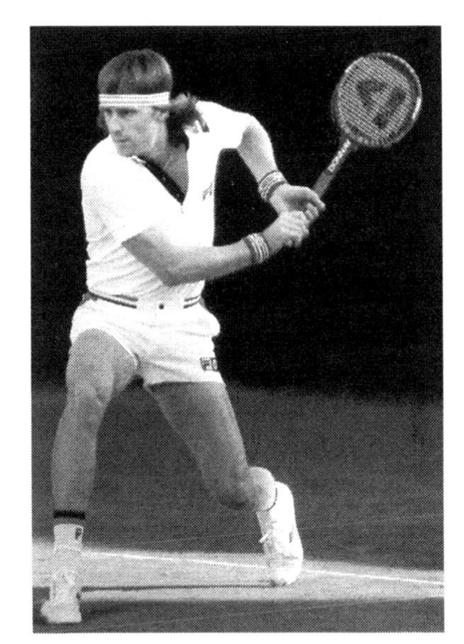

Swedish tennis legend Bjorn Borg vanquished many opponents with his devastating, spiraling strokes which generated enormous topspin, power and accuracy.

> *Sitting with spine erect & weight equally balanced on your sitz bones (your derriere's bony parts), begin to move your pelvis in a gentle spiraling motion, starting in the center of an imaginary spiral and unwinding 3 times, tracing an expanding Golden Spiral. Then spiral back to the center by reversing the exercise. Note that the Golden Spiral moves up through the spine and entire body, even though it's initiated in your pelvis. As you spiral back to center, the spiral's center may feel like a gentle still point. Pause and enjoy the feeling for a few moments.*

When you move in Golden Spirals, you're moving along *Nature's Path of Least Resistance & Maximum Efficiency & Performance.* And like a Bjorn Borg or a Roger Federer, graceful,

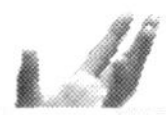

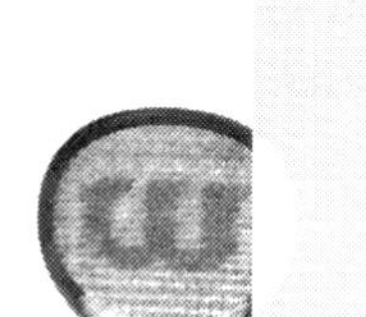

Roger Federer's Golden Ratio ADvantage

Seen and unseen Golden Ratios abound in the work of geniuses everywhere, including Swiss tennis great Roger Federer. Renowned for his fluid grace, a 2016 injury imposed a first-ever 6-month rest/recovery period, reducing his usual heavy training/tournament schedule towards more Golden Ratio balance—*leading up to his 18th Grand Slam title at the 2017 Australian Open.* More Golden Ratio links arise from Mark Hodgkinson's statistical analysis in his fantastic book *Fedegraphica: A Graphic Biography of the Genius of Roger Federer.* For example: Among current and past tennis greats, only Roger's career first serve percentage is **exactly 62%**, with **62%** of his aces landing in the ad court; **38%** in the deuce court. **62% & 62:38 = the Golden Ratio,** Game, Set and Match. *Tennis anyone?*

more effortless movement flows forth. Let your body sense this natural unity of form and function. Learn to recognize spiral tendencies in your movements. Whenever Golden and other spirals become conscious parts of your movement, a powerful message flows through your body. Sports like golf and tennis contain multidimensional spiral motions, as do the movements in many sports and exercises like yoga and tai chi. Spiral motions naturally correct structural problems such as back pain and other joint ailments. Improved posture, balance, coordination and timing will positively impact any sport or movement routine you enjoy. *Awareness that spirals are Nature in motion reminds us to integrate them into our daily life.* Spiralic movement helps you move through life and sports with least resistance and most efficiency—which also reduces chances of injury.

> *Exercise to stimulate, not annihilate.*
>
> **Lee Haney, 8-time Mr. Olympia**

Rob Moses & David Carradine: Spiral Fitness & the Human Gear

Sifu Rob Moses is the Kung Fu wizard behind the cutting-edge Spiral Fitness System, whose movements mirror the Nature's Golden Ratio geometry found in Nature. In his

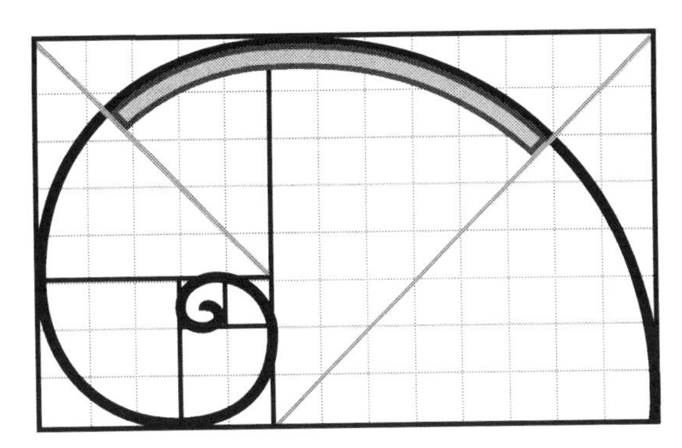

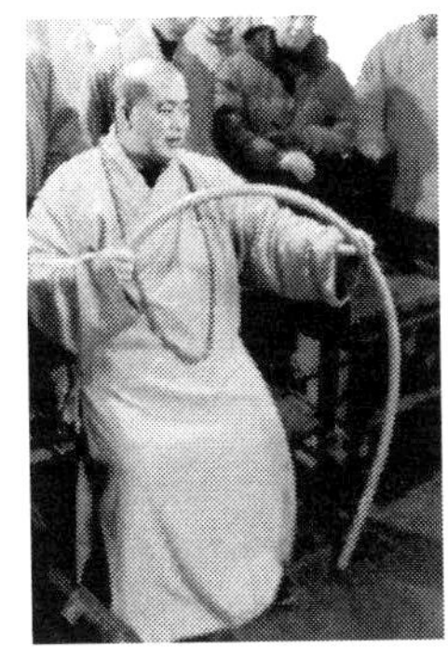

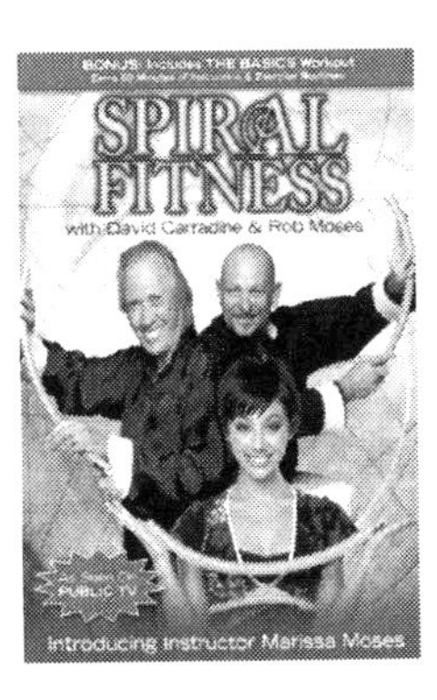

(*L*) The PhysioStix's design is a section of the Golden Spiral. (*C*) Shaolin Monk with PhysioStix long version. (*R*) ***Spiral Fitness*** DVD cover, showing actor David Carradine, Rob and Marissa Moses.

system, Kung Fu's aggressive animal archetypes are transformed into gentler, peaceful movements. Rob's best-known student was *Kung Fu's* **David Carradine**, who he trained for 25 years and on 3 movies: *Kung Fu, The Legend Continues* and Quentin Tarantino's *Kill Bill I & II*. Moses took Nature's invisible Path of Least Resistance and manifested it in his **PhysioStix—a Fibonacci-based fitness/workout stick**—which he describes as follows:

> *Humankind has harnessed natural movement for exercise, healing and survival. Throughout history movement has evolved by emulating Nature. The Fibonacci Spiral represents a prime way Nature expands and contracts; it is Nature's formula for beauty and strength and the ultimate* **Human Gear**. *The PhysioStix design is based on the Fibonacci Spiral in order to tap into this universal dynamic of movement-alchemy. It helps you activate your highest potential by enhancing your circulation, articulation and breathing. Movement becomes free flowing, like liquid. It offers a perpetual approach to the martial arts while minimizing bloodshed imagery. This truth holds up at all velocities, allowing the practitioner to resonate at a frequency close to that of plant growth, shaping itself like infinite seashells expressible in all directions.*

The evolution of the martial arts has taken a quantum leap with Sifu Rob Moses' Spiral Fitness system, of which David Carradine was a leading proponent. The heretofore-invisible secret of martial arts, the Golden Spiral, has been distilled into a visible and fun guidance tool, through which healing and transformative movement flows. The PhysioStix training tool is designed with Nature's intelligence in mind and makes a great addition to your Golden Ratio Workout gym bag. **GoldenSpiralWellness.com**

WrightBalance® for Peak Performance in Golf & All Sports

Golf professional and biomechanics expert **Dr. David Wright** discovered that restoring Golden Ratio postural relationships in the body ensures a balanced symmetrical core, essential for deriving maximum ground force from your golf swing. Optimal balance is determined by your stance width, hip and shoulder alignment, ball position and grip size. A golf swing tracks the natural anatomical Golden Spirals in the body: function following form. The slightest deviation at the beginning of the swing is amplified as the swing progresses, resulting in both power loss and outside-in or inside-out distortions. Such small initial perturbations which lead to large effects downstream are similar to the **Butterfly Effect**: *When a butterfly flaps its wings in one part of the world, a hurricane can result thousands of miles away.* The pressure plate measurements from a golfer's feet Dr. Wright uses in his analyses look uncannily like the designs on a butterfly's wings. Any perturbations or symmetrical imbalances are easy to identify and correct. Since all golfers wish to avoid the dreaded slice, hook or shank, great benefits can be enjoyed from Dr. Wright's approach, aka the WrightBalance® system; this easy-to-learn Golden Ratio postural restoration method also applies to many sports. **wrightbalance.com**

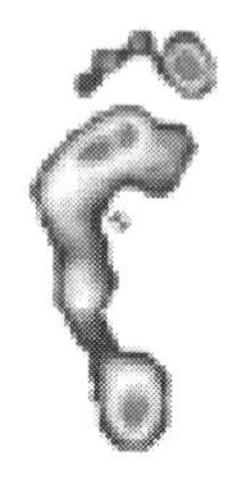

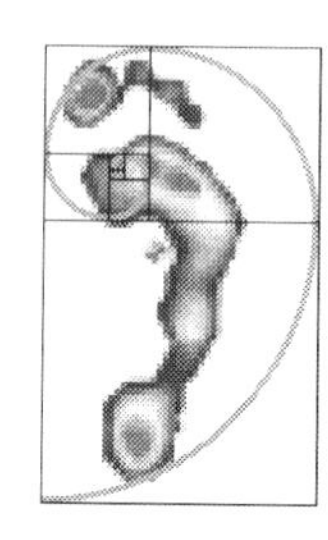

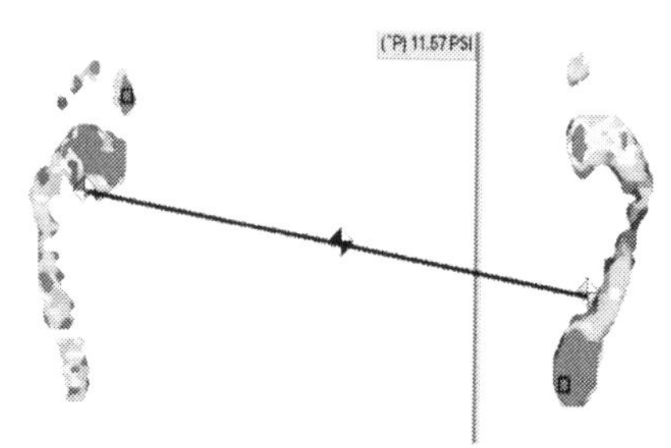

(*L*) Pressure plate imagery of a golfer's feet resembles a butterfly's wings, revealing a perfectly balanced, symmetrical stance. The butterfly effect of Golden Ratio symmetry can then move through the entire swing. (*R*) Asymmetrical pressure plate imagery of an imbalanced golfer's stance, likely to increase the chance of a slice, hook or shank. Line connecting the feet represents the degree that the pelvis is torqued.

SECTION 4: Golden Ratio Cardiovascular Dynamics

Golden Ratio Blood Pressure Decreases Death Risk

In a ground-breaking scientific discovery, Austrian statistician **Hanno Ulmer, Ph.D.**, and his research group confirmed our Golden Ratio hypothesis that having one's systolic:diastolic blood pressure in Golden Ratio is *highly* beneficial to your health and longevity. They evaluated a substantial primary care-based patient cohort of 166,377 people and found that the systolic:diastolic blood pressure ratio was 1.618—the Golden Ratio—in participants who *didn't* die during the 20 year study and 1.745 in people who did die during that same period. They concluded that,

> *...blood pressure values in 'well' individuals, but not in those who are at risk of dying, exhibit the* ***Golden Ratio.***

This is a staggering confirmation of the Golden Ratio's heretofore unrecognized power to promote great health and longevity. We must always consider both quality *and* quantity when looking at physiological parameters, such as blood pressure; **maintaining quality in this case means keeping your systolic and diastolic pressures in Golden Ratio.** Maintaining quantity is making sure that blood pressure doesn't get too high, even though the systolic and diastolic pressures may be in Golden Ratio. For example, a blood pressure of 160/100 (a 1.6 ratio), although typically considered high, is in Golden Ratio and will afford some level of protection against death as evidenced by Dr. Ulmer's study. However, a greater level of health and survivability could be obtained by having both an overall lower blood pressure in addition to being in Golden Ratio, e.g., in the range of 120/75 (a 1.6 ratio). **The power of viewing and fine-tuning key physiological parameters through the Golden Ratio is being validated before our eyes, unleashing nothing less than a Copernican revolution in health and medicine.** How? By revealing a simple low-tech yet high-impact method to: 1. Reconceptualize valuable diagnostic information about our bodily systems; 2. Allow us to harness its therapeutic power in rebalancing out-of-ratio physiology through the simple application of the Golden Ratio/NSN.

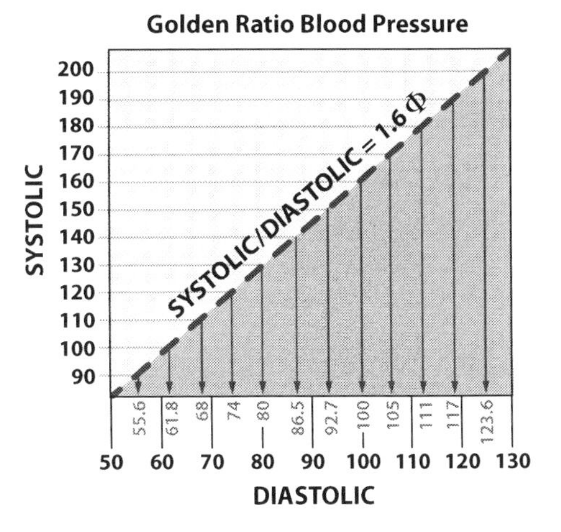

6

Balancing Blood Pressure the Golden Ratio Way

Since the blood pressure cuff's invention in 1881, physicians have missed the crucial observation that blood pressure readings often reflect the Golden Ratio. Our bodies have a finely-tuned homeostatic mechanism that strives to maintain the Golden Ratio with respect to systolic and diastolic blood pressure. For example, a so-called normal blood pressure has been typically reported as 120/80: a ratio of 1.5. **Viewed through the Golden Ratio lens, a truly normal blood pressure reading would be in the range of 120/75: a ratio of 1.6.** You could have numerous other normal Golden Ratio readings, as long as the ratio of the systolic to diastolic is around 1.6. Even if a person has high blood pressure, the body's wisdom still strives to maintain the Golden Ratio. A blood pressure reading of 160/100, though high, gives a ratio of 1.6. This Golden Ratio compensation keeps the physiology efficiently functioning through a wide range of bodily stressors, even though the long-term deleterious effects of hypertension may still occur. Once the Golden Ratio of systolic to diastolic blood pressure is lost, general adaptation is compromised and the individual may begin suffering a more rapid downward spiral in their health. In the future, blood pressure measuring devices (sphygmomanometers) may well have a window that calculates the ratio of systolic to diastolic pressure to inform the user how close to the more optimal Golden Ratio they are.

Your Speedometer: An Easy Golden Ratio Blood Pressure Gauge

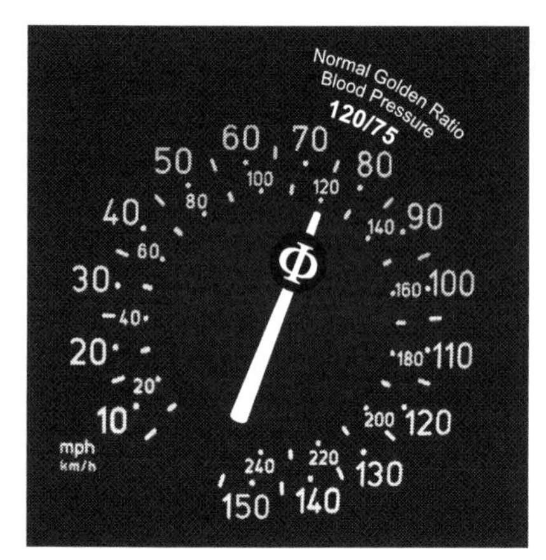

You can use your speedometer to determine Golden Ratio Blood Pressure.

An fun Golden Ratio conversion method also allows for quick plotting of your blood pressure readings to see how close they are to the Golden Ratio: an automobile speedometer, showing miles per hour (mph) alongside kilometers per hour (km/h). The speedometer's scale reveals an open secret: **the ratio of mph to km/h is very close to the Golden Ratio—and can also be used to evaluate blood pressure readings,** e.g., you'll notice that the following Golden Ratio readings are plain to see on your speedometer, and resemble various possible blood pressure readings:

100 km/h = 60 mph
120 km/h = 75 mph } **Φ 1.6 Golden Ratio**
160 km/h = 100 mph

To see if your blood pressure readings are in Golden Ratio range, find your systolic reading (the higher of your two blood pressure numbers) on the kilometers/hour (km/h) line. Then look directly across at the miles/hour (mph) line and plot your diastolic reading (the lower of your two blood pressure numbers) in miles/hour (mph). If your systolic reading is directly across from your diastolic reading, then they are in Golden

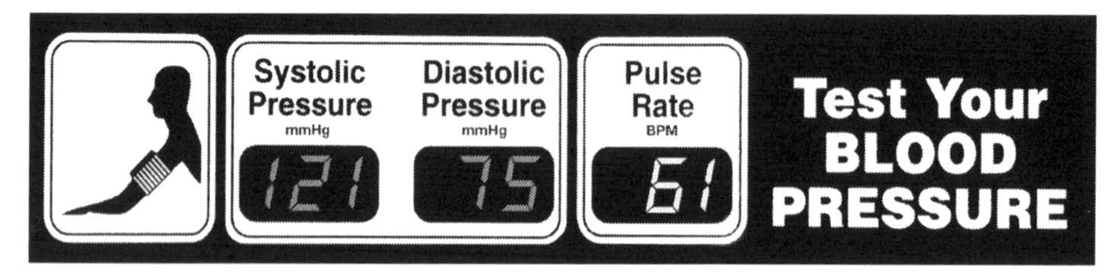

Automated blood pressure device showing a perfect Systolic:Diastolic Golden Ratio of 1.6.
Simply divide the larger number (Systolic) by the smaller number (Diastolic) to calculate your ratio, e.g., 121/75 = 1.61. Easy-use home blood pressure monitors are reasonably priced and available online.

The Golden Ratio Heart of the Matter

ECG Form and Function: In a healthy heart's Electrocardiogram (ECG), contraction (QRS) and relaxation (T) waves are in Golden Ratio to one another. Many other Golden Ratios and their harmonics can be found between the electrical signatures in a healthy ECG. In unhealthy and disease states these Golden Ratio relationships are invariably lost.

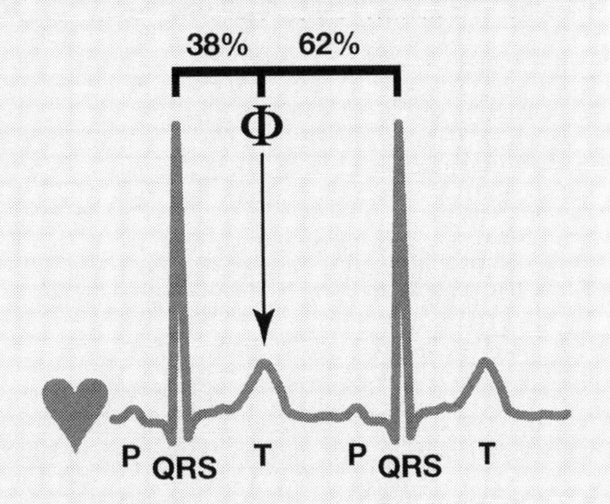

6

Our hearts are aligned structurally and functionally with the Golden Ratio.
Note the multiple Golden Spirals in our hearts design.

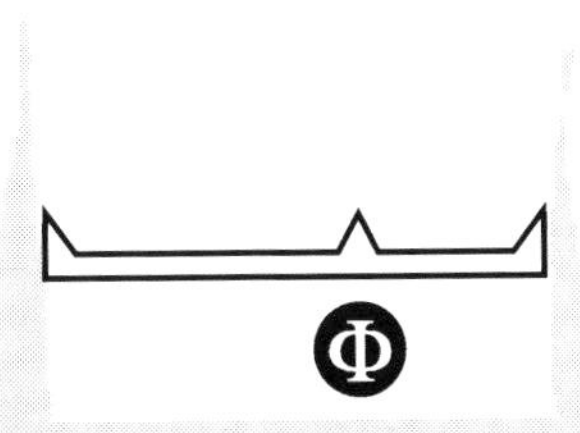

The human heart is located ***off-center*** at the horizontal Golden Ratio point of the chest.

Ratio. Golden Ratio blood pressure evaluations always look at *quality* and *quantity*. Whether or not the systolic and diastolic readings are in Golden Ratio determines the *quality* of the reading. How high or low the readings are determines the *quantity*. In the speedometer examples above, 100/60 is considered borderline low blood pressure, yet still maintains a Golden Ratio. 120/75 is in the normal range and is also in Golden Ratio. 160/100 is considered high blood pressure, yet still maintains the Golden Ratio. Even if a blood pressure reading is too high or too low—*quantity*—there is still a presumed physiologic advantage if it's in Golden Ratio—*quality*. If your blood pressure readings are either too high or too low and/or aren't right across from one another on your speedometer, start incorporating the Nature's Secret Nutrient recommendations into your life, in addition to consulting with your physician or health care professional.

Golden Ratio Resting Heart Rate & Longevity

A 2014 study by **Mark Woodward**, et. al., in the *European Journal of Preventive Cardiology* revealed a strong association between elevated **resting heart rate** over 65 beats min. and both overall mortality and stroke. **Each 10 beats/min increase in *resting heart rate* resulted in a 10%-20% increase in mortality risk.** By keeping your resting heart rate low over time, the number of beats allotted to you at birth can be used up at a slower rate—resulting in a lengthening of your life expectancy. By preventing or reversing resting heart rate increases over time, you can lower your mortality risk and add years to your life. All mammals, including humans, have about 1.5 billion allotted heart beats in their lifespan; it's just a matter of how fast they're used up.

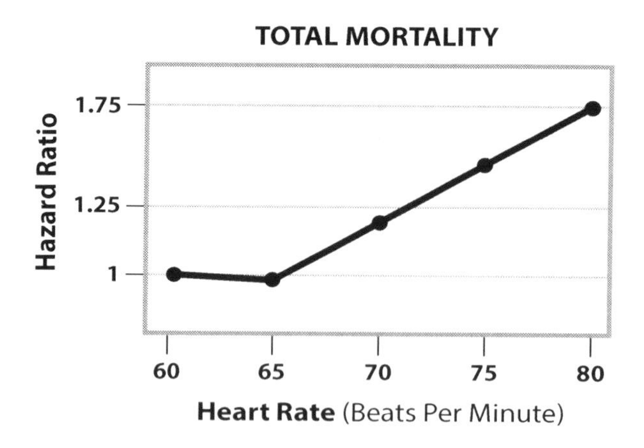

The powerful correlation between elevated heart rate and increased mortality can point us towards NSN exercise training Rx's designed to increase heart pumping efficiency and decrease resting heart rate. Other NSN Rx's are designed to decrease resting heart rate through stress-reducing exercises and behaviors. *(Adapted from: Woodward, Euro Journal of Preventive Cardiology, 2014 21: 719).*

For example, a giant tortoise with a heart rate of 6 beats/min. might take 177 years to use them up, while a mouse with a heart rate of 240 beats/min. takes only 5 years to burn through them. Humans are no different in how fast or slow we use up our allotted total heart beats. The difference is *we get to choose how we want to "spend" our heart beats—fast like a mouse, slow like a tortoise, or somewhere in between.* There is a Golden Ratio Heart Dividing Point which we can effectively use as a simple yet powerful longevity hack. By superimposing resting heart rate over Golden Ratio divisions on a 0-100 scale we see that 62 beats/min is a convenient dividing point (*adjusted down slightly from the Heart Rate/Mortality graph*), above which overall mortality risk increases. Other studies use 62 beats/min as a dividing line for coronary event risk. Approaching the lower and upper extremes on the line—0 beats/min on the low end; 100 beats/min on the top end—are both very high risk areas best avoided; obviously, heading towards 0, the heart beats too slowly to pump enough blood to sustain life, with sure death as a lower end point. On the upper end, approaching or exceeding 100 beats/min, too rapid a heart rate prevents the heart from efficiently filling with blood between beats; if the heart rate elevates to a critical level, sure death will result as an upper endpoint. **We're interested in the range of moderation, the Golden Mean of not too much and not too little, where peak performance *and* longevity coincide.** That's the ***Golden Ratio Heart Rate Dividing Point***, that point we want to stay at or below, recognizing that above the dividing point, mortality increases 10%-20% for every 10 beats/min.

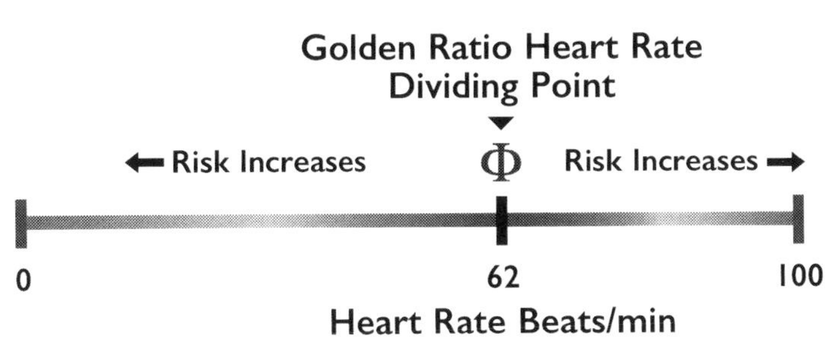

Below 62 beats/min we find the realm of highly conditioned athletes, whose hearts beat slower than the normal person—some even down to 28 beats/min, as did 5-time Tour de France champion Miguel Indurain. You don't have to lower your heart rate to that of an elite athlete to avoid the increasing mortality risks associated with higher heart rates. Being within 5 or 10 beats above or below the *Golden Ratio Heart Rate Dividing Point* of 62 beats/min is a reasonable marker to keep for longevity insurance. Many recreational and competitive athletes will be in the 50's or even 40's, yet that may not possible for the fitness exerciser who works out for the recommended 55 minutes/day. Remember, the target is just being at 62 beats/min or below. In addition to exercise for lowering your heart rate, anything that facilitates stress reduction will also have a corresponding slowing effect on your heart rate. Meditation, naps and sufficient nighttime sleep all have a direct effect on the autonomic nervous system that results in a slower heart rate. The best approach is to use both exercise (up to 55 minutes/day) to tonify the heart, coupled with relaxing activities that slow heart rate through nervous system regulation. **NOTE:** Sometimes it's not recommended for certain people to have slow heart rates, as it can increase the chances of heart rhythm disturbances, e.g., atrial fibrillation (rapid, irregular beating). Check with your doctor to verify your best resting heart rate range and configure your exercise and stress reduction activities accordingly.

The Golden Ratio Dance of Heart, Breath & Mind

Blood does not flow in a straight line as it courses through your arteries and veins; it actually flows in a multitude of spirals and vortices. Likewise, your heart doesn't pump in an up-and-down bicycle pump fashion as you might have thought. Instead, your heart contracts and relaxes in twisting, Golden Spiral-like motions. Your heart's electrical signature directly reflects the Golden Ratio as well, as its contraction and relaxation phases delineate Golden Ratios, clearly seen on an electrocardiogram ECG, aka EKG. During the contraction phase, blood moves into your body and lungs. When your heart relaxes, blood moves from your body and lungs back to your heart. A dynamic interaction between lung and heart activity is required for efficient oxygenation and release of carbon dioxide to occur. At rest the approximate ratio of respirations to heartbeats also reflects the Golden Ratio:

6

(Respirations/Heartbeats) x 10 = 1.6 Φ

Two clear examples showing this Golden Ratio respiratory/heartbeat relationship are: A person with a respiratory rate of 10 breaths/min. and resting heart rate of 60 beats/min. would have a Golden Ratio (1.6) of respirations to heartbeats:

10 ÷ 60 x 10 = 1.6 Φ

A person with a respiratory rate of 12 breaths/min. and resting heart rate of 75 beats/min. would also have the same ratio:

12 ÷ 75 x 10 = 1.6 Φ

We don't often appreciate how amazing it is that our Golden Ratio designed hearts are pumping away in perfect physiologic Golden Ratio harmony with each breath—until that balance is lost. Anyone who's ever hyperventilated or had a panic attack knows how it feels to have their breathing and heart rate fall out of Golden Ratio. Such out-of-control episodes are very unnerving and affirm how the body and mind are intimately connected and integrated into one elegant

The amazing Golden Ratio correlation between your heart and brain: 60-65% (Golden Ratio range) of your heart's total cells are specialized neural cells, which are very similar to those found in your brain.

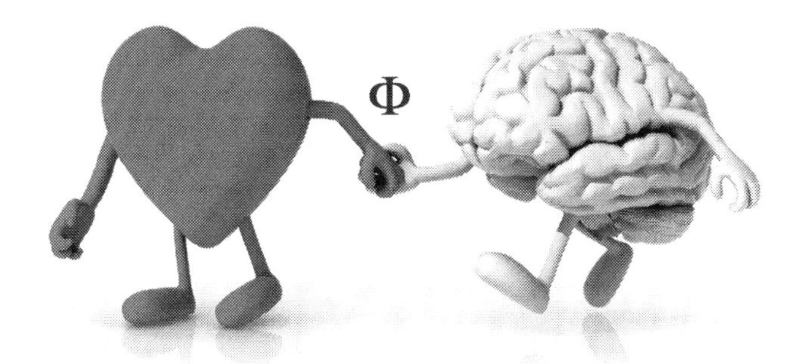

system. Referring to recent research in neuro-cardiology, **Joseph Chilton Pearce**, in *The Biology of Transcendence*, notes that,

> *About 60–65% of all the cells in the heart are neural cells, which are precisely the same as in the brain, functioning in precisely the same way, monitoring and maintaining control of the entire mind/brain/body physical process as well as direct unmediated connections between the heart and the emotional, cognitive structures of the brain.*

Of course, the 60–65% of heart cells which are neurons frames the 62% Golden Ratio. **This maximally efficient communication pathway between our holographic heart/mind is made possible by none other than the embedding of the Golden Ratio in numerous structural and functional layers throughout our entire cardiovascular and nervous systems.**

When you start fully appreciating the vital role the Golden Ratio plays in your body's form and function, you step into greater harmony and power in all movement, exercise and performance. This sets the stage to enjoy more of the *Flow state* in both your exercise *and* life—that timeless, transcendent state typical of the Golden Ratio in action, unifying mind, body and motion in the *present moment.* Nature's Path of Least Resistance in movement and exercise turns out to be a Golden Path to Flow.

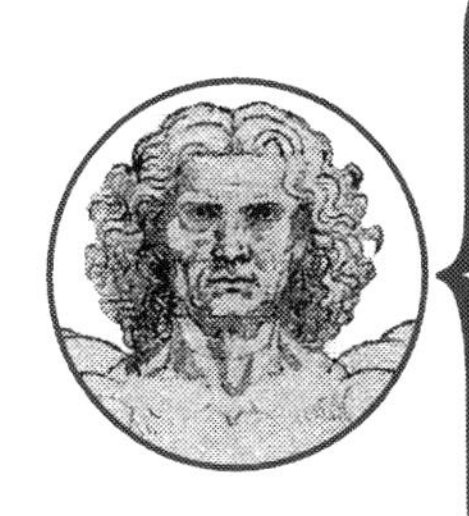

Remember, you're only as ***Fit*** *as your last* ***EXERCISE***. So be sure to get Golden Ratio exercise at least 3-4 times/wk. Add FIT intervals 1-2 times/wk to release Human Growth Hormone (HGH). Use the 40/30/30 Golden Olympic Training (GOT) ratio for Endurance, Strength & Flexibility. Strengthen your Golden Ratio Core Zone as a foundational priority. And last yet not least, one of the best mood elevators bar none is—Exercise!

Detox: #7 driver for maintaining vibrant health

Deep breathing–health driver #1–is one of your most powerful cleansing practices that supports access to Nature's Secret Nutrient/NSN.

With the ongoing Fukushima, Japan radiation disaster **protecting against** ionizing **radiation** sources is crucial.

Which two fruits have a Golden Ratio (1.6:1) of insoluble to soluble fiber? **Apples & Pears**. As we say, *an apple a day keeps the toxins away.*

Did you know that most Americans are **70,000 bowel** movements short over a lifetime? This is due to a fiber-poor Western diet.

Increasing dietary soluble & insoluble **fiber** is essential for keeping your entire digestion system clean & flowing.

Sweating via exercise, sauna or steam bath & alternating with cold water therapy is a powerful regular detox practice.

What's the most important nutrient to detox your body? Water! It's Nature's **universal solvent**, purifying your body from metabolic wastes & toxins.

Did you know that warm/hot **Epsom salt** baths both relax and detoxify your body? Add them to your regular detox regimen.

Every single chronic insidious disease process is related to one word: Toxicity.

Dr. Rashid Buttar

7

Detox

Elimination of undigested food and other bodily waste is just as important as the proper digestion and assimilation of food.

Dr. Norman W. Walker, nutrition & health pioneer

Detoxification is becoming more important every day, as we are constantly bombarded with increasing toxins from within and without. Luckily, our livers have the intelligence to detoxify metabolic waste products as well as environmental toxins and transform many of them into water-soluble substances that can be excreted in urine, bile, stool, sweat and breath. Water is the universal solvent that enables this process to occur. It's only when the degree of detoxification can't keep up with the amount of internally and externally generated toxins that problems arise. Our bodies have the ability to store toxins when we can't detoxify fast enough. However, at some point the storage capacity fills up and the toxins begin to inhibit efficient functioning of our metabolic machinery. Opportunistic microbes and parasites often arrive on the scene to feed on the sludge, which only complicates the situation. Then, varying degrees of unwellness begin to manifest: vague, low-grade symptoms like fatigue, headaches, insomnia, depression and subpar performance. Left unchecked, these low-grade symptoms can progress to actual pathologies like heart disease, asthma, cancer, diabetes, arthritis, Alzheimer's, Parkinson's or various immune system problems. However, by regaining Golden Ratio balance within each of the 10 MegaNutrient drivers of the NSN system, you can rev-up your detoxification processes, eliminate the backlog of toxins and support the restoration of your health. Starting with Breathing and Hydration, we'll see how Air and Water are two of our most powerful detoxification agents.

Breathing as Detoxification

The category of detoxification is woven through each of the top drivers in the Nature's Secret Nutrient System. Each of the top categories has within it a detoxification phase in order to maintain Golden Ratio balance of intake and output. In the case of driver #1, Breathing, respiration brings fresh oxygen/O_2 into our bodies and also removes carbon dioxide/CO_2. The exhalation phase of breathing both gets rid of carbon dioxide and helps to regulate acid/alkaline balance. Without adequate respiration, we would see many adverse health effects due to lack of oxygen and accumulation of metabolic acids. Breathing rate is dependent on activity demands and O_2/CO_2 levels at any given time. Our body's innate intelligence can dynamically shift in response to demands of the moment, e.g., when exercising we naturally breathe faster; at rest we breathe slower.

Most of us get into trouble when we're at rest: we tend to hypoventilate or under-breathe. Over-breathing or *hyper*ventilation is a less common occurrence and is typically caused by anxiety. Under-breathing or *hypo*ventilation is usually exacerbated by poor posture, where rounded shoulders and a caved-in chest inhibit deep and adequate breaths. When you're not breathing deeply enough, acidity develops in your blood which then forces your kidneys to get rid of excess acids. Over time, this stress moves even deeper into your physiology, putting stress on your endocrine glands and even dips into and depletes mineral stores in your bones to buffer and keep your acid/alkaline balance in check. Your body is programmed with the homeostatic ability to maintain many different physiologic Golden Ratio set points. We're constantly striving to keep all of our set points in Golden Ratio balance, including O_2/CO_2, acid/alkaline, blood sugar levels, hormones, blood pressure, temperature, hydration, etc. A good first step for correcting hypoventilation—under-breathing—is to set up some constant reminder to scan your breathing and posture on a regular basis.

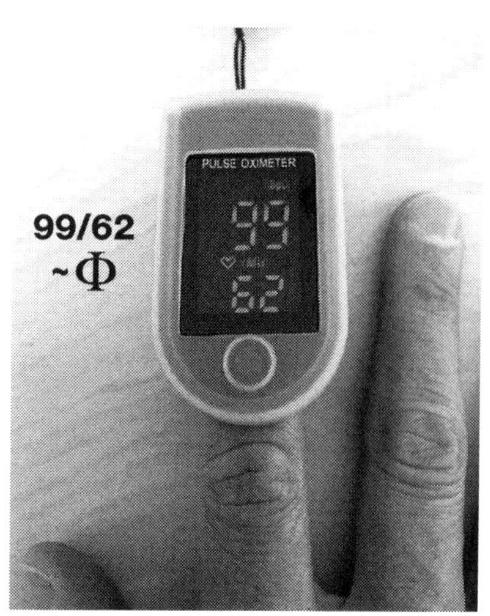

A Pulse Oximeter monitors oxygen saturation (top) and heart rate (bottom).

You might want to set up a timer to stand up, stretch and do a few cycles of Golden Ratio Breathing every hour. An easy way to measure hypoventilation is to get a Pulse-Oximeter, a simple device that clips on your finger and measures both blood oxygen saturation and pulse rate. It does this by shining red and infrared light through the skin and measuring the difference in absorption between oxygenated and deoxygenated hemoglobin. It then displays the oxygen saturation level along with pulse rate. You'll be amazed at how quickly your oxygen saturation increases after just a few rounds of Golden Ratio Breathing.

Water, the *Alkahest*: Nature's Universal Solvent

When your fish are sick, first change the water in the tank. Likewise, when YOU are sick, change the water in YOUR tank by flushing your body with clean water.

Robert D. Friedman, M.D. & Matthew K. Cross

Classical alchemists believed that there was a universal substance that had the ability to dissolve all other substances, gold included. They called this magical substance the *Alkahest*, a word coined by Renaissance physician and alchemist **Paracelsus**. Alchemists were especially interested in its medicinal potential and projected onto this hypothetical substance the label of the much sought after *Philosopher's Stone*. Like the ancient alchemists, we too are interested in the medicinal potential of the Alkahest, except in our case the universal solvent is the ubiquitous compound of water. Water—commonly known as H_2O—has chemical properties that make it a true universal solvent. On a practical level, although water can't dissolve all substances as the Alkahest theoretically could, it has the ability to dissolve enough substances that our physiology has taken advantage of this property to assist with bodily detoxification. Toxic substances from both external sources like environmental pollutants and internal metabolic waste products are dissolved in water so that they can be excreted through urine, breath, sweat, bile and stool.

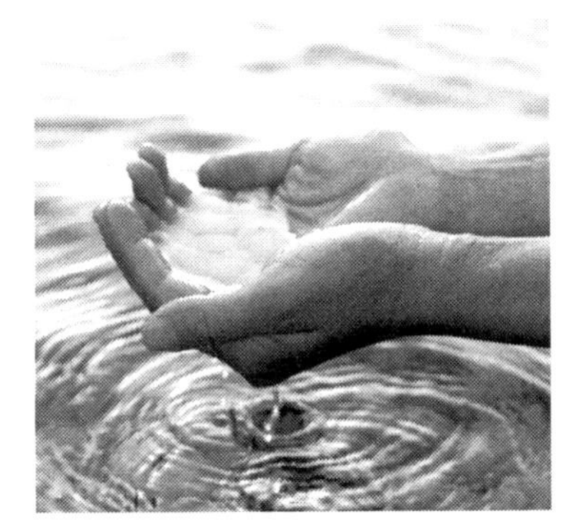

Water, Nature's universal solvent.

7

It makes sense that we would want to give our system enough fresh water to keep up with detoxification demands. In this day and age, the importance of adequate water intake cannot be overemphasized. As **Dr. Rashid Buttar, D.O.**, Vice-Chairman of the

American Board of Clinical Metal Toxicology states,

> *I can now very comfortably and definitively state to you that, in my opinion, based on the evidence, every single chronic insidious disease process is related to one word: toxicity. You cannot address the issues of aging unless you address detoxification.*

Dr. Buttar's insights into toxicity are all the more relevant when we take an honest look at sources of toxicity that are less apparent. The Associated Press reported in their 5 month investigation that over-the-counter and prescription drugs have been found in the drinking water supplies of 24 metropolitan areas across the United States. Drugs including antibiotics, antiepileptics, antidepressants, steroid hormones, acetaminophen and ibuprofen, among others, were found in trace amounts in all drinking water samples. The public at large is being continually poisoned with micro-doses of medications. It so happens that water is a bipolar molecule (although it's neither manic nor depressed) with a net negative charge near the oxygen end and a net positive charge at the polar hydrogen end. This is what accounts for its universal solvent properties. Luckily, water's bipolar structure assists our detoxification mechanisms in getting rid of these and other unwanted pollutants. The Center for Disease Control's (CDC) landmark study in 2003 identified 116 chemicals in blood and urine samples from hundreds of Americans. The toxicology screens identified significant levels of heavy metals, secondhand smoke residues, plastic residues, pesticides and herbicides in *all* subjects. This sobering study highlights the pervasive degree of environmental toxicity in virtually the entire U.S. population. It also can redirect our focus to learn about detoxification protocols and remind us of the importance of the universal solvent, water—the Alkahest—in regularly flushing these toxins from our bodies.

Water's near-miraculous ability to dissolve so many substances allows our lungs, liver, kidneys, intestines and sweat glands to eliminate these toxins. All we have to do is make sure that we are drinking enough pure water throughout our day to satisfy this demand. Water intake varies according to age, size, activity level, temperature and health. Everyone has an ideal amount of fluid intake. We can think of this ideal amount as each person's Golden Ratio quantity where not too much and not too little water intake will facilitate optimum functioning. This ideal amount changes from day to day and hour to hour depending on the circumstances. As we learned in Ch 2 Hydration, just following your thirst impulse isn't accurate enough to monitor your body's water requirements, as there is a lag time between dehydration and the awareness of thirst. So, you have to *anticipate dehydration* and always be rehydrating even when you're not actually thirsty. In addition, as we age the thirst mechanism may become blunted, making our awareness of thirst even slower and duller. Ask yourself throughout the day if your hydration level is at the Golden Ratio point: not too dry/not too wet. For a review of optimal hydration techniques, see the Rx's for Ch 2 Hydration.

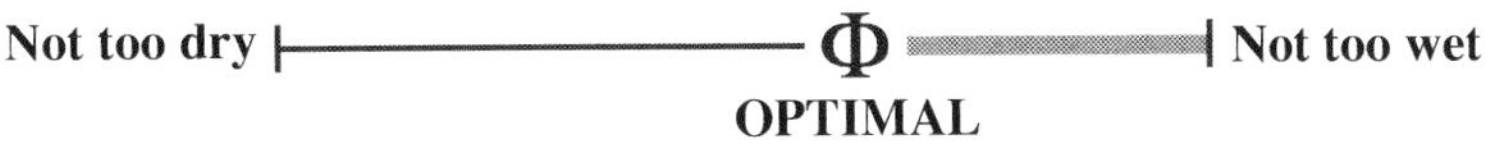

Not too dry |———————— **Φ** ————| **Not too wet**
OPTIMAL

This diagram shows how the Golden Ratio can be applied to optimize any health situation where there are opposing polarities, in this case the *just right* point between dehydration and over-hydration. Over-hydration is rare yet can occur in marathon runners who drink too much or in certain medical conditions.

The Bowels: A 2-Way Street For Absorption & Elimination

Ultimately, optimal nutrient absorption at the cellular level is dependent on how many nutrients are absorbed through your intestinal lining into your bloodstream. If your intestines are chronically constipated and clogged with excess debris and biofilm—an all-too-common condition for many—then no matter what great nutrients you eat, it's impossible for them to be fully absorbed into your bloodstream and nourish your cells. Simply put, to increase and optimize nutrient absorption, you must reduce the waste in your system.

> *It's not what we eat, but what we digest that makes us strong.*
> **Francis Bacon**

Der Goldene "Schnitt": The Golden Bowel Movement = 1.6x/day

Der Goldene "Schnitt" is German for the Golden Cut or Golden Ratio and also just happens to rhyme with the English word *Sh–t*. Nevertheless, the concept of the Golden Ratio can be applied to the subject of intestinal detoxification to give us some valuable insights. A study of bowel movement frequency in over 20,000 people in *Public Health Nutrition*, 2004, by **Miguel Sanjoaquin**, et. al., revealed that vegan (a vegetarian who eats no animal or dairy products) males had an average of 11.6 bowel movements per week. That averages 1.6 bowel movements per day, or what we call the Golden "Schnitt" (recall that 1.6 is the Golden Ratio in two digits). Meat eaters fell significantly short of the Golden "Schnitt" at around 9.5 bowel movements per week, with an average of only 1.35 bowel movements per day. The amount of fiber of eaten directly impacts the frequency of bowel movements. The average American only gets about 15 grams of fiber per day in their diet, whereas a vegan can get upwards of 50 grams of fiber per day. When bowel movement quantity is low, it's likely that bowel movement frequency will be low and out of Golden Ratio. One is then subject to a backup of toxic waste with a high likelihood of various maladies manifesting. Regarding the out-of-ratio bowel movements of modern Americans, renowned naturopath **Dr. Richard Schulze** remarked with his typical incisive wit,

> *They will have an average of 2-4 bowel movements a week coming up 70,000 bowel movements short in their lifetime, definitely having diverticulosis and digestive and elimination problems.*

Quality of bowel movements is influenced not only by *how much* fiber is in your diet, but also by the *type* of fiber—a critical distinction. The two classes of dietary fiber are known as soluble and insoluble, both indigestible. Soluble fiber is able to absorb water and is fermentable by intestinal bacteria. These fermentable by-products are known as SCFA (short-chain fatty acids) and are important due to their ability to regulate blood glucose, lipids and cholesterol. **They also favorably modify the milieu and microbiome (bacterial population) of the total intestinal environment,** including the pH, reducing the risk of polyps and colon cancer. Insoluble fiber doesn't absorb water, but is mainly responsible for speeding the transit of toxins from the colon. Increasing both soluble and insoluble fiber in one's diet can either resolve or have a favorable impact on many conditions, including:

acne	*diabetes*	*hemorrhoids*
anxiety	*diarrhea*	*IBS (irritable bowel syndrome)*
arthritis	*diverticulosis*	*immune dysfunction*
bloating	*eczema*	*indigestion*
brain fog	*fatigue*	*insomnia*
constipation	*gas*	*obesity*
depression	*heart disease*	

Simply increasing the amount of fiber in your diet to the point where your bowel movement frequency approaches or exceeds the Golden "Schnitt" range—**a minimum** of at least 1.6 per day—can be a major contributing factor in its own right in restoring

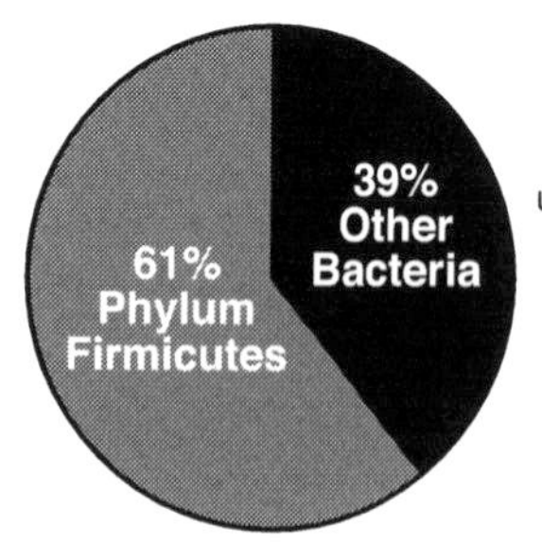

The Optimal Intestinal Microbiome Ratio. In normal populations of uBiome laboratory studies, bacterial populations comprising the intestinal microbiome amazingly hover around Golden Ratio distribution, with Phylum Firmicutes comprising around 61% of the entire intestinal bacterial population. Lactobacillus acidophilus, commonly used in yogurt and keifer culture, is a well-known member of Firmicutes.

healthy immune function and healing disease. The ratio of soluble to insoluble fiber varies greatly among foods, however there are no unprocessed whole foods with just one type of fiber. All fruits and vegetables have a mix of soluble and insoluble fiber, with some having soluble/insoluble ratios in near-perfect Golden Ratio balance. Both types of fiber have the ability to increase the speed of bowel movements, thereby getting rid of toxic waste products faster. So if you want to approach the Golden "Schnitt," averaging or exceeding 1.6 bowel movements per day, just increase both your soluble and insoluble fiber intake gradually until you reach that target. Due to individual variations, many people may average more than 1.6 bowel movements per day. Soluble fiber has the special property of being able to bind toxins and bile acids in order to sequester and remove them from your body.

Lower Cholesterol with Soluble Fiber

A safe alternative to using dangerous statin drugs to lower cholesterol is simply to eat more soluble fiber in your diet. Soluble fiber binds bile acids and prevents their reabsorption, thereby preventing the bile from being re-synthesized into cholesterol. Oats, grapefruit, orange and asparagus are particularly high in soluble fiber.

Quality of a Golden Schnitt

In addition to consuming enough dietary fiber to get the average number of daily bowel movements to at least 1.6 per day, we can consider other factors that contribute to the consistency or quality of a normal stool. Ideally, a Golden Schnitt should resemble a smooth or slightly wrinkled banana, being not too hard or too soft, along with being low odor. Both adequate fiber and good hydration are foundational conditions that allow a normal microbial flora, or microbiome, to flourish, resulting in optimal elimination. We've seen that urine color—ideally a chardonnay hue to clear—is a key indicator of healthy hydration. Stool consistency is another. Dehydration causes stools to be dried out and leads to constipation, as does inadequate or imbalanced fiber intake. Only when these basic conditions are established can a normal quality and quantity of stool and bowel movements occur. There are other factors that come

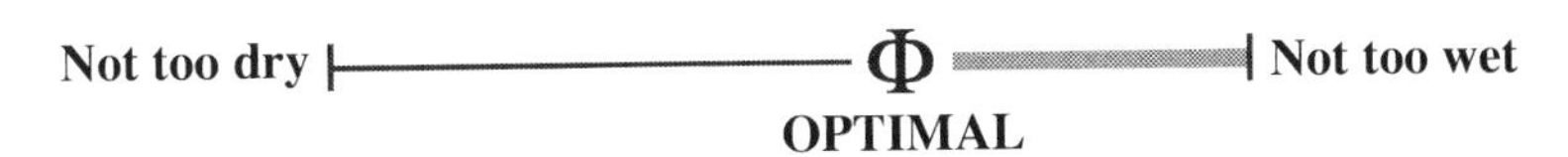

Normal stool consistency or quality is determined by both fiber content and hydration level. The optimal stool is not too dry (constipation) nor too wet (diarrhea)—but just right (*Golden Schnitt*).

In Search of the Golden Schnitt

Renowned herbalist **Dr. Richard Schulze** was curious as to exactly what a Golden "Schnitt" was, so he set off on a world-wide journey to answer that question, since he hadn't been able to find one in America. Schulze reported:

> *I have traveled the world in search of the perfect bowel movement. I have traveled to the jungles of Central America and to China, India, Africa, and Asia. I wanted to see primitive, rural people living simple, natural lives, and I wanted to find out what their bowel habits were like, because I wasn't going to find normal and natural anywhere in America. Simple and natural people, who gather wood, eat natural food, and have relaxed, unstressed lives have between two and three bowel movements a day. They eat, and within 15 to 30 minutes after their meals, they wander off to their spots, squat, and have bowel movements. These are usually light in color, soft, and unformed, and they come out easily, with no straining, grunting, pushing, or meditation.*

Schulze discovered that these "primitive, rural people" were having up to twice as many bowel movements than the average American vegan. They were super-vegans, in that they were consuming enough fiber to account for their increased stool volume and frequency. A possible side effect of consuming too much fiber is that some of the nutrients might not be absorbed since they would be bound-up in the fiber and excreted too rapidly. This malabsorption effect is probably of no consequence with the amount of fiber consumed by most American vegans.

into play as well, such as stress levels and exercise frequency. People who sit at their desks or in front of the TV for extended periods are at a higher risk of colon cancer. Regular movement breaks at least hourly can offset these risks and contribute to healthy bowel function. Stress reduction is a positive side effect of exercise and both can be used as interventions for improving bowel health.

Golden Insoluble/Soluble Fiber Ratios

Ample quality and quantity of fiber is clearly a vital dietary and internal cleansing requirement. Apples, pears, grapefruit, oranges and asparagus have insoluble/soluble fiber ratios in near-perfect Golden Ratio balance. These are contrasted to examples like brown rice and pinto beans, which have higher ratios of insoluble/soluble fiber. Wheat bran can be an overly harsh fiber to eat and has the most lopsided insoluble/

Food	Insoluble/Soluble Fiber Ratios	
Wheat bran	11.3:1 *(wheat bran is overly processed and thus at the extreme end of the spectrum)*	
Brown rice	8.0:1	
Beans (pinto)	3.36:1	
Flax seeds	2.0:1	
Apple	**1.61:1**	**Golden Ratio/NSN Φ**
Pear	**1.63:1**	
Strawberries	1.55:1	
Beans (black)	1.55:1	
Cauliflower	1.5:1	
Celery	1.5:1	
Sesame seeds	1.5:1	
Sunflower seeds	1.5:1	
Grapes	1.5:1	
Sweet potato	1.44:1	
Carrots	1.38:1	
Broccoli	1.3:1	
Oats	0.92:1	
Grapefruit	0.61:1	
Orange	0.61:1	**Golden Ratio/NSN 1/Φ**
Asparagus	0.64:1	

More Insoluble Fiber ↑ ↓ More Soluble Fiber

soluble fiber ratio. This comes as no surprise, as wheat bran is a very refined food, lacking the vital nutritional components of the whole grain. Eating more Golden Ratio fiber-balanced foods will improve digestion, immune function and will shift bowel movements into the healthy 1.6+/day range.

In actuality, both soluble and insoluble fibers work together through both binding power and elimination speed to detoxify your system and fine-tune your intestinal environment. So, if you want to better detoxify yourself simply increase fruits and vegetables to get both more soluble and insoluble fiber. Some people get fiber benefits from grains, however a growing body of evidence points to the possible negative immune-modulating and allergenic effects of grains. If you feel that you're not getting enough fiber through your diet, a wide variety of fiber supplements are available to augment your fiber intake. Remember to always increase your water intake when you use fiber supplements, since these products are dehydrated.

The Average American is a Toxic *Waist* Dump

America's increasing obesity epidemic is multifactorial, with increased sedentariness, poor nutrition, sleep and emotional stress among the key causes. However, there is a huge elephant in the room rarely talked about as a leading cause of excess weight—toxins. **Obesity must also be recognized as one of the body's clever survival mechanisms to deal with the onslaught of environmental and food pollutants.** Once our normal detoxification functions become overwhelmed by an excess of environmental poisons, the body has no choice but to store the toxins wherever it can. This mechanism gets them out of circulation, preventing cellular damage and compromised organ function. Fat tissue is an ideal location for toxin storage for so many environmental pollutants including auto exhaust, pesticides and heavy metals.

If more storage space for toxins is needed in the body, an ingenious method to generate extra storage space has been developed. The brain simply increases hunger signals, which leads to more food consumption and eventually more fat accumulation. More fat accumulation equates to more storage space for toxins. Bitcoin aficionados would recognize this as a metabolic *Segwit* adaptation for extra fat storage facilitated by a hungry *soft-fork*. The belly is usually the first place where this process begins. Unless you're pregnant, a growing abdomen is a clear sign that you've been adding more storage space for toxins. This endless loop produces more fat to store more toxins and until the input of further toxins is stopped, this process continues. It's apparent that the obesity epidemic and deterioration of our environment and poisoning of our food with deadly toxins are all intertwined. Government regulations have proven worthless when it comes to dealing with the increasing environmental pollution that's poisoning the entire population. The only thing to do is to take matters into your own hands by becoming your own doctor and begin self-healing by cleaning up both your external and internal environments (terrains). As **Louis Pasteur** purportedly remarked on his deathbed,

The microbe is nothing... ***the TERRAIN is everything.***

Pasteur had dramatically changed his opinion in his later years about microbes or germs as being causal to the origin of disease, agreeing with researchers Antoine Béchamp and Claude Bernard on their theory that **it's the body's internal milieu or terrain that sets the stage for either health or disease to manifest.** In our time, we must be concerned with both our internal and our external milieu, otherwise known as the environment; yet our foundational health driver is always our internal terrain. The only solution is to declare our bodies as EPA Superfund cleanup sites and begin immediate remediation and detoxification. The easiest and quickest way to begin to eliminate the fat-embedded toxins is to begin a multi-faceted approach; exercise and increased water intake to mobilize toxins, followed by sauna sweating to discharge them. The great benefit of adding sauna sweating following exercise is that it prevents the released toxins from being reabsorbed into the fat before they're eliminated from your body. Remember to go easy in the beginning, as the released toxins can cause uncomfortable symptoms until they're discharged from your body. As you lose fat, you're simultaneously getting rid of years of accumulated toxicity and cellular garbage. Just like the good feeling you get when you clean out your storage locker, so too will you begin to feel the hum of health as all of your physiologic functions begin to normalize and come back into Golden Ratio. Please refer to the Ch 7 Detox Rx section for detox protocols designed to optimize and flush out your internal organs. Many of the Rx's cover multiple drivers, such as Dave Asprey's Bulletproof® Coffee which serves as an energizing AM circadian wakeup and also doubles as a mini-liver/gallbladder flush.

Radiation Protection/Detoxification 101 & Tips

Doctors know there is NO such thing as a "safe" dose of radiation☠.
Helen Caldicott, M.D., co-founder, Physicians for Social Responsibility

Since March 11, 2011, radiation from the Fukushima, Japan nuclear disaster has been spreading across the Earth, affecting everyone alive, including generations to come. Radiation from Fukushima and other sources is cumulative and *there is no "safe" radiation level for humans.* While everyone's immune system is unique, there is always a threshold level of radiation that triggers disease and premature death. Avoidance and targeted detoxification must now become a way of life for every sane person as a matter of survival, let alone for optimal health and longevity. This will give your body the best shot at dealing with this latest deadly, conspicuously under-reported radiation source, added to the "normal," increasingly toxic mix that's in our 21st century air, water, food and environment worldwide. On the next page are key tips on what you can do to help protect and detoxify yourself and your family from the growing menace of man-made radiation.

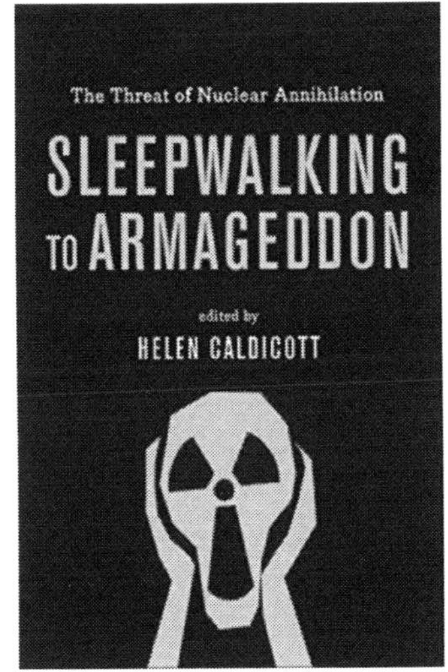

Sleepwalking to Armageddon, edited by Helen Caldicott, M.D. The trefoil cover design ***Screams*** the deadly dangers of radiation (see next page for more on the trefoil symbol).

7

Key Radiation Protection/Detoxification Practices & Tips

- **Radiation alert websites:** www.blackcatsystems.com/RadMap/map.html www.nuc.berkeley.edu/UCBAirSampling • www.radiationnetwork.com
- If airborne radiation levels are elevated, stay inside & avoid going outside, especially in the rain; exercise indoors & drive with windows closed.
- Take a shower & do sinus irrigation with salt water after being outside in questionable air. Refrain from bathing in or drinking rainwater.
- Use a True HEPA air filter, change filter regularly & dispose of properly/safely.
- Ideally, use a 3-stage water filter with activated carbon, R/O & ion exchange.
- Wash vegetables & fruits with biodegradable soap or baking soda.
- Take frequent detox baths with Epsom salts, sea salt or baking soda.
- Practice regular oral chelation & intestinal detox with EDTA, garlic, chlorella.
- Take extra antioxidants to prevent cellular damage: Vitamins A-B-C-D-E, Spirulina, R-lipoic acid, turmeric, green tea extract, grape seed extract, sea vegetables, including brown seaweed (fucoidan).
- Avoid seafood & seaweed if from a radiation affected area.
- Take iodine supplements daily to replenish body stores; more if higher radiation levels warrant it.
- Reduce or eliminate animal & milk products, as they are more concentrated radiation sources. Avoid seafood if it's from a radiation affected area.
- Follow the Japanese custom of removing your shoes before entering your home. This simple practice prevents tracking radioactive particles into your house.
- Preliminary research shows that ionizing radiation exposure can be ameliorated with exogenous ketones and/or a ketogenic diet.

Ionizing Radiation Radiation that damages living tissue by disrupting and destroying individual cells at the molecular level. All types of nuclear radiation—x rays, gamma rays and beta rays [and extreme UV, UltraViolet light closest to X rays]—are potentially ionizing. Sound waves physically vibrate the material through which they pass, but do not ionize it.

Non-Ionizing Radiation Electromagnetic radiation, the photons of which lack the energy required to ionize atoms or induce ion formation. Non-Ionizing Radiation includes sound, ultraviolet [near UV, the light closest to visible light], visible, and infrared light, microwaves and radio waves.

Hidden Innocent Origins of the Radiation Symbol

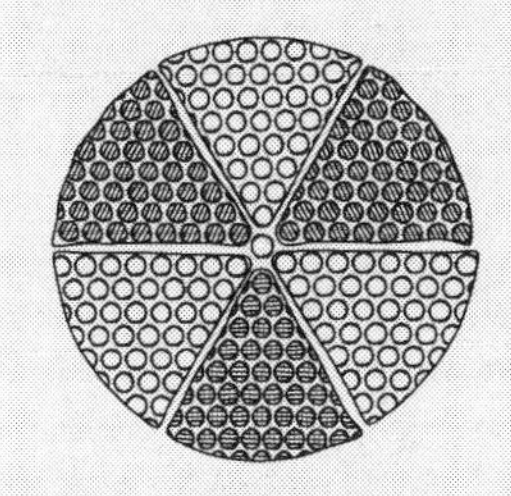
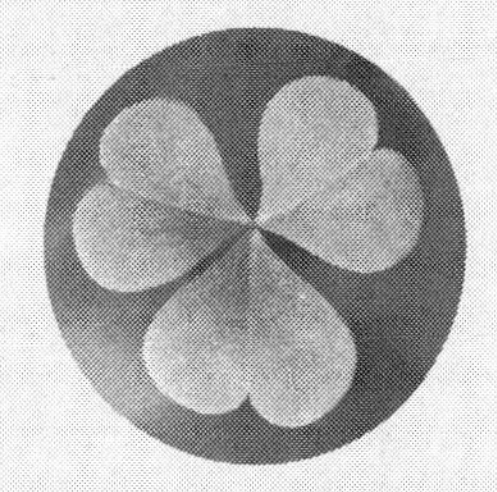

The international radiation hazard symbol (*L*) is a trefoil (3-leaf) design, often used in architectural design, ornamentation, coats of arms and warning symbols. Nature's trefoils predate human-designed trefoils, as seen in the diatom plankton species (*middle*) and in a 3-petaled clover leaf (*R*). It's ironic that the impression conveyed by these beautiful life forms is in stark contrast to the radiation symbol's dire warning. Both diatoms and atoms use fission and fusion; diatoms for reproduction and atoms for energy production and destruction. It makes one wonder if the diatom pictured above was the inspiration for the radiation symbol's design. Additionally, *clover* contains the word *love*—the opposite message to that of the radiation symbol. How ironic that Nature's lovely trefoil design was co-opted for use as a danger symbol—yet not really all that surprising when we remember the sage words of George Orwell in *1984*: *War is Peace. Freedom is Slavery. Ignorance is Strength.*

- Decrease exposure to *all* sources of both ionizing and non-ionizing radiation as much as possible. Avoid airport radiation scanners and microwave ovens. Keep cellphones as far from your body as possible; always use either the speakerphone or a headset. **Again, ionizing radiation from radionuclides is a CUMULATIVE deadly toxin, thus there is NEVER a "safe" daily radiation exposure dose.**

7

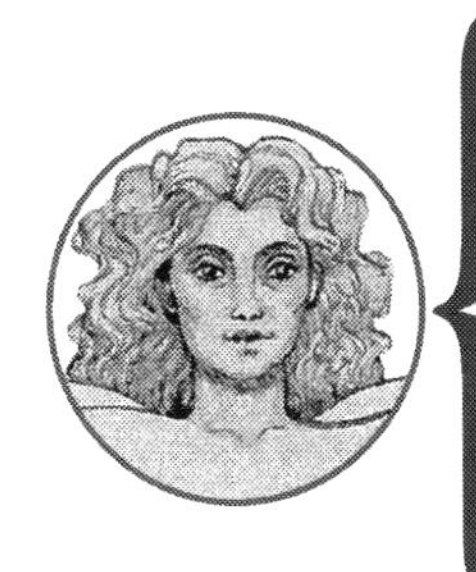

Remember, you're only as ***Clean*** *internally as your last* ***DETOX****.*
So be sure to establish daily bowel movements in the Golden Ratio range of at least 1.6 x/day or at least 11 times/wk. Increase fiber intake and exercise your Golden Ratio Core Zone to support healthy elimination. Improve detoxification with deeper breathing, increased hydration & sweating and periodic colon & liver cleanses. Avoid all radiation exposure.

Happiness: #8 driver, a cause & effect of vibrant health & longevity

Most people instinctively view the world through a **62/38 Golden Ratio lens** of positive to negative thoughts.

What is a major cause of depression & unhappiness? Sleep deprivation, which is **easily treatable** with NSN Rx's.

Your emotions naturally orbit around your ***happiness set point,*** which is upgradable via simple changes in perspective.

Did you know that you have ***molecules of emotion*** that play with your DNA? They can trigger either health or disease, depending on your attitude.

Activate your latent **happiness genes** through gratitude, positive focus & serving others.

Applying the Golden Ratio in your life can deepen wonder, happiness & **inner peace**.

Decrease stress & balance your immune system by adjusting **work to personal time** towards the Golden Ratio.

Stress kills. Like chronic inflammation, chronic stress is a hidden grim reaper. Reduce key stressors, **practice mindfulness** & invite NSN into your life.

Happiness is determined 60% by genetics & life circumstances and 40% by our **behavior & thoughts**.

Keep a **positive attitude** at least 62% (Golden Ratio) of the time & upgrade your DNA.

Happiness is the meaning and the purpose of life, the whole aim and end of human existence.

Aristotle

Happiness

Genes that govern happiness must exist latently within everyone.
The genes are just waiting to be switched on.

Kazuo Murakami, Ph.D., leading geneticist
& author of *The Divine Code of Life*

DNA & the Golden Ratio of Happiness & Inner Peace

The Golden Ratio can be discovered in virtually every scientific discipline, including the field of human behavior. One of the more fascinating insights relating to the Golden Ratio is in the understanding of factors that determine happiness. In **Sonja Lyubomirsky's** book, *The How of Happiness*, she summarizes the general consensus of psychological research as to what are the most important determinants of happiness. Everyone has a happiness "set point" around which contentment hovers during their lives. Many longitudinal twin studies reveal that approximately 50% of our happiness is dependent on genetic inheritance from our parents, 10% due to life circumstances and a remarkable 40% is due to our behavior and thoughts. Surprisingly, life circumstances such as socioeconomic status, educational attainment, family income, marital status and religious commitment had minimal effect on one's overall well being. Even for people blessed with favorable circumstances—such as wealth or exceptional beauty—happiness is not guaranteed.

8

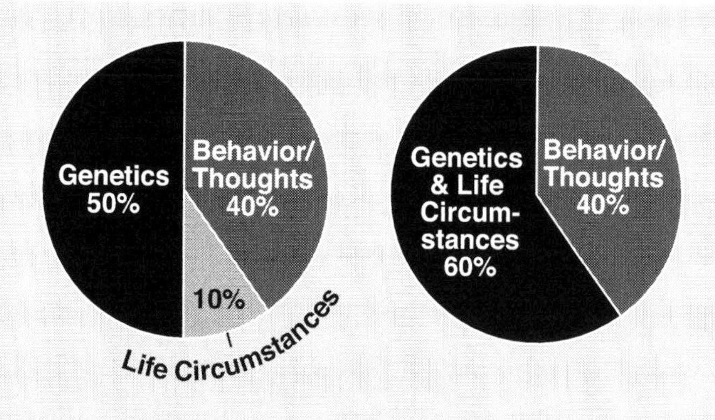

Slicing the Pie of Happiness in Two Different Ways

L: Happiness' causal factors have traditionally been divided into three categories which divide the Pie of Happiness into three seemingly independent and unrelated slices: 50% Genetics, 40% Behavior & Thoughts and 10% Life Circumstances.

R: The causal factors of Happiness can be consolidated and regrouped into two slices, 60% & 40%, divisions that approach the Golden Ratio. 60% of total Happiness is then seen as based on Genetics & Life Circumstances and the remaining 40% on Behavior and Thoughts. Only when parts are in Golden Ratio is the relationship of the whole pie to the large slice similar to the relationship of the large slice to the small slice. This implies that there is a dynamic, interactive relationship between the 60% and 40% divisions. With respect to these causal factors, strengthening the positive aspects of our Thoughts and Behaviors can epigenetically positively modify our Genetic set point for Happiness and also counter-balance disrupting influences of unexpected Life Circumstances. Without seeing these factors through the lens of the Golden Ratio, they would each appear to exist in a vacuum and not have any effect on each other. Positive Thoughts and Behavior can be extremely powerful agents for increasing your **Happiness Set Point**; in this chapter and its Rx section, you'll find some powerful Golden Ratio tips and practices to activate them.

A phenomenon called *hedonic adaptation* seems to effectively neutralize these fortunate life circumstances over time. We become accustomed to the same input over time, no matter how wonderful, and invariably gravitate back to our natural **Happiness Set Point**. Conversely, Lyubomirsky says that a saving grace of hedonic adaptation is that in times of the reverse—such as illness or accident—adaptation also occurs, returning us to our genetic **Happiness Set Point**. According to Lyubomirsky, paying attention to and cultivating positive, life-affirming behaviors and thoughts can make up for poor

DNA: Golden Ratio to the Core

As Above, So Below. Jean-claude Perez, Ph.D. identified a unified field of biology: the DNA Supracode, a fractal-like Golden Ratio & Fibonacci Sequence pattern principle. DNA's building blocks (G,C,T,A) exhibit Fibonacci Ratios between one another and between triplets or codons. Even so-called "junk" DNA has heretofore unseen complexity and information carrying ability. As complex systems organize via the Golden Ratio & Fibonacci Sequence, we look for universal patterns first; then fill in the gaps with details to complete the picture; it's like having a birds-eye view of a finished jigsaw puzzle before assembling the pieces. Absent a guiding macro vision, completing the puzzle is far more difficult. This *Secret Hidden in Plain Sight* can transform scientific and medical research. NSN Rx's mirror this ***As Above, So Below*** principle. Since Fibonacci & Golden Ratios are integrated in the Rx's, via fractal harmonics the ***Above*** (your daily thoughts, feelings & actions) resonate with and impact the ***Below*** (the epigenetic level of your DNA).

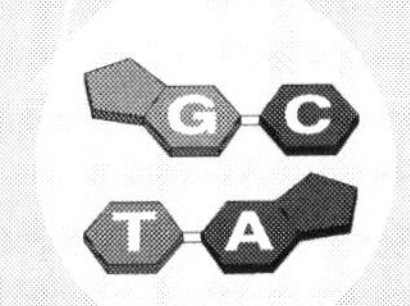

predispositions in our genetic Happiness Set Point as well as "bad luck" in life circumstances. For people who are naturally blessed with a sunny disposition, cultivating positive behaviors and thoughts can lead to especially fulfilling lives. For those less fortunate, cultivating such behaviors can be nothing short of transformational. If we look at this 50/40/10 distribution a little closer, we can see an opportunity to tap the hidden transformational power of the Golden Ratio in this data, as the breakdown can be regrouped as follows:

Genetics 50% + Life Circumstances 10% = 60%;
Behavior & Thoughts = 40%

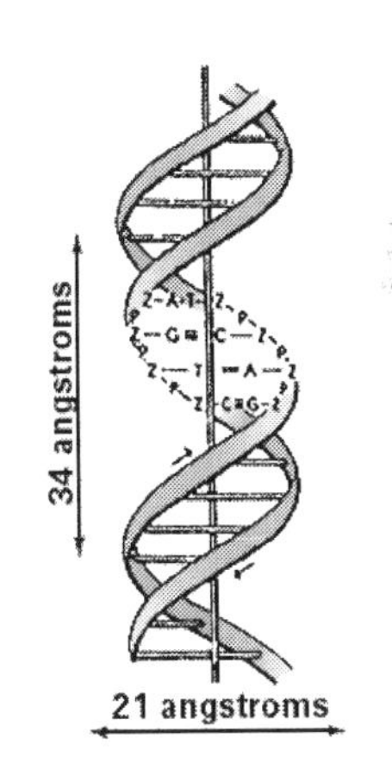

Our Golden Ratio shaped DNA (34 by 21 angstroms) is epigenetically modifiable through our thoughts and behavior.

This gives a 60/40 ratio—which approaches the Golden Ratio. In other words, one's tendency towards happiness falls under the influence of the Golden Ratio. This is not surprising, since even our genetics are based on the precise, Divinely-Coded shape of our DNA: the primary structure of DNA's double helix has a length/width ratio of 34/21—Fibonacci Sequence numbers—angstroms, which approximates the Golden Ratio of 1.618.

Our Hardwired 62/38 Golden Ratio Perspective

[Psychologist] **B.A. Kelly** proposed in 1955 that everyone evaluates the world around them using a system of bipolar constructs. When judging others, for instance, one end of each pole represents a maximum positive trait; the other a maximum negative trait, such as honest/dishonest, strong/weak, etc. Kelly had assumed that average responses in value-neutral situations would be 0.50. He was wrong. **Experiments show a human bent toward favor or optimism that results in a response ratio in value-neutral situations of 0.62—the Golden Ratio.** Numerous binary-choice experiments have reproduced this finding, regardless of the type of constructs or the age, nationality or background of the subjects... When [psychologist] **Vladimir Lefebvre** asked subjects to choose between two options about which they have no strong feelings and/or little knowledge, answers tend to divide into the Golden Ratio proportion: 62% to 38%... When subjects are given scenarios that require a moral action and asked what percentage of people would take good actions vs. bad actions, their answers average 62% [towards the good actions]. **'When people say they feel 50/50 on a subject,' says Lefebvre, 'chances are it's more like 62/38.'** Lefebvre's provocative Golden Ratio-revealing research resonates perfectly with the sage insight of Eastern spiritual authority **Alan Watts:**

> *In the ancient Hindu creation of life mythology, the forces of the dark side are operative for 1/3 of the time, the forces of the light side 2/3 of the time. And this is a very ingenious arrangement, because we are seeing here the fundamental principles of drama [and life].*

When people aren't aware of or forget the Golden Ratio's power, they commonly default to the more easily remembered 1/3 to 2/3 distribution. For example, a common default is regularly seen in the field of photography, where photo viewfinders divide the screen into thirds, i.e., the "**Rule of Thirds**." We can upgrade this rougher notion by simply using Nature's more accurate natural division of 62% to 38% Golden and Fibonacci Ratios (vs. the usual 66% to 33%) to more accurately conform to Nature's design. Instead of using 1/3 to 2/3 to divide viewfinders or anything else, use 2/5 and 3/5 (both Fibonacci Ratios) for more natural and higher resonance. **This intriguing research indicates that our general default ratio of positive opinions/perspective vs. negative reflects the Golden Ratio of 62% positive to 38% negative.**

Source of Kelly/Lefebvre data: *The [Elliott] Wave Principle of Human Social Behavior*, by **Robert R. Prechter, Jr.**

8

Your DNA is Modifiable & Upgradable—by YOU

One of the world's top geneticists, **Kazuo Murakami, Ph.D.**, has proven that our DNA is not just a static data bank. On the contrary, it has the dynamic potential to have desirable latent regions activated—or active, undesirable regions silenced—*by psychological input alone*. For example, Dr. Murakami proved that diabetics could lower their blood sugar simply by watching comedy movies. The molecular mechanism had to do with the activation via laughter/good emotions of 23 genes that have roles in controlling blood sugar. This calls to mind journalist and world peace activist **Norman Cousins**' successful treatment of his heart disease and arthritis through comedy movie laughter therapy (and mega-doses of Vitamin C). Cousins explored the biochemistry of emotions in his best-selling book *Anatomy Of An Illness*. The modification of gene expression by conscious psychological input has revolutionized traditional concepts of our DNA as being a static, unalterable destiny control system. In essence, this research shows that we are *not* held hostage by our family's genetic heritage. Dr. Murakami says that we can epigenetically activate our beneficial genes through positive or "genetic thinking," as he states in his book *The Divine Code of Life:*

> *My hypothesis is that an enthusiastic approach to life leads to success and activates the genes that make us experience happiness.*

Among the methods for activating and amplifying the good or positive genes in your DNA, Dr. Murakami suggests:

> ***Keep your intentions noble... Live with an attitude of thankfulness... Keep your thoughts positive*** [which he believes is the most important]. *The trick is to take a broader perspective... we need to see the bigger picture and endeavor to see the positive in everything that happens to us in life... Let yourself be inspired. If nothing inspires you in the moment, think back to a time when you were deeply moved... I believe that when we are inspired, our genes never move in an adverse direction...* [*another method is to*] *shake up your habits regularly to become refreshed and invigorated—mentally and physically. A change in environment can also make you see new things and become the start of a new life...* ***Our genes can even make possible those things we think are impossible... We are all born with the strong potential to become living miracles.***

Sleep Deprivation: A Surprising Major Cause of Unhappiness

When PBS talk show host **Charlie Rose** asked **Derek Bok**, author and former Harvard University president (1971-1991), what causes people the most unhappiness, Bok replied that there are three afflictions that seem to cause real unhappiness, as long as they persist: *1. Clinical Depression 2. Chronic Pain 3. Sleep Disorders* (deprivation or sleep apnea). Nature's Secret Nutrient provides a solid framework for addressing all three of these conditions. Note: Derek Bok is the author of *The Politics of Happiness: What Government Can Learn from the New Research on Well-Being.* Excerpt from *The Charlie Rose Show*, PBS, 4/30/10.

Dr. Murakami's inspiring work underscores the value of consciously, daily increasing the ratio of one's positive to negative thoughts. It calls to mind the importance of strengthening our ability to dwell at or above the 62% Golden Ratio point of positive, inspiring thoughts and feelings. This is especially true in light of the prevailing blizzard of negativity we are subjected to on a daily basis. Indeed, even the negative-to-positive ratio of emotion words silently conspires to pull us into the negative, as **Chip and Dan Heath** point out in their book *Switch: How to Change Things When Change is Hard:*

> *In an exhaustive study, a psychologist analyzed 558 emotion words—every one that he could find in the English language—and found that* ***62 percent of them were negative vs. 38 percent positive****. That's a pretty shocking discrepancy. According to an old urban legend, Eskimos have 100 different words for snow. Well, it turns out that negative emotions are our snow* [note the 62/38 Golden Ratio at work in plain sight].

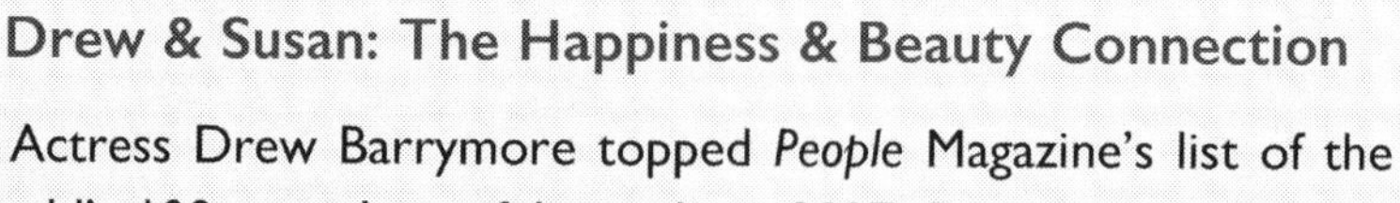

Drew & Susan: The Happiness & Beauty Connection

Actress Drew Barrymore topped *People* Magazine's list of the world's 100 most beautiful people in 2007. Barrymore attributes her beauty to her happy frame of mind and fun-loving approach to life: *Cheerfulness helps you look and feel pretty. People with a joyful nature always look beautiful.* It's no surprise that Barrymore's face also features Golden Ratio beauty in abundance. Oscar-winning actress (and ping-pong enthusiast) Susan Sarandon echoes Drew's happiness and beauty mindset: *At the heart of looking good is, more than anything, having fun and greeting each day saying 'Yes.'*

In the above example, it is clearly imperative that we consciously focus on the "meaningful minority" 38% positive words in our daily language. This example highlights the major disconnect between our 62% predominantly positive perspective and the 62% *reverse* negative predominance of the emotionally charged words available to us to express our positive outlook on life. This creates a cognitive dissonance in our society, an unrecognized source of stress and unhappiness. Dr. Murakami says that we can dramatically improve the quality and perhaps even the quantity of our life through conscious activation of the Divine Code of Life within us all. This means we must choose to minimize or even avoid exposure to the way-out-of-ratio negativity of mainstream media and language. It ought to also cause us to healthfully reduce the amount of time we spend around negative people and situations. Regarding the unlimited wonder of genes and DNA, Dr. Murakami's work highlights the sublime role of what he calls *Something Great* plays in the evolution of humanity and the Universe.

Reclaiming Your Health & Happiness

In **Bruce Lipton, Ph.D.'s** book, *The Biology of Belief*, he makes the case that our DNA only *indirectly* controls what happens in our life. He proposes that environmental and/or psychological inputs—by their molecular interactions with cell membranes—have the power to modulate how various genes are turned on or off. By becoming aware of what our psychological state is at any given time, we can reclaim control over how our DNA is expressed. In essence *everything* we ingest, feel and think—from food, drink, drugs, sounds, emotions and thoughts—can and does have incredibly strong influence over our DNA expression. The end result of these combined inputs has enormous, immediate and ongoing impact on our health, happiness and longevity. Psychological inputs are what **Candice Pert, Ph.D.**, calls *Molecules of Emotion*, which is also the title of her landmark book on the subject. Pert, one of the featured speakers in the film *What the Bleep Do We Know!?* states that molecules of emotion are peptides that circulate in our blood in response to mental-emotional activity. In other words, our beliefs and emotions can generate molecules that can interact with our cell membranes causing an intracellular cascade effect that can turn various DNA switches on—or off. There is in actuality a push-pull relationship going on between our genes on the one hand and environmental factors and psychological inputs

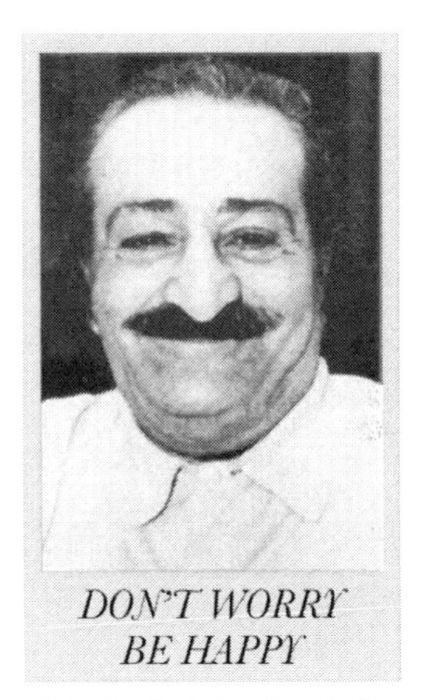

Words of wisdom from Indian mystic Meher Baba (1894-1969), which inspired Bobby McFerrin's 1988 hit *Don't Worry, Be Happy.*

on the other. This scenario is in accordance with Dr. Murakami's "genetic thinking" concept, and reminds us that we have more power than we realize to alter and upgrade our life perspective and experience, thereby resetting our happiness set point to an upward, expanding Golden Spiral. Since our genes (DNA) structure is designed with Golden Ratio parameters, we can surmise that DNA may functionally and epigenetically operate by Golden Ratio principles as well. The more conscious alignment we have with the Golden Ratio, the more positive resonance will be possible with our DNA. That is why by incorporating the easy-to-apply Rx's within this book, it's possible to access more of Nature's Secret Nutrient/NSN to turn on and light up those genes that are linked to your maximum happiness, health, longevity and life potential.

> *Happiness depends upon ourselves.*
>
> **Aristotle**

The Golden Ratio Happiness Zone

Happy For No Reason author **Marci Shimoff** shows how happiness manifests along a spectrum. We've reinterpreted her concept with the Golden Φ Ratio, as seen below.

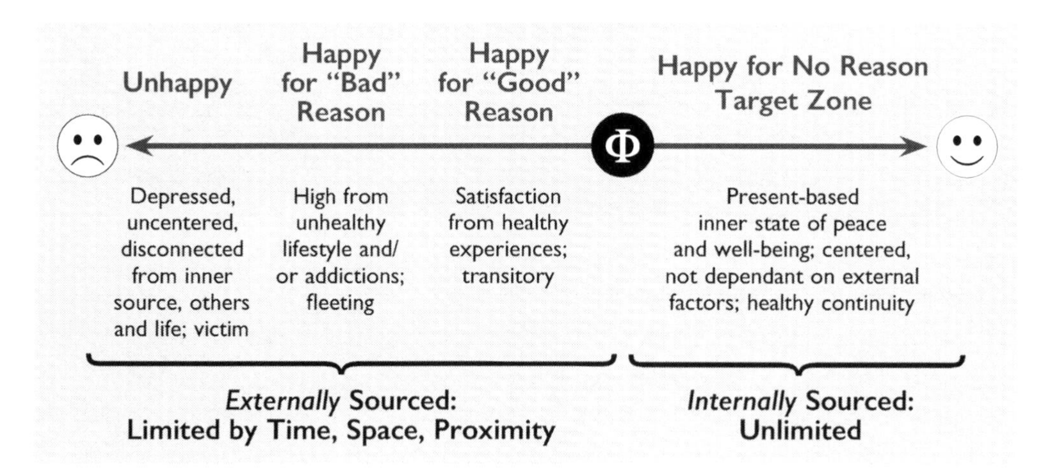

The ultimate goal is Happy for No Reason, or the state of Inner Peace. The distinction between happiness for any reason and Inner Peace is highlighted by this insightful quote Marci shares from the Upanishads:

Happiness for ANY reason is just another form of misery.

By activating Golden Ratio Biomimicry in your daily practices and life, you will increasingly radiate and attract greater happiness, contentment and Inner Peace. Perhaps as more people become aware of this unifying power and begin to implement it in their lives, the state of Inner Peace will become more frequent and lasting. As we'll see in the following section, this is exactly what seems to be happening with many people, as they seek and find increasing Golden Ratio balance between their work and personal lives.

De-stress for More Happiness: *The 4-Hour Workweek (4HWW)*

There is no lack of time–only a lack of priorities.
Tim Ferriss, author of *Tools for Titans*

For many, the word **Work** is similar to the word **Diet** in its negative connotations. While most people spend an extreme ratio of their waking hours at, travelling to or thinking about work, far too few would describe their work as a source of happiness, fulfillment and inner peace. Clearly there's room for improvement in the quality *and* quantity of work time for many. Taking work quantity to an intriguing opposite extreme, visionary anti-workaholic author and lifestyle designer Tim Ferriss has developed paradigm-shifting ways of whittling down one's working time to as little as 4 hours a week. How? In his bestselling book *The 4-Hour Workweek*, Ferriss explores the time we routinely waste in our work and life and shows how to ruthlessly reclaim it. His innovative time reclamation strategies can rapidly revolutionize your work-to-personal-time ratio. To begin reclaiming wasted time, we've applied the Golden

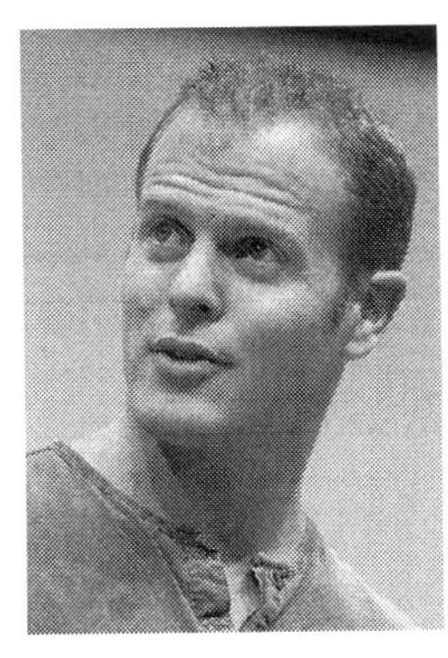

Lifestyle Design pioneer Timothy Ferriss, author of *The 4-Hour Workweek* (4HWW).

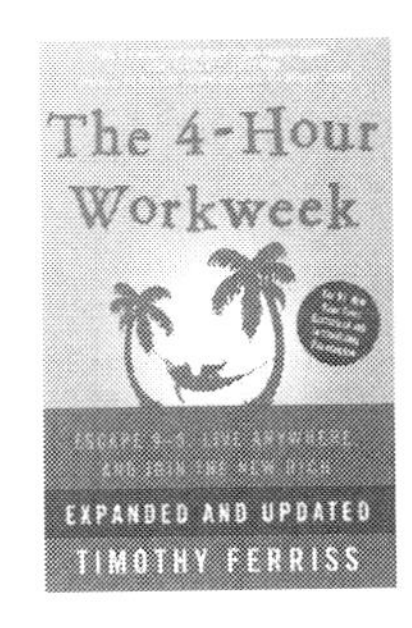

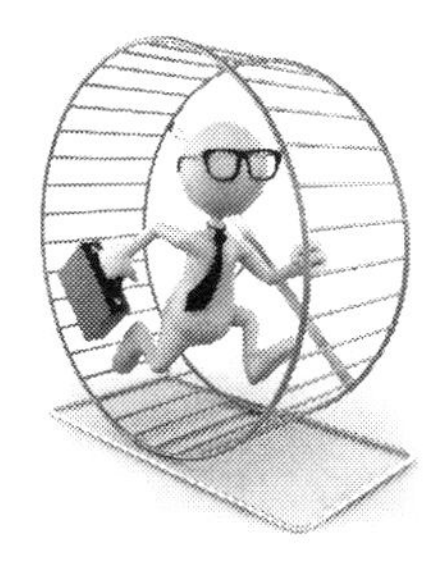

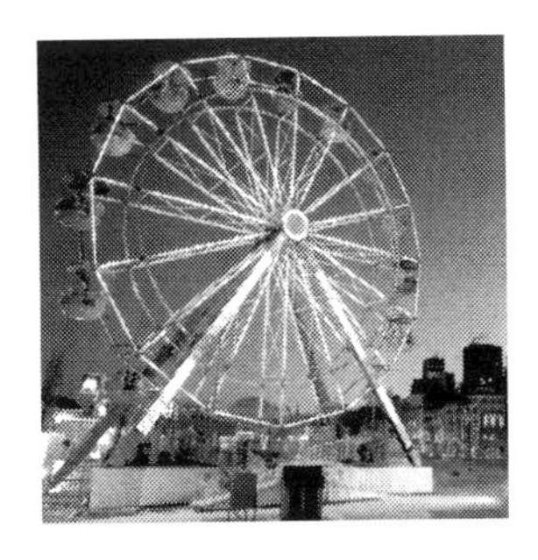

(*L*) *The 4-Hour Workweek*, Tim Ferriss' bestselling manifesto for life/work fulfillment and success. (*Center*) While running on a hamster wheel might be fun for hamsters, humans generally prefer more stimulating and enjoyable pursuits. If you've ever felt like this in your work life, know that there *is* another way. (*R*) By applying the 4-Hour Workweek principles, you can begin to step off the traditional work hamster wheel and onto the more fulfilling and fun *Tim Ferriss Wheel*.

The 4-Hr. Workweek Reduction Graph: To reduce your workweek start with whatever # is closest to the hours you're currently working. At your own pace, continue down towards a 4-HWW. Each reduction is a Golden Ratio drop following a reversed Lucas Sequence, similar to the Fibonacci Sequence, except it begins: 2, 1, 3, **4, 7, 11, 18, 29, 47, 76**... In addition to excess hours, most people are also working too many *days* per week, as 4.3 days is the Golden Ratio of workdays in a week (7/4.3=1.62).

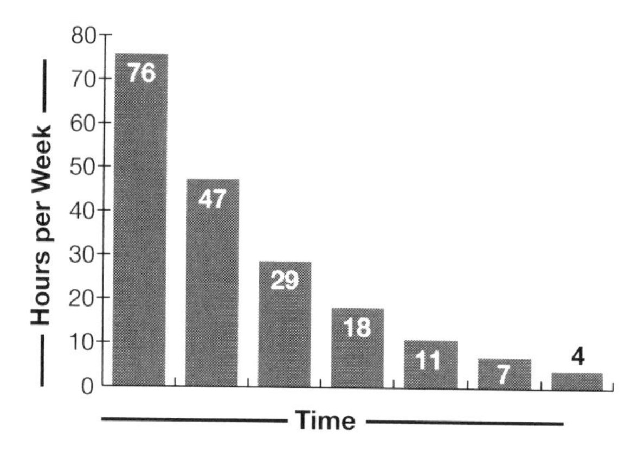

Ratio to a work-reduction graph to highlight how you might begin to move towards a 4-hour workweek. While you may not want to go down to 4 hours a week (or initially feel capable of it), you can use this Golden Ratio work reduction graph to gauge your decremental progress towards a healthier work/personal time ratio. As many people are working in excess of 45 hours a week, this means they're still working outside of the first Golden Ratio reduction, with insufficient personal/recharge time. Invariably we end up *robbing Peter to pay Paul*, compromising our sleep, grooming, eating and personal time. If this describes you, take a closer look at how you could reduce your work time towards healthier, lower Golden Ratios of work to personal time. Start by including more **white space** in your daily schedule—rest, relaxation, recharge and personal/family time. While it's possible to burn the candle at both ends for years—working 50–70+ hours a week at work you may not enjoy, the long-term effects on your health, happiness and longevity can be far more serious than you allow yourself to think.

> *Get satisfied with doing less of what matters least,*
> *and more of what matters most.*
> **Frank Sabato, philosopher**

Enhancing Healthy Work/Life Ratios

Like an athlete who overtrains without sufficient rest and recovery (leading to poor performance, burnout or injury), poor work/life ratios invariably lead to under performance and unhappiness, not to mention potentially deadly health challenges. One study of 7,095 British civil servants revealed that long/overtime working hours increase the risk of coronary heart disease by a whopping 67%. **Mika Kivimaki**, professor of epidemiology and public health at University College London and lead author of the study published in the *Annals of Internal Medicine* put it this way:

We knew there was an association between working long hours and coronary heart disease, but we were really surprised that it was such a strong predictor.

Clearly, maintaining a healthy work/life ratio is crucial for health, happiness and longevity. While everyone's work/life ratio needs are unique, many are both overworked and insufficiently fulfilled, with inadequate personal/recharging time. Whether you're interested in a 40+ hour, 4-Hour or a Golden Ratio 4 days out of 7 workweek, the following strategies offer support for achieving your own ideally fulfilling work/life ratio.

Adding Time To Your Life & Life To Your Time

We all get the same gift of 168 hours per week: 7 days x 24 hours/day. If you figure the Golden Sleep Ratio of about 9 hours of sleep/rest for every 24 hours (63 hours/week), 3 hours/day for meals prep/eating (21 hours/week), and 1.5 hours daily for bathing/bathroom/grooming (10.5 hours/week), it adds up to 94.5 hours/week—for just the basics. This leaves 73.5 hours/week of waking time for work, commuting, exercise and all personal activities. It's logical that in order to improve the quality of your life, you'd want to increase your personal time ratio in order to arrive at your individual healthy ratio of work to personal time. Of course, everyone's idea of the ideal ratios will vary, depending on the rewards obtained from work vs. personal activities.

Hours worked per day and week through the centuries (US and Europe)			Avg. hours worked per week in different countries (2008/pre-recession data)	
Time Period	Work hours per day	Work days per week	Country	Work hours per week
Middle Ages	8	6	USA	35
1800	14	N/A	Poland, Czech Republic	38
1840	10	N/A	South Korea	44
1919	8-9	N/A	Spain, Denmark, Ireland	31
1936	8	5	France, Belgium	30
2010	5-8	4-5	Netherlands, Norway	27
Ferriss 4HWW	<1	.5	Ferriss 4HWW	4

Life is precious and our days are numbered. We have a total of about 29,000 days to live at birth, assuming an 80 year lifespan. If you're 40, this means you have around 14,500 days to go—14,500 sunrises and sunsets. It goes pretty fast, especially if you fail to be fully present and appreciate the moment—it's said that dwelling more consciously in the **Now** is key to happiness, inner peace and agelessness. To top it off, none of us knows for sure when the screen of our life will read: *Game Over.* **But hold on, here's**

the great news: when you engage the Nature's Secret Nutrient System, you can vastly increase the quality of your life along with your odds of living 100+ healthy years. This translates into enjoying 36,500 days of life from birth or about a 25% increase above the "norm" of around 29,000 days. Since most people spend the majority of their waking time working, doing work that's fulfilling and meaningful ought to be high on everyone's list, whether it's for 4 or 40+ hours a week. Along with upgrading the quality of your work to be more enjoyable, de-stressing by upgrading your work-to-personal time ratio is clearly a major modifiable happiness/longevity behavior you *can* control. Greater happiness, health, inner peace and longevity are among the inevitable results.

> *We hold these Truths to be self-evident, that all Men are created equal,*
> *that they are endowed by their Creator with certain unalienable Rights,*
> *that among these are Life, Liberty, and the Pursuit of Happiness...*
>
> **Thomas Jefferson**

Kaizen: Small Steps for Greater Happiness & Life Quality

A journey of a 1000 miles begins with the first step.

Lao Tzu

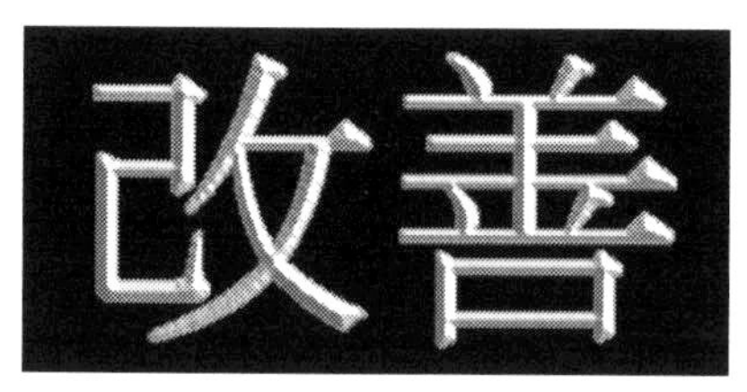

Kaizen (*Continuous Improvement*) in Japanese, a key facet of Quality.

The Hoshin North Star process and The First 15%, as inspired by **Dr. W. Edwards Deming,** are at the root of *Kaizen* (Japanese for Continuous Improvement), consisting of taking small, sure steps of improvement towards a goal. In his Deming/Kaizen-inspired book *One Small Step Can Change Your Life*, **Dr. Robert Maurer** shows how taking small steps invariably leads to big progress, as large steps often cause a fear-of-change, shut down reaction in the brain. Kaizen's small steps approach are at the heart of this book's Action Rx's & 21-Day Priority Coach System.

By taking small daily steps in support of the key NSN health & longevity driver MegaNutrients, the butterfly effect of increasing returns is activated. Like the ripples in the surface of a lake after a skipping stone is launched, the waves start small—yet grow exponentially. Energy and momentum builds in a cross-reinforcing chain reaction. Kaizen's power is that the steps need not be big ones; again, the most effective steps are paradoxically often the smallest. In the work arena for example, if your current job is unfulfilling, you're more likely to take the small step of 5 minutes of reading a chapter in **Richard Bolles'** *What Color Is Your Parachute* or polishing up your resume vs. taking the bigger step of quitting your current job today. Such small steps invariably set the stage for the big changes and upgrades desired; they prime the pump and get you in the game. The key to Kaizen's success is to take *meaningful* small steps aligned with your key priorities. This strategy works well with Tim Ferriss' 4-Hour Workweek approach, and is a key element for more fulfillment and happiness in life and work. So, *Banzai Kaizen!*

The 80/20 Principle: Work Smarter (& Happier) vs. Harder

> *Anyone can be more effective with less effort by learning how to identify & leverage the 80/20 principle—the well-known, unpublicized secret that 80 percent of all our results* [and happiness] *in business & life stem from a mere 20 percent of our efforts.*
>
> **Richard Koch, author, *The 80/20 Principle***

First observed in 1906 by Italian economist **Vilfredo Pareto** and later championed by Romanian quality genius **Dr. Joseph Juran**, the 80/20 Rule (aka the **Pareto Principle**) can positively transform your work and life. Pareto initially observed that 80% of the land in Italy was owned by 20% of the people, closer to home noting that 80% of the peas in his garden came from 20% of the pods. Eight words summarize this principle: *80% of results come from 20% of actions.* This dynamic of uneven cause/effect distribution is at play everywhere in the Universe. **Whether the 80/20 Pareto Ratio or the 62/38 Golden Ratio, the Universe seems to operate according to a seesaw of unequal, yet dynamic ratios of causes to effects, actions to results:**

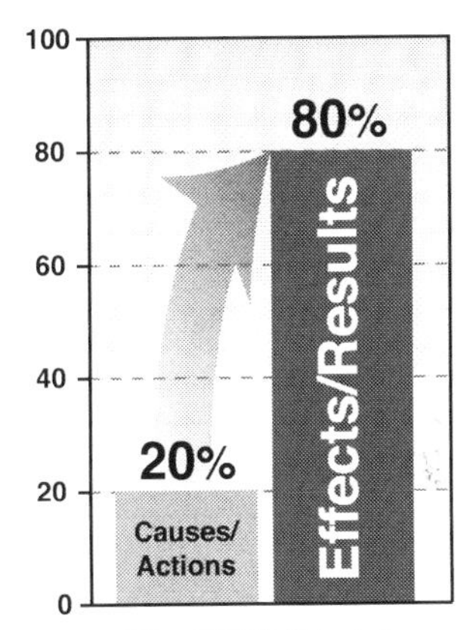

The 80/20 Principle: 80% of the results come from 20% of the actions. What are the key 20% of actions that lead to 80% of *your* desired results?

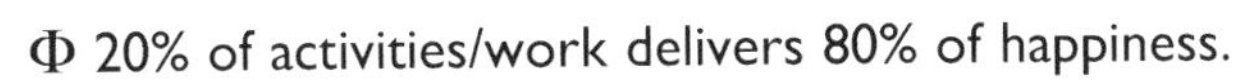

- Φ 20% of activities/work delivers 80% of happiness.
- Φ 20% of customers generate 80% of business.
- Φ 20% of people = 80% of fulfillment in relationships.

Identifying and enhancing the 20% "vital few" minority causes and/or actions leads to the majority of desired outcomes. Even a little more focus on the 20% of your daily activities which deliver 80% of the desired/necessary results can greatly multiply your productivity and value. Author **Richard Koch** calls applying this principle to life and work *80/20 Thinking* and it's magic for supporting greater fulfillment and happiness.

Order From Chaos: A Human-Scaled System for Enhanced Productivity

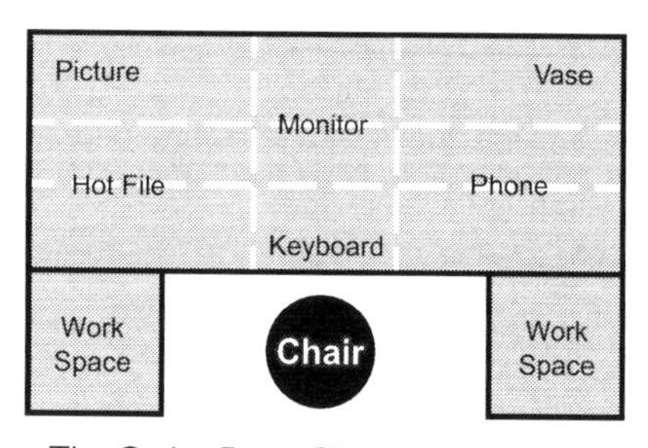

The Order From Chaos system upgrades work space to enhance productivity. Positioning key desk items using a Golden Ratio grid (like a camera's Golden Ratio viewfinder grid) can provide an added boost.

Order from Chaos: Six Steps To Personal & Professional Organization is organizational expert **Liz Davenport's** system for increasing the ratio of creativity and productivity to chaos. Some of Liz's research reflects the Golden Ratio, e.g., mistakes increase about 40% when most people try to do multiple things at once, aka multitasking, and a U.S. survey revealed that 60% of people are habitually disorganized. While chaos and creativity often go hand-in-hand, the challenge comes when the *ratio* of creative chaos to productivity/fulfillment falls out of proportion; frustration and stress rises and inner peace and happiness inevitably suffers. Liz's system integrates you into your work environment, enhancing confidence and calm. Your desk and work space gets tuned to human scale, e.g., items used daily are placed in hand's reach; weekly, arm's reach; monthly, in the room (out of hand's/arm's reach). This supports the 80/20 Principle at work: on average, 80% of the time you work with 20% of your papers/files. The system includes optimizing your to-do list and calendar systems. Integrating Golden Ratio dynamics boosts the system further, e.g., the small step of positioning key objects on your desk (monitor, phone, pen cup, picture, etc.) according to general Golden Ratio grid points. Greater productivity and happiness—Nature's Path of Least Resistance and Maximum Performance—are more predictable results of this easy-to-implement system.

Stress: Disarming the Hidden Grim Reaper

Stress is the #1 health epidemic of the 21st century.

The World Health Organization

8

Chronic mental and emotional stress often leads to chronic cellular inflammation—a silent and insidious grim reaper smoldering slowly over time, leading to reduced life quality and often, illness and premature death. **In short, stress kills—but first it warns you—via various pains, illnesses, diseases, fatigue, etc.** Some signs of excess stress are obvious—fatigue, anxiety, poor sleep or digestion, any persistent health, discomfort or pain challenges—while others are insidious and largely unknown or unnoticed, e.g., high blood pressure, hormonal imbalance, chronic inflammation, persistent excessive mental/emotional stresses, etc. Even though mental and emotional stress may appear to be on a purely energetic level, concrete physiologic changes can be seen with targeted blood testing, e.g., C-Reactive Protein (CRP) is a common blood test that identifies non-specific inflammation from any source. Stress can also cause abnormalities in vital body systems which can also often be identified via blood testing (see blood tests in Ch 6 Rx section). Blood sugar, cholesterol and even immune and hormonal abnormalities can be caused by stress, as can heart attacks, strokes and very possibly even cancer. With both chronic mental and emotional stress, an honest assessment is the first step in identifying the primary causes. The next step is to commit to a steady campaign to both reduce key stressors and adopt proven stress reduction practices—such as meditation and breath awareness—presented in this book. **The research confirms the bad news: stress kills. The good news? You can step in and disarm this hidden grim reaper with the Nature's Secret Nutrient system.**

Inner Peace Leads to Outer Peace: Imagining a Golden Ratio Renaissance

Imagine all the people, living life in peace.
You may say I'm a dreamer, but I'm not the only one...

John Lennon

In October 2005, the New Jerusalem Foundation in Israel unveiled a Golden Ratio-based 50-ton sculpture called *Ratio* in Jerusalem. Thirty-two 1.5-ton limestone blocks modeled after key stones in the Western Wailing Wall were arranged in Golden Ratio formation. The vertical arrangement of the blocks in the sculpture mirrors the beginning numbers in the Fibonacci Sequence, edges beautifully gilded with gold to catch the rays of the rising and setting sun. Sculptor **Andrew Rogers** of Australia had this to say about

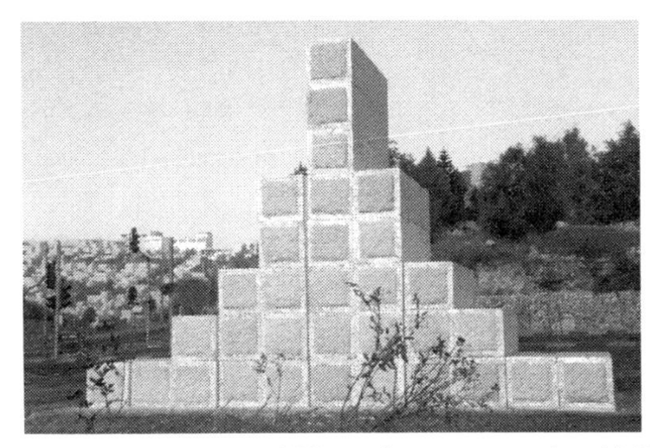

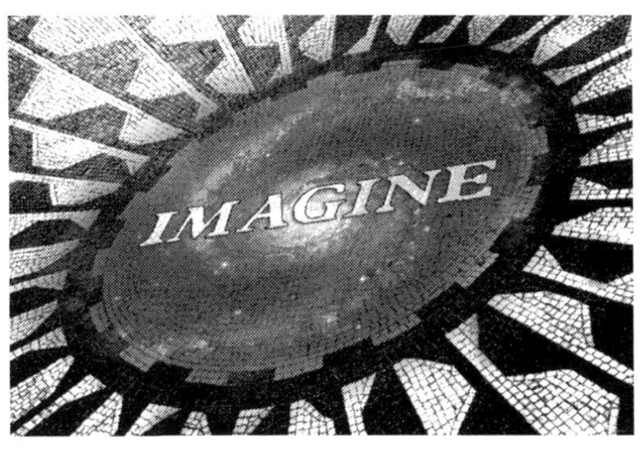

(*L*) Andrew Rogers' 50 ton *Ratio*, a stone & gold Golden Ratio sculpture in Jerusalem. The number of stones in each column are stacked vertically in a numerical *palindrome* of a rising and falling Fibonacci Sequence: 1-1-2-3-5-8-5-3-2-1-1. (*R*) ***Imagine*** mosaic on the ground at the center of New York City's Central Park John Lennon memorial; custom Golden Spiral galaxy enhancement by the authors.

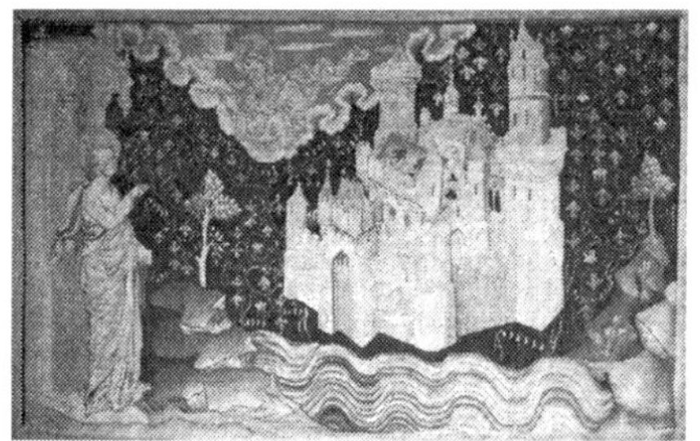
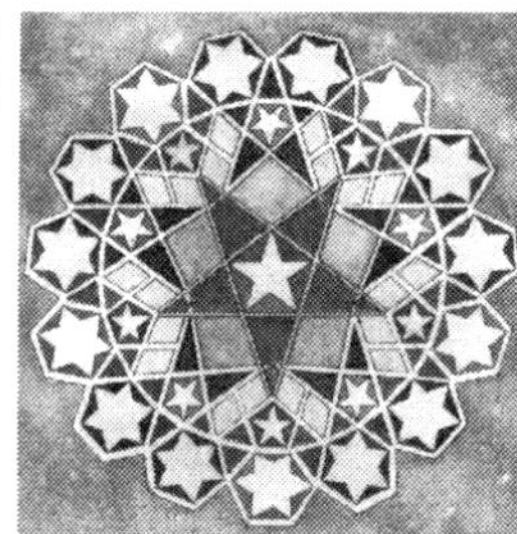
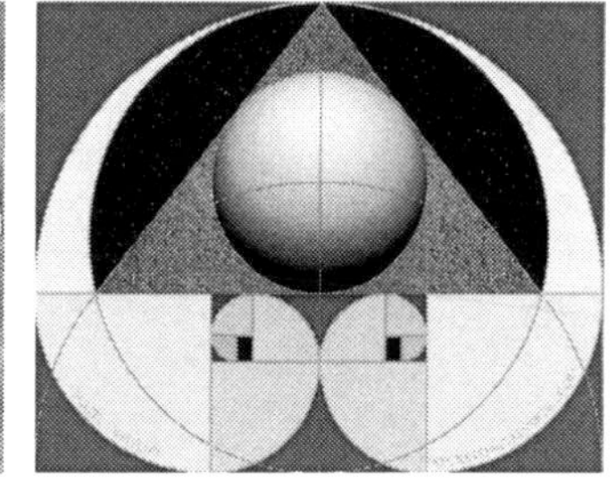

(*L*) John of Patmos watches the descent of the New Jerusalem from God in a 14th century Golden Rectangle tapestry. (*C*) John Michell's *New Jerusalem* pentagonal Golden Ratio diagram. (*R*) Scott Onstott's visionary Golden Ratio art and books explore the unifying micro/macro expressions of the ratio throughout mathematics, art and nature (visit: SecretsInPlainSight.com)

his unique work of gold-fringed stone:

> *I came at the invitation of the New Jerusalem Foundation. This is a very special city for me. I came here to create a stone sculpture called "Ratio"... "Ratio" demonstrates a mathematical formula, which helps us understand the compositions of plants and how they grow, the proportions of plants and the human body. In everyday terms it helps explain the curve of a snail shell or seashell, the sections on a pineapple, the proportions of our body, and it helps explain in my case a lot of sculptures that I'm creating around the world. I started a project in contemporary art initially in the Arava desert, and to explain this project, we set out the mathematical formula in stone... I thought that because this is such a universal city and the Golden Ratio is such a universal explanation that there was a synthesis and symbolism of having it here... after all, it's one of the cradles of civilization and the Golden Ratio is one of the universal theories...*

Jerusalem is a city where three major world religions and cultures intersect. In our current era, this intersection has been one of ongoing war, separation and chaos. The principle of the Golden Ratio—of parts coming together in such a way as to form a harmonious, greater whole—can be seen as a key principle of the New Jerusalem concept. Prophecies in the Bible describe New Jerusalem as a place of peace and harmony that will descend from the heavens. English author **John Michell** writes eloquently about the New Jerusalem concept, offering a visionary template for its re-establishment on Earth in *The Dimensions of Paradise: The Proportions and Symbolic Numbers of Ancient Cosmology*. Canadian author and architect **Scott Onstott** echoes similar resonant themes in his fascinating books *Taking Measure* and *Tripartite*. This emerging global consciousness, grounded in the science of sacred geometry inclusive of the unifying Golden Ratio, would serve to unite the discordant fragments of world culture and religion, reorganizing them into a peaceful, inclusive whole. As a timeless symbol of unity, the sculpture *Ratio* may

The Golden Ratio & Peace Symbol Connection

The Peace Symbol is a creative adaptation from semaphore signaling designed by Gerald Haltom in 1958. The semaphore signals for **N** & **D** stand for **N**uclear **D**isarmament, and when superimposed on one another form the universally recognized icon. The semaphores divide the circle into near-Golden Ratio angles of 137.5° & 222.5°. The unification principle is at the heart of a true peace symbol, heralding a hunger for peace in our time *and* the re-emergence of Golden Ratio unity consciousness.

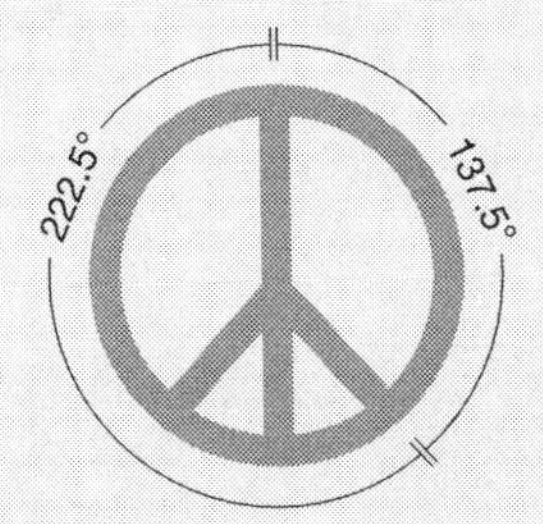

Peace Symbol with Golden Ratio angles.

Semaphores "N" and "D" are the original inspiration for the peace symbol.

act as a catalyst for the New Jerusalem to rise again in our time. For those not living in Jerusalem, the concept of the New Jerusalem is synonymous with awakening to a deeper sense and enjoyment of the sacred, of the Divine Proportion which links and unifies us with one another and with all life and creation. Identical Golden Ratio sculptures are being established by Andrew Rogers in twelve countries worldwide, in conjunction with UNESCO's World Heritage project. Other countries that will have their own Golden Ratio sculptures include Peru, Great Britain, America, Australia and Iceland. As more people become aware of their divine nature and interconnectedness with all life, the positive effects will naturally ripple outward and become evident throughout the world. Visionary artisans like John Michell, Andrew Rogers and Scott Onstott are among the modern-day Golden Ratio Renaissance pioneers, helping people reawaken to their personal sense, restoration and stewardship of the New Jerusalem, within and without.

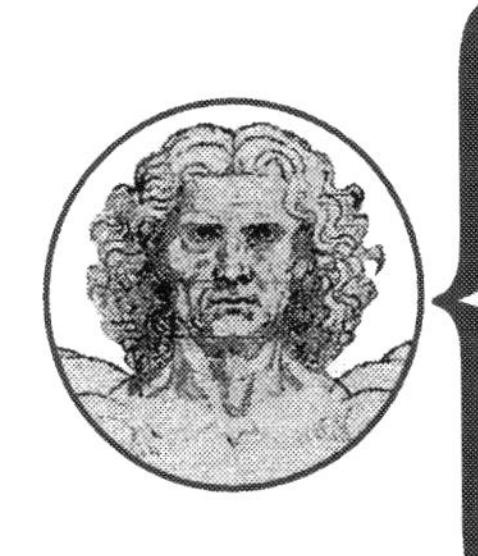

Remember, you're only as ***HAPPY*** *as you feel in any moment.*
If you're feeling blue, activate your latent Golden Ratio-blueprinted Happiness genes by practicing gratitude & giving & doing more of whatever makes you happy & strengthening intimate connections and social networks. Last yet not least, turn on your Mona Lisa Smile and take time to meditate daily for even 5–8 minutes, until you're *Happy For No Reason.*

Anastasia Soare's eyebrow sculpting method enhances your **natural beauty** by accentuating the Golden Ratio symmetry in your face.

Our **facial features** are designed around the Golden Ratio. Learning how to enhance these Golden Ratio relationships is the secret.

Did you know that dentists are able to **restore oral beauty,** form & function by realigning jaw & teeth to the Golden Ratio?

Studies show a direct connection between a strong **immune system** & facial & body symmetry.

Enhancing your personal appearance with Nature's Secret Nutrient/ NSN improves self-confidence & **sexual attractiveness.**

Beauty/ Relationships: #9 driver, Golden Ratio secrets of beauty & attraction

Did you know that your life has a Golden Ratio Prime Zone? It's **between ages 19–31**. NSN can reactivate this vitality zone in your life.

Enhance **love & intimacy** in your relationships by balancing the spaces in your togetherness as a reflection of the Golden Ratio.

The mathematics of the Universe are visible to all in the form of Beauty.

John Michell

Beauty/Relationships

...it can be said that wherever there is an intensification of function or a particular beauty and harmony of form, there the Golden Ratio will be found.
Robert Lawlor, author of *Sacred Geometry: Philosophy & Practice*

Reactivating Your Golden Prime Zone Years: Ages 19 to 31

From ages 19 to 31, Nature ingeniously fine-tunes hormonal physiology and sexual attractiveness to maximally reflect the Golden Ratio. Nature's elegant Golden Ratio engineering has designed the attraction of the opposite sexes to be a force that is too strong to resist, thus ensuring the passage of one's DNA to the next generation. **Thus the numbers 19 and 31 define the boundaries of your prime physical 13-year lifecycle phase and are also known as "prime" numbers.** Prime numbers are numbers that are only divisible by themselves and the number 1. However, 19 and 31 are special prime numbers known as *Golden Primes,* as 31 divided by 19 approximates the Golden Ratio 1.6. In essence, your most robust years—those between ages 19 and 31—comprise your "**Golden Prime Zone.**" This double entendre highlights the fact that the physical robustness and sexual vitality that almost everyone experiences in their Golden Prime Zone is the ideal state to which all health, exercise, diet and lifestyle programs aspire—the Nature's Secret Nutrient System included. Maximizing natural beauty, attractiveness and intimacy are some of the desirable outcomes resulting from aligning with the Golden

9

Ratio, converting them into a potent **Meta**Nutrient. Your inherent genetic potential is optimized once the primary drivers of the Nature's Secret Nutrient system are aligned and activated. Yet the external beauty associated with the Golden Ratio doesn't stop with appearance and physiology. It can powerfully manifest in character, behavior and creativity as well. The Golden Ratio attributes of "beautiful people" are only an external hint of the excellence that anyone can display in any of the multitude of human endeavors. As a reminder of how beautiful the Golden Ratio can be manifested in human form, let's look at a few iconic examples and some reasons underlying their natural beauty and charismatic power of attraction.

Marilyn Monroe & Sean Connery: Divinely Proportioned Sex Icons

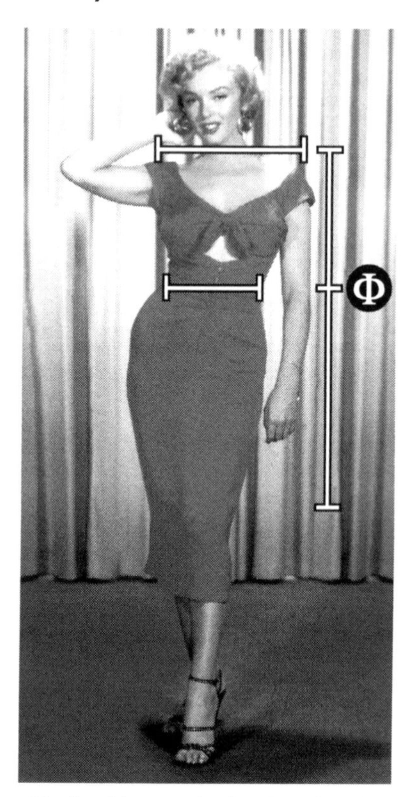

Marilyn Monroe displays her shapely Golden Ratio attributes in this publicity portrait from *Niagara* (1953). Shoulder width/waist width = the Golden Ratio, and her elbow and waist are also at the vertical Golden Cut point between shoulders and knees.

Marilyn Monroe and Sean Connery are two of the 20th century's best known sex icons. They epitomize Divine Proportions in their archetypal physical attractiveness and magnetism. Monroe's Golden Ratio attributes are very apparent in the accompanying photo from the 1953 film *Niagara*. One's attention is immediately drawn to her shapely hourglass figure and bustline. Her waist accentuates the Golden Ratio dividing point between her shoulders and knees, while the width of her shoulders to waist displays Golden Ratio proportions as well. Monroe's ability to arouse the opposite sex was no doubt based on a subconscious Golden Ratio recognition by her fans. In spite of her short career, she won the 1960 Golden Globe Award for Best Actress for *Some Like It Hot*. Her image is forever etched into America's collective unconscious as the archetypal beautiful and sexy female of her generation.

Sean Connery developed his rugged masculinity early in his career by sculpting his body with serious weight training. He also learned to master and express graceful movement, which set him apart from other actors. All of these techniques complemented his innate animal magnetism to

9

produce one of the era's most iconic sex symbols. As *GQ* magazine describes Connery:

> *All the actors who have inhabited the role of James Bond have enjoyed the trapping of style—killing bad guys in Savile Row bespoke—but only one of them can truly be said to have style... Sean Connery is still the yardstick by which all other Bonds are measured—the arched eyebrow, the dry wolfish smile. But we at GQ think it mostly has to do with the way he moved. It only looked effortless: Before he was cast in Dr. No, Connery was an ardent student of the Swedish movement teacher* **Yat Malmgren,** *whose book on body technique became Connery's bible. That's how the former bricklayer from a hardscrabble section of Edinburgh learned to walk with (in one observer's memorable phrase) 'the threatening grace of a panther on the prowl.' Read it as a gloss on his penchant for violence or his sexual prowess: It works both ways.*

Sean Connery used his Divinely Proportioned attributes to great advantage, from his legendary James Bond role to many other films, including his 1987 Academy Award-winning performance as Best Supporting Actor in *The Untouchables*. Many critics and fans have said that the quality of Connery's acting, like fine wine, only improved with time. Certainly his personal appeal has. In 1989, at nearly 60, he was voted *People* Magazine's Sexiest Man Alive; in 1999, at 69, he was voted Sexiest Man of the Century. He has also received a Crystal Globe for outstanding artistic contribution to world cinema.

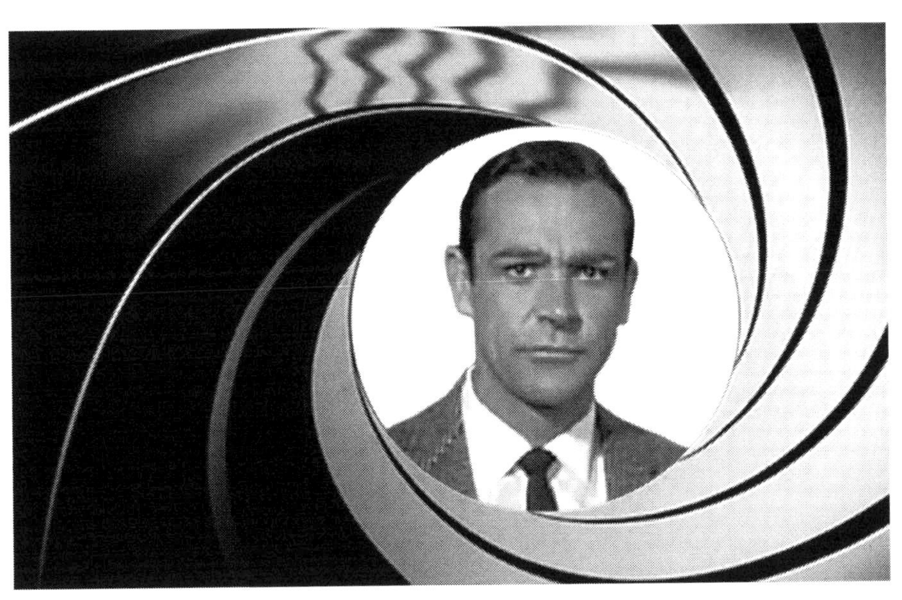

Sean Connery, the ultimate, suave and debonair ***Bond... James Bond*** personifies the Golden Ratio in style, movement and charisma. Note that every Bond film since 1962's *Dr. No* also highlights the Golden Ratio's open-secret cultural presence: 007 begins each film framed by the multiple Golden Spirals inside a gun barrel. See the Rx in Ch 8 Happiness for the custom Bond Golden Ratio Aston Martini.

9

James Bond's Ultra Cool Performance & Longevity Weapon: Ice-Cold Scottish Showers

Alternating hot and cold showers was one of James Bond's secret techniques for quick rejuvenation and looking cool and suave after fighting the likes of Dr. No, Goldfinger or Blofeld. Bond took "Scottish Showers" in virtually all of the original James Bond novels. The alternating hot and cold showers would leave him refreshed, invigorated and ready for his "undercover" work with the likes of Pussy Galore, Tiffany Case and Solitaire. Here's one of author Ian Fleming's excerpts from *Casino Royale*, the first in the Bond series:

> *Bond walked up to his room, which again showed no sign of trespass, threw off his clothes, took a long hot bath followed by an ice-cold shower and lay down on his bed. There remained an hour in which to rest and compose his thoughts before he met the girl in the Splendide bar, an hour to examine minutely the details of his plans for the game, and for after the game, in all the various circumstances of victory or defeat.*

Brad Pitt's Golden Ratio Facial Score

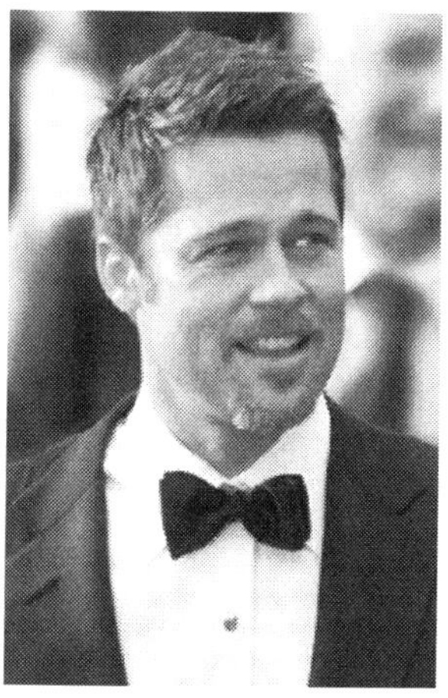

Brad Pitt scored 9.3 out of 10 on Oprah Winfrey's *Laws of Attraction* special with Golden Ratio beauty expert Dr. Kendra Schmid.

America's famous television host and media mogul, **Oprah Winfrey**, has discovered the science of the Golden Ratio. In March, 2009, she presented a series of shows on the *Laws of Attraction*, on which she hosted biostatistics professor **Dr. Kendra Schmid**. By using 29 precise facial measurements, including several Golden Ratio parameters, Dr. Schmid is able to assess anyone's level of essential attractiveness. For example, to get a higher score, the length of the face compared to the width should be 1.6,—the Golden Ratio. Dr. Schmid then takes other key measurements of proportion and symmetry to come up with a composite score on a scale of 1–10, with 10 being the ideal. Two of the highest scoring celebrities, Brad Pitt and Angelina Jolie, scored 9.3 and 7.7 respectively. Brad Pitt's 9.3 is the highest score received by any celebrity thus far. Dr. Schmid noted that Angelina's famous "full lips," [although voluptuous], were what lowered her score. Dr. Schmid said that *the width of a mouth should be twice the height of the lips.* Other notables: Halle Berry at 7.4 and Hugh Jackman at 6.5.

Anastasia Soare: Golden Ratio Natural Beauty Master to the Stars

Taking all the knowledge I learned from Leonardo da Vinci and Leonardo Fibonacci, I was able to consistently create the perfect Golden Proportion on anybody's face.
Anastasia Soare

A Golden Ratio Genius is someone who has been inspired by and applied the Golden Ratio in a unique and original way in their work and life. In our first book, *The Divine Code of Da Vinci, Fibonacci, Einstein and YOU*, we featured some of the more prominent Golden Ratio Geniuses in history, including Da Vinci, Fibonacci and Einstein. We are always pleasantly surprised when a new and innovative Golden Ratio Genius arrives on the scene. Anastasia Soare, Hollywood's Golden Ratio natural beauty master, has joined the ranks of history's Golden Ratio Geniuses with her breakthrough Golden Ratio-inspired innovations in the fields of beauty, aesthetics and cosmetology.

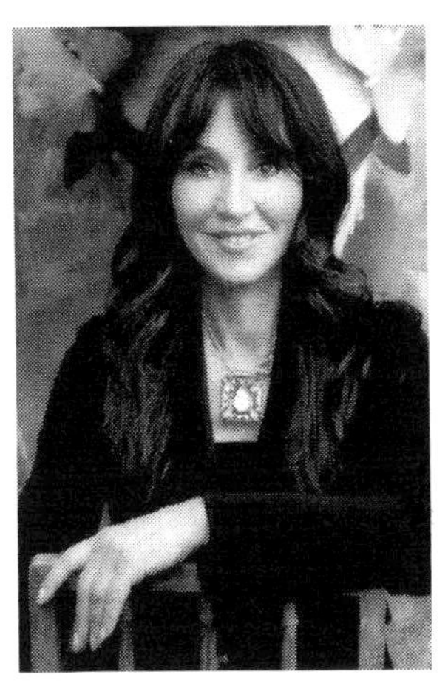

Anastasia Soare, Golden Ratio beauty master to celebrities worldwide. Her work has transformed the art and science of natural beauty enhancement.

Anastasia and her family emigrated from Romania to America in 1989. Despite not yet speaking English, she soon found work in a Los Angeles salon as a cosmetologist. In 1997 she opened her own salon, with an emphasis on eyebrow sculpting. As a result of her innovative approach, she quickly became the rave of Beverly Hills, in high demand by the world's top celebrities. Some of her notable clients include Oprah Winfrey (whose eyebrows Anastasia sculpted live on Oprah's show), Madonna, Jennifer Lopez, Heidi Klum, Jennifer Aniston, Kim Kardashian, Reese Witherspoon and Ryan Seacrest. What was it that compelled Hollywood's most beautiful and influential people to have Anastasia sculpt their brows and upgrade their look and appearance? While it's true that Anastasia has an eastern European flair to her personality and work, **what really distinguishes her peerless approach is her underlying mastery of the Golden Ratio**. In Romania, Anastasia studied architecture, engineering, drawing and mathematics, including an emphasis on the works of the two Leonardo's: Da Vinci and Fibonacci. These were the seminal imprints that would later inspire her breakthrough insights as an aesthetician and cosmetologist. While studying proportions of the human face, she had the intuitive flash to apply Golden Ratio proportions to achieve optimal eyebrow sculpting results. **This simple yet profound Golden Ratio upgrade enhances the intrinsic beauty inherent in anyone's natural facial proportions and bone structure**, and became the underlying concept that led Anastasia to revolutionize the field of aesthetics and cosmetology and create the **Anastasia Beverly Hills** beauty empire. She discovered that anyone's eyebrows could be sculpted to Golden Ratio proportions by determining three key landmarks:

1. An imaginary line running vertically through the middle of the nostril determines the medial eyebrow border.
2. The high point on the eyebrow arch can be found on a line connecting the tip of the nose to the center of the iris. The high point divides the eyebrow into Golden Ratio proportions.
3. The point that lies on a line running through the edge of the corresponding nostril through the outer edge of the eye determines the lateral eyebrow border.

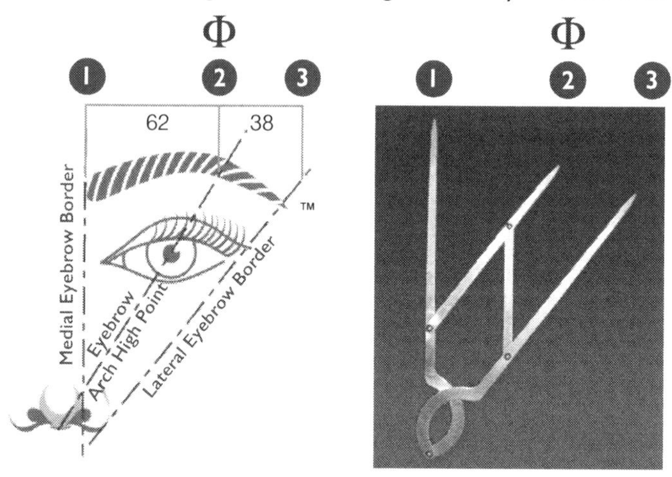

(*L*) Detail from Anastasia of Beverly Hills' educational materials, illustrating her patented formula for Golden Ratio eyebrow sculpting. (*R*) Authors' comparison of how Anastasia's dotted facial lines mirror the Golden Ratio calipers' design.

Although most people's facial proportions deviate to varying degrees from the Golden Ratio, **Anastasia's eyebrow sculpting and makeup application techniques easily reorients anyone's facial features back towards Divine Proportion.** This supports the revelation of their unique natural beauty and attractiveness, cross-reinforcing an upward spiral of enhanced inner and outer self-esteem. Regarding the universal applicability of her discovery Anastasia said,

> *Studying technical design and art in Romania gave me the ability to see things in 3-D. Back then, we didn't have computers—we figured things out with pencils. Once I became an aesthetician, I took that knowledge and studied the bone structure of every ethnic group. It helped me to find the perfect shape for anyone's bone structure. I became really obsessed with the eyebrow, because nobody thought that it was important... My goal is to make the eyebrows beautifully symmetrical and proportionate to a person's own natural symmetry and bone structure, because even when features are asymmetrical—as they often are—* ***well-shaped brows will bring a harmony, proportion and balance to the face.***

Anastasia's genius was to superimpose Golden Ratio caliper geometry over the nose, eyes and brow in order to find the precise Golden Ratio divisions of the brow. Golden Ratio calipers have two arms that are parallel and one arm at a variable angle. Looking at Anastasia's facial lines graphic you can see that, just as with Golden Ratio calipers, two lines are parallel and one line is at an angle. In addition, the three lines running from the nose to the eyebrow do not originate from a single point, just as the three arms of Golden Ratio calipers don't originate from a single point. This unique linear array makes it possible to integrate and enhance nasal, eye and eyebrow features within the unifying, beautifying context of Golden Ratio proportions.

Beauty is not Perfection. Real beauty is Proportion.

Anastasia Soare

When you make contact with anyone, your attention first goes naturally to their eyes. If their eyes are framed by the eyebrows above and the nose below—all in Golden Ratio proportion—the beholder receives the message that the Golden Ratio always conveys, that of beauty, harmony, unity and attractiveness. Anastasia's profound epiphany was to fuse the Golden Ratio with the insight that the eyebrow is the single most impactful feature to upgrade total facial symmetry towards Divine Proportion. Essentially, Anastasia created a universal, noninvasive, high-impact method for restoring and accentuating anyone's natural beauty and attractiveness, male or female. In the process, she revealed a profound new beauty truism and created the remarkable method to bring it to life:

Beauty is in the eye of the beholder—and in the eyebrows of the beheld.

Not only has Anastasia's day-to-day salon practice benefited from her breakthrough insights into the Golden Ratio, she also reaps the growing business and achievement rewards that inevitably follow aligning one's work and passion with it. Her expanding line of products are featured in over 400 locations in the United States, including Nordstroms, Sephora and Ulta, as well as globally. While Anastasia's natural beauty empire grows in a graceful upward Golden Spiral, she also keeps giving and receiving in Golden Ratio: she is associated with many charitable foundations, including *Oprah's Angel Network* and *The Blue Heron Foundation,* which benefits Romanian orphans. Anastasia's story is a classic case of the vast power of the Golden Ratio to transform the lives, beauty and fortunes of those who seek and apply its secrets in plain sight.

Beauty & the Golden Dental Ratio

In order to optimize the appearance, structure and function of their patients, more leading-edge doctors are incorporating Golden Ratio principles in their treatments. **Dr. David Frey** is a top Beverly Hills-based dentist who creatively utilizes the Golden Ratio to restore healthy proportion to his patient's teeth. This results in increased bite efficiency, more relaxed jaw, face and head muscles and enhanced beauty and appearance. In his book *Revitalizing Your Mouth*, Dr. Frey notes,

> *Combining the Golden Proportion with modern-day full mouth restoration techniques enables you to find the smile that is in proportion to your face. For example, the Golden Proportion can be applied to your two front teeth by measuring their width and mathematically determining the proper length. If the teeth have worn down, porcelain veneers can add the necessary length to restore them to Golden Proportion. It has been discovered that when your mouth is positioned in the physiologically correct bite, your top and bottom teeth can generally be placed in Golden Proportion—or Golden Vertical Dental Index—when the teeth are closed together.*

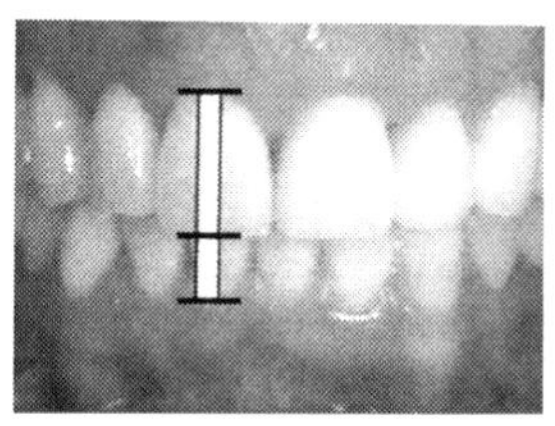

The Golden Ratio Vertical Index illustrates the Golden Ratio relationship between upper and lower incisors.

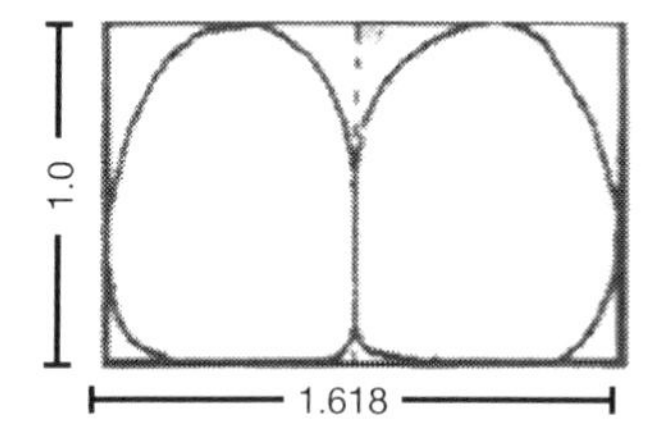

Front teeth in height-to-width Golden Ratio.

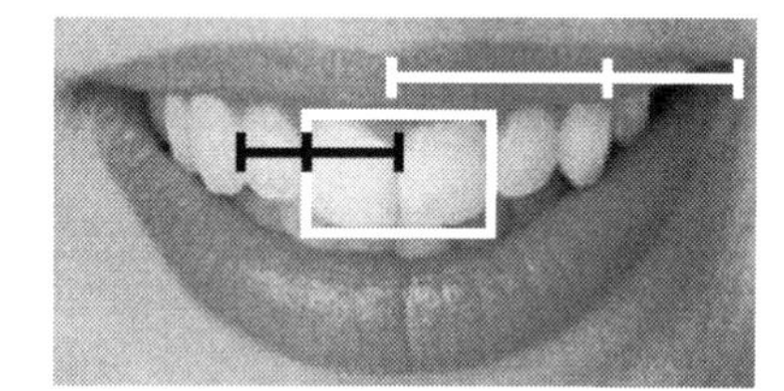

Your teeth have multiple Golden Ratio relationships.

New Jersey-based Orthodontist **Dr. Yosh Jefferson** is a Golden Ratio medical pioneer focusing on orthodontics. He developed a standardized system for the ideal position of the jaw and facial bones and a temporomandibular joint (TMJ) realignment therapy based on the Golden Ratio. Such realignment has been shown to alleviate a host of conditions such as chronic headaches, mouth breathing, myofascial pain, TMJ dysfunction, scoliosis, skin disorders and chronic fatigue syndrome. It can also improve respiration, memory, mental and hearing acuity, as well as lessen depression.

Dr. Jefferson's breakthrough Golden Ratio approach is described in the *Journal of General Orthodontics* (June 1996), for which he wrote the cover article, *Skeletal Types: Key to Unraveling the Mystery of Facial Beauty and its Biologic Significance.*

Whole-Body Dentistry, Xylitol & the Health & Beauty Connection

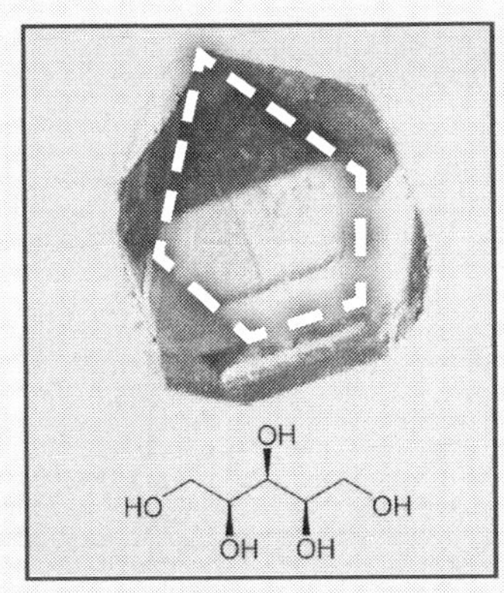

(*Top*) Xylitol crystal magnified, showing pentagonal structure. In addition to having a pentagonal-shaped crystal face, Xylitol also expresses its Golden Ratio "fiveness" by being a 5-carbon sugar alcohol (pentane-1,2,3,4,5-pentol) structure (*Bottom*).

Maintaining a healthy mouth environment is a vital cornerstone supporting your total health, beauty and a long and vital life. Not only is your mouth the First 15% of healthy digestion, due to proper mastication (chewing), it turns out that the same bacteria which cause tooth decay and gum disease can migrate to the heart, directly leading to increased inflammation and heart disease—the #1 cause of death in America (another vital reason to regularly brush, use dental floss and reduce sugar consumption).

Dr. Mark Briener, a Connecticut-based dentist and author of *Whole-Body Dentistry*, reveals how the health of your teeth and mouth is directly connected to the health (and by extension the beauty) of your whole body. Essentially, healthy teeth and gums are a fractal predictor of total health. Dr. Briener's visionary work has received extensive media coverage and is endorsed by many leading health authorities, including Nicholas Perricone, M.D., Bernie Siegel, M.D., Stephen Sinatra, M.D., and Gary Null, Ph.D. Reducing or eliminating white sugar and refined and processed foods along with practicing healthy oral care, including flossing daily, is of course vital. Dr. Briener points out that including the naturally occurring sugar substitute xylitol in your oral health regimen adds another clinically proven support factor for tooth and total health. Xylitol, a unique 5-sided sucrose-free crystal originally discovered in 1896, is available in toothpaste, gum, mints and as a sugar substitute. What makes xylitol special is that it tastes as sweet as sugar yet at the same time it neutralizes the bacteria which causes tooth decay and gum disease—unlike regular refined sugars, which accelerate tooth decay and wreak havoc with our health. Xylitol also does not cause blood sugar levels to spike, so it's safe for diabetics and hypoglycemics. To learn more about xylitol's proven dental and health benefits and the teeth–total health connection, see Dr. Briener's book *Whole-Body Dentistry*; also visit www.WholeBodyMed.com www.EpicDental.com and www.XylitolUSA.com

In that article, Dr. Jefferson speaks on the Golden Ratio beauty connection:

All living creatures, including man, are intimately connected by a biologic phenomenon known as Divine Proportion [Golden Ratio]. We are all genetically encoded to develop into this ideal shape and form for many reasons.

Dr. Jefferson further states that individuals who conform to the Divine Proportion/ Golden Ratio are more likely to be biologically and physiologically efficient and healthy. In his view, most physical variations from Divine Proportion, especially extreme ones, are environmentally induced—which explains why most people tend to deviate somewhat from the ideal. Restoration therefore should closely approximate the biological standard that is both aesthetically pleasing and physiologically healthy. He observes that all living things, including humans, are genetically encoded to develop into an ideal and defined proportion. **This proportion is universal, applying to all individuals regardless of race, age, sex, and geographic or cultural variabilities.**

The Universal Golden Beauty Ratio

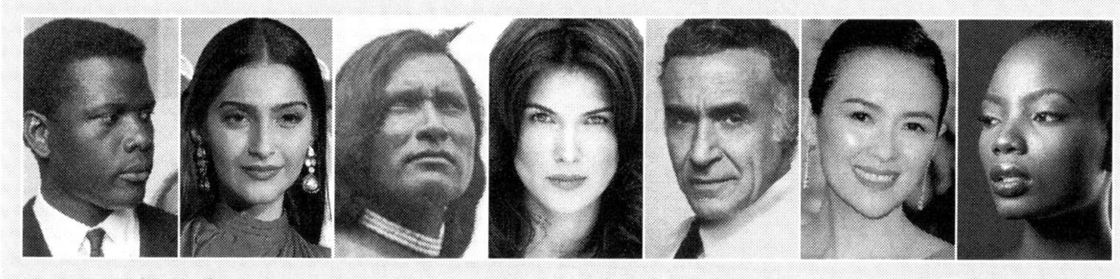

(*L–R*): Sydney Poitier, American Actor; Aishwarya Raj, Indian actress; Nez Pierce, American Indian warrior; Monica Birladeanu, Romanian model/actress; Ricardo Montalbán, Mexican actor; Zhang Ziyi, Chinese actress; young African woman.

At first glance, you might think that you're looking at a random gallery of beautiful faces from around the world. While on the surface that's true, looking deeper you're also looking at **the common, timeless thread which makes the recognition of beauty possible in all faces across time.** This thread is the Golden Ratio—the universal template through which all facial features are integrated into a divine unity—which registers as beauty to our innate Golden Ratio recognition system. And while some may visually reflect this biological truth more closely than others, we all naturally dance around it throughout our lives in form, function and spirit.

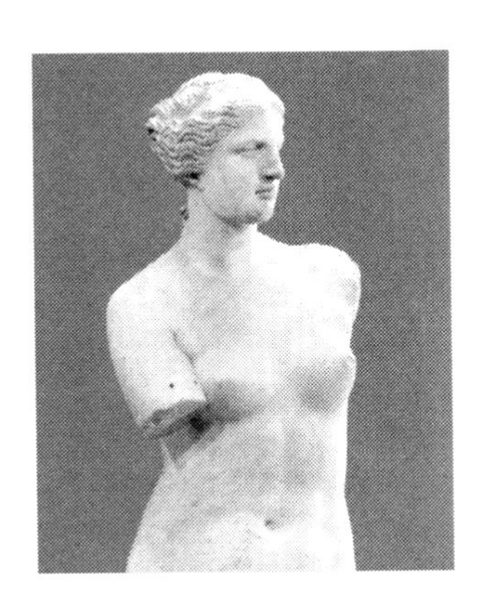

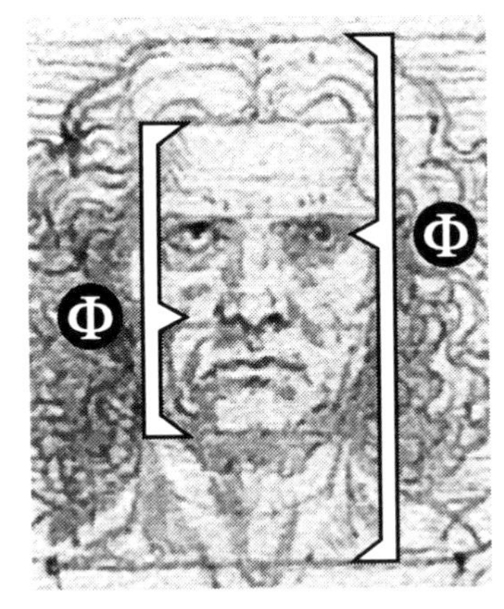

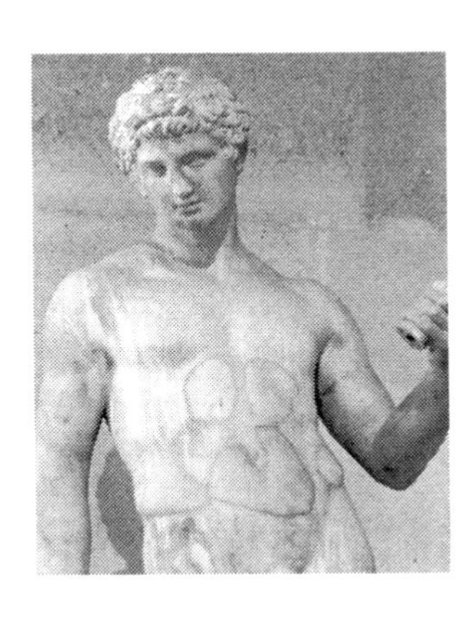

The ancient Greek icons Venus de Milo (*L*) and Adonis (*R*) set the Golden Ratio bar for timeless beauty which continues to this day. Leonardo Da Vinci continued this tradition with respect to Golden Proportions, right down to the precise Golden Ratios evident in the face of his classic Vitruvian Man.

Bottle-fed babies also tend to be mouth breathers, which can lead to various types of facial and dental abnormalities. Artificial influences during the First 15% of early childhood such as the above can obviously cause development away from the Golden Ratio. In a perfect world, free of extreme environmental conditions such as high stress, abnormal biomechanical habits, pollution, toxins, radiation, allergens, and latex bottle nipples, etc., most people would naturally develop closer to the Golden Ratio. Dr. Jefferson also notes that many studies have proven the universality of beauty:

> *A number of recent cross-cultural researchers have shown that the basis for judging facial attractiveness was consistent across cultural lines. Furthermore... babies as young as three months can distinguish between attractive and unattractive faces. Because babies at this age are deemed too young to be substantially exposed to cultural standards of beauty, these studies indicate an innate ability of all human individuals to appreciate facial form and balance that have universal appeal.*

Dr. Jefferson believes this carries enormous social implications: We are instinctively inclined to search for mates whose features conform more closely to the Golden Ratio. By looking for partners that are Divinely Proportioned, we are at the same time unknowingly looking for partners who are vibrantly healthy, thereby ensuring the health and survival of our offspring. We are all apparently predisposed to the lifelong appreciation of and search for beauty. The social implications of being perceived as beautiful are staggering, as **Diane Ackerman** describes in *A Natural History of the Senses:*

> *Attractive people do better: in school, where they receive more help, better grades and less punishment; at work, where they are rewarded with higher pay, more prestigious jobs and faster promotion; in finding mates, where they tend to be in control of the relationship*

Elizabeth Hurley's Golden Ratio Beauty

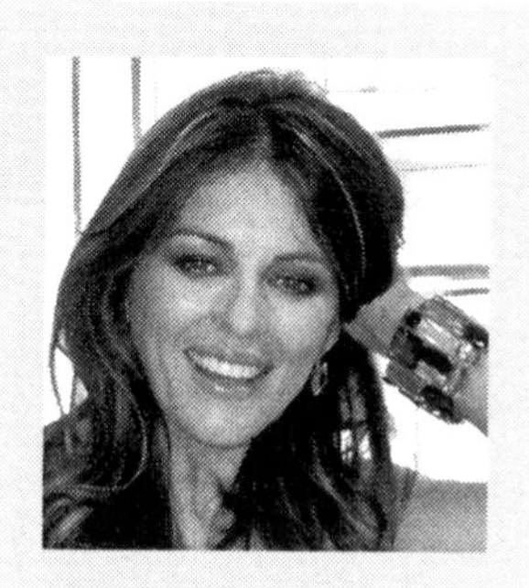

Actor and author **John Cleese** (of *Monty Python* and *A Fish Called Wanda* fame) wrote and presented a fascinating program for the BBC called *The Human Face*, which showcases the secrets of the Golden Ratio and beauty. It features model and actress Elizabeth Hurley as a timeless example of Golden Ratio facial proportions.

and make most of the decisions; and among strangers, who assume them to be more interesting, honest, virtuous and successful.

A brain imaging study led by **Dr. Hans Breiter**, published in the November, 2001 issue of *Neuron*, revealed that when men were shown pictures of various faces, only female faces deemed beautiful triggered activity in brain centers previously associated with food, drugs and money. With one group of men, studied via a brain imaging procedure known as functional magnetic resonance imaging (fMRI), researchers found that only attractive female faces set off the brain's reward circuitry. **Dr. Nancy Etcoff**, a coauthor of this study, noted that the research echoes previous work suggesting that the human perception of beauty may be inborn. Dr. Etcoff added:

While we know that experience, learning and personal idiosyncrasies all have an impact on attraction between particular individuals; these results show that this basic reward response is deeply seated in human nature.

> *It is impossible to join two things in a beautiful manner without a third being present, for a bond must exist to unite them, and this bond is best achieved by a proportion.*
>
> **Plato**

9

Clearly, our responses to beauty and Divine Proportion are more instinctive than conscious. We have been programmed to recognize, love and delight in that which reflects our universal, divinely inspired Golden Ratio design. California-based **Dr. Stephen Marquardt** has taken practical advantage of our natural instinct for beauty. In his work as a leading maxillofacial plastic surgeon, Dr. Marquardt developed male and female "beauty mask" facial overlays utilizing the Golden Decagon (a ten-sided Golden Ratio-based geometrical shape) and its application to facial beauty. Faces that

Golden Φ Ratio Facial Proportions

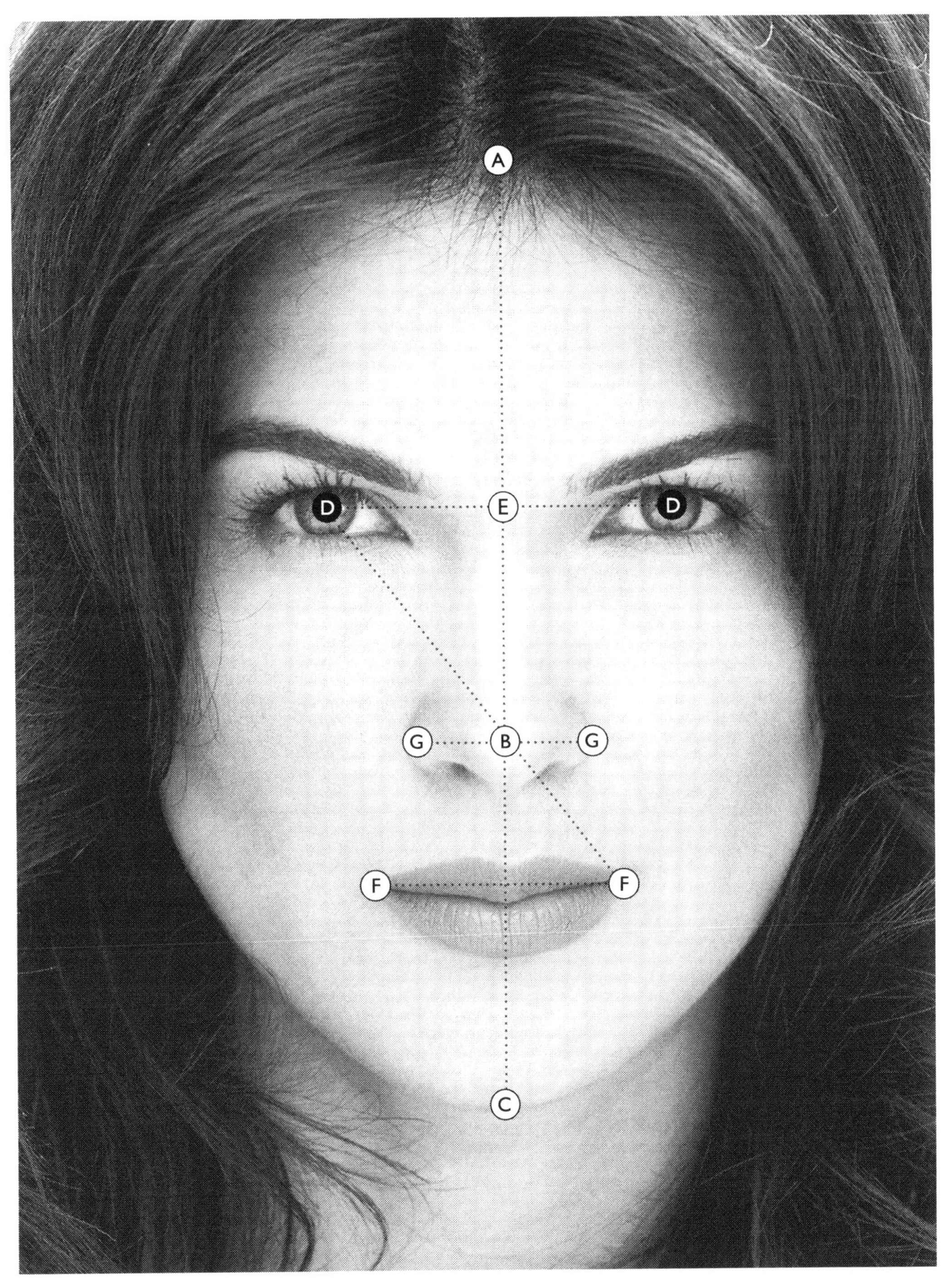

The human face is endowed with numerous Golden Ratios. In the beautiful face of actress Monica Birladeanu, we highlight four. Line segments shown are in Golden Φ Ratio to one another.

1. (A)(B):(B)(C)=1.618 2. (E)(C):(D)(D)=1.618 3. (D)(B):(B)(F)=1.618 (*diagonal*) 4. (F)(F):(G)(G)=1.618

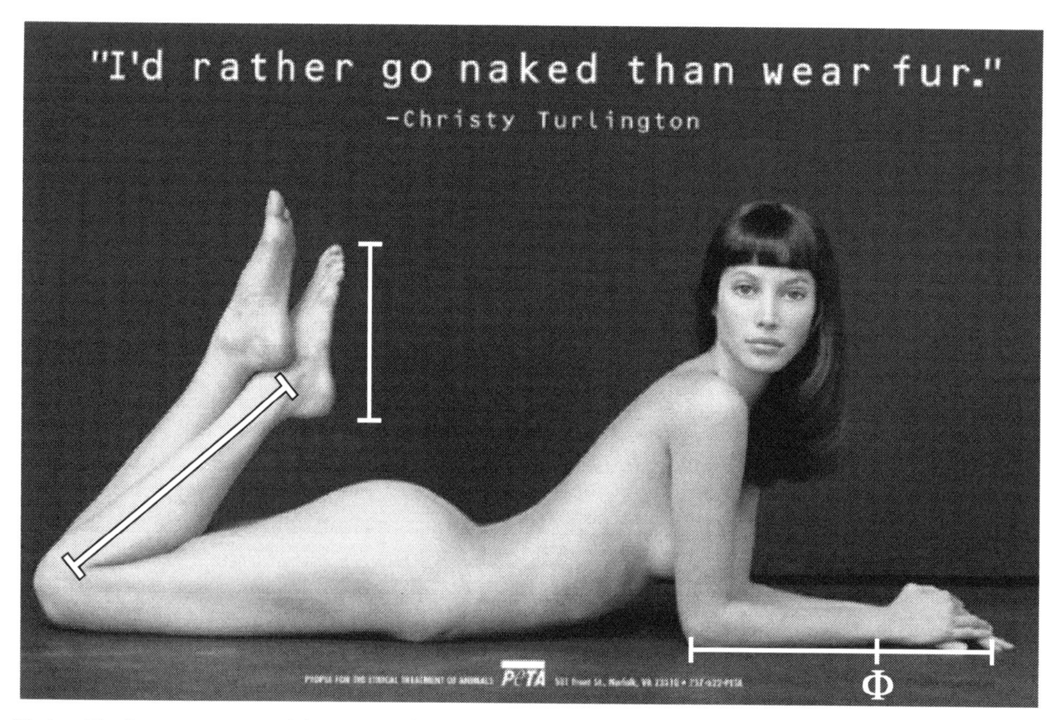

"I'd rather go naked than wear fur."
-Christy Turlington
PETA
Φ

Christy Turlington, supermodel, yogini and author (***Living Yoga***) exhibiting some of her furless Golden Ratio proportions for PETA (*People for the Ethical Treatment of Animals*). Golden Ratio bars added by the authors.

conform to the mask will be universally perceived as beautiful, regardless of race, age or nationality. His beauty mask can be utilized to guide the application of makeup, to aid in the evaluation of a face for orthodontic or dental treatment or facial surgery, or simply to see how closely a face conforms to the Golden Ratio. Dr. Marquardt's beauty mask and work has attracted international attention, validating yet again the universality of the Golden Ratio as a touchstone of beauty.

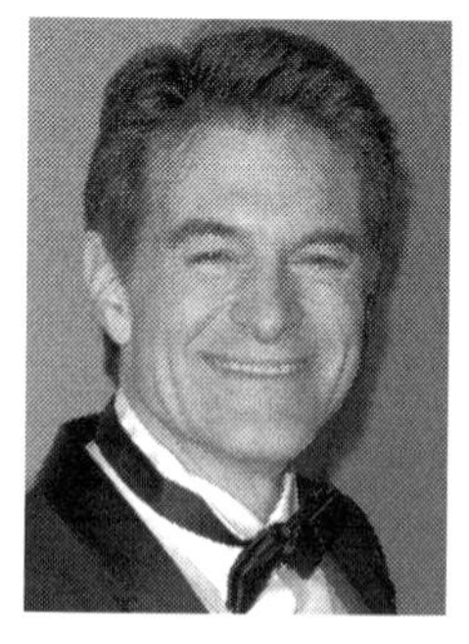

Dr. Mehmet Oz.

Drs. Mehmet Oz & Michael Roizen: Beauty, Your Immune System & the Golden Ratio

Cardiothoracic surgeon, author and TV personality Dr. Mehmet Oz shares some of his insights on the Golden Ratio's connection to beauty, healthy immune function and genetics. Dr. Oz is co-author with Michael Roizen, M.D., of the popular *YOU: The Owner's Manual* health book series and is one of *Time* magazine's *100 Most Influential People* (2008) and *Esquire* magazine's *75 Most Influential People of the 21st Century*. From *YOU: Being Beautiful:*

The theory is that the more symmetrical a face is, the healthier it is… the formula for beauty is that precise Golden Ratio (go ahead and pull a ruler and a calculator on your next date). The same ratio holds for the width of the cheekbones to the width of the mouth… [similarly] the width of the mouth should be roughly 1.6 times the width of the bottom of the nose… Scientists also believe that symmetry is equated with a strong immune system—indicating that more robust genes make a person more attractive. Of course, that's the element of beauty that you typically can't control. You have what you were born with. But that doesn't mean that you can't make changes—changes to enhance your beauty and, along with it, the way you feel about yourself.

Michael Roizen, M.D., author of the award-winning *RealAge* book series and Dr. Oz's co-author in the *YOU* health book series, shared these insights on the Golden Ratio's beauty connection in the audiobook *YOU: Being Beautiful*,

The omnipresence of phi [the Golden Ratio] throughout our world creates a sense of balance, harmony and beauty in the designs we see naturally and artificially. Phi is also a driving force in human attraction—men and women around the globe prefer a mate whose face is symmetrical and follows this ratio (more than 2,000 years ago, Pythagoras developed a formula for the perfect female face, which included such stats as this one: The ratio of the width of the mouth to the width of the nose should be—ta-da!—1.618 to 1).

The Fashion Code's Golden Ratio Magnetism

The Fashion Code is based on the timeless secret for beauty [the Golden Ratio] *that has inspired everyone from Da Vinci to today's top fashion icons. Once women know what this secret is and how to use it, they will have the power to create the perfect outfit everyday.*

Sara and Ruth Levy, developers of The Fashion Code

In one of our previous books, *The Divine Code of Da Vinci, Fibonacci, Einstein and YOU*, we described the two complementary aspects of the Golden Ratio known as The Golden Twins. Dual aspects of the Ratio allow it to be seen alternately as 1.618:1 and other times as 0.618:1, depending on the context. The Golden Twins are like two sides of a coin, their complementary natures forming a unified whole. Likewise, in the world of haute couture, twins Ruth and Sara Levy, both beautiful brunette fashion designers, have taken a

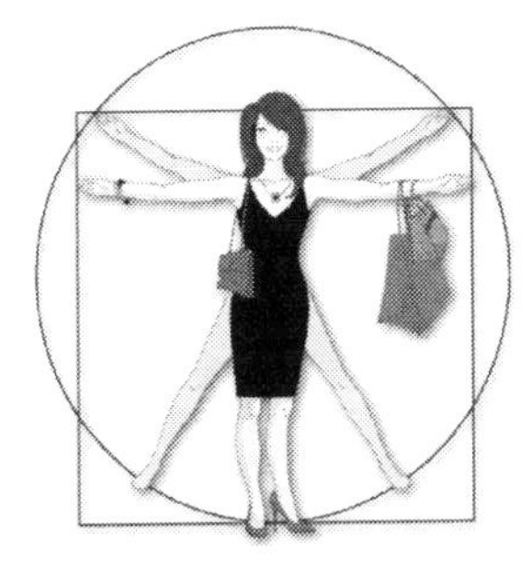

The Fashion Code's logo, with a Vitruvian flair.

9

Golden Ratio Magazine Cover Design

Michael Trott, chief scientist at Wolfram Research, Inc. discovered that throughout the last century, human face positioning on magazine and internet publications worldwide *consistently dances around the Golden Ratio and affiliated Rule of Thirds.*

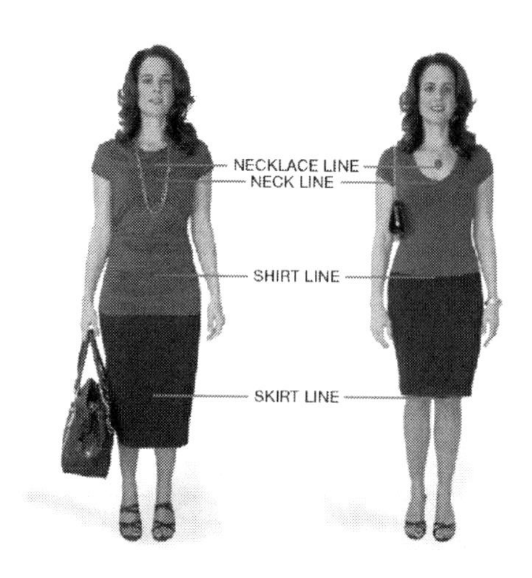

Golden Ratio makeover; before (*L*) and after (*R*) application of the Fashion Code.

hint from Da Vinci's *Vitruvian Man* and created a breakthrough in the art and science of fashion. Ruth and Sara discovered that 10 Golden Ratio division points—superimposed over a client's body—reveal the most flattering clothing lengths and proportions, from necklines to hemlines. As these Golden Ratio Fashionistas say,

> *These days, there's an instruction manual for everything—except how to dress... Sure, there are tips and tricks for looking good, but nowhere is there an actual foolproof formula for dressing beautifully... until now.*

On their debut on the *Rachel Ray Show* on April 15, 2010, the twins said that with the Fashion Code any woman can instantly... *look 10 pounds thinner, 10 years younger and 10 times more stylish.*

> *It's a real jaw-dropper* [the Golden Ratio Fashion Code]... *I'm a believer!*
>
> **Rachel Ray, commenting on Sara & Ruth Levy's Fashion Code.**

Several models, including the twins, showed how Golden Ratio Fashion makeovers accent anyone's hidden Divine Proportions. A visibly impressed Rachael Ray noted that the ***Fashion Code is where the Da Vinci Code meets fashion***. This is a universal truism, since the simple mathematics of the Golden Ratio work on virtually everyone. Not to worry—the twins have taken care of the math. To apply the twin's Golden Ratio knowledge of dress and fashion, you need only enter your height on their website—www.TheFashionCode.com—and they'll supply you with an elegant, customized chart of the magical necklines and hemlines for all of your outfits and accessories.

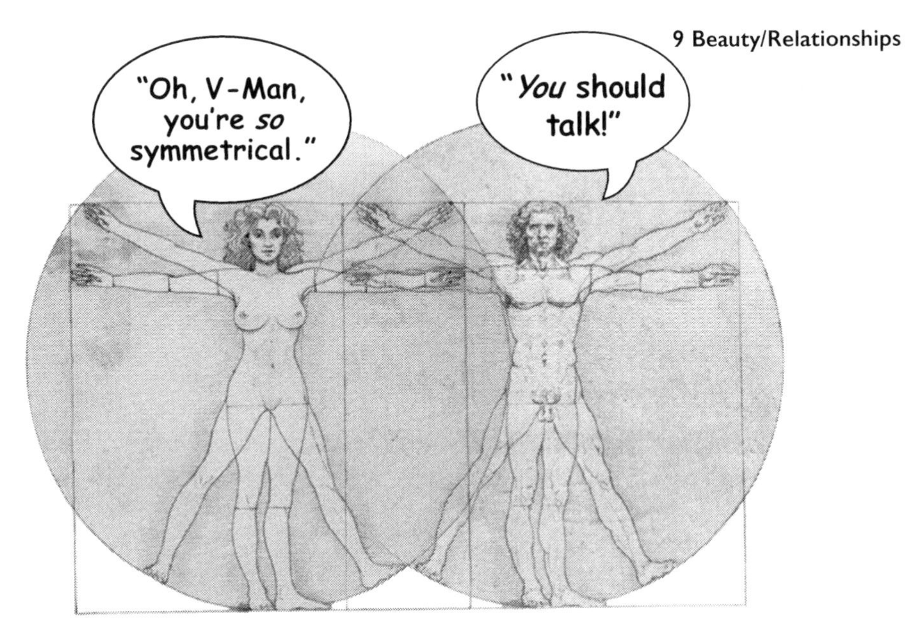

Vitruvian Woman and Man comparing notes.

Julia Roberts & the Mona Lisa Smile

At the front end of the 21st century, Julia Roberts was one of the highest paid actors in the world, commanding twenty-five million dollars for her starring role in 2003's *Mona Lisa Smile*. In our time, Julia Roberts' trademark smile easily rivals Da Vinci's *Mona Lisa* smile in recognition, however different they may be. What Julia and the *Mona Lisa* have in common is their ability to encompass and express many quantifiable as well as unquantifiable aspects of the Golden Ratio. In the *Mona Lisa*, Da Vinci masterfully embedded the Golden Ratio in many levels of the painting's geometrical composition. First coming to global prominence in the hit 1990 film *Pretty Woman*, Roberts revealed a rarely seen charm that only enhanced her broad, dazzling smile. Actor Tom Hanks commented on her remarkable stage presence, as reported by HollywoodReporter.com:

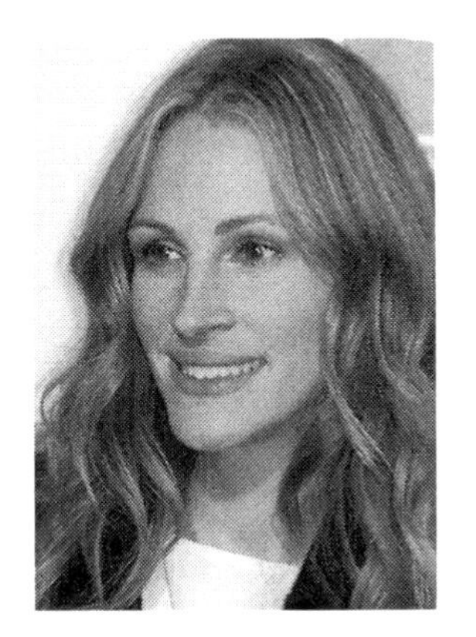

Julia Roberts.

> *When you share the screen [with her], you might as well be a waffle iron in a tree... No one is ever looking at you... Everybody loves Julia Roberts, absolutely everybody.*

Winner of the 2001 Academy Award for Best Actress for *Erin Brokovich*, Roberts has been voted to *People* magazine's list of the world's "*Fifty Most Beautiful People*" eleven times. Julia Roberts reminds us that the Golden Ratio shows up not only in quantifiable physical appearance, but also in many immeasurable and intangible personal qualities.

George Clooney had this to say in 2010 about Robert's secret to staying lovely:

It has nothing to do with the way she looks. It has everything to do with who she is.

> *What I study is photographic, two-dimensional attractiveness, photos with no dimension or sense of time or personality... In the real world, beauty has to do with elegance, sense of humor, how a person carries herself. It's something completely different.*
>
> **Mounir Bashour, M.D., Ph.D., plastic surgeon and author of** ***Is an Objective Measuring System for Facial Attractiveness Possible?***

George Clooney: An Ideal Male Face

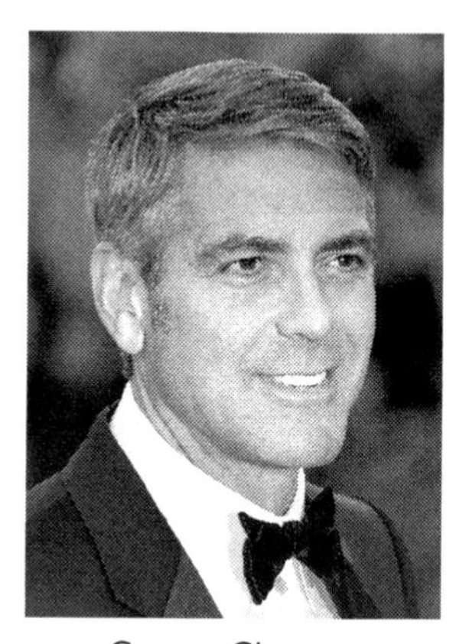

George Clooney.

In 2003, the American Academy of Facial Plastic and Reconstructive Surgery polled its membership to learn which stars embody present-day appeal and timeless allure. Twenty-five percent of the plastic surgeons selected actor George Clooney as the male "modern-day ideal face of beauty" (Brad Pitt and Mel Gibson were tied for 2nd place, at twenty percent each). Plastic surgeon and AAFPRS President **Dean M. Toriumi, M.D.** was quoted on www.aafprs.org:

George Clooney was selected because he possesses a strong jaw, deep brown eyes, an "ever-perfect" olive complexion, and a strong and straight masculine nose... Clooney is known for his sense of humor, often seen in interviews making wry comments, jokes, and pulling pranks, thus, his appeal seems partially to stem from a persona, which is a blend of warmth and humor.

Like his friend and co-star Julia Roberts, Clooney's appeal is a mix of physical attractiveness, wit and charm. His Golden Ratio-chiseled good looks also got him honored as *People* magazine's *Sexiest Man Alive* (twice) and as one of *People's Most Beautiful People* (2007). In 2005, Clooney won an Academy Award for Best Supporting Actor for *Syriana*. Clooney's career showcases in dynamic proportion his multifaceted talents, which include acting, directing, screenwriting and producing.

> *Beauty is the splendor of truth.*
>
> **Plato**

Divine Symmetry & Graceful Movement

We are clearly predisposed to the appreciation of and the search for beauty, and the Golden Ratio is beauty's foremost blueprint. Those whose appearance and movements more closely mirror the Golden Ratio/Spiral inevitably attract more attention and interest from the world at large, and the opposite sex in particular. The following excerpt from Jeanie Davis' *WebMD* article *Men Who Dance Well May Be More Desirable As Mates* (December, 2005) describes the research of **William M. Brown, Ph.D.** This study highlights the importance of bodily symmetry in dance as it relates to mate selection:

> *Dancing is believed to be important in the courtship of a variety of species, including humans, writes researcher William M. Brown, Ph.D., an anthropologist with Rutgers University. Mating studies revealed that women seek out males with bodily symmetry. If the potential mate has a great degree of asymmetry, he or she is judged to be less than optimal. In numerous species, asymmetry is linked to greater rates of disease and early death, and lesser success in fertility—all-important to their selection as mates. A guy's or girl's symmetry (or lack of it) affects their attractiveness in other ways, too—like odor, voice, and facial appearance... Why is symmetry so important? 'We do not know,' writes Brown: 'Perhaps it indicates good coordination or good health, including freedom from parasites. Attractive dances may be more difficult to perform, more rhythmic, more energetic, more energy efficient, or any combination of these factors.'*

Golden Ratio of Attraction

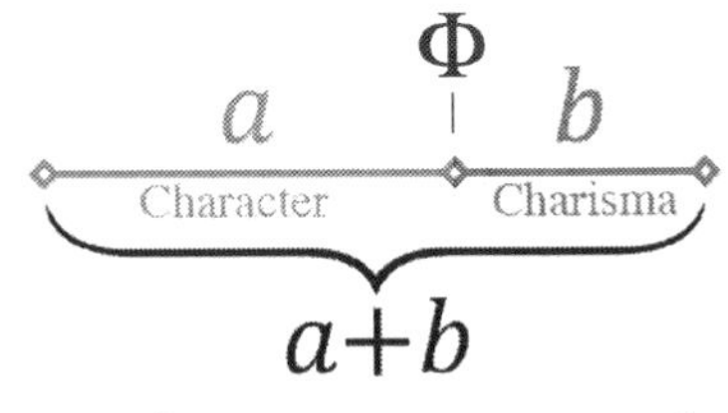

Jackie Summers' Golden Ratio synergy of Character and Charisma.

Jackie Summers is the founder of Jack from Brooklyn (purveyors of Sorel® liqueur) who also writes poetically and frankly on love, passion and life. His engaging blog post about the Golden Ratio of character and charisma in relationships caught our eye:

> *Charisma makes us swoon but might lead us to disaster. Character is steadfast and honorable but often wooden, and dull. How do we resolve this? With Phi Φ (an irrational number along with its more famous cousin, π Pi). If you think you're unfamiliar with the concept of phi, you're mistaken. The equation which represents perfect symmetry is everywhere you look, if you're looking. Ratios can be defined as the proportion of one thing to another; it's knowing how much Jack Daniels to add to a Coke to have just the right balance of sweetness and potency. Phi, the aptly named Divine Proportion, is simply the best ratio to combine any parts.*

So, why not apply the concept of ideal proportions to a lover? When set upon a predominant base of character, charisma provides the stage to perform its seduction over and over. The ability to identify these qualities and their relative proportion to each other is key, not just in seduction but in securing healthy, stable, sustainable relationships. The capacity for character and charisma exists in each of us, as does their right ratio to one another. Instead of simply searching for an ideal mate, begin by adjusting the sliding scale in yourself to ideal proportions. Souls of a like nature seek each other out, so if you truly want to find The One, start by becoming The One.

> *An Archives of Sexual Behavior study reveals that woman are most attracted to muscular men whose shoulders measure 1.6 times* [the Golden Ratio] *the size of their waist.*
>
> **John Barban, *The Perfect Body Formula*; *Men's Health* Magazine, July/August 2008**

Jackie's message is simple yet profound: **if we wish to attract (and keep) a special "One" in our lives, we must start with the First One—ourselves—first.** Most people focus on the movie, the projection on the other One, instead of on the projector (ourselves), which invariably leads to chasing shadows. If you're looking for *The One*, try this: make a short list of the key qualities you desire in another. Then focus with care and frequency to cultivate and refine those same qualities within yourself. Get ready: Like attracts like, or as the ancients said, *As Above, So Below.*

The Prophet of Golden Ratio Relationships

Khalil Gibran wrote in his timeless classic *The Prophet:*

Let there be spaces in your togetherness, and let the winds of the heavens dance between you... Love one another but make not a bond of love: Let it rather be a moving sea between your shores... Sing and dance together and be joyous, but let each one of you be alone, even as the strings of a lute are alone though they quiver with the same music... And stand together, yet not too near together: For the pillars of the temple stand apart, and the oak tree and the cypress grow not in each other's shadow.

As Gibran beautifully illustrates, a dynamic balance, a ratio, must exist in space, energy and time in order for relationships to become fulfilling and ultimately unifying states. Interpreting his wisdom through the lens of the Golden Ratio, we can see that harmonious relationships require a dynamic symmetry—a ratio or proportion—and it's not a static 50:50 ratio. For example: Consider the possibility that a healthy relationship might benefit with 62% of total time being spent with a partner, and 38% spent apart. This could set the stage for you to better enjoy the "spaces in your togetherness" and thus better appreciate one another, especially over time. The ratio could of course be flipped or modified in those relationships where people want to spend either more time together or more time apart.

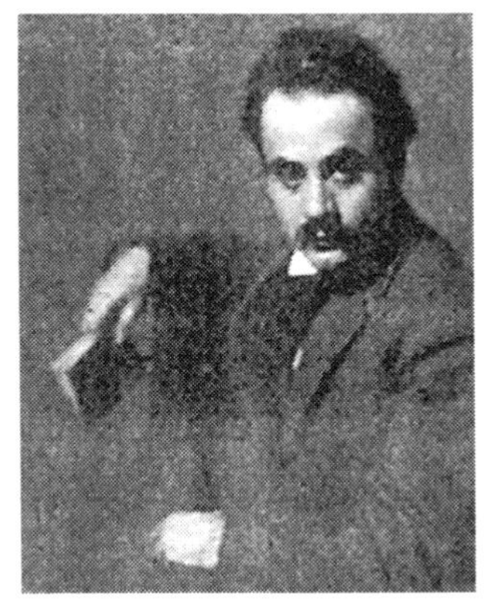

Khalil Gibran (1883-1931) hints at Golden Ratio relationships in *The Prophet.*

One must also consider the balance or ratio of power in relationships of every kind. For example, our world is now struggling to reestablish a dynamic divine balance by moving away from near-total male dominance in the areas of leadership, business and decision making. Yet this can only occur when the feminine perspective is restored to its proper proportion. The key word here is *dynamic.* Like the play of the tides, the various ratios of interactions within healthy relationships manifest and move through endless expressions of the Golden Ratio. These include time together vs. time apart, giving vs. receiving, action vs. rest, etc. These cycles naturally flow between the Golden Ratio's "low tide" side (38%) to its "high tide" side (62%). In reality, all relationships reflect this continuous dance, and all relationships can benefit from greater conscious sensitivity to these natural ebb and flow cycles.

Golden Intimacy: The Feel-Good Health & Longevity **Macro**Nutrient

An orgasm a day keeps the doctor away.
Mae West, Legendary (and Long-Lived) Hollywood Actress

It should come as no surprise that lovemaking reduces stress, boosts immune function, promotes sounder sleep, increases optimism and releases hormones beneficial for health, happiness and longevity. Countless studies confirm that lovemaking offers so many health benefits it could literally qualify as a supernutrient. Regular doses of this feel-good nutrient may even save your life: in 2002, the *Journal of Epidemiology and Community Health* reported that 914 U.K. men were monitored for 20 years. At the end of the study, those who'd enjoyed lovemaking at least twice a week had a 50% less chance of having a fatal heart attack, compared to those whose lovemaking frequency was once a month. From Golden Ratio aficionado **Dr. Michael Roizen**, author of *RealAge: Are You as Young as You Can Be?*:

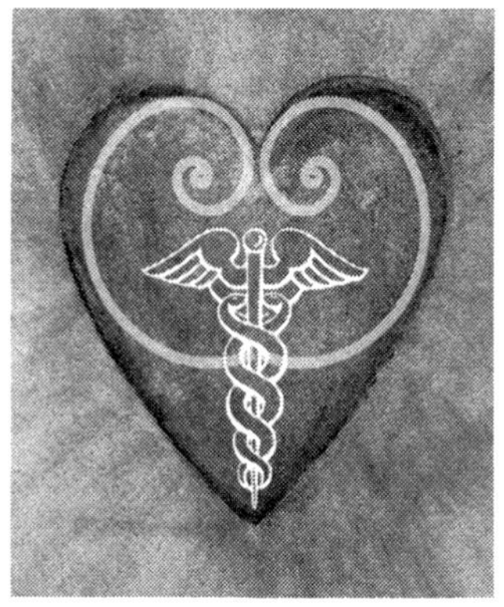
Every heart is composed of two Golden Spirals.

Having sex at least twice a week can make your RealAge 1.6 years younger than if you had sex only once a week.

Dr. Roizen defines 'real age' as *an estimation of your age in biological terms, not chronological years.* Other studies reveal sexual dissatisfaction as a predictor of the onset of cardiovascular disease. For example, a study published in the November-December 1976 journal *Psychosomatic Medicine* compared 100 women with heart disease with a control group. Sexual dissatisfaction was found in 65% of the coronary patients, yet in only 24% of the control group. In a long-term study of 3,500 people ages 30 to 101, published in his book *Secrets of the Superyoung*, Scotland's **Dr. David Weeks** revealed the age-reversing power of intimacy. In his study, he discovered that those who were enjoying satisfying intimacy with the same partner about 4 times a week on average were perceived by others to be 4 to 7 years younger than their actual age. This was arrived at through impartial ratings of the study subject's pictures. This is interesting data, as the Golden Ratio point falls at approximately 4.3 times per week (7 days ÷ 4.3 = 1.62, the Golden Φ Ratio). Dr. Weeks, a clinical neuropsychologist at the Royal Edinburgh Hospital, attributed the perceived age reversal to significant stress reduction, greater contentment and sounder sleep, stating that:

The key ingredients for looking younger are staying active...
and maintaining a good sex life.

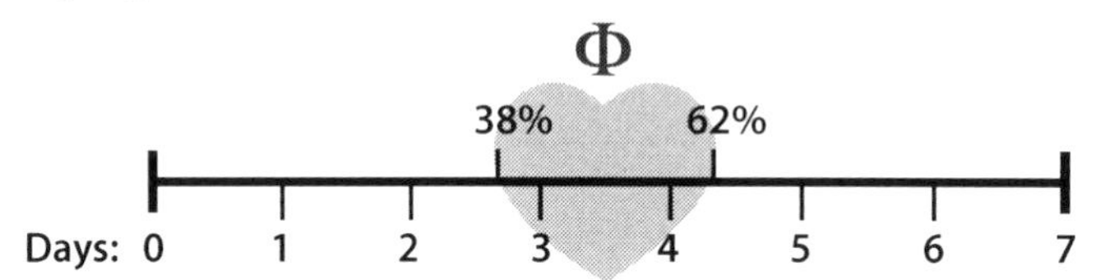

The 4 times per-week lovemaking frequency found in *Superyoung* people falls within the Golden Lovemaking Ratio range of 2.6 to 4.3 times a week, which frames the 38% to 62% range within a 7-day week.

Since everyone's libido is unique and tends to rise and fall over time, no one can say for sure what a "perfect" regular lovemaking frequency is. Everyone must find their own Golden/Divine Ratio in this personal life area based on desire, condition and of course, your partner. **Yet the above data highlights the critical importance regular intimacy plays in a healthy and happy lifestyle.** In light of this, you might consider adding intimacy as a tracking category to your 21-Day Priority Coach.

The Golden Intimacy Rati-O

The lover is drawn by the thing loved, as the sense is by that which it perceives.

Leonardo da Vinci

The ultimate purpose of sexual union, as **Dr. Wilhelm Reich**, 20th century sexual psychology and life energy pioneer proposed in *The Function of the Orgasm*, is a loving communion. The divine sharing of intimacy is meant to result in both partners experiencing a full and ecstatic energetic release, renewal and union with one another. Reich, a one-time protégé of Sigmund Freud, theorized that a lack of healthy sexual intimacy is a root cause behind much of humanity's dysfunction, repression and dis-ease. Orgasm can be likened to a strong outgoing wave or tide of energy, followed by a natural resolution or afterglow stage when the tide comes back in. The post-orgasmic afterglow time allows us to integrate the vital regenerative energies of which Dr. Reich spoke. Early scientific research by Masters & Johnson and others into the physiology of the human sexual response identified five primary stages of lovemaking:

1. Foreplay > 2. Excitement > 3. Plateau > 4. Orgasm > 5. Afterglow

When the Golden Ratio is superimposed over the idealized graph (below) of these 5 stages of lovemaking, we find that the onset of orgasm occurs at a point approximately 62% of the way through lovemaking. This indicates that in order for enjoyable lovemaking and mutually fulfilling orgasms to occur, both partners can much benefit from honoring lovemaking's first phase: foreplay. Chaos theory pioneer Professor Edward Lorenz could easily have been referring to the divine importance of foreplay when he said,

When a butterfly flutters its wings in one part of the world [if the initial conditions are right] it can eventually cause a hurricane in another.

As if to reinforce the importance of a healthy, foundational ratio between foreplay and orgasm, *Esquire Magazine* conducted a survey of 2000 women in 2003. Given a choice

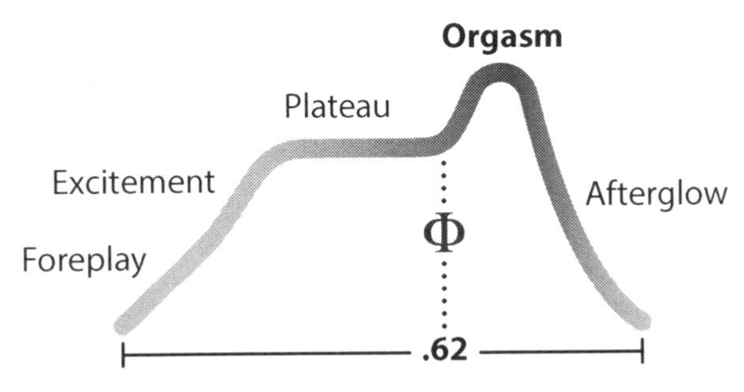

Idealized five-stage sexual response graph, with orgasm onset at the approximate Golden Ratio point.
Note: this graph is a stylized version of how an orgasm could be represented graphically.

The Golden Ratio Code of Love and Creation

The Golden Ratio plays a ubiquitous and fascinating role in every aspect of humanity, from creation through all stages of development and life to the stairway to heaven. As seen throughout this book and below, the ratio magnetically unifies form and function at every stage of the human experience and beyond. For as author Robert Lawlor said, *...wherever there is an intensification of function or a particular beauty and harmony of form, there the Golden Ratio will be found.*

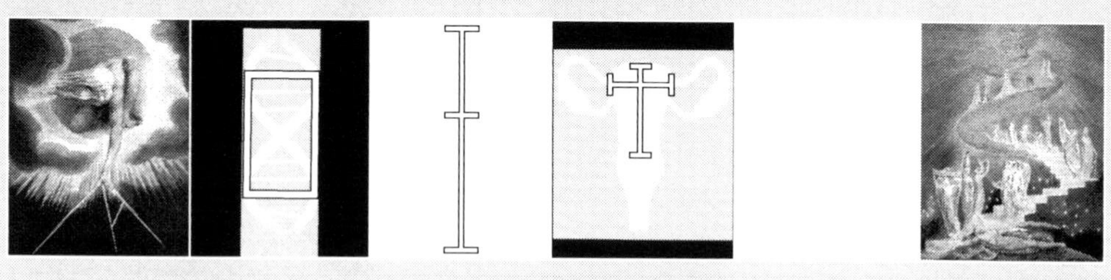

The following images exhibit various aspects of the Golden Ratio, from creation to ascension (*L–R*): *The Ancient of Days* (God Creating the Universe with Golden Ratio Calipers), by William Blake (1794); DNA; Vitruvian Man & Woman; the Golden Womb/Uterus) (as verified by J. Verguts, M.D., et.al.); Spiral Fetus; *Jacob's Dream* (Golden Spiral Stairway to Heaven), by William Blake (1805).

between cuddling and making love, 62% preferred to cuddle while 38% preferred to more immediately make love. Healthy foreplay is the stimulus for Oxytocin release, the trust-building and bonding neurohormone that supports a loving and mutually fulfilling union. Lastly, prolonging the resolution or afterglow phase of lovemaking allows energies to rebalance and harmonize.

Chocolate: Golden Ratio Aphrodisiac & Life Extender

All you need is love... but a little chocolate now and then doesn't hurt.

Charles M. Schulz, master cartoonist and creator of *Peanuts*

Look on most dark chocolate bar ingredient labels and you'll find that 62% of chocolate's fat is saturated and the remaining 38% is polyunsaturated and mono-unsaturated, as stated in **Dr. Peter D'Adamo's** bestseller *Eat Right For Your Type*. This 62% to 38% distribution falls exactly into Golden Ratio proportions. One of chocolate's main psychoactive chemicals is theobromine—literally "Food of the Gods"—with an antioxidant profile higher than red wine or green tea, it certainly qualifies for such a lofty title. Chocolate also contains small amounts of the marijuana-like chemical (cannabinoid) anandamide. Phenethylamine, otherwise known as the "love chemical" is also present in small amounts in chocolate. The combination of these elements, along with tryptophan and trace amounts of caffeine, give chocolate its characteristic addicting flavor and powerful mood elevating and aphrodisiac qualities. Some have questioned chocolate's purported aphrodisiac effects. Yet the popularity of movies such as *Like Water for Chocolate* and *Chocolat*, starring Juliette Binoche and Johnny Depp—to say nothing of Chocolate's well-known connection to Valentine's Day—suggest that the amorous effects of chocolate are undeniable.

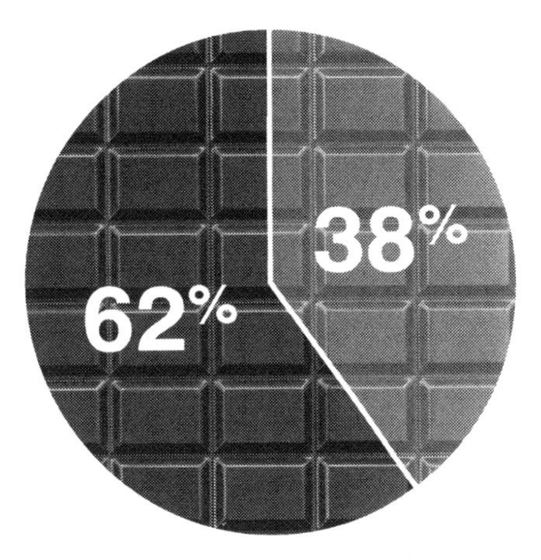

Chocolate is truly a Food of the Gods, with a Golden Ratio of 62% saturated to 38% unsaturated fat composition and more health and longevity enhancing antioxidants than red wine or green tea.

With its mix of Divinely-Proportioned components, it's no wonder that so many people become chocoholics—which may actually be a healthy addiction, in moderation. A growing number of studies are revealing that minimally processed, dark chocolate (cocoa with a higher ratio of polyphenols) is very beneficial for the prevention of heart disease, high blood pressure and stroke—and may in fact enhance longevity. Review the Chocolate Rx in Ch 10 Longevity section for more sweet data and a delicious recipe incorporating the Food of the Gods.

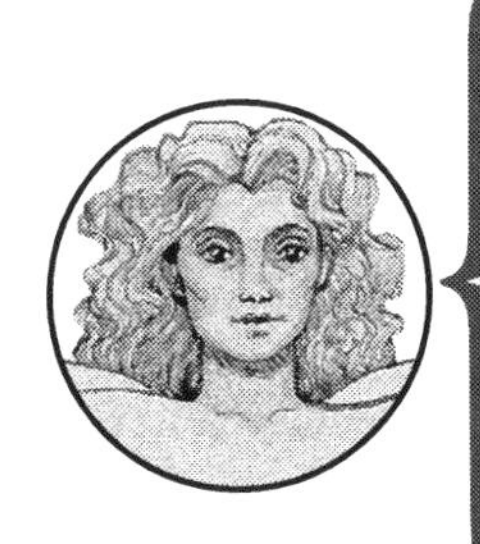

Remember, you're only as ***BEAUTIFUL*** *as you feel.*
So use all of the Golden Ratio beauty enhancements you desire, yet know that true beauty starts from within. Cultivate your Golden Ratio sense of beauty and passion within and without. Learn to appreciate the uniqueness and special nuances that only your face reflects. Remember that seeing beauty in others enlivens *your* inner feeling of beauty & your relationships as well.

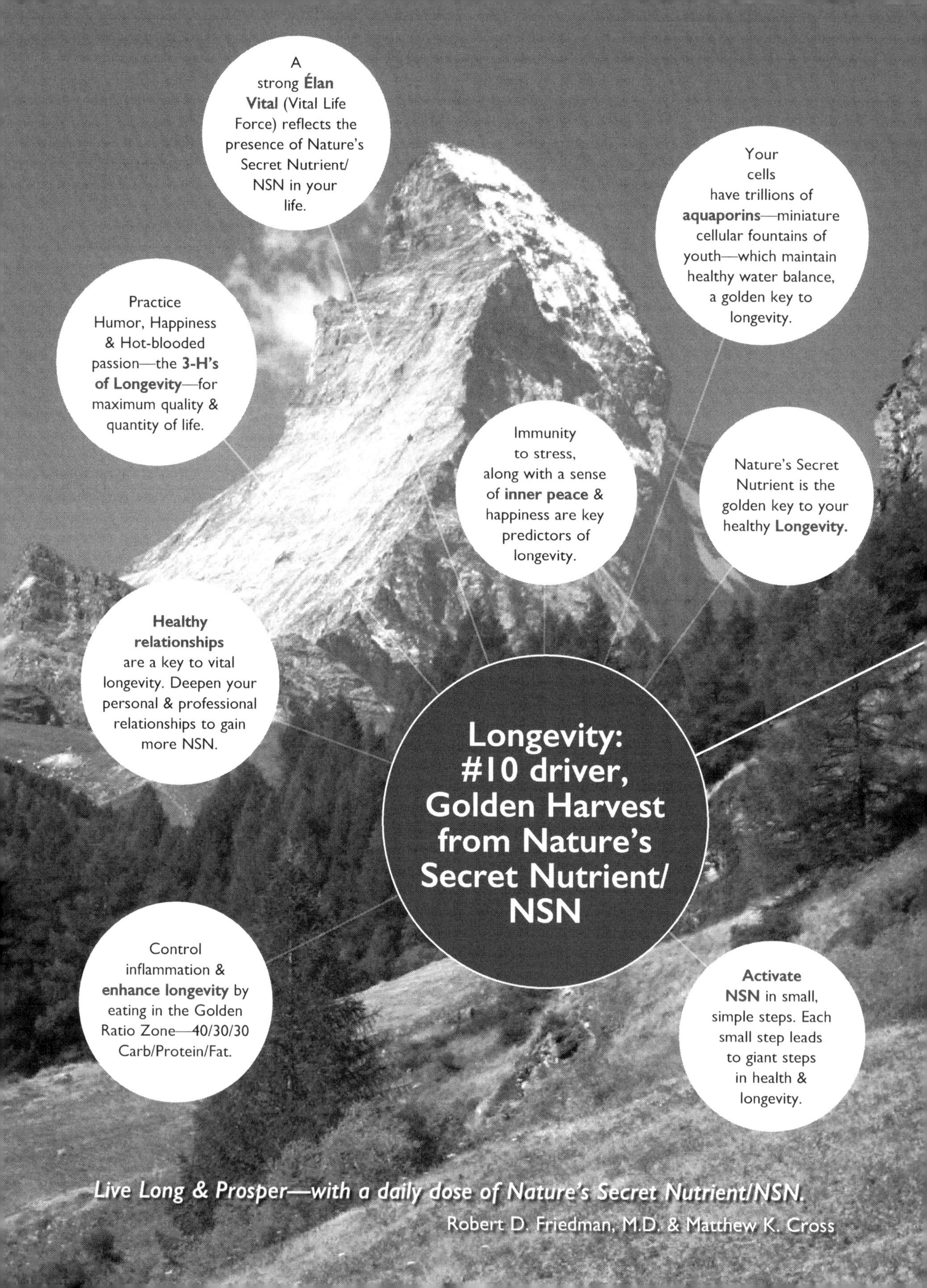

Longevity: #10 driver, Golden Harvest from Nature's Secret Nutrient/ NSN

A strong **Élan Vital** (Vital Life Force) reflects the presence of Nature's Secret Nutrient/ NSN in your life.

Your cells have trillions of **aquaporins**—miniature cellular fountains of youth—which maintain healthy water balance, a golden key to longevity.

Practice Humor, Happiness & Hot-blooded passion—the **3-H's of Longevity**—for maximum quality & quantity of life.

Immunity to stress, along with a sense of **inner peace** & happiness are key predictors of longevity.

Nature's Secret Nutrient is the golden key to your healthy **Longevity.**

Healthy relationships are a key to vital longevity. Deepen your personal & professional relationships to gain more NSN.

Control inflammation & **enhance longevity** by eating in the Golden Ratio Zone—40/30/30 Carb/Protein/Fat.

Activate NSN in small, simple steps. Each small step leads to giant steps in health & longevity.

Live Long & Prosper—with a daily dose of Nature's Secret Nutrient/NSN.

Robert D. Friedman, M.D. & Matthew K. Cross

10

Longevity

The water you touch in a river is the last of that which has passed and the first of which is coming. Thus it is with time present. Life, if well lived, is long.

Leonardo da Vinci

Biomimicry & the Golden Ratio Fountain of Youth

Tapping Nature's Secret Nutrient/NSN has the ability to lift you to a level of extraordinary health, happiness and wellness heretofore unobtainable by any other means. By learning how to easily access NSN vast *free energy* becomes available. The concept of free energy, usually thought of in the context of quantum physics, is focused here on **optimizing your physiology and augmenting your energy—and thus your total life force**. As you practice charging up each MegaNutrient health priority with NSN, you gain access to your internal Fountain of Youth—the ultimate biohack. The elusive Fountain of Youth is reputed to have restorative powers that confer eternal youth on anyone drinking its waters. *In our case, NSN confers its profound health-giving and life-extending waters on all who apply its principles.* How is it possible to increase your energy and vital life force—your *élan vital*—to optimize the quality *and* quantity of your life? One simple answer: the art and daily practice of Golden Ratio **Biomimicry**—mirroring Nature, whose efficiency and dynamism is unparalleled and which operates with the Golden Ratio both structurally *and* functionally at every scale.

Thus a unified field appears throughout Nature where the resulting whole is *greater* than the sum of the parts—the very definition of *synergy*. This is where free energy or élan vital appears. When two complementary elements of any system are brought into Golden Ratio balance, a unified relationship emerges. This opens the door to a new realm of energetic efficiency, robust health and maximum longevity. In the NSN system, there are always opposing yet complementary polarities that can be tuned to Golden Ratio balance for optimal results. For example, as you've learned, by tuning your sleep/wake cycle closer to the Golden Ratio of about 9 hours of sleep/rest and 15 hours of wakefulness at least 3-4 nights/week, you superboost your body's regenerative powers. You get more energy out of your days—and nights—than you would have otherwise. The increased energy obtained simply by optimizing your sleep/wake ratio then combines with other Golden Ratio-adjusted drivers to support ultimate lifestyle synergy and increased free energy. **This enhanced synergy/energy is at the core of longevity.**

Looking at the longest-lived cultures in the world, such as the Hunzans in northern Pakistan, the Okinawans in Japan, the Vilcabambans in Ecuador and the Abkhazians in the Caucasus mountains, we see that their lifestyle naturally includes all critical aspects—in healthy ratios—of the Nature's Secret Nutrient approach. Reviewing NSN's top health drivers, fresh air is abundant in their isolated and thus more pristine environments, as is pure water. In many of the isolated mountainous valleys which are longevity hotspots, electricity is limited or unavailable, so people aren't disposed to late nights or light in their sleeping environments. They are therefore more likely to maintain healthier Golden Ratio sleep/wake cycles. Due to recurring lean times, abundant food may not be available all year; thus, people are subject to unavoidable periodic caloric reduction—one of the scientifically proven methods of immune restoration and life extension.

The mineral-rich water in the remote mountainous valleys of some of the longevity hotspots is known as "glacial milk," and has been found by researcher **Dr. Patrick Flanagan** to have an extremely low surface tension. This low surface tension allows for easier absorption and may improve cellular hydration. As we have seen in chapter 2/Hydration regarding total body composition, a decreasing percentage of body water accompanies aging, obesity and many disease states. Mineral-rich glacial water prevents chronic dehydration from occurring. In addition, due to the low surface tension of the water, bodily toxins are more easily dissolved and excreted, thereby enhancing detoxification. Detoxification is one of the pillars of the NSN system, to which these centenarians are naturally adhering. Another promising scientific discovery supporting our emphasis on detoxification is from Polish and Danish studies that found the main detoxification enzyme in the body—glutathione reductase—to be higher in centenarians.

Aquaporins: Your Molecular Fountains of Youth

Aquaporins are microscopic openings in your cellular membranes where water molecules move in and out of cells. **Dr. Peter Agre** won the 2003 Nobel Prize in Chemistry for his discovery of aquaporins. In an interview with *The New York Times* by Claudia Dreifus, 1/26/09, Agre said that on the suggestion of his old hematology professor Dr. John Parker, he should consider that his unidentified protein fragment could possibly be "the long-sought water channel." The scientific search for this cellular water channel is reminiscent of the legendary search for the elusive Fountain of Youth. These searches are actually quite similar, although on different scales of magnitude. Dr. Agre is a modern-day Ponce de Leon, who focused his vision down to the cellular level and actually discovered molecular-sized Fountains of Youth *within* the human body. When water molecules move through aquaporins in an unimpeded manner, like the water coming from a fountain, your body's total cellular processes have a greater chance of flourishing—and flourishing health is always about abundant, consistent energy.

Aquaporins

Free-flowing aquaporins help maintain your intracellular-to-extracellular Golden Ratio water balance. About 62% of your total body water is intracellular, 38% is extracellular. If aquaporins aren't freely flowing, then this delicate Golden Ratio is upset, with resulting metabolic inefficiency and aging.

Over time, aquaporins are vulnerable to becoming damaged by free radicals or clogged with debris, such as heavy metals, environmental toxins or metabolic by-products. Just as a clogged fountain ceases to produce a strong flow, the same can happen to aquaporins. When the aquaporins of millions of cells degenerate, we experience decreased performance, aging and ultimately death. Perhaps the secret to high-level wellness and longevity is to keep our molecular Fountains of Youth clean and freely flowing. All preventive measures are critical, such as eating organic food and avoiding exposure to environmental toxins. Detoxification procedures are vital for eliminating cellular toxic debris and restoring aquaporins to full function. Cellular detoxification is augmented by optimizing blood flow, lymphatic drainage, urination, defecation, breathing and sweating. More extensive detoxification therapies can include chelation, colonic irrigation, liver and kidney flushes, the use of digestive enzymes and avoidance of allergic foods.

Jeanne-Louise Calment (1875-1997): Longevity Torch Bearer

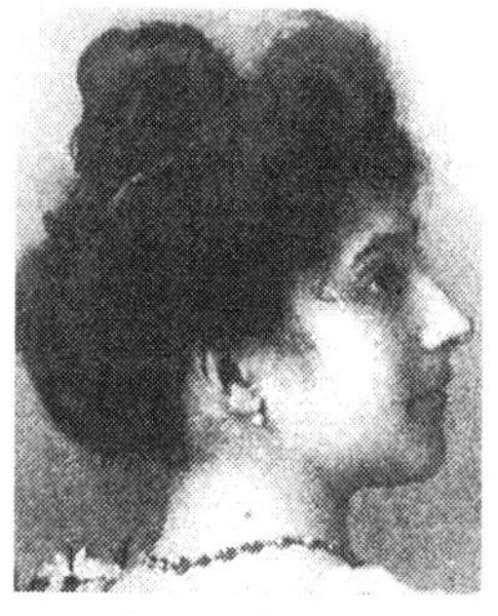

Jeanne-Louise Calment of France at 20. Calment lived to be 122, the world's oldest documented supercentenarian.

Get Busy Living—or Get Busy Dying.

Tim Robbins (as Andy Dufresne),
The Shawshank Redemption

Although many societies like the Hunzans, Vilcabambans, Okinawans and Abkhazians claim supercentenarians (someone over 110 years old), Jeanne-Louise Calment of France, who lived to be 122, is the only supercentenarian whose age has been verified by official documents. In a *New York Times* article (8/5/97) Craig Whitney quotes French author and public health researcher Jean-Marie Robine regarding insights on Mrs. Calment's longevity:

> *The French, who celebrated her as the doyenne of humanity, had their theories about why she lived so long, noting that she used to eat more than two pounds of chocolate a week, enjoyed a regular glass of port wine, poured olive oil on all her food as well as rubbing it onto her skin, rode a bicycle until she was 100, and only quit smoking five years ago… 'I think she was someone who, constitutionally and biologically speaking, was immune to stress,' he said in a telephone interview. She once said, 'If you can't do anything about it, don't worry about it.'*

Clearly, one of Jeanne-Louise's most notable longevity factors was her "immunity to stress" and sense of inner peace. This attribute was likely a combination of genetic predisposition, epigenetic influence of behaviors and thoughts as well as favorable life circumstances. However, as explored in chapter 8/Happiness, this quality of stress resistance can be cultivated through various methods. Your entire physiology can be modulated in a new, positive direction by reprogramming your reactions to stress. Jeanne's orientation to humor was also very strong and though hard to measure or quantify, was probably a key factor enhancing her "immunity to stress." Here are a few of Jeanne's most memorable quotes which illustrate her positive, long-life attitude:

- *I think I will die laughing.*
- *I never wear mascara;*
  I laugh until I cry too often.
- *I see badly, I hear badly and I feel bad, but everything's fine.* *(see p. 238, The Golden Ratio Happiness Zone)*
- *Always keep your smile.*
  That's how I explain my long life.
- *I'm not afraid of anything.*
- *I took pleasure when I could.*
  I acted clearly and morally
  and without regret. I'm very lucky.
- *I'm interested in everything*
  but passionate about nothing.
- *Not having children is one less worry.*
- *I've only got one wrinkle–and I'm sitting on it.*

U.S. Longevity Champions Hall of Fame

Every culture has its own Longevity Champion's Hall of Fame. These are celebrated individuals who productively made it into their 89-144 Fibonacci Golden Years. Even without knowledge of the Golden Ratio, they most likely excelled at one or more of the Nature's Secret Nutrient health drivers. Here we present a few notable longevity examples from America:

Name	Career	Age lived to	Noted longevity support factor(s)
Dr. John Harvey Kellogg	Breakfast cereal pioneer, Loma Linda founder	91	Moderation in everything; glass of water w/ lemon juice every morning, solar therapy, hydrotherapy
Dr. W. Edwards Deming	Quality leadership & management genius	93	Strong life purpose, joy in work, learning, & teaching
Dr. Linus Pauling	Chemist, peace activist, two-time Nobel Prize winner	93	Vitamin C, great curiosity
Katherine Hepburn	Legendary actress	96	Cold showers/baths/ocean swims; exercise, positive attitude
Jack LaLanne	Father and face of the modern fitness revolution	96	Exercise/weight-lifting in moderation, raw juicing, health pioneer
Kitty Carlisle	Singer, actress, ***To Tell The Truth*** panelist	96	Humor (stress reduction), dance/exercise
John D. Rockefeller	Oil magnate & philanthropist	97	Ample sleep; always eating to less than fullness; avoided worry
Norman W. Walker	Raw food and juicing pioneer	99	Raw juicing, detoxification
Bob Hope	Comedian, philanthropist	100	Daily massage, humor (stress reduction)
W. Clement Stone	Businessman, philanthropist, self-help guru	100	Positive attitude (stress reduction)
George Burns	Comedian, actor, writer	100	Humor, positive attitude (stress reduction)
Irving Berlin	Composer, lyricist	101	Music (stress reduction)
Dolores Hope	Philanthropist, wife of Bob Hope	102	Deep spiritual faith
Joseph M. Juran	Quality management genius and 80/20 pioneer	103	Married 81 yrs./Single 22 yrs. (80/20 rule in action); loved work
Rose Kennedy	Mother of President John F. Kennedy	104	Deep spiritual faith; cold ocean swims
Roy Neuberger	Financier, art patron	107	Business, art collecting, philanthropy; loved his work
Bernando LaPallo	World's oldest blogger; born between 1901–10	104-114	Colon cleansing, raw diet/pescetarian (fish for protein)
Leila Alice Denmark, M.D.	Pediatrician	114	Whole foods, low sugar diet, healthy hydration
Walter Breuning	Railroader	114	Healthy hydration habits, exercise

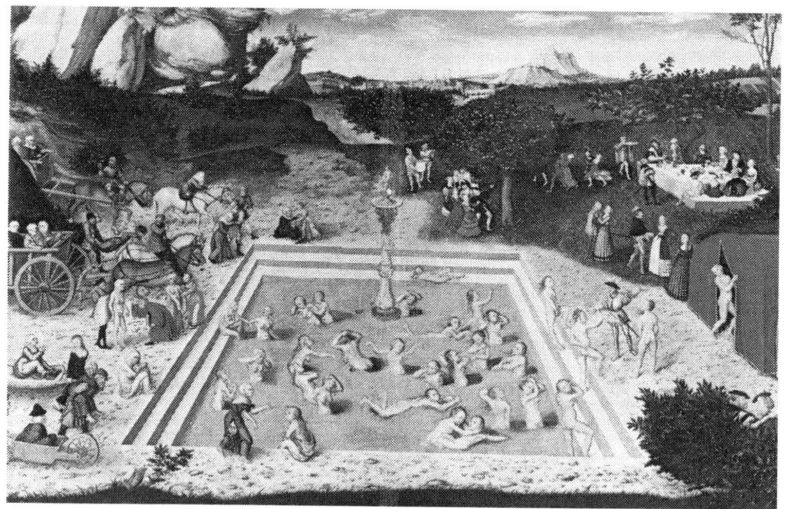

The Fountain of Youth, by German artist Lucas Cranach (1546). Note how the people enter the fountain pool as elders on the left and emerge on the right with their youth restored. Engaging the Nature's Secret Nutrient system is your lifetime VIP ticket to tapping your own Fountain of Youth.

Supercentenarian & World's Oldest Blogger Bernardo LaPallo

Bernando LaPallo of Mesa, Arizona (born August 17, between 1901–1910; died December 19, 2015) was a retired master chef, podiatrist, herbalist, massage therapist, entrepreneur and at an age between 104-114, the world's oldest blogger. A selection of Bernardo's key quotes offers a window into his healthy longevity:

> *HEALTH should be your FIRST PRIORITY, and in order to do that, you have to eat properly—not a bunch of stirred up, boiled-to-death food—and keep your colon clean. I was a protege of Dr. Richard Schulze's mentor, Dr. John Christopher; I and most of my family have been using Dr. Schulze's SuperFood since the 1980's.*

His longevity practices included:

- Ate mostly raw fruits, vegetables and soups; didn't eat at night
- Pescetarianism (fish for protein)
- Drank cinnamon tea for blood sugar control
- Ate only two meals a day
- Ate dinner around 4-5 pm
- Walked 1.5 miles daily
- Rubbed olive oil on his body and face daily to prevent wrinkles (*just like 122 year-old Jeanne Calment*)
- Took Echinacea every morning
- Ate Dr. Schulze's SuperFood daily

See Bernardo's book *Age Less, Live More* here: http://agelesslivemore.wordpress.com/

Telomeres: Biomarkers for Optimal Life Quality & Length

Telomeres are the DNA-protein caps at the ends of your chromosomes that protect them from deterioration with age. With each cell division telomeres continually shorten, until the DNA in the chromosome isn't protected anymore and begins to unravel, like a frayed shoelace whose plastic tip or aglet has deteriorated. At a critical point the cell approaches its **Hayflick Limit**: its maximal number of cell divisions (after **Leonard Hayflick**, DNA research pioneer). As more and more cells lose their telomeres aging begins, with disease and ultimately death the result. Scientists conclude that shorter telomeres = shorter life expectancy. Telomeres have a repair process that's controlled by the enzyme telomerase, yet this enzyme is usually dormant in adult cells. Some cells do have active telomerase, like stem cells, reproductive cells—and unfortunately cancer cells. Telomerase is a double-edged sword: just enough can promote normal cell division and regeneration, but too much can enable cancerous cells to proliferate. Cancer cells have learned how to rebuild their telomeres by activating their telomerase enzyme—becoming essentially immortal. Scientists have perpetuated a particular line of aggressive, immortal cancer cells for medical research from a woman named **HE**nrietta **LA**cks, who died of cancer in 1951. These so-named "**HeLa**" cells have become a standard cancer research cell line worldwide. HeLa cells have become so prevalent it's estimated that the total mass of this immortalized cell line weighs more than 100 Empire State Buildings. *The Immortal Life of Henrietta Lacks* by Rebecca Skloot and the film starring Oprah Winfrey offers added insight into telomeres, cancer and the ordeal Henrietta's family endures by having their mother's cells dispersed in laboratories worldwide.

In 2009 **Elizabeth Blackburn, Ph.D.**, of pure air haven Tasmania (p. 309), won the Nobel prize in Physiology or Medicine for her co-discovery of how chromosomes

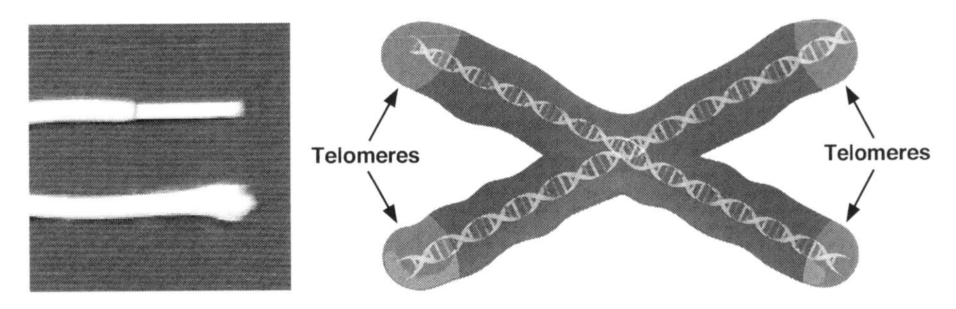

(*L*) Shoelace aglets: normal (top) and frayed (bottom). (*R*) Chromosome capped by telomeres. The telomeres are DNA-protein complexes that function like protective shoelace aglets, preventing degeneration and aging. Professor **Ramin Farzaneh-Far, M.D.** of UCSF correlated higher levels of omega-3 fatty acids with a slower rate of telomere shortening in patients with coronary heart disease. This finding may translate to a slowdown in overall cellular aging simply by increasing one's intake of omega-3 oils.

can be protected against degradation during replication by telomeres and the enzyme telomerase. Her bestselling book with **Elissa Epel, Ph.D.**, *The Telomere Effect*, explores the fascinating interplay between telomere length, length and quality of life and our ability to positively influence all 3 factors. A few summarized highlights from their excellent book include the following:

> Φ *Telomeres are an integrative index of many lifetime influences, both the good, restorative ones like fitness and sleep, and also bad ones like toxic stress, poor nutrition or adversities.* Φ *Telomere length may be the "Holy Grail for cumulative welfare" and while there will be no one biological indicator of human lifetime experience, telomeres are among one of the most helpful indicators.* Φ *Telomeres do not simply carry out the commands issued by your genetic code. Your telomeres are listening to you.* Φ *The way you live can tell your telomeres to speed up the process of cellular aging—but it can also do the opposite.* Φ *The food you eat, responses to emotional challenges, amount of exercise, childhood stress, neighborhood safety—all of these factors and more influence your telomeres and can prevent premature aging at the cellular level.* Φ *Your genes affect your telomeres, both their length when you're born and how quickly they dwindle down.* Φ *The great news is that you can step in and take some control of how short or long and robust your telomeres are.*

Blackburn and Epel's telomere-strengthening regimen includes mindfulness meditation, QiGong, avoiding excess stress and fried foods, healthy exercise and other key lifestyle upgrades resonant with many of those in this book. For example, their keen observation that your telomeres *actually listen to you* beautifully aligns with geneticist Dr. Kazuo Murakami's research as explored in ch 8, Happiness. There is now a telomere length test which can approximate one's longevity, a test reminiscent of Andrew Niccol's classic 1997 film *GATTACA*, starring Ethan Hawke and Uma Thurman. The film explores a future where one's vitality and longevity—and correlated social standing—is validated at birth via a blood drop. GATTACA is a creative rearrangement of DNA's prime letter code—the four DNA nitrogen bases (A,T,C,G). The film's clever tagline, *There is No Gene for the Human Spirit* brings up a provocative question to ponder: *who or what actually controls and modulates our telomeres, DNA and epigenetics...?*

Jeanne Calment's Secret: Stress Reduction ➨ Long Telomeres ➨ Longevity

If you can't do anything about it, don't worry about it. **Jeanne Calment**

There's often a hidden message in a name. In Jeanne Calment's case, her first name is a homonym for *Gene* while her last name, *Calment* is a conjunction of two words: Calm + Ment (or mind). Together, the alternate translation is *Gene for a Calm Mind.*

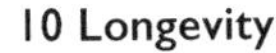

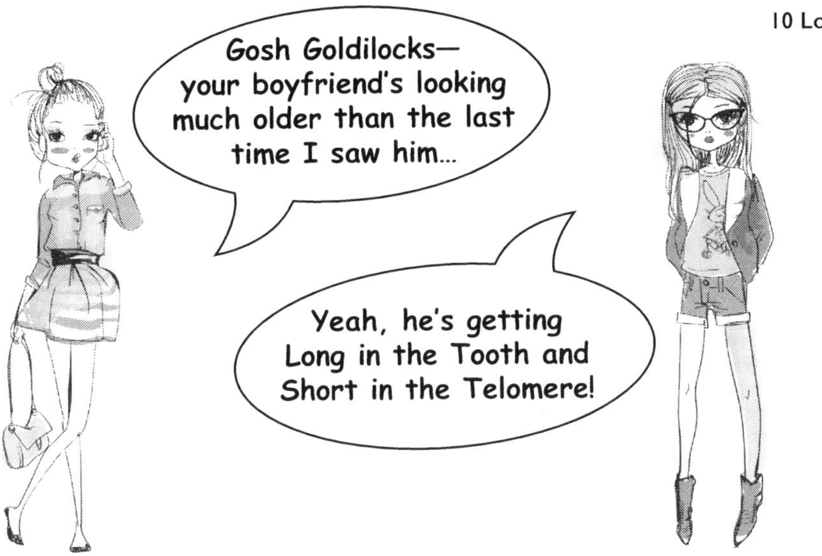

Goldilocks [see pgs. 28-29] wants a boyfriend with "Just Right" Golden Ratio telomeres—neither too long (predisposing to cancer) nor too short (predisposing to aging, immune dysfunction and disease, including cancer). Keeping your telomeres in Golden Ratio range is a self-led genetic key to peak health and longevity. Many NSN drivers and Rx's in this book are resonant with Nobel prize-winner Elizabeth Blackburn, Ph.D., and Elissa Epel, Ph.D's (*The Telomere Effect*) recommendations for easy lifestyle upgrades that protect and restore telomeres for robust longevity. As a side note, tooth-length age estimation works for horses and some animals, not humans; telomere length test kits for people are available via online labs.

Jeanne Calment clearly had the Gene for a Calm Mind, making her more immune to stress, contributing to her amazing longevity. As Elizabeth Blackburn and others have shown, stress is a major factor in telomere degradation and thus premature aging. **Dr. Herbert Benson**, founder of the Mind/Body Medical Institute at Boston's Massachusetts General Hospital, has also taken stress pioneer **Dr. Hans Selye's** (*The Stress of Life*) fight-or-flight discoveries down to the genetic level. Benson's stress reduction research via the Relaxation Response has been proven to favorably alter gene expression and possibly even affect apoptosis—programmed cell death. In his book *Relaxation Revolution,* Benson shows that various genes responsible for high blood

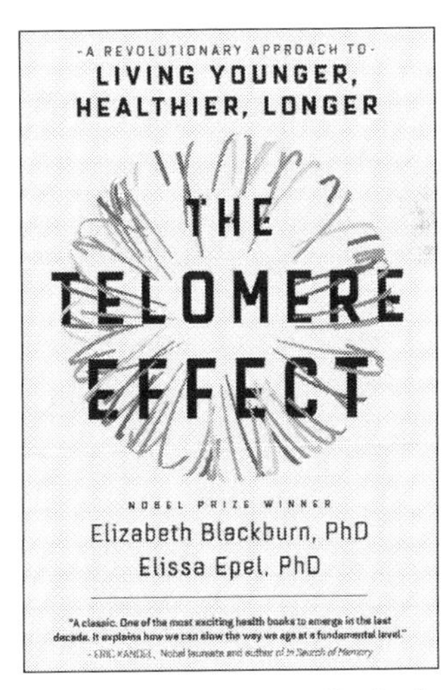

The Telomere Effect, by Elizabeth Blackburn & Elissa Epel.

> *The Ageless Body bears a quality of emotions that are light and joyous, willing to experience ecstasy and the richness of life at any moment.*
>
> **Chris Griscom, *The Ageless Body***

pressure, anxiety, depression, back ache, infertility, insomnia, headache, hot flashes and even phobias can be down-regulated (reduced) via the Relaxation Response. Scientists hypothesize that increasing telomere length may be the genetic mechanism through which stress reduction has its remarkable positive effects on longevity. In a related study, cardiologist **Dean Ornish, M.D.** showed that telomerase enzyme could be increased by 29% in prostate cancer patients, simply by instituting a series of lifestyle upgrades, including a diet low in refined sugars and fat and rich in whole foods, fruits and vegetables; aerobic exercise; breathing exercises and meditation. Dr. Ornish concluded that increasing telomerase through lifestyle modification may not be specific to just prostate cancer patients—it may have similar powerful benefits for the total population. **Drs. Ornish, Benson, Blackburn, Epel, et al, have shown that stress reduction and lifestyle modification practices can favorably influence gene expression and potentially preserve/restore healthy telomere length, thus increasing life expectancy.** Working with the sequenced health priorities combined with NSN builds on the work of these longevity pioneers. It offers us a head start into the research of modulating gene expression for optimizing telomere/life length in simple ways. Living well into the next Fibonacci Sequence life stage, Golden Ratio Years 89 to 144+, is now close at hand. To ensure that you reach this next Fibonacci lifespan zone healthy and intact, be sure to metaphorically "tie your shoes"—with your telomere's aglet shoelace ends intact—by consistently supporting or "tying up" your key NSN health priorities, including reducing stress and increasing your inner peace and happiness.

Cross-Cultural Longevity Research Supports Nature's Secret Nutrient

Scientific corroboration of key factors in the Nature's Secret Nutrient System are described by author **Dan Buettner**, whose cross-cultural research into the secrets of longevity led him to many of the Earth's centenarian hotspots, aka ***Blue Zones***: Sardinia, Italy; Okinawa, Japan; Nicoya, Costa Rica; Loma Linda, California; Ikaria, Greece; Abkhazia, Caucasus Mountains; Hunza Valley, Pakistan and Vilcabamba, Ecuador. In his great book ***The Blue Zones:*** *Lessons for Living Longer From the People Who've Lived the Longest* and in *National Geographic Adventure Magazine*, Buettner shares the key consistent factors leading to healthy longevity, after which we list some correlating NSN priority drivers and chapters. While not the last word on longevity, Dan's research provides a framework for writing and living your best health and longevity lifescript. As he suggests,

> *Set up your life, your home environment, your social environment and your workplace so that you're constantly nudged into behaviors that favor longevity* [e.g., conditions conducive for the daily generation of Nature's Secret Nutrient].

Some Blue Zone Longevity Factors & NSN Health Priority Correlations

- Φ A key Ikarian longevity secret is clean, fresh air. ***Ch 1 Breathing, 7 Detox***
- Φ Centenarians cultivate kindness, humor, altruism. ***Ch 8 Happiness, 10 Longevity***
- Φ Over 80% of Ikarian men nap daily. ***Ch 3 Sleep***
- Φ Happier people tend to live & laugh longer. ***Ch 8 Happiness, 10 Longevity***
- Φ Okinawan centenarians get exercise through gardening; reduces stress, source of fresh air, sunshine/vitamin D & source of fresh herbs & vegetables. ***Ch 3A Sun, 4 Nutrition, 6 Exercise, 8 Happiness***
- Φ Reconnect with & strengthen your Faith. ***Ch 8 Happiness***
- Φ Unhappiness can be as harmful as smoking. ***Ch 7 Detox (Fibonacci's smoking reduction technique), Ch 8 Happiness***
- Φ Longevity is more a function of what you *don't* eat than what you do eat. Use a smaller plate like the Okinawans. ***Ch 4 Nutrition/Caloric reduction slows aging. Intermittent fasting. Not eating over 2/3 full***
- Φ Ikarians observe about 150 days of religious fasting/year, stay up late, sleep late & nap. ***Ch 3 Sleep, Ch 4 Nutrition, Alternate Day Diet, Caloric Reduction***
- Φ Eat a predominantly plant-based diet; eat meat infrequently. ***Ch 4 Nutrition, 40/30/30 Golden Ratio Nutrition; Vegans good to supplement vit. B-12***
- Φ Ikarians eat a diet high in leafy greens. ***Ch 4 Nutrition/Green Foods, Smoothie***
- Φ Hydrate w/ ample pure water; fill & flush regularly. ***Ch 2 Hydration, Ch 7 Detox***

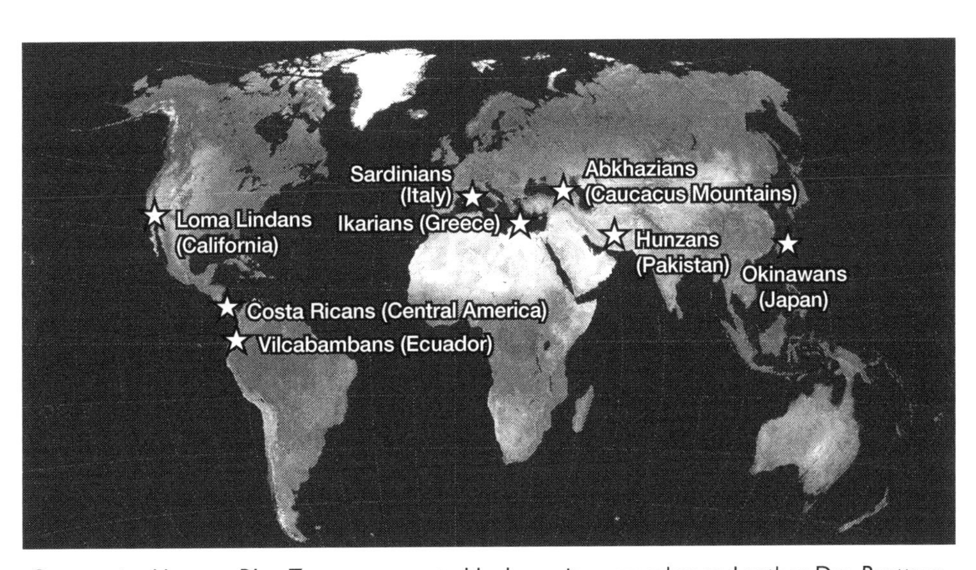

Centenarian Hotspot *Blue Zones*, as reported by longevity researcher and author Dan Buettner.

10

- Φ A daily glass of wine is medicinal, e.g., Sardinian red wine has 3x the antioxidants of other wines. ***Ch 4 Nutrition; resveratrol, gene silencing SIRT-1 gene***
- Φ Ikarians pick garden herbs, steeping them for evening & breakfast tea. Diuretic herbs normalize blood pressure, prevent heart attacks, strokes & dementia. Herbs & green tea have high antioxidant levels protecting against premature aging. ***Ch 2 Hydration, 6 Exercise/Golden Ratio blood pressure, 7 Detox***
- Φ Invest in family & nurture **Strong Social Relationships**. ***Ch 8 Happiness***
- Φ Cultivate a sense of Life Purpose—Okinawans call it *Ikigai;* Costa Ricans call it *Plan de Vida.* ***Ch 8 Happiness/Dr. Murakami, Ch 10 Longevity***
- Φ Take breaks & allow for ample Rest, Relaxation & Recharge. ***Ch 3 Sleep***
- Φ 95% of Ikarians live in their own homes, 85% of men are married. ***10 Longevity***
- Φ Lead an active life with regular *yet low-stress* Lifestyle Exercise, e.g., walking, biking, gardening. ***Ch 6 Exercise***

> *Age is a question of mind over matter. If you don't mind, it doesn't matter.*
>
> **Mark Twain**

Dr. Ellen Langer: Mindfulness, Time Travel & Longevity

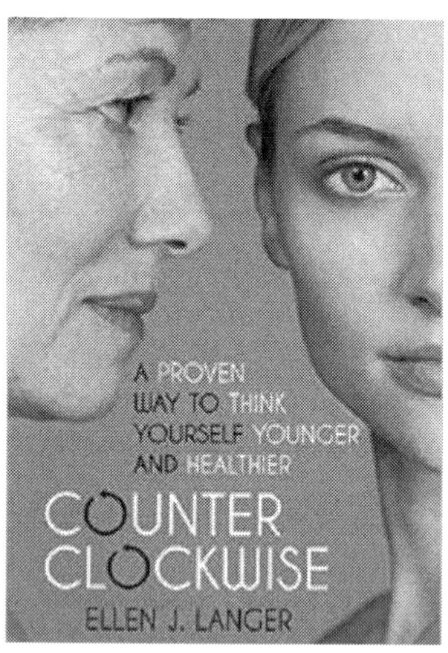

Dr. Ellen Langer's ground-breaking book on age reversal, *Counterclockwise: A Proven Way to Think Yourself Younger and Healthier.*

Mindfulness—the simple act of noticing new things— is crucial to our health in several ways. First, when we're mindless, we ignore all the ways we could exercise control over our health...

Ellen Langer, Ph.D.

Harvard psychologist and professor Ellen Langer, Ph.D., author of *Counterclockwise: A Proven Way to Think Yourself Younger and Healthier*, performed a landmark study in 1979 that opened new frontiers into the science of longevity. In her fascinating experiment, Langer psychologically time-shifted a group of 70-80 year-olds back in time 20 years—to the year 1959—by designing a totally realistic, isolated residential setting in rural Peterborough, New Hampshire that mimicked the visual, auditory and tactile detail of that bygone era. **Every on-site detail—from the selection of television**

programs, magazines, radio and music, clothing—even the topics of their daily conversation reflected the ambiance of the late 1950's and no later. Amazingly, *after just one week* of living in this immersive time warp, the men showed the following significant improvements in key biomarkers of aging:

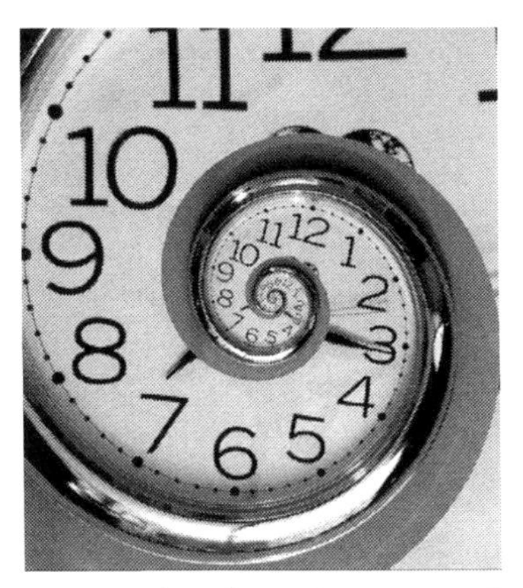

The benefits of mental & emotional time travel include tapping into your inner Fountain of Youth.

- Φ Weight loss
- Φ Key physiologic improvements, including decreased blood pressure
- Φ Less arthritic symptoms, with better dexterity & decreased inflammation
- Φ An overall sense of enhanced wellbeing.
- Φ Gait & posture improvement; height increases
- Φ Brain & sensory improvements in memory & hearing
- Φ A more youthful appearance post-study, via before-and-after photo comparison

Langer's intriguing research challenges us to reevaluate our concepts of the blurry division between mind and body, and the multi-directional flow of time. While many may not make the effort to recreate physical stage sets of times past as Langer did in her study, we can still easily apply her work to our lives. How? By practicing mental/emotional time travel: revisiting our 19–31 Golden Prime Zone years when we were exceptionally happy, healthy and robust. **By being mindful of and strategically revisiting Golden Prime Zone memories that were especially invigorating to body, mind and spirit, we can support the re-release of those same enlivening neurotransmitters and hormones—and thus experience their powerfully rejuvenating, healing effects *now*.** As 1964 Olympic Gold Medal 10k Champion Billy Mills says, *the subconscious mind cannot tell the difference between "reality" or imagination*. You can time travel into your past and enjoy the regeneration and rejuvenation benefits via the Ch 10 Longevity Rx section. There you'll find easy instructions in Rx 1: **Power Up Your Golden Prime Zone Age-Reversing Holodeck**.

> *What you want to do is to regenerate and return*
> *to your* **true** *genetic blueprint—which has* **no** *age.*
> *(see p. 291, the work of anti-aging scientist David Sinclair)*
>
> **Janet Krier**

10

Golden Ratio Oldies: Activating Your Golden Prime Zone Through Music

Music is the primary sense which both anchors and activates emotion
and can literally, physiologically, transport us back in time.
Michael Rossato-Bennett, director of *Alive Inside, A Story of Music & Memory*

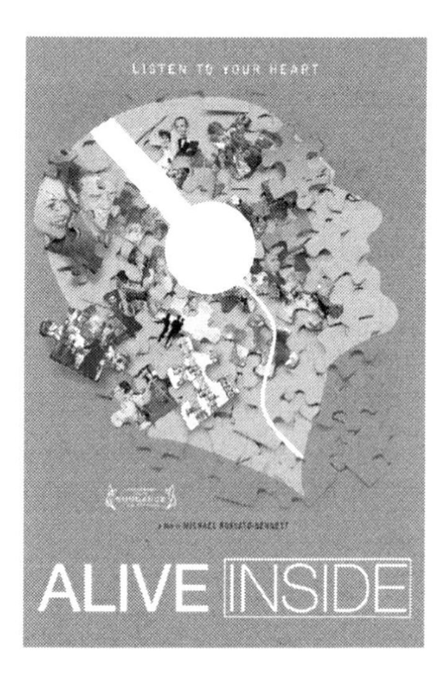

The remarkable film *Alive Inside* explores the vast therapeutic power of music to help restore memory and youthfulness.

At the 2014 Sundance film festival a most inspiring film premiered that's igniting a revolution in the way music can be used to revive nursing home patients with various types of dysfunction or dementia, including Alzheimer's disease. *Alive Inside, A Story of Music & Memory* by Michael Rossato-Bennett chronicles **Dan Cohen's** (Music & Memory^{SM}) journey into old-age-homes with a magic sound bullet: an iPod with headphones. Music played to patients who had been withdrawn and unengaged for years spurred unexpected and almost instantaneous awakening and emotional responses when they listened to favorite music from their youth. Even though dementia had decimated parts of their brains, other deep memory and emotional areas of their brains were still intact and capable of near-instant recognition and reactivation in response to the music. Patients once written off as mentally unretrievable had an essential part of themselves miraculously restored, simply by listening to meaningful music from their youth. Nursing home staffs were delighted to discover that there was a non-drug, non-invasive method that dramatically improved interaction and engagement with these seemingly lost souls. Director Michael Rossato-Bennett noted,

> *When you lose [frontal lobe function], there are deep primal parts of the brain that are activated by music. They're co-located with emotion, so when emotion is stirred in you these pathways are awakened and, literally, function that people thought is gone is rekindled.*

In the film, noted neurologist Oliver Sacks validates Rossato-Bennett's theory that music has more ability to activate more parts of the brain than any other stimulus. This is stunning. When drugs fail, the therapeutic ability of music to rekindle and harmonize brain activity is near-miraculous. Dormant memories of youth have unrecognized power to reactivate not just emotions and improve social interaction in the aged, but can also be harnessed by the average baby boomer who wants a resurgence of neurotransmitter and hormonal activity that was once overflowing and

The Golden Prime Zone: 31 ÷ 19 = 1.6 Φ

Age 19 20 21 22 23 24 25 26 27 28 29 30 31

The **Golden Prime Zone (GPZ)** is the natural state of peak health and performance enjoyed by virtually everyone between ages 19-31. In math, 19 & 31 are known as **prime numbers** and remarkably are also in Golden Ratio to each other: 31 ÷ 19 = 1.6 Φ. Reactivate your GPZ with Ch 10 Rx #1, the **Golden Prime Zone Holodeck Meditation**.

responsible for the vigor of their youth. As we saw in the previous section, Dr. Ellen Langer proved in her landmark 1979 Counterclockwise study that a group of men put into a 1959-appearing environment significantly regressed their biologic age. One of the factors that had the power to transport the men back in time in mind and body was listening to vintage music and radio broadcasts from decades earlier. These men didn't have dementia, yet like their nursing home counterparts dramatically benefited from the power of targeted musical input to reawaken and realign with the physical and emotional vitality of times past. As Dr. Langer said, ***Wherever you put the mind the body will follow.*** Considering that sage advice, let's take a tip from our institutionalized elders who have benefitted so much from targeted music therapy. Get your iPod or smartphone and download and listen to your favorite Golden Ratio Prime Zone "Oldies" and watch what happens. Remember that **the years from 19–31 are your Golden Prime Zone years** (31÷19= 1.6; 1.6 = Φ Phi). Music from other non-Prime Zone eras in your life is also enhancing of course, yet there is a deep subconscious imprint from your Golden Prime Zone years that's particularly strong. *The goal is simple: to reactivate and resonate with that Prime Time Zone when your life force or élan vital was at its peak.* As you deploy this simple strategy, note how you feel, look and function. Don't be surprised if you start catching glimpses in the mirror of that robust, super-healthy 19 to 31-year old version of yourself! See Rx 1 on this subject in Ch 10 Rx's.

Demographics of Longevity

By looking at the life expectancies of inhabitants of the longest-lived cultures in the world—the Blue Zones—we can see that the tendency to take a quantum Fibonacci jump in life expectancy is already happening. The number of centenarians in Okinawa is the highest in the world, at a rate of 50 per 100,000 population. The U.S. has a considerable number, yet lags behind, having a rate of around 18 per 100,000 population in the year 2000. However, the absolute number of centenarians will skyrocket to 834,000 by the year 2050, according to U.S. Census Bureau projections. Interestingly, the demographics of this exponential rise in the number of centenarians has some Golden Ratio aspects, as can be seen in the accompanying diagrams. The demographics of longevity graphs on the next page are alarming, especially in the areas of disability, marital status, poverty and living situation. It may be hard to imagine yourself living to 100+, yet if these U.S. Census Bureau data are accurate, many of us will become centenarians or supercentenarians and may have to confront living with disabilities, poverty, loneliness and compromised living quarters. Perhaps the NSN system can both help us become centenarians *and* overcome the challenges that longevity can present as we age. By applying the sequenced drivers in this book, you now have the ability to make a quantum evolutionary jump into *healthy* longevity. Can you imagine yourself transcending the accepted limit of an 80 year lifespan or becoming a parent in your 70's or 80's? The possibilities of what can be accomplished at any age expand preconceived lifecycle limits and need to be reevaluated and reimagined.

Red Wine & the Art of Moderation for Maximum Health & Longevity

God in his goodness sent the grapes, to cheer both great and small; great fools drink too much, and little fools not at all—and Golden Ratio fools drink just the right amount.
Robert D. Friedman, M.D. & Matthew K. Cross, adapted from anonymous

Every centenarian and supercentenarian has arrived at their Golden years by practicing the principle of moderation, either consciously or unconsciously. So, how can you become more moderate in everything you do and thus increase *your* health and longevity? It's as simple as discovering a Golden Ratio balance in all facets of life. **The Golden Ratio, after all, is Mother Nature's inherent principle of moderation.** One simple and enjoyable way to practice moderation is by having a glass of full-bodied red wine with your dinner. The French have incorporated wine drinking into their daily lifestyle for centuries. In spite of the fact that French people have an extremely high fat intake, their rate of coronary heart disease is a remarkable 40% less than that of Americans. This discrepancy between high fat intake and lower rates of coronary heart disease, known as the "French Paradox," has been explained by the offsetting benefits obtained from consuming increased amounts of red wine polyphenols. Research has shown that wine has cardio-protective effects *when consumed in moderation.* We see the same beneficial effects from wine consumption in many other areas of the world, including the so-called Blue Zones. These are specific areas identified by researcher Dan Buettner where the inhabitants routinely live to 100 years or more, such as in Sardinia. Residents of the island of Sardinia, Italy

MAGA: Make Aging Great Again

The data below reveals the paradox of increasing life quantity and decreasing life quality in the US. There are more centenarians than ever, dealing with increased poverty, compromised living and worsening morbidity. The dichotomy in quantity and quality of years isn't what Biblical Longevity Legends like Adam, Noah and Methuselah likely experienced in their presumed near 1000-year lifespans (p. 298). They undoubtedly unlocked anti-aging secrets that made life bountiful in both years and pleasure. The humane goal in the current aging paradigm? Be like a Longevity Legend: *Make Aging Great Again* by living a long, healthy life followed by a quick transition—*without a lingering period of poor health and suffering.*

Every problem contains an answer and the solution for the coming rise in centenarians lies in the area of anti-aging research. A leading scientist in this field is David Sinclair, Ph.D., who theorizes that it may be possible to access and activate an unrecognized and uncorrupted "backup disk" of our pristine DNA. If successful, Sinclair and colleagues will usher in a new era of age-reversing and regenerative techniques just in the nick of time to meet the rising tide of new centenarians. While most people don't have access to a high-tech genetics lab like Sinclair, we can use NSN Rx's as an advanced, truly natural approach for optimal rejuvenation and cellular regeneration. Nature's Secret Nutrient/NSN is the perfect solution to match the anticipated increase in the quantity of our years with an equally robust quality.

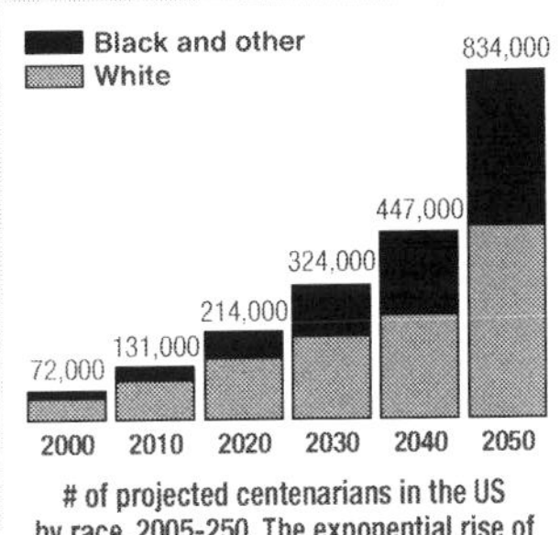

\# of projected centenarians in the US by race, 2005-250. The exponential rise of centenarians conforms to the Golden Ratio.

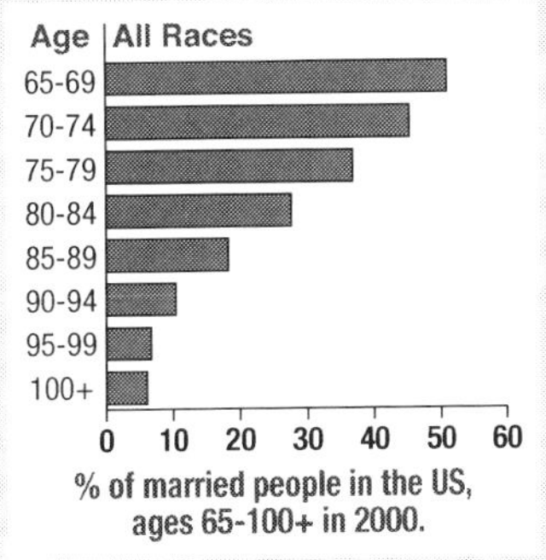

% of married people in the US, ages 65-100+ in 2000.

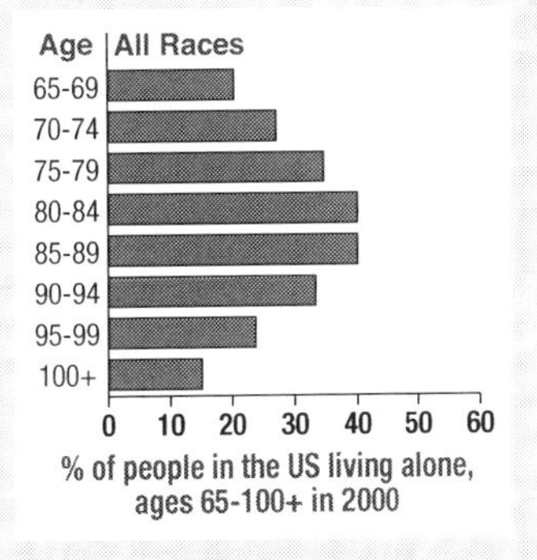

% of people in the US living alone, ages 65-100+ in 2000

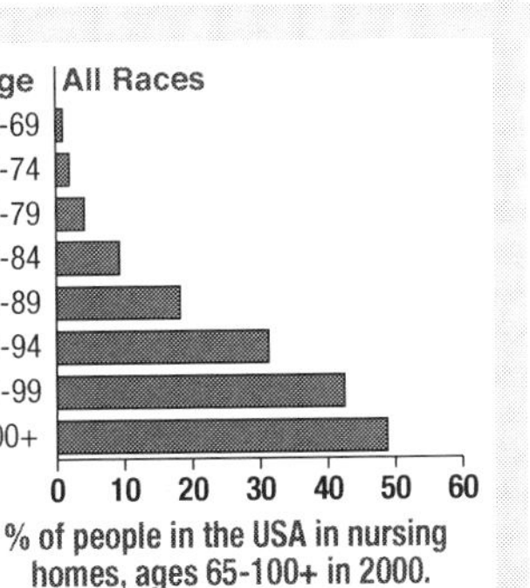

% of people in the USA in nursing homes, ages 65-100+ in 2000.

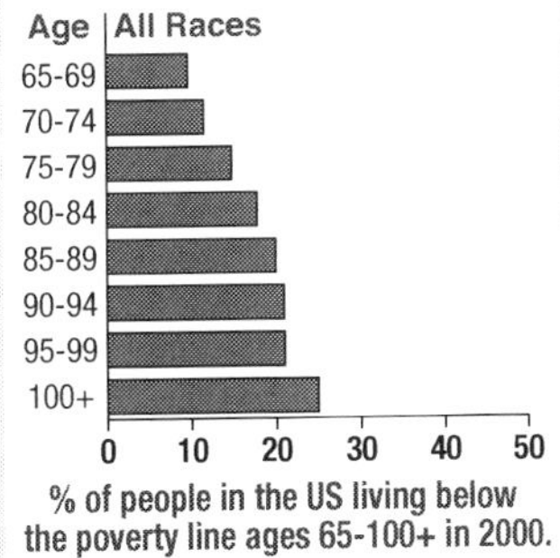

% of people in the US living below the poverty line ages 65-100+ in 2000.

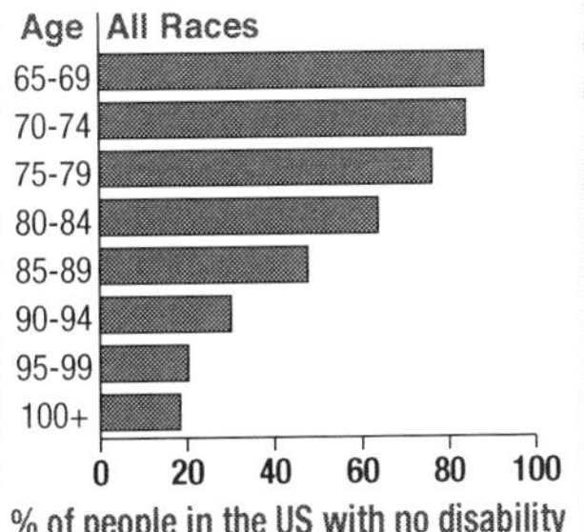

% of people in the US with no disability limitations, ages 65-100+ in 2000.

One of the World's Oldest Human's Longevity Secrets

As we've learned, Jeanne-Louise Calment (1875-1997) lived to the ripe old age of 122 and is purported to have been the oldest documented human, even having known Vincent Van Gogh in the late 1800's. As one of her life-extending practices, she cultivated the daily habit of enjoying a glass of Port wine. Although she wasn't focused on its life-extending properties, she enjoyed her glass of Port for the simple *joie de vivre.* The Port also gave her a regular dose of life-extending nutrients like resveratrol and other flavonoids found in grape seeds and skins. Port wine is produced in the Duoro region of Portugal, hence the name Port. Calment presumably would have consumed unfiltered Port, which contains more of the nutrient rich sediment, where the highest concentration of resveratrol and flavanoids reside.

drink locally grown, full-bodied red wine called *Cannonau* that also has unusually high levels of polyphenols. These cardio-protective compounds have favorable effects on cholesterol levels, blood vessel integrity, blood vessel relaxation, beneficial effects on blood clotting as well as anti-inflammatory and anti-oxidant effects. **However, one of the most important nutrients obtained from drinking wine is largely overlooked. Nature's Secret Nutrient can be obtained from wine, but only through moderate consumption.** Drinking not too little nor too much, but just the right amount allows you to hit the Golden Ratio target for your body size and physiology. Drinking the Golden Ratio amount allows you to obtain all the benefits of wine without adverse side effects, e.g., compromised thinking, DWI, hangovers, liver and brain damage, etc. Yet what is the right amount of wine to drink? Studies show that a J-Curve emerges

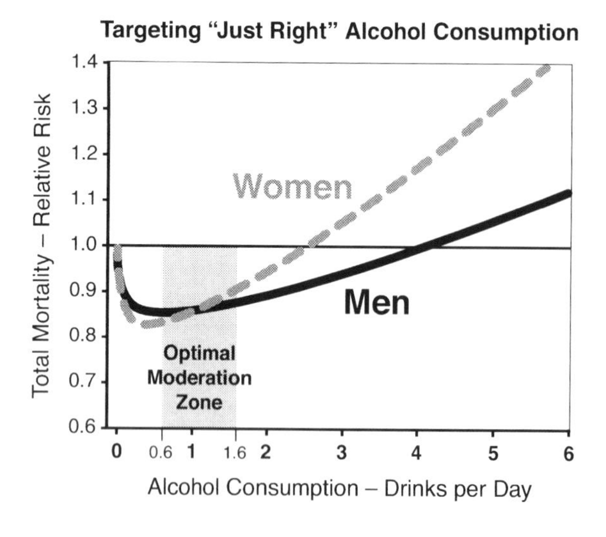

To avoid increased mortality from excess alcohol consumption, keep number of glasses per day in the Optimal Moderation Zone/Golden Ratio range of 0.6 glasses to 1.6 glasses. Note that wine is used in this graph; if stronger liquor is consumed, adjust quantities downward.

when plotting mortality vs. number of drinks consumed per day. Not surprisingly, the lowest mortality rates occur when moderate alcohol consumption is followed. Due to body size variance, this comes out to around 1 drink a day for women and 1 to 2 drinks for men. On closer inspection of the J-Curve, we can refine the estimates to Golden Ratio values: around 0.6-1.0 drinks per day for women and 1.0-1.6 drinks per day for men. The J-Curve shows that drinking Golden Ratio amounts confers a low mortality risk, lower than that of heavy drinkers and surprisingly, even lower than that of teetotalers. Through the effect of moderation in alcohol consumption, NSN appears and bestows long life to the one who knows the perfect amount to imbibe.

Iceman Wim Hof: Cold Therapy + Yogic Breathing as Adaptogenic, Healing & Longevity Nutrients

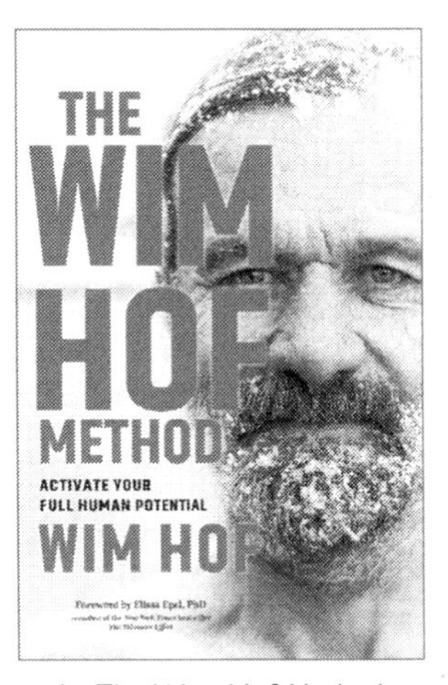

In *The Wim Hof Method*, Wim shares his proven Iceman training method and how anyone can transform their health, performance and potential—and become their own Iceman.

Most people would cringe at the thought of deliberately subjecting themselves to extreme cold, yet that's exactly what Dutchman Wim Hof does with regular ease. Aka The Iceman, Wim routinely swims in Arctic lakes, runs half-marathons barefoot in sub-zero conditions and sits cross-legged on glaciers while meditating. **Hof has great reverence for the cold, referring to it as a *Noble Force*.** The Noble Force taught him the secrets of cold adaptation in a continuing one-on-one partnership, resulting in a synergistic breathing process and immune boosting system which underlies his superhuman feats. Wim broke through the once-thought-to-be exclusive realm of Sherpas and Tibetan yogis, who can withstand prolonged extreme cold exposure. Through ancient yogic breathing practices, force of will and persistence, Hof biohacked his way to metabolic high performance. He's been studied by doctors who discovered that he has the remarkable ability to shift from burning mainly WAT (White Adipose fat Tissue) to burning BAT (Brown Adipose fat Tissue) for high-efficiency thermogenesis (heat production). **Wim learned how to tap into a seldom-used ancient biochemical pathway in the body** that preferentially burns stores of BAT, which is high-octane fat. Babies and infants naturally burn high-efficiency brown fat to stay warm, yet gradually shift to burning white fat (WAT, White Adipose Tissue) as they age. By shifting into brown fat burning at will Wim increases his metabolic rate, enabling him to healthfully endure record-setting extreme cold, a skill he teaches via WimHofMethod.com (Breath Control + Cold Training + Commitment = Empowerment, Healing & Transformation).

From Iceman to Newman

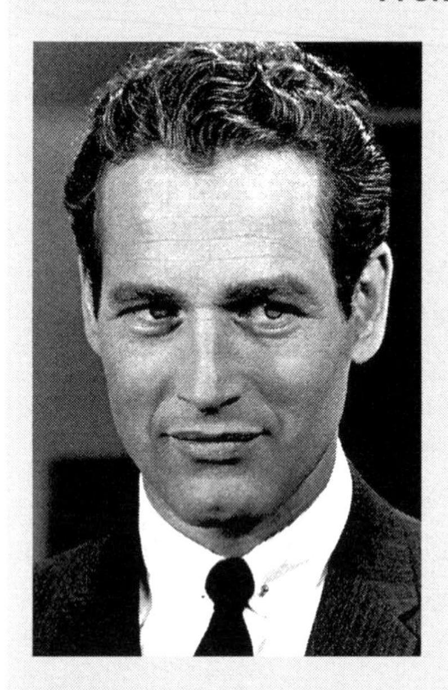

In 1967 Hollywood legend **Paul Newman** shared a little-known secret daily ritual of his with host Johnny Carson on *The Tonight Show*: Every morning Paul immersed his face in a basin filled with ice water for 30 seconds to give himself an invigorating wake-up. The icy water would contract the capillaries in his skin, eliminate puffiness and keep his Golden Ratio face glowing and youthful. In addition and perhaps unknown to Newman, the practice also triggers a primitive involuntary reflex in sea mammals and humans known as the *Mammalian Diving Reflex.* Initiated by cold water on the skin, the reflex enhances one's ability to breath-hold underwater for extended periods by reflex action on the autonomic (involuntary) nervous system. Yet these adaptive effects aren't just reserved for seals, dolphins and whales—and any humans interested in extended breath-holding—they also offer powerful benefits for modern-day, over-stressed humans.

The reflex also causes blood in the extremities to be shunted to the lungs, heart and brain as well as inducing a bradycardia (slowing down) of the heart. The result? **A calming effect that permeates the entire body, as more oxygenated blood is shunted to the brain for greater emotional equanimity and sharper thinking.** Paul Newman upended the negative connotation that to throw cold water on something was to dampen one's enthusiasm, and turned it around into a positive invigorating daily practice. And who knows, perhaps his daily ritual had something to do with the title of one of his blockbuster films: *Cool Hand Luke.*

Instant Superstar Cold Water Rx: To practically harness the power of this innate yet little-known reflex, World Free-Diving Champion Stig Severinsen recommends covering your face with an icy cold, wet towel for 30 seconds before any appearance, presentation or meeting to activate the diving reflex and infuse you with a lasting, cool calm. This easy practice calms your nerves, sharpens your mental and emotional acuity and reduces or even eliminates performance anxiety. For a feet-first variation, try Russian kinesiotherapist **Sergey Bubnovsky's** recommended feet ice water dip (in a bucket or basin) for 30 seconds daily to boost and tune your immune system.

Katharine Hepburn & the Proven Power of Cold-Water Therapy

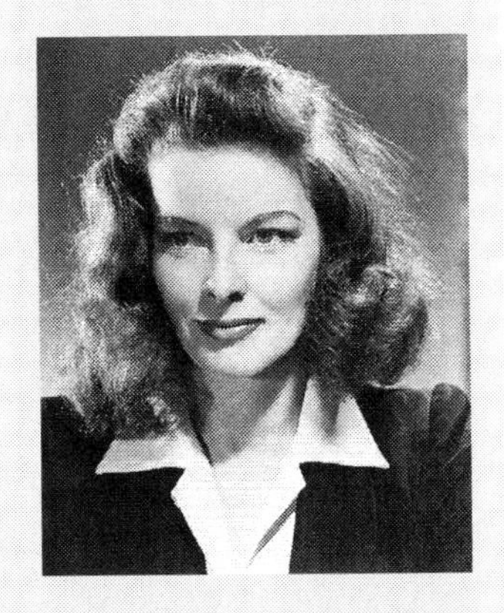

One of many great examples of the cold-water therapy, robust health and longevity connection was nonagenarian and 4-time Oscar-winner Katharine Hepburn, who lived to the ripe age of 96. Hepburn was raised in a strict Connecticut Yankee home, where morning cold showers were part of the family's daily health regimen. "Health is Youth" was her physician father Thomas' guiding motto, which inspired young Hepburn to follow a lifestyle that emphasized exercise and natural hygiene. In addition to her daily cold shower regimen, she enjoyed cold-water ocean swimming as well as cold-water morning baths, which she claimed built character, discipline and drive. **Hepburn unequivocally stated that cold-water therapy was responsible not only for her boundless energy, it was also her #1 beauty secret.** Katharine fervently believed that *the bitterer the medicine, the better it was for you*—and cold water therapy certainly fit the bill. While there's no guarantee that cold-water therapy will make you a legendary, long-lived movie star, it can certainly invigorate your body, mind and spirit as well as give you a regular dose of character-building medicine.

My mission is to show that everybody through their mind can reach more depth within themselves and tap their real inner healing power.
Wim Hof, The Iceman, master teacher of how to utilize cold exposure & the breath as a synergistic healing force

Hof has conclusively shown that exposure to extreme cold goes more than skin deep, repeatedly demonstrating underlying super adaptations in immune, hormonal and nerve function, all verified in impeccable laboratory conditions. *Cold acts as a super-metabolic stimulant and immune system strengthener when applied in controlled adaptation over time.* This unusual method of metabolic tonification activates latent, ancient cellular pathways that can raise total health & performance to peak levels. Wim has shown that the ability to utilize cold as a thermogenic adaptogen is a skill that anyone can learn and master—providing they have the frosty determination to activate their inner Iceman.

Another pioneer in the study of Cold Thermogenesis (CT) is **Jack Kruse, M.D.**, neurosurgeon, biophysicist & neopaleo-photon-*bayouhacker* (see page 104 for more on this peak health genius). Dr. Kruse's personal research revealed that it takes around 30 days of cold training to achieve metabolic adaptation to extreme cold exposure. Kruse lost 77 pounds in only 3 months and 133 pounds over a year by taking daily ice baths. He reports that as a result of his Iceman-like activities, he dramatically increased his metabolic rate, balanced his thyroid, hypothalamus and regulated his entire endocrine system. His leptin (hunger satiation hormone) and insulin resistance also resolved, thereby ending persistent hunger and food cravings that contributed to his overeating and obesity. The front end—or First 15%—of Dr. Kruse's protocol takes a cool cue from Paul Newman: it begins with acclimating just your face to ice water, which triggers the diving reflex and resets your body's homeostatic set points. It gradually advances to putting ice packs on your body and finally to immersing yourself in an ice bath for up to an hour. Cold thermogenesis is a dramatic treatment that produces dramatic results, yet it's not for everyone. For those with cryophobia (fear of cold, not fear of crying), there are more gradual low-intensity methods for achieving similar yet less dramatic results over a longer period of time. See Ch 10 Rx's for additional Cold + Hot Therapy practices to access extra life-boosting/extending NSN, via what Iceman Wim Hof calls the Noble Force of deep cold.

The Time Of Our Lives

Kay Gardner (1941–2002) was a world-renowned musician, composer and author, who had an insightful view into the stages of life that interestingly correlate with numbers from the Fibonacci Sequence. The Fibonacci numbers in the standard Fibonacci Stages of Life chart delineate the stages of life as would be expected with a standard lifespan up to 89 years. However, since the human lifespan has increased over the millennia and quite dramatically in the last 100 years, we can project an expansion in the Standard Fibonacci Stages of Life to the next higher numerical range in the Fibonacci Sequence, 89-144. Imagine an ever-expanding Nautilus shell and you'll see that there's always another arm of the spiral to move to. Applying this to the standard Fibonacci Stages of

Standard Fibonacci Life Stages		Expanded Fibonacci Life Stages	
Childhood	8	Childhood	8
Puberty	13	Puberty	13
Full Sexual Blossoming	21	Full Sexual Blossoming	21
Motherhood/Fatherhood	34	Motherhood/Fatherhood	**21–89**
Menopause/Andropause	55	Menopause/Andropause	**89–144**
Elderhood	89	Golden Ratio Elderhood	**144+**

10

Life, we see that the end of the lifecycle wouldn't be at 89 years, it would expand to the next Fibonacci number, 144+. Likewise, Motherhood/Fatherhood could have a range of 21-89 years and Menopause/Andropause a range of 89-144. This seemingly dramatic increase in lifespan may be something of a stretch to contemplate at first. Yet with the rapid advances in nutrition, mind and brain enhancement, medical technology and the applied art and science of NSN it's entirely possible, even if it requires an upgrade to an elevated level of consciousness.

Aubrey de Grey, Ph.D.: Living Well to Fibonacci Ages 89–144–233...

Just as landing on the moon or running a sub four-minute mile were once "impossibilities," extending human lifespan well beyond current accepted limits is one of mankind's new frontiers. Considering that human lifespan has been on an upward curve over time, especially in the last few centuries, it's not unreasonable to expect that we could see healthy triple-digit birthdays becoming the norm in the not-so-distant future. **Imagine turning a healthy 162!**

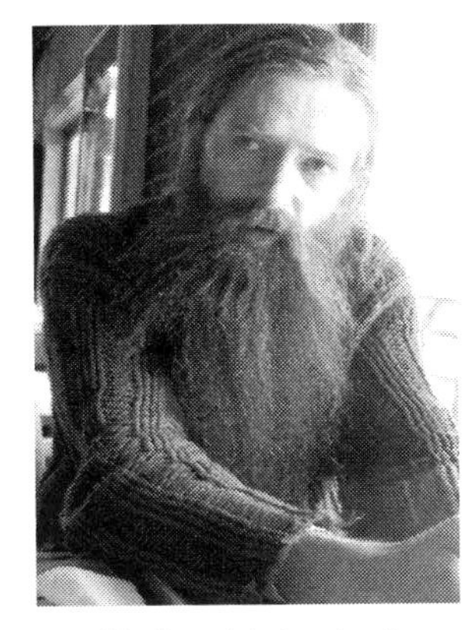

Methuselah-inspired maverick English longevity researcher, Aubrey de Grey, Ph.D.

Human Life Expectancy at Birth Over the Centuries

Year	Age
2000 BC	18
500 AD	22
1400	33
1790	36
1850	41
1900	50
1946	67
1991	76
2009	80 Women (USA)
	75 Men (USA)
	32 (Swaziland, Africa)

Maverick English researcher Aubrey de Grey is one of many pioneers pushing this longevity frontier forward. De Grey challenges us to expand our paradigm of possibility into the radical notion that *aging is optional*—and may instead actually be a culturally accepted disease. Called "The Prophet of Immortality" by *Popular Science* magazine, de Grey is a gerontology theoretician and co-author of *Ending Aging*. He works on the development of Strategies for Engineered Negligible Senescence (SENS), a tissue-repair strategy for human rejuvenation, prevention of age-related decline and extended lifespan. To this end, De Grey identified seven types of molecular and cellular damage caused by metabolic processes. SENS is a therapeutic protocol to repair '*the set of accumulated side effects from metabolism that eventually kills us.*'

> *True health is an ageless, painless, tireless body.*
>
> **Paul Bragg, health pioneer**

Through regenerative medicine negating the deleterious effects of metabolism and a challenge to the "global pro-aging trance," de Grey champions research to reach "lifespan escape velocity." He submits there is a serious gap in understanding between scientists and biologists studying aging and those studying regenerative medicine. Through the application of leading-edge approaches like the Nature's Secret Nutrient system, SENS and others, the celebration of triple-digit birthdays may well become as common as running a sub-four minute mile is today.

Longevity Legends: Biblical Myths... or Actual Reality?

Peppered throughout the Bible are dozens of examples of longevity superheroes, pointing to the possibility of "extreme" longevity. They are grouped here into their respective "Generation Phi" categories by sequential Fibonacci Sequence number divisions. Methuselah is the Bible's archetypal elder... Enoch's son, Lamech's father and Noah's grandfather. Maybe longevity researcher Aubrey de Grey's supposition that *aging is optional* has some basis in the historical record (de Grey's longevity prize, with an award amount over $1 million dollars, is named the Methuselah Prize). Visionary *Star Trek* creator Gene Roddenberry referenced Methuselah in the *Star Trek* episode *Requiem for Methuselah*, which first aired in 1969. Most ironically, the last three digits of that year match Methuselah's reported life years reached: 969. The episode's main character, Flint, shared this provocative pearl of longevity wisdom:

Death, when unnecessary, is a tragic thing.

Biblical/Generation Φ Longevity Legends, Grouped by Adjacent Fibonacci Numbers

Ages 89–144		144–233		377–610	
Joseph	110	Jacob	147	Salah	433
Joshua	110	**Abraham**	**175**	Eber	464
Rebecca	120	Isaac	180	Shem	600
Moses	**120**	Terah	205		
Aaron	123	**Job**	**210**	**610–987**	
Miriam	125	Serug	230	**Lamech**	**777**
Sarah	127			Mahalalel	895
Deborah	130	**233–377**		Enos	905
Kohath	133	Reu	239	Adam	930
Ishmael	137	**Enoch**	**365**	**Noah**	**950**
Levi	137			**Methuselah**	**969**

10

Generation PHI Φ

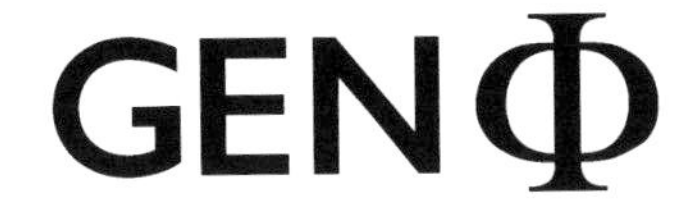

In the next several decades we may well see the emergence of generations of people with the ability to healthfully access their higher Golden (Ratio) Years—89 to 144 and beyond—**Generation PHI Φ**. In addition to the many personal implications of living longer, there will be profound social, political, environmental, global and extraterrestrial implications of extending our lifespan into the next, higher Fibonacci Spiral of life. The current near-universally accepted paradigm is that aging is an inevitable, downward spiral to eventual death. In contrast to that rather depressing prognostication is a more optimistic paradigm-stretching option: perhaps one day soon we will be able to fully access Nature's Secret Nutrient in all areas of life and dwell within our 19-31 Golden Prime Zone years in perfect health, for as long as desired, until our Earthly mission feels complete. This upgraded paradigm is echoed by longevity researcher Aubrey de Grey:

> *I think we're in striking distance of keeping people so healthy that at 90 they'll carry on waking up in the same physical state as they were at age 30 [Golden Prime Zone], and their probability of not waking up one morning will be no higher than it was at 30.*

> *Consider growing younger—instead of growing older.*
>
> **Jeff Goldblum, actor**

Never has there been a greater opportunity to live well past longevity "norms" into realms stretching beyond present imagination. In this vibrant spirit we wish for you a level of youthful agelessness that echoes the immortal words of Buzz Lightyear:

To Infinity... and Beyond!

Robert D. Friedman, M.D. & Matthew K. Cross

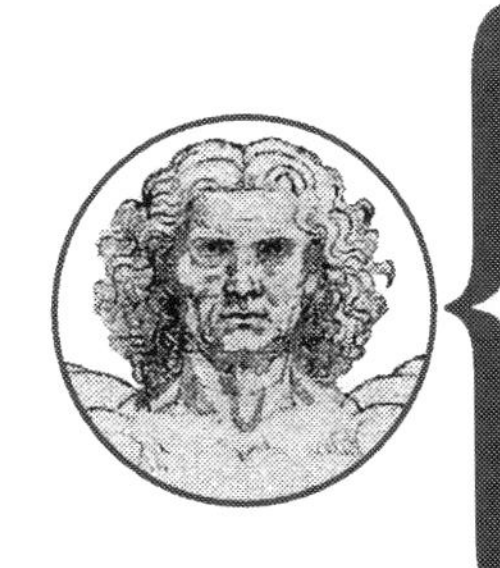

Remember, you're only as ***YOUTHFUL*** *as you feel.* So if you don't feel as vibrant as you did in your Golden Ratio Prime Zone (ages 19-31), revisit & reignite the energy of those years via the Golden Prime Zone Age-Reversing Holodeck Rx. When used with the other NSN Rx's in this book, you can reactivate your internal Fountain of Youth and kickstart the hormonal cascade to regenerate & rejuvenate your mind, body, spirit, and life!

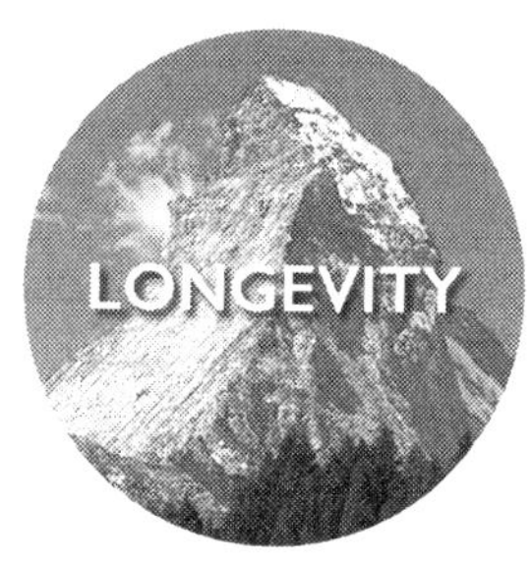

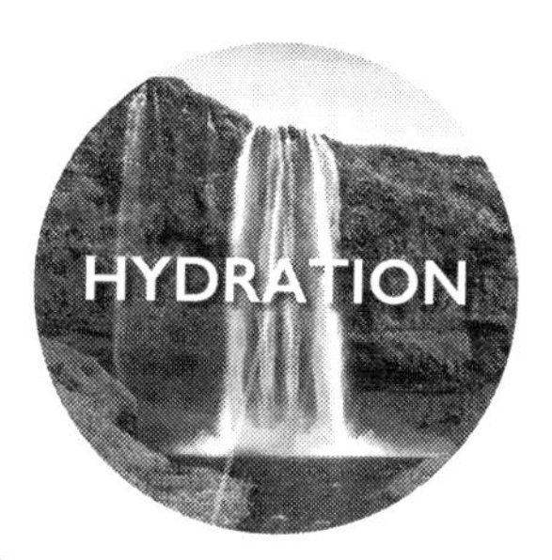

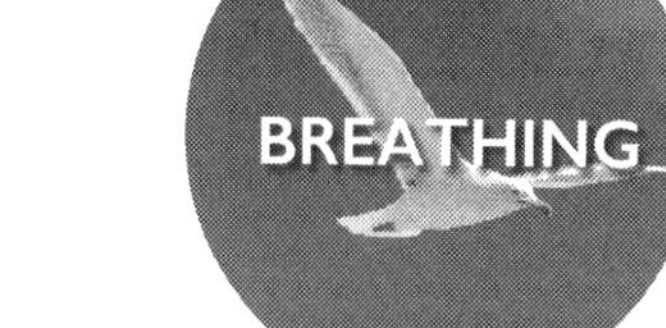

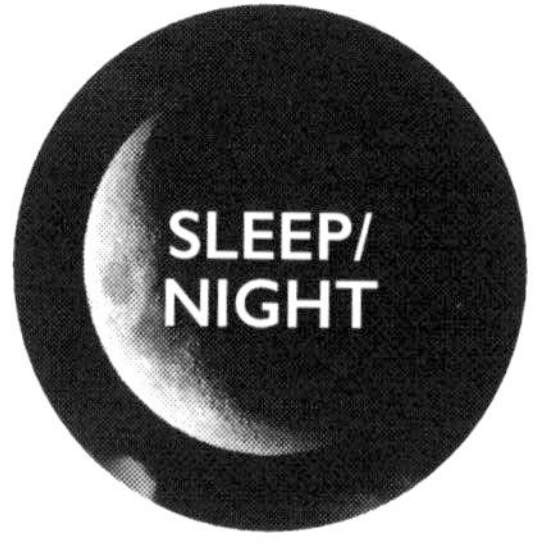

BEAUTY/
RELATIONSHIPS

Nature's
Secret Nutrient/
NSN Action
Rx's

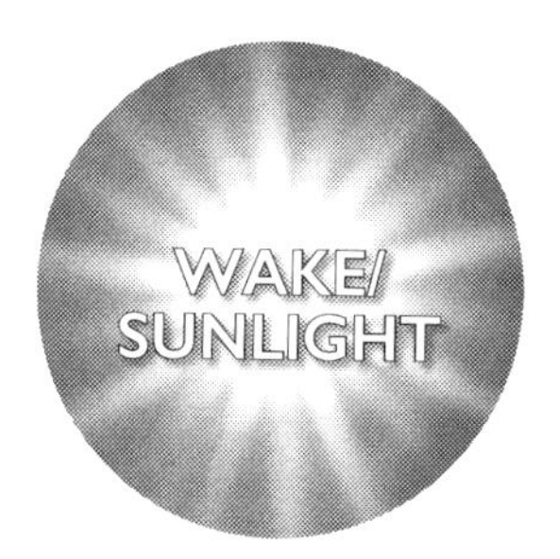

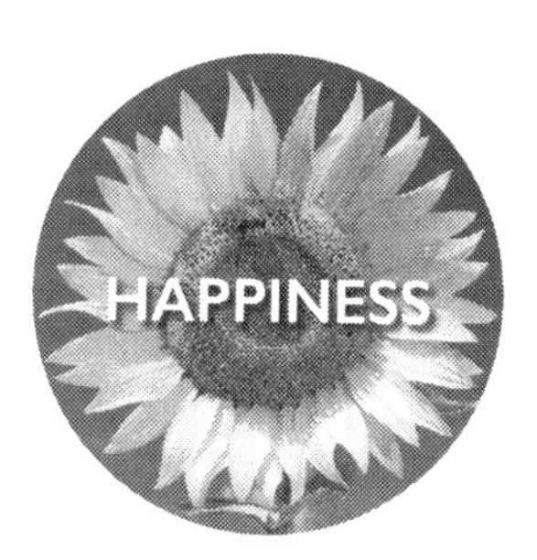

NUTRITION

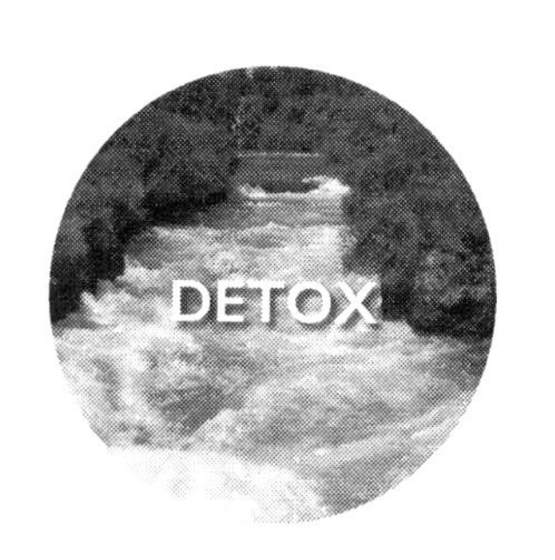

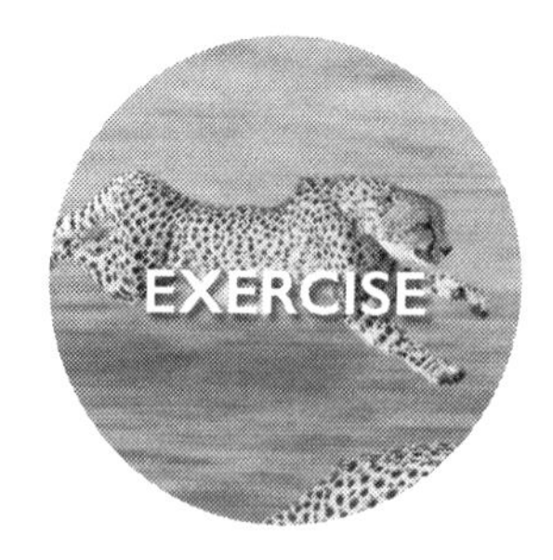

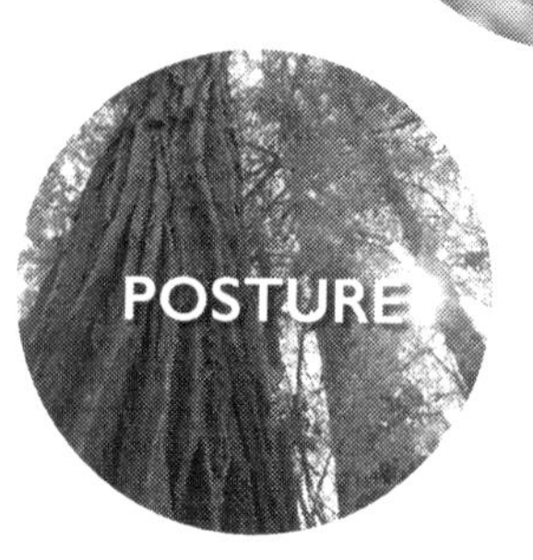

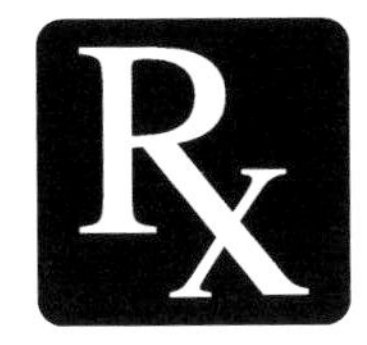

Section II: NSN Action Rx's

We call the simple practices in the section ahead, which activate and sustain Nature's Secret Nutrient, **Action Rx's**. They are easy "Prescriptions" that help you extract and enhance NSN, whether from the air you breathe, the food and water you consume, your exercise routine, your posture, a good night's sleep, etc. **Most are simple Golden Ratio adjustments to what you're already doing every day in your life. Essentially, NSN Action Rx's are actions designed to move the ratios within each of your primary nutrient sources into the more optimal Golden Ratio zone.** You only need to select a few Action Rx's to start.

For example, in Ch 1 Breathing, Rx #1 is an easy NSN breathing technique where you inhale to a count of 3; exhale to a count of 5. This ratio of using the Fibonacci numbers 3 and 5 results in a Golden Ratio of inhalation to exhalation. Your total physiology is thus gently led into Golden Ratio synergy and function via this one simple yet powerful practice. **All NSN Action Rx's revolve around this one Principle:** By aligning with **Nature's Biomimicry Code**—the Golden Ratio—you'll extract maximum NSN from your daily lifestyle practices, e.g., breathing, sleeping, eating, exercising, etc. It's like lining up the right numbers on the combination lock to the vault of vibrant health, happiness and performance. With NSN at your side, the vault door opens wide.

To see how quickly you can begin to enjoy the benefits of Nature's Secret Nutrient/NSN in each of the key health, performance & longevity drivers, look for this Stopwatch in the Rx's in the 10 Rx sections ahead.

To successfully access Golden Ratio Biomimicry, remember this easy 3-A sequence:

1. **FOUNDATION**: Open your eyes to the Golden Ratio's ubiquitous presence in Nature all around you, including in your own body and life. Consider that Nature has already solved virtually every problem over eons of her evolutionary genius. You need only mirror and realign with Nature—via the magic of Golden Ratio Biomimicry—to receive the best solutions for your health and life. *When solving a design problem look to Nature first,* says Biomimicry pioneer Janine Benyus.

2. **ACTION**: Use the NSN Rx's to begin integrating Golden Ratio Biomimicry principles into your daily lifestyle habits, via the Priority Coach tracking system.

3. **RESULTS**: Celebrate and deepen your embodiment of Nature's Golden Ratio Biomimicry Code in your lifestyle and life.

Great news for the mathematically disinclined—you won't need to do *any* calculations to use the Action Rx's. The abundance of Action Rx's that follows allows you to choose from many easy ways to activate NSN in your daily life. Not every Rx will appeal to everyone, nor is every Rx required. For example, some people have an aversion to alcohol, so they can skip the Rx on the benefits of moderate red wine consumption. For others, just the thought of taking cold showers to increase their metabolic rate for enhanced health, weight loss and longevity sends shivers up their spines. No problem—simply skip any Rx that doesn't resonate with you.

This NSN Action Rx section is designed to be a practical handbook with varying degrees of redundancy. This means that you only need choose just a ***vital few*** Rx's to reboot your system and reap NSN's benefits. We know from the 80/20 Pareto principle that 80% of the effects usually come from just 20% of the causes. So, if you were to select 10 Rx's to work with, it's likely that most of the health promoting effects will come from the vital few—in this case the vital 2 or 3—of your chosen Rx's.

The Vital Few principle is amplified by the fact that we used the Hoshin GPS™ method to prioritize which of the Rx's have the most wide-ranging influence on health, peak performance and longevity. Each of the 10 Rx sections that follow are organized with the most foundational, impactful Rx's at each section's start. Everyone has their own unique biochemical and environmental makeup, so the relative importance of the Rx's will naturally be different for each person. For best results you'll want to select the Rx's that can be the best catalysts for your own health and lifestyle upgrades. **Or you can simply start with our suggested top-10 Rx selections if you like,**

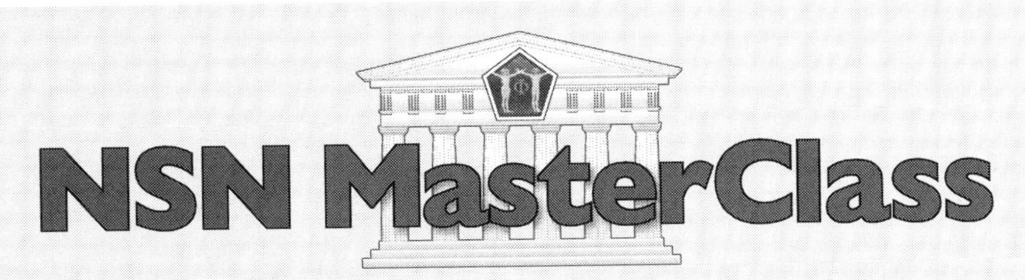

NSN MasterClass is the interactive online course with the authors, Robert D. Friedman, M.D. and Matthew K. Cross. NSN MasterClass fast-tracks your learning and integration of the NSN Action Rx's and brings the complete Nature's Secret Nutrient system to life for maximum benefits and momentum. *See p. 484.*

which are pre-filled in as a fast-start Priority Coach option on page 452. One caveat: You usually won't initially know which of your selected Rx's are the most impactful until you've test driven them for a few weeks. That's why it's important to assume the role of Doctor, as well as patient, while you're learning to integrate NSN principles into your daily routine. The daily tracking and feedback from the Priority Coach system greatly enhances your learning in support of fine-tuning and progress. With an ample selection of NSN Rx's to choose from, you can change them up as desired on a trial-and-error basis. So have some fun selecting the 5-10 Rx's that will open the vault to the vital health and healing power of Nature's Secret Nutrient.

Little-known Fun Fact: *Leonardo Fibonacci originated the ℞ symbol, which he used for square roots; it later became the standard global symbol for prescription writing.*

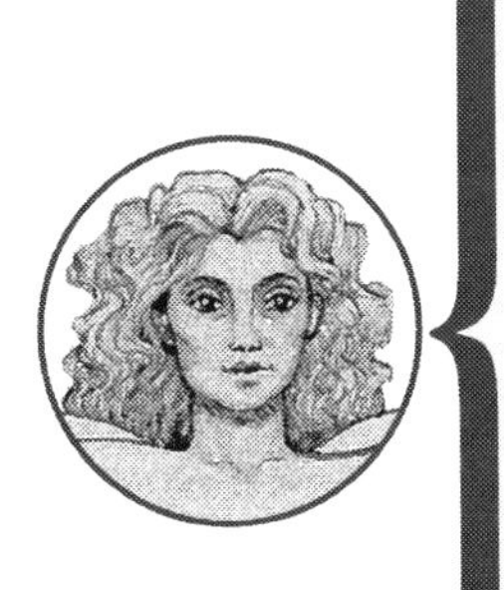

Remember, your ***RESULTS*** *are only as impressive as your daily practice & follow-through on what you've learned.*
So select the NSN Action Rx's that most align with your goals; then monitor your progress with the Priority Coach system. Go easy if you have periodic slips or think you're losing ground, as the Golden Ratio works in a 5 steps forward : 3 steps back catapult manner.
And as Irish playwright **Samuel Beckett** eloquently stated:
Ever Tried. Ever Failed. No Matter.
Try Again. Fail Again. Fail Better.

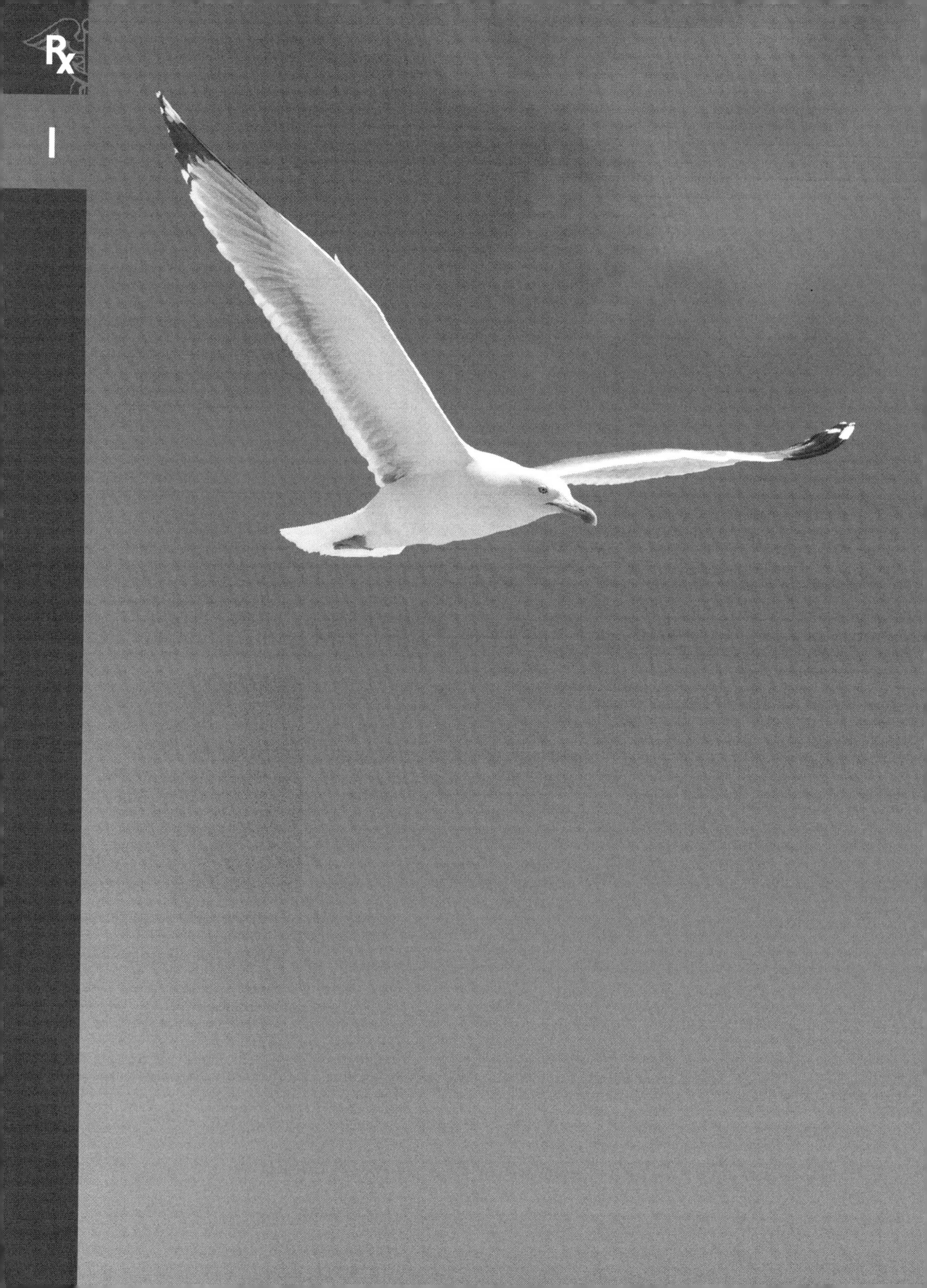
Rx
I

I

Breathing Rx's

Add one or more of the following Rx's to your NSN daily health regimen.

1 Breathing Out of the Box: Golden Ratio Breathing

Time To BeneFIT 3 Seconds

Since we know that deeper, more efficient breathing is the #1 factor that can improve your immediate and long-term health and increase your longevity, it's imperative that the biomechanics of your breathing be correct. A key vertical Golden Ratio division point of the body is at the navel level; internally this is at the same general level where the tendons of the muscular diaphragm attach to anterior longitudinal ligaments of the spine. Due to these anatomical relationships, every breath actually originates as a subtle yet strong reminder of the Golden Ratio's critical design role in your body.

When we tune any aspect of our MegaNutrient intake to the Golden Ratio we generate Natures Secret Nutrient in our body. Golden Ratio Breathing is the fastest and easiest way to activate Nature's Intelligence (NI). Many breathing techniques utilize *Box Breathing*, i.e., equal duration of inhalation to exhalation, e.g. 5 seconds inhalation to 5 seconds exhalation. Box Breathing □ assuredly leads to unimaginative Box Thinking. The only way to *Think Out of the Box* is to *Breathe Out of the Box*—and the only way to

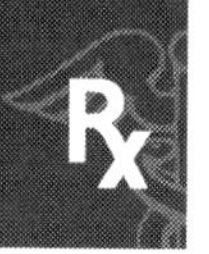

Breathe Out of the Box is by adjusting inhalation and exhalation to the Golden Ratio. As an example, breathe in for 3 seconds and out for 5 (as your breath capacity increases you can try 5/8, 8/13, 13/21...). This simple yet ingenious breath adjustment generates a synchrony and dynamism that pervades your entire body/mind & spirit. The Golden Ratio is instantly recognized by your body's intelligence as Nature's Intelligence (NI). The process of cellular reorganization and regeneration aligned with the Golden Ratio begins immediately. In addition to physical invigoration, noticeable improvements in mood, out-of-the-box clear thinking, improved creativity, peace, equanimity and joy follow.

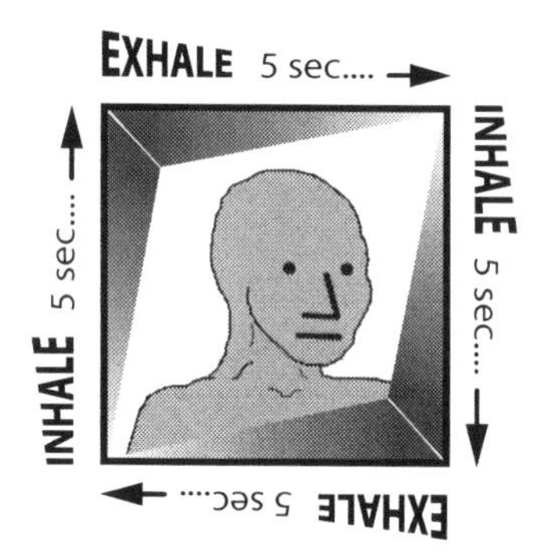

Box Breathing
In-The-Box | Sub-optimal Breathing

In and Out breaths equal, but duration optional. Equal length pauses optional. Box breathing is non-dynamic and can't generate NSN.

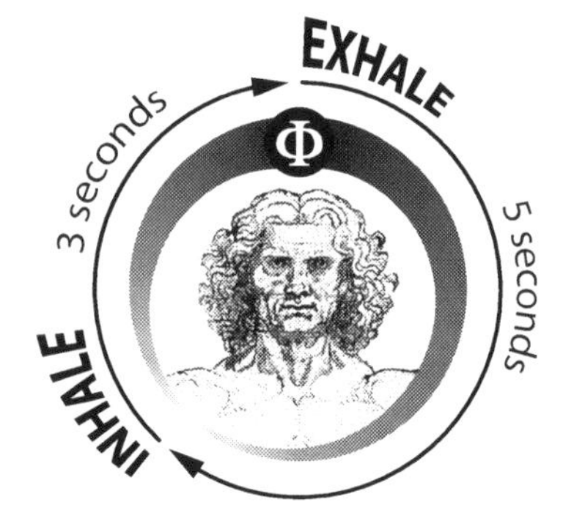

Golden Ratio Breathing
Out-Of-The-Box | Super-optimal Breathing

Circular breaths tuned to the Golden Ratios (3/5, 5/8, 8/13). Use Fibonacci numbers (3, 5, 8...) for optional pauses. *Golden Ratio Breathing is dynamic and is the only way to generate NSN.*

2 The Art and Science of the Full Buddha Breath

Let's relearn the basics of full, deep breathing. Many people breathe with low/no awareness and have fallen out of healthy breathing habits. The following full breath cycle restores healthy breathing. Try practicing this breath throughout your day. Every breath is fact a never-ending, continuous, flowing movement— a recharging of life-enhancing energy.

This example of a healthy full breath is broken into four basic parts: a two-stage inhalation, followed by a two-stage exhalation, with pauses inserted as desired. Breathing through your nose is recommended, as it activates and synergizes your brain, body and mind.

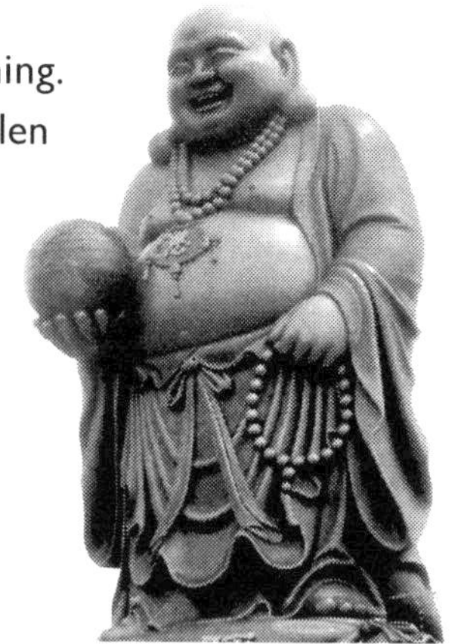

Buddha, demonstrating how his belly moves out during the first phase of a full inhalation.

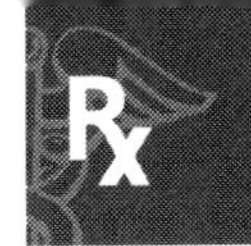

The breath begins with:

1. A relaxed, full Buddha-belly inhalation, into…
2. A full chest inhalation that gently lifts your chest, shoulders and head. When you've inhaled just the right amount of air, you will feel a sense of satisfaction and relaxation moving through your whole body. You might choose to linger and enjoy this for a moment, before cresting the breath wave and…
3. Letting your breath go completely, through your nose, allowing your lungs' naturally loaded elasticity to effortlessly contract and exhale, leading into…
4. Reverse Buddha-belly, by pulling your navel towards your spine to complete the full exhalation. When your lungs feel empty, your belly naturally relaxes and returns to a neutral position, pausing as desired, naturally flowing into…
5. Your next breath, starting over at #1 above.

Many people have a contrary or paradoxical respiratory motion, where the movement of the diaphragm is reversed. By placing your hand over your navel and assuring its outward, expansive movement (Buddha-belly) as you breathe in and its inward movement (reverse Buddha-belly) as you breathe out, you will know that your respiratory efficiency is being optimized. To regularly recharge your system, it's a good idea to take a series of deep, Golden Ratio Breaths at least hourly. This breath is also an excellent compliment to all meditation, mindfulness and movement practices.

3 Practice Golden Ratio Lung Yoga

Golden Ratio Lung Yoga stretches and strengthens your breathing capacity with deeper inhalations and exhalations. On the lung volume graph below, note the dotted lines extended over the top line and below the bottom line of the example Vital Capacity curve. You can expand your Vital Capacity (VC), thereby increasing your health and longevity, by including this easy practice in your normal breathing several times a day.

- Φ Take 3 small extra sips of air at the end of a full inbreath, through your nose. This extra small volume of air gently stretches your lungs and chest cavity and expands lung capacity over time.
- Φ Exhale 3 extra puffs at the end of a full exhalation, through your nose. These tiny extra expiratory efforts strengthen your chest and diaphragmatic muscles, enabling them to get rid of stale air at the end of each breath.

You can increase your respiratory efficiency, stretch and strengthen your respiratory muscles, regain lost Vital Capacity and increase your vitality, performance and longevity by doing this several times a day. Increased Vital Capacity shifts you towards the left on the Longevity & Breath graph below; by regaining as little as 250-500 ml. of lung volume (1-2 cups), you may enjoy a reduction in physiologic age of as much as 5-10 years.

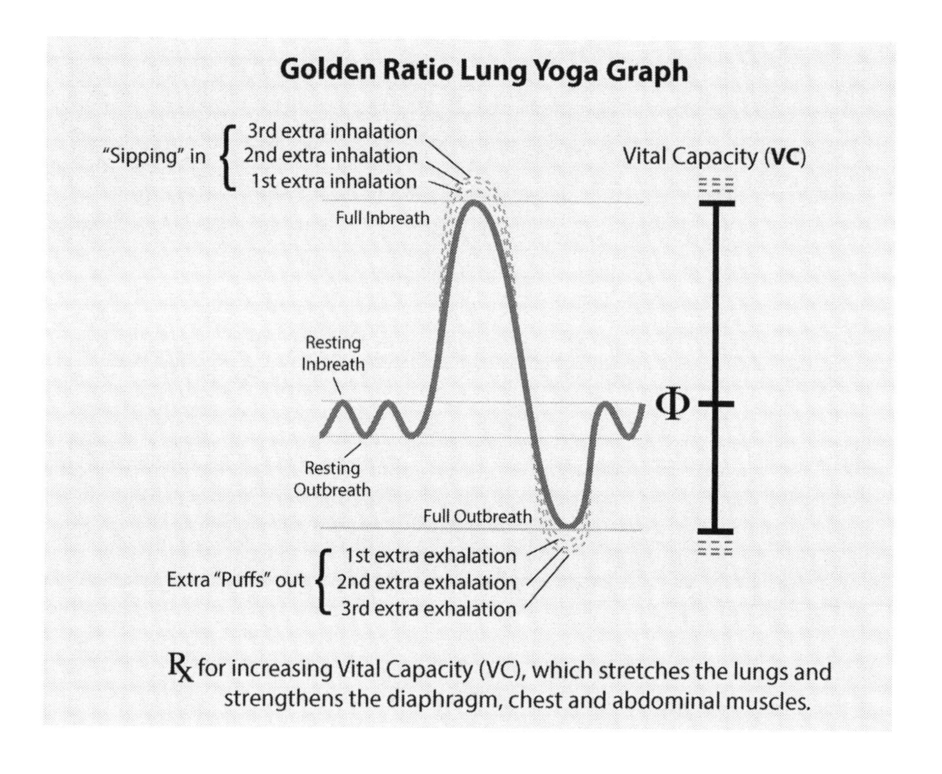

℞ for increasing Vital Capacity (VC), which stretches the lungs and strengthens the diaphragm, chest and abdominal muscles.

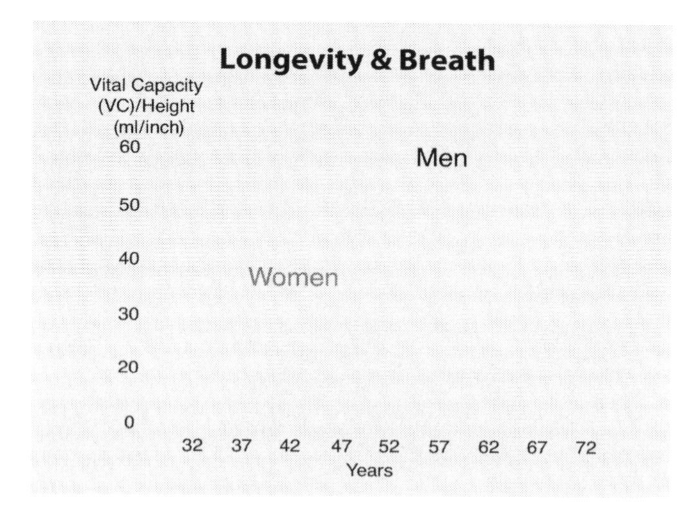

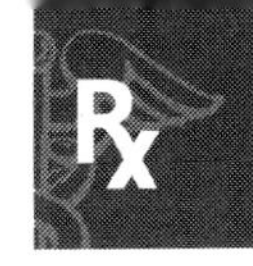

All You Need Is The Air You Breathe: Upgrade Your Air *Quality*

The quality of the air you breathe contains a powerful yet invisible ingredient with a visible and profound impact on your health. There are two critical elements which must be considered regarding the quality of the air in every breath. First is the purity of the air and absence of pollution. Second is the air's vibrance or élan vital, rarely considered yet crucial for optimal health and state of mind. **A strong component of air's vitality is a healthy, natural balance of negative and positive ions—micro particles carrying either a negative or positive charge, aka VITA—*Vitamins In the Air.*** The optimum ion content and balance is found in natural settings with an abundance of pure air, water and often wind—at the ocean, near lakes, waterfalls, forests and mountains. It's no accident that we visit such places in Nature for REcreation on the weekends and during holidays and vacations. The ion balance/life charge of the air we breathe is tuned by Nature in pristine settings, where air pollution is very low or virtually nonexistent. Yet such places on the planet are increasingly rare and shrinking, due to mankind's relentless technological progress-at-any-cost mind-set.

In cities, ion concentration is severely reduced as the ions precipitate out particulates and various toxins in polluted city air. This loss of natural ionic charge and invisible life force energy is the norm in both outdoor and indoor city air, where artificial, hermetically sealed indoor environments are contaminated with toxic off-gases produced by synthetic carpet, paints and indoor building materials, not to mention heating and cooling systems.

Here are three air enhancement and purification Rx's you can use to improve the quality of The Air You Breathe as well as overall Breathing—NSN's #1 health driver:

- Φ **Bring Nature Inside**: Some easy ways that can help purify your indoor air and restore the natural ion balance include: • Open a window if not hermetically sealed. • Escape outside regularly to breathe fresh air, even if for a short walk. • Plants. • Mini fountains or waterfalls. • Himalayan pink salt lamps. • Ozone air purifier—ozone is one of Nature's top air purifiers and disinfectants; run it when you're away from your space for a few hours; upon return, open windows or run ventilation system to air out space; best not to breathe ozone directly.
- Φ **Location is Everything:** How's the outside air quality where you presently live? If unhealthy, seriously consider moving to a cleaner environmental location. Aim to spend more time in Nature in a healthier air quality environment, since Breathing is NSN's #1 health and longevity driver. To support your body's powerful natural air purification and air vitalizing systems, follow the other key Rx's

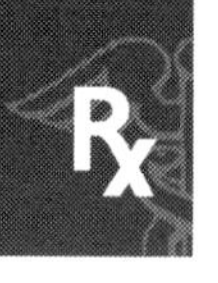

in this book, especially those in Ch 7 Detox, e.g., cold water therapy, epsom salt bath soaks and Triangulation Detox, which includes regular therapeutic sweating.

Φ **Take a Pure Air Respiration Inspiration Vacation** by visiting one of the rare places on earth with pristine air. Ten such remaining places on earth were profiled in the excellent *Travel & Leisure* article, *World's Cleanest Air*, by Adam McCulloch. They include: Tasmania, Hawaii's Big Island (upwind from the Vog/Volcano Smog), Iceland, South Africa's Cape Peninsula, Tahiti, Samoa, Antarctica, Easter Island, Argentina's Patagonia Lakes region and New Zealand's South Island. *Ahhhhhhhh.....*

In addition to the above recommendations, **begin upgrading the unconscious habit of shallow, auto-pilot breathing to breathing deeper, with conscious gratitude for every breath.** By integrating easy Fibonacci Breathing techniques, e.g., inhaling to the count of 3 and exhaling to the count of 5—you further enhance the impact the Vital Force of Air has on your total health, performance and longevity. Remember the sage words of yogi and healthy lifestyle master **Gurumarka Khalsa**: *Breath Is Life!*

5 Golden Ratio Breathwalk

As you walk, try synchronizing your steps and breaths with numbers from the Fibonacci Sequence: 1, 2, 3, 5, 8... For example: two steps forward equals one full inbreath—the next three steps, one full outbreath, for a 2:3 ratio. Try experimenting with longer inhale-to-exhale ratios, like 3:5 (three steps forward equals one full inbreath, the next five steps equal one full outbreath) or even 5:8 as your lung capacity grows. The ratio may change from moment to moment, depending on your oxygen and carbon dioxide levels. The Golden Ratio breathwalk is an easy way to synchronize breathing with exercise and tap the power of Nature's Secret Nutrient.

6 Breathing With Awareness for Better Awakening, Energy & Calm

Although your breath, like your heartbeat, is an automatic and generally unconscious bodily function, conscious breathing offers an opportunity to enhance this continuous pulse of life. Breathing with awareness is like investing in a compounding health and longevity annuity. It also gently tunes you back into the natural rhythms of life—the wind in the trees, ocean waves and tides. So become more aware of your breath's depth, breadth and quality. It is both the foundation of health and longevity and the fastest way to change or upgrade your energy and state of mind and body.

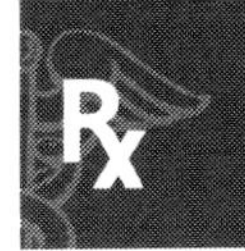

The fastest way to change your neurobiology is through your Breath.
Dr. Phil Nuernberger, author of *The Warrior Sage*

As an added bonus, when you consciously enhance your breath with the Golden Ratio, you instantly access Nature's Secret Nutrient and its health bestowing powers. Following are some easy Breathing With Golden Ratio Awareness exercises to play with. Remember to breathe through your nose and to breathe with full presence and gratitude for each breath.

Φ **AM Breathing Wake Up:** Upon awakening, find a warm, comfortable place to sit with a straight spine. Inhale fully through your nose and into your abdomen to the count of 3; then exhale to the count of 5. Repeat this breathing pattern for 8 cycles. Keep breathing slowly and deeply. As your breathing capacity improves, try inhaling to the count of 5 and exhaling to the count of 8. You might eventually try inhaling to the count of 8 and exhaling to the count of 13. Go only as far as is comfortable for you. Now your blood is super-oxygenated and you're ready for your day. Feel free to add pauses between inhalations and exhalations, as desired.

Φ **Too tired or fatigued? Breathe with Phire for an Energy Supercharge.** This breath combines breaths in Fibonacci Ratio with an ancient yogic technique that uses quick powerful inhalations and exhalations to stoke your inner Phire and revitalize a tired and fatigued body and mind. Here's how:

- Inhale and exhale through your nose 8 times, rapidly, deeply and forcefully; 1 second inhale to 1 second exhale.
- Then, take a slow recovery breath IN—still through your nose— to the count of 3 and OUT to the count of 5. Repeat for 3 breaths.
- Repeat the total cycle 2 more times.

This stimulating breath immediately awakens your nervous system and delivers a strong boost of life-giving Oxygen to your brain and body. Use this breath instead of caffeine anytime you need a quick energy boost.

Φ **Too wound-up, anxious or needing greater calm and focus?** With eyes closed, try tuning your breath to higher sequential Fibonacci numbers, e.g., inhale to 5..... exhale to 8........ or inhale to 8........ exhale to 13............ Keep your breath gentle, strong and steady; inhale peace and calm.....exhale stress and tension. Try this relaxing breath for 8 to 13 repetitions. Observe how you feel.

As with these and all Golden Ratio breathing exercises, play and experiment. **The important thing is to simply start becoming more aware daily of the gift, power and potential of each breath.** Your life will flourish to the degree that you allow your breath to be conscious, full and free. ***To Life!***

7 The Art & Benefits of the Deep Yawn & Stretch

Don't like yoga? While you may never have thought of it this way, the yawn and stretch that many of us do when waking up or during the day when we're tired is the most natural form of yoga stretching (asana) and breathing (pranayama). Yawning is a built-in reflex that automatically resets your oxygen and CO_2 levels and equalizes ear pressure. The accompanying slow, slight resistance stretch also lengthens and tones your muscles, relieves stiffness and increases blood and lymphatic circulation. There's even a word for this built-in yawn and stretch reflex: *Pandiculation*. Pandiculation is a Golden Ratio reset. How? Your system is programmed to re-establish internal balance or homeostasis whenever it goes too far out of balance. Think of pandiculation—a yawn accompanied by a deep, refreshing breath and slow, extended stretch—as a type of primal, restorative yoga. All of the other yoga poses and breathing techniques developed over time are simply more complex variations on the basic yawn and stretch.

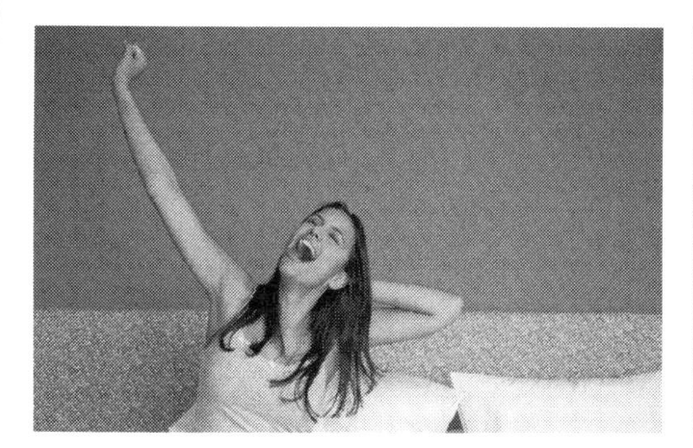

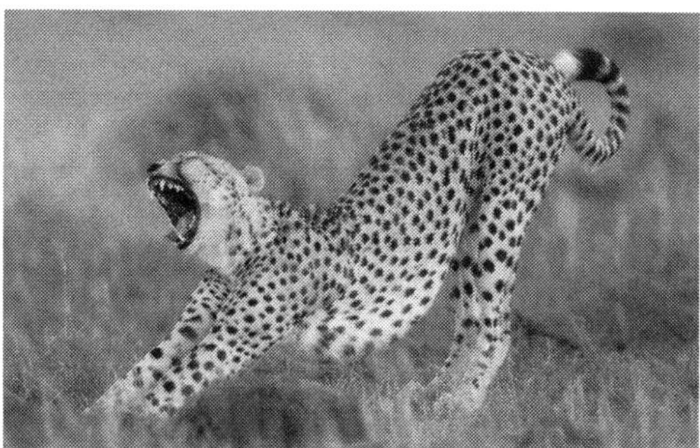

(*L*) The essential yawn and stretch reset, aka *Pandiculation*.
(*R*) Animals are natural pandiculation masters, including this lightning-fast cheetah.

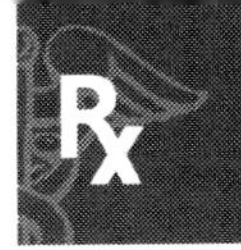

8 Enhanced Breathing Through NSN Resistance Training

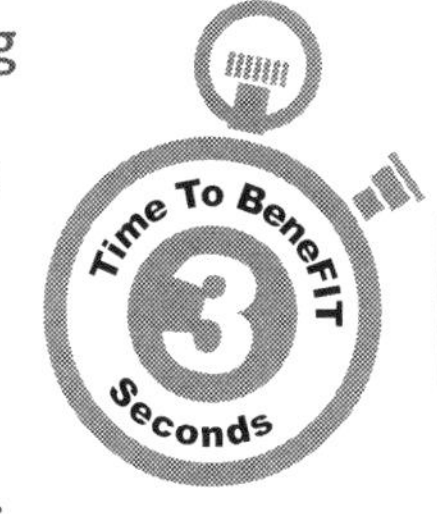

By pursing your lips during in and out breaths you can increase the airway resistance and strengthen your diaphragm and total breathing muscles. Also try this exercise by closing your mouth and gently squeezing your nostrils partially closed with your thumb and finger. This simple practice increases the depth and efficiency of your breath. When paired with Fibonacci breathing ratios, you have a simple and highly effective method to amp up NSN and super-charge your entire system. Try this:

1. Sit or stand with your spine straight.
2. Purse your lips and breathe in deeply to the count of 5.
3. Hold your breath to the count of 3.
4. Exhale through pursed lips to the count of 8.
5. Repeat the above cycle 5 times. After you get the hang of it, increase to 8 or 13 times.

Experiment with the extent of lip pursing or mouth closed/nostril squeezing so you can feel the resistance, yet still breathe fully without getting light-headed. Open your lips more or stop the exercise immediately if you start to feel light-headed. Try this NSN Über-Breath every morning to jump-start your day. It's also great to use before workouts or races to give your system an added boost.

You can also purchase a specially designed breathing resistance device called the Expand-a-Lung Breathing Fitness Trainer, which has an easy-adjust resistance valve. It's used by Navy Seals, divers and athletes to enhance and strengthen lung function and improve O_2 & CO_2 exchange. Those with compromised lung function (asthma & COPD) can also benefit, but due to increased lung pressures involved should consult their physician before using.

Expand-a-Lung adjustable breathing fitness trainer.

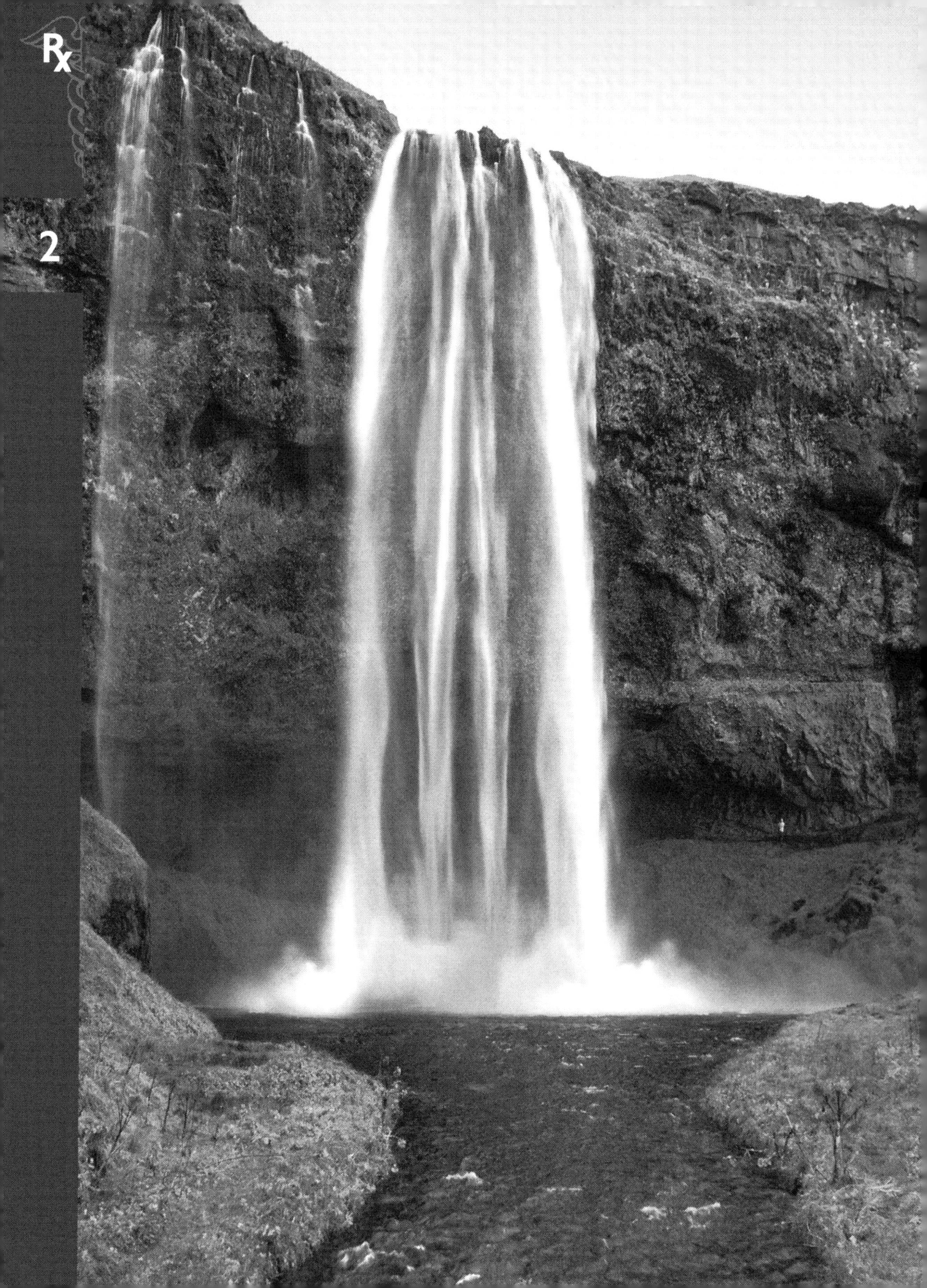
Rx
2

Hydration ℞'s

Pick one or more of the following Rx's to add to your NSN daily health regimen.

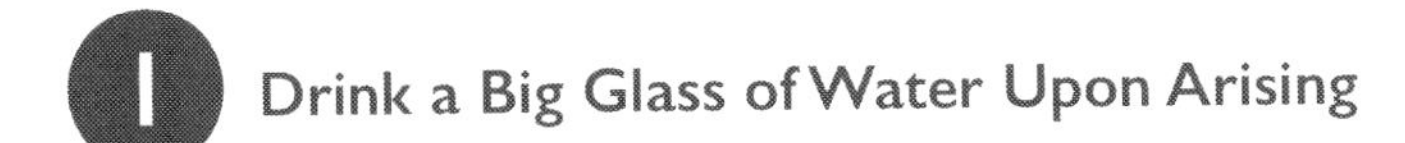

1 Drink a Big Glass of Water Upon Arising

Water is critical for the efficient functioning of your whole system. When you awaken in the morning, all of the toxins produced during sleep and filtered through your kidneys must be eliminated through urination. The fluid lost through urination, plus additional night time fluid lost through breathing and sweating **must be replaced ASAP.**

This is a metabolic priority falling into the First 15% Percent of your body's daily requirements. The best way to facilitate morning fluid replacement is to drink one or two large glasses of pure water within 5 minutes of arising. This simple step at the start of your day will help maintain your body's water percentage near its optimal Golden Ratio level.

2 Color of Chardonnay as Healthy Hydration Gauge

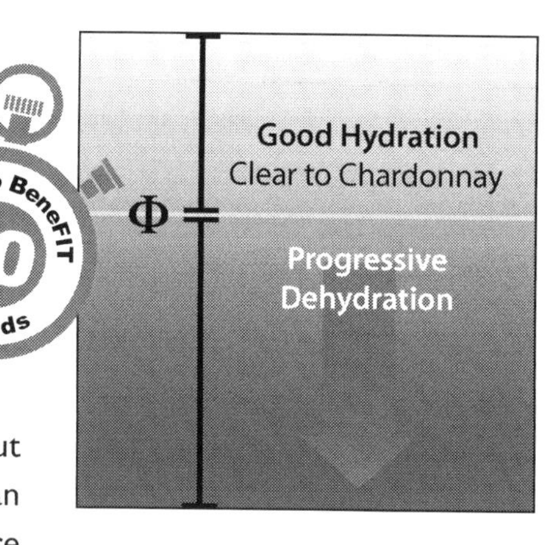

The Golden Ratio Urine Color Chart shows your relative hydration status: Φ and above indicates good hydration; below PHI indicates progressive dehydration. Note: Kidney, bladder or systemic diseases, B-vitamins & some drugs can change urine color & invalidate this test.

It's often recommended to drink a certain number of glasses of water per day to replenish and maintain your hydration. However, it's difficult to tell if you're actually getting enough water without some feedback mechanism. Here's an easy, low-tech way to gauge if you're meeting your body's daily hydration requirements. This method adapts to individual variations such as gender, Body Mass Index (BMI) and activity level. By looking at your body's actual physical signs, you can get customized, real-time feedback on whether you're hydrated or dehydrated. The most logical symptom to look at first is your sense of thirst. Yet you need to understand that your sense of thirst is often blunted and also has a delay from when your body is actually dehydrated to the time you're thirsty. **One of the easiest ways to monitor your hydration is by looking at the color of your urine.** Your kidneys filter your blood, getting rid of toxins and at the same balancing fluid levels, mineral levels and blood pressure. By simply gauging the color of your urine, you can quickly tell if you need to drink more water. The more dehydrated you are, the darker your urine. It can range from clear to various shades of yellow, with deep amber indicating more severe dehydration. Ideally, try to keep your urine in the range of clear to a light **Chardonnay**—pale yellow. If your urine is darker, you need to drink until it clears. **Dark urine is your body's silent cry for water. You may not feel thirsty, yet the darker your urine is, the more water you need to drink.**

> **Note:** *Various substances including drugs, vitamins and certain medical conditions can also cause urine to be various colors—red, bright yellow, orange, green, blue or brown. If you notice any unusual urine color, you need to see your physician for evaluation. Also, if you have any heart, liver or kidney disease or hormonal abnormalities, you should be under the guidance of your physician to monitor your fluid intake, so as not to overload your system.*

3 Upgrade Your Water Quality

It's of course critical that the water you drink be as pure as possible. Short of having access to fresh spring water, the best way to ensure that you have clean water is to either buy filtered water or better yet do it yourself with a home filter. Your filter should remove both man-made and naturally occurring toxins, e.g., chlorine, fluoride, excess minerals, organic toxins, heavy metals including lead, drugs, microbes and radiation. A *triangulation of fire* (a minimum of three different yet complimentary actions) water filter consisting of activated carbon, reverse osmosis and ion exchange is an excellent choice; another solid option is a top-rated water pitcher filter such as the Zero Water 5-stage filter system. Dispose of used filters as per your local health department.

Note: Glass or stainless steel bottles are recommended to avoid hormonally disrupting plastic toxins like phthalates and BPA. While plastic is never recommended for water or food storage, *safer* plastics have the recycling numbers 1, 2, 4 & 5 on the bottom within a triangle; unsafe numbers are 3 & 6. More sophisticated water purification systems include distillation, UV, ozonation, oxygenation, alkalinization and water structuring properties.

Φ Freshen Your Water with Lemon Juice

Lemon juice has high concentrations of both citric acid and vitamin C. These tart substances will revive any flat tasting water in seconds. Added benefits of lemon water are its cleansing and detoxification effects—a flush for your kidneys and a peristaltic activation for your intestines.

Φ Yogi Pure Water

A quick way to oxygenate your water is by using an ancient yogic technique. Get two glasses, one full and one empty. Pour water from one glass to the other 5, 8 or 13 times to oxygenate the water. As you pour the water from one glass to the other, gradually increase the distance between the glasses. Drink the water immediately while the oxygen is still in solution. For an added energetic boost, do the pouring in direct sunlight.

Φ Optimize Water Absorption with Salt

A simple way to enhance the absorption and assimilation of your drinking water is to add a small pinch of sea salt or Himalayan pink salt to an 8 oz. glass of water. This optimizes the water for quicker absorption and assimilation (not recommended for those who need to restrict sodium intake).

4 Drink Fresh LIVE Juice, Nature's Perfect Water

One of the best ways to get the ultimate in purified water is to drink fresh, *unpasteurized* vegetable juices (even "gently pasteurized" kills all of the enzymes and vital live factors present in truly fresh juice). Nature has already ultra-purified and supercharged the water in vegetables. As they grow, they slowly draw water, molecule by molecule, from the earth up their stalks, into the leaves and finally into the vegetables. This water is among the purest water you can get, yet is often overlooked as a source of purified water. For more information on the remarkable health benefits of juicing see **Jay Kordich's** *The Juiceman's Power of Juicing: Delicious Juice Recipes for Energy, Health, Weight Loss and Relief from Scores of Common Ailments* and **Joe Cross**' inspiring film and book *Fat, Sick & Nearly Dead.*

When juicing it's best to use predominantly vegetables, as fruit juice has a high glycemic index and thus raises havoc with blood sugar levels. Ideally, rather than juicing your fruit, eat your fruit. This allows the natural fruit fiber to slow down the absorption of the fruit sugar. Low glycemic fruits like blueberries, strawberries and raspberries are more favorable choices as opposed to high glycemic, sweeter fruits like mangoes, bananas, papayas, pineapple and melons. Also, remember that beets and carrots, although vegetables, have a high glycemic index and should be juiced sparingly; the Golden Ratio Glycemic Zone index data on pages 134-6 provides a measure of how quickly blood sugar levels rise after eating a particular type of food.

Fibonacci's Easy Five-to-Three Juice Recipe

Whenever you need a pick-me-up in the mid-afternoon, there's nothing like a fresh vegetable juice to recharge body and mind. The best time of the afternoon to recharge your system is around five to three. 5 to 3 is also the perfect Fibonacci Ratio of greens to roots & fruits to conjure up a delicious fresh and raw delight. It also packs a potent punch Golden Ratio punch, otherwise known as Nature's Secret Nutrient/NSN.

Juice the following and enjoy; remember to always use organic produce for your juice:

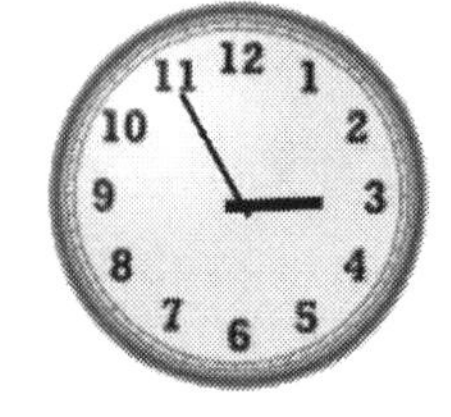

- Φ **5 handfuls of a mix of: Romaine Lettuce, Kale (Dino/Lacinato) & Cucumber**
- Φ **3 handfuls of a mix of: Apples, Beets & Carrots**

  An optional ginger slice adds a healthy, anti-inflammatory spice. If you're sugar sensitive or are carb reducing, substitute more cucumber in place of apples, beets & carrots.

> *Even if you improve your diet radically and take all the right supplements, while you'll be getting some measure of preventive benefit, you still won't be doing enough to reverse existing damage. Add juicing to the mix, though, and you can actually begin to repair damage. Juicing is the key to reversing the progress of disease.*
>
> **Gary Null, Ph.D., health authority & author of *The Joy of Juicing***

5 Do the Prune/Plum Skin Pinch Test

Time To BeneFIT 10 Seconds

Skin hydration is another way to get information on how hydrated or dehydrated you are. It complements both your degree of thirst and color of your urine as dehydration indicators. There's also a critical time lag between being dehydrated and feeling thirsty. We need as many easy dehydration cues as possible to remind us to drink—including the skin pinch test. Here's how to do it:

Simply pinch the skin on the back of your hand and see how rapidly it returns to its original state. If you're dehydrated it will look more like dough, slowly falling back to normal. This test can be confounded by loss of natural elastin in your skin. Elastin is the natural protein that gives your skin its elasticity, yet is lost with the aging process or skin damage through excess sun exposure. You'll have to figure out if you're dehydrated or have skin damage or both. With a little practice you'll get the hang of it. Use the skin pinch test along with your sense of thirst, the dizziness upon-standing-test and the Chardonnay urine color test to see if you're dehydrated. Remember that rehydrating your entire system may not happen overnight. **You may have to start a new habit of drinking before you're thirsty in order to reconstitute yourself from that dry prune back into a nice, juicy plum!**

6 Enjoy Alcoholic Beverages Without Dehydrating Hangovers

Drinking alcohol is an enjoyable experience for many people. Yet one of the banes of alcohol consumption is the dreaded hangover. This nasty side effect can be easily reduced or even eliminated once you understand some basic physiology of alcohol's impact on your brain and body. Alcohol blocks the pituitary's secretion of antidiuretic

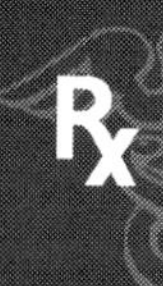

hormone (ADH), resulting in your kidney's inability to retain water as it filters the blood. Hence the frequent urination that accompanies alcohol consumption. Depending on the amount of alcohol consumed, you can lose up to 1 or 2 quarts/liters of water an evening—which exacerbates the fact that alcohol also requires ample water to process it through your body. In addition to causing unpleasant side effects like headaches, fatigue, nausea and malaise, alcohol's extreme dehydrating effect distorts your body's natural ability to maintain a healthy Golden Ratio water balance. If people were cognizant of this one fact, alcohol's after-effects could be easily mitigated.

An easy practice to offset the dehydrating effects of alcohol is to drink 2-3 ounces of water for every ounce of alcohol you're consuming. It's always best to be proactive and ahead of the game when drinking alcohol, so preempt its dehydrating effects by pre-loading your system with one or two glasses of water before you imbibe. During alcohol consumption, always have a *water back* (tall glass or bottle of water on the side). To keep up with the emerging water deficit caused by alcohol, a water back could be something like a liter bottle of Perrier or Pellegrino, with lemons and/or limes on the side. If you follow this simple Rx, you'll be amazed that you don't have a hangover when you awaken the next morning. You will have thoroughly enjoyed the beneficial effects of alcohol without the nasty side effects, and the British bulldog spirit of **Sir Winston Churchill's** witty wisdom will toast you:

I have taken more out of alcohol than alcohol has taken out of me.

 Hydrate When Eating Dehydrated Foods

Dehydrated/dried food has only a fraction of the water volume of the original food. Depending on the amount of dehydrated food you're eating, you could be setting yourself up for a sizeable water deficit. During digestion, a lot more water in the form of digestive juices is needed to process dehydrated, highly concentrated dried foods than if you were to eat the original food in its natural state. Imagine the difference between eating a juicy grape vs. a raisin. Due to extreme water loss, dried fruit is also far higher in sugar/carbs by weight compared to fresh fruit and thus plays havoc with your blood sugar and insulin levels. This principle applies to *all* concentrated foods, including all energy/food bars and drinks. When eating dried food, be sure to consume sufficient additional water to balance out the difference. Pasta lovers are well aware of this; that's why dry pasta is inedible and needs to be reconstituted in boiling water before eating. This will help keep your body fine-tuned hydrodynamically.

2

8 Keep Your Largest Organ Hydrated

When most people think about hydration, they think about drinking enough water to keep *internal* fluid levels in a healthy range. Yet hydration of your largest organ—your skin—is also of vital importance. In addition to keeping it supple and youthful, *external* hydration of your skin strengthens its role as a temperature modulator, a resilient barrier to infections and environmental toxins and especially dehydration. Depending on your environment, moisturizing your skin will have variable importance. If you live in a high-humidity environment, moisturizing is less important, while in a drier or arid environment, skin moisturizing not only maintains the suppleness of your skin, but also prevents significant fluid loss through cutaneous transpiration. Perspiration is noticeable as sweat, while transpiration is the insensible evaporation of water vapor through your skin. It's hard to imagine that a significant amount of water could be lost through the skin, but that's the reason that produce managers put wax on cucumbers and apples. There's nothing less appetizing than seeing a cucumber that's dehydrated and shriveled up. You can easily lengthen your shelf life and avoid the insidious and ongoing process of dehydration with daily skin moisturizing.

Select a quality moisturizer without toxic ingredients, as creams and lotions can be absorbed into your blood to varying degrees. Try simple organic oils in your skin hydration regimen, e.g., almond, olive or coconut. Ideally, your moisturizer should be pure enough to eat—if not, it doesn't belong on your skin, e.g., avoid mineral oil, a toxic petroleum by-product that doesn't belong on or in your body. Many toxic ingredients are easily identified by being multi-syllabic, hard-to-pronounce and/or have CAPITALS or numbers in their names, e.g., PEG-13. Visit the Skin Deep website: www.cosmeticsdatabase.com to evaluate the safety of many cosmetic personal care products or ingredients. Proper skin hydration is basic common sense, yet is often not common practice. It's no accident that Frenchwoman **Jeanne Calment**, at 122 the world's longest-lived person (thus far), hydrated her skin regularly with pure olive oil. Apply moisturizer as needed morning and evening. Anti-aging authority and dermatologist **Nicholas Perricone, M.D.** confirms the importance of proper hydration for both your skin and your body as a whole, revealing the critical connection between dehydration and inflammation. In Dr. Perricone's view, chronic inflammation is a key factor in cellular aging and disease. **Essentially, proper hydration is also a simple way to reduce premature aging:**

> *Logic tells us that when we have an unwanted fire, we throw water on it to put it out. Therefore it makes perfect sense that water would help quell the cellular inflammation that goes on in our bodies. In fact, this is true.* ***Water will decrease inflammation in the body.***

2

9 Revitalize Your Water with the TC Fibonacci Carafe & Bottle

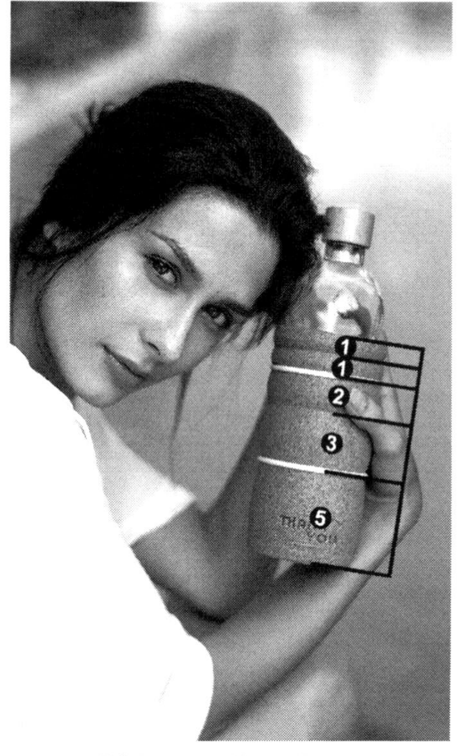

TC Fibonacci Water Bottle,
with removable natural cork sleeve.

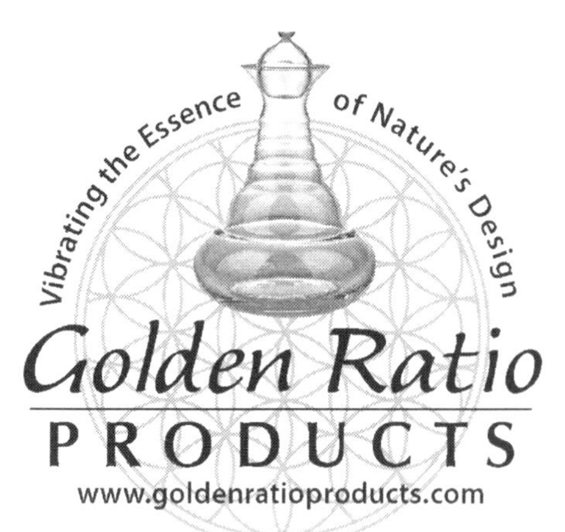

Vibrating the Essence of Nature's Design
Golden Ratio
PRODUCTS
www.goldenratioproducts.com

TC Fibonacci Water Carafes,
available in six sizes.

Through his research on musical form and composition, composer and engineer **Thomas Chochola** (TC) developed a novel approach to design: creating form from sound. Chochola composes on piano and then converts the music into beautiful glassware that reflects musical harmonics. His beautiful glass carafes and water bottles feature multiple Fibonacci Sequence progressions in their elegant designs. Water contained in such vessels assumes the energetic signature of the container, revitalizing the water molecules with a Fibonacci imprint. This process is similar to what happens as water is naturally recharged and invigorated as it rushes down a mountain stream.

It follows that water charged with the Fibonacci imprint contains Nature's grand design and vitality. Chochola effectively developed an easy way for people to bring the revitalizing quality of a mountain stream into drinkable water in their homes. Utilizing the same knowledge as the legendary architects of Europe's great cathedrals, he created powerful glass forms which enhance water's bioenergetic vitality. Visit: www.GoldenRatioProducts.com

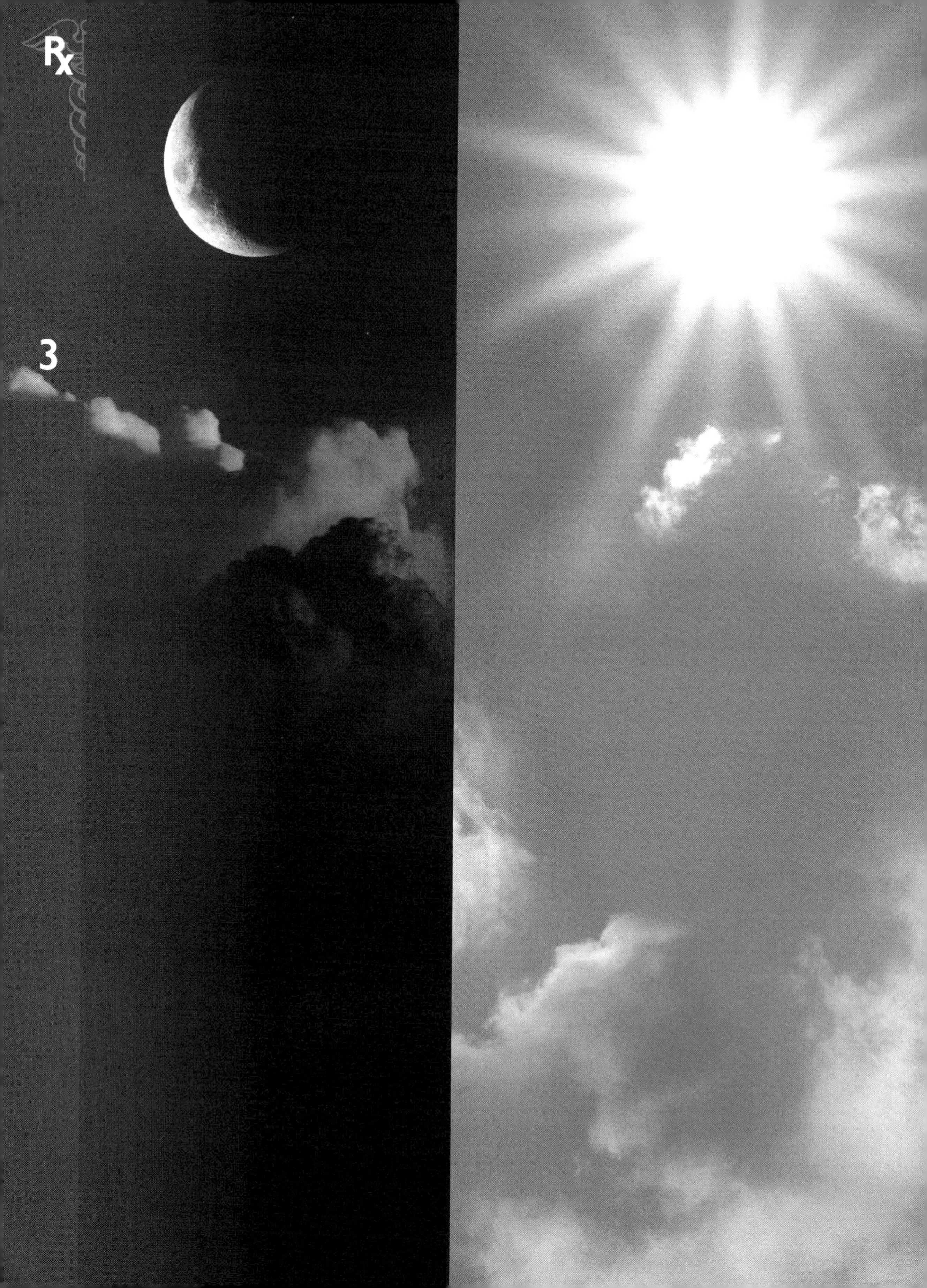
Rx
3

Rx

3

Sleep~Night & Wake~Sunlight Rx's

Pick one or more of the following Rx's to add to your NSN daily health regimen.

The Sleep~Night & Wake Sunlight Rx's are complementary to one another, so make sure you select at least one Rx from each section. Each aspect of sleep that you improve acts as a springboard or opportunity to improve elements of your waking hours. For example, if you get a Golden Ratio amount of quality sleep, your cells will have had an adequate amount of time to regenerate so that they'll be ready to hit the ground running when the sun hits your retinas in the morning. Then, the entire cascade of hormones and neurotransmitters will be optimally functioning and be at your beck and call to optimally support all your daytime endeavors.

Great news for insomnia sufferers: the following Rx's offer simple, effective and drug-free practices to address and ameliorate poor quality and/or quantity sleep. As with all NSN Rx's, the secret is to pick at least *one* from each of the two sections ahead to start with and put them into regular practice. To jump start, enter your selected Rx's into the Priority Coach self-coaching system (p. 449). Then you can step right into the tracking and habit reinforcing phase of the system when you're finished reviewing the NSN Rx's.

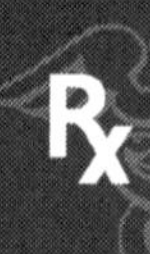

SECTION 1: Sleep~Night Rx's

1 Rejuvenate with Golden Ratio Sleep at least 3–4 Nights out of 7

Since restorative sleep is the #3 NSN driver, it's crucial to keep a Golden Ratio of sleep/rest to waking time, or about 8-9 hours of combined sleep/rest at least 3 to 4 nights per week. Everyone's biology is different, so the Golden Ratio recommendation of 8-9 hours can be taken as a general range, depending on genetic, environmental, differing schedules and other life factors. 8–9 hours of sleep/rest at least 3–4 nights/ week acts as a Golden Ratio "fudge factor," allowing your body to better catch up on any sleep deficits incurred during the week. 3–4 nights/week approximates a 38%–62% Golden Ratio range. If you fall below 3 out of 7 nights/week for any length of time, you are putting yourself at risk of increased physiologic stress, poor physical and mental performance, all leading to potentially disastrous outcomes. Adequate also sleep gives your brain enough time to rebalance neurotransmitters, eliminate brain waste products and consolidate mental and emotional processes from the day. Many people struggle to get enough hours of sleep and the proper ratio of REM to non-REM sleep at night, however they can make up the deficit by adding in an afternoon nap or siesta. Many types of relaxation or chill time can also help to balance out sleep deficits. Remember that the 8-9 hrs. of sleep/rest 3 to 4 nights per week need not be in one continuous block of time, although the majority of it should be. Before the Industrial Revolution, segmented or biphasic sleep was the dominant form of human slumber in Western civilization, so it's not unusual and in keeping with our ancestry to get your sleep and rest in segmented blocks and not all at one time. So... ***Let Golden Slumbers fill your eyes, so that smiles awake you when you rise...*** The Beatles, *Abbey Road.*

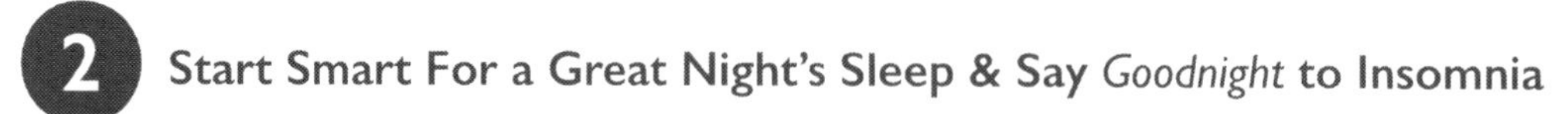

2 Start Smart For a Great Night's Sleep & Say *Goodnight* to Insomnia

To set the stage for the deepest and healthiest sleep, review and begin to incorporate the following easy upgrades into your sleep regimen:

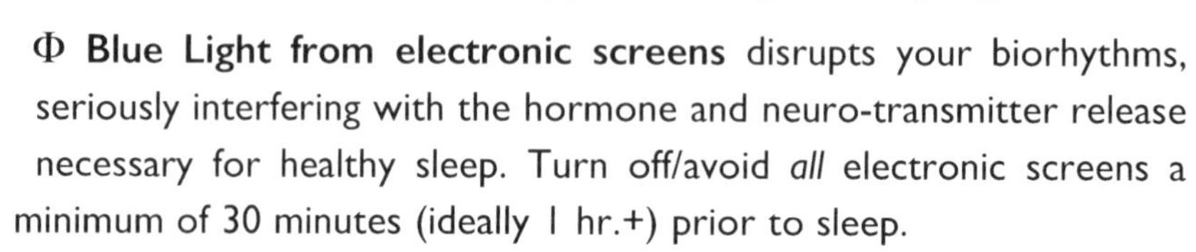

Φ **Blue Light from electronic screens** disrupts your biorhythms, seriously interfering with the hormone and neuro-transmitter release necessary for healthy sleep. Turn off/avoid *all* electronic screens a minimum of 30 minutes (ideally 1 hr.+) prior to sleep.

Φ **Prepare for Sleep with Brief Moon/Star Gazing**. Night sky light frequencies have undefined yet beneficial circadian resynchronization impact on health & sleep.

Φ **Make your Room as Dark as possible,** which signals your brain to begin secreting melatonin (natural sleep hormone). Consider using eyeshades if you can't get your room totally dark. Unplug clock radios and any other light sources, however faint.

Φ **Keep your sleeping room within a 60-65°F temperature range.** Research shows that a cool sleeping environment best supports a healthy drop in core body temperature, which in turn supports both sleepiness *and* deeper sleep.

Φ **Tap the soothing magic of an Epsom salt bath before bedtime.** Deeply relaxes your muscles with a rich dermal dose of magnesium, calming body, mind and soul. Use 2-3+ lbs. Epsom salt in comfortable hot water; add essential oil as desired.

Φ **Turn off the WiFi transmitter in your home just before going to sleep and remove or unplug all electric devices in your sleeping room** that produce light or electromagnetic fields (EMF's): Cell phones, cordless phones, computers, clock radios, electric blankets—*anything* you'd plug into an electric outlet or which is battery powered that can interfere with sound, healthy sleep (EMF's are also being implicated as a causal/contributing factor in many common diseases). **Remember that sleep is the primary time when your body heals and regenerates,** so the less toxic EMF's you let interfere with your night's sleep and restoration the far better off you'll be, both short *and* long term.

Φ **Many people take over-the-counter Melatonin** (natural sleep hormone) about 30 minutes before bed to help them sleep when nothing else works. Low dosages are better (from 0.5mg up to 3mg). Too high a dosage can trigger intense dreaming, so start on the low end. People with autoimmune issues or asthma should avoid melatonin as it has immune stimulating properties.

Φ **Make sure that your Mattress is made of organic material** like cotton, wool or similar natural material. Avoid toxic mattress materials, e.g., petroleum derived or synthetic foam. Unnatural mattress materials disrupt the natural electromagnetic field of your body. It's also best not to sleep on metal spring mattresses, as they interfere with your body's natural energy flow and can also impinge circulation.

Φ **Wake up Naturally—Without an Alarm—as often as possible.** *Think about it: waking to an alarm almost always means you're shortchanging you body's natural sleep requirements,* in addition to starting your day off on an *alarming* note. The word "alarm" literally means *Sudden fear, danger, warning; to fill with alarm or anxious concern;* ***a call to arms!*** Not the best way to begin your day. So give yourself the gift of waking up naturally on at least 3 days out of 7. If you feel you need an alarm clock on some mornings, consider upgrading to an elegant Fibonacci Alarm Clock by Now & Zen, which awakens you to gentle chime tones synchronized to the Fibonacci Sequence. Available at: www.Now-Zen.com

3 Regulate Your Nighttime Blue Light Screen Exposure with f.lux & NightShift

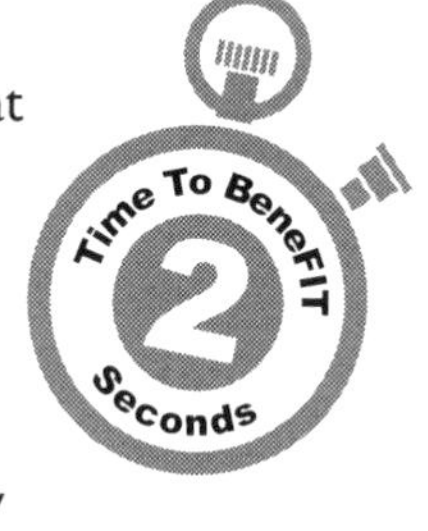

Yankee ingenuity seems to arise just at the right time in order to save humanity from itself. The invention of the personal computer is one of the greatest innovations ever created for the advancement of mankind. Most new inventions are initially embraced with enthusiasm—only later do we recognize their downsides. Scientists have only recently learned that the blue light emitted by electronic screens desynchronizes our biorhythms. Humans are designed to accommodate blue light as part of the solar spectrum—*yet only during daylight hours.* By exposing ourselves to the blue light from our computer/phone/tablet screens at night, we've overridden our innate circadian signaling system which tells our brain and body which neurotransmitters and hormones to release after sundown, and in which order. Sleep onset and numerous other downstream signals are disrupted, becoming causal factors for many modern diseases seen today.

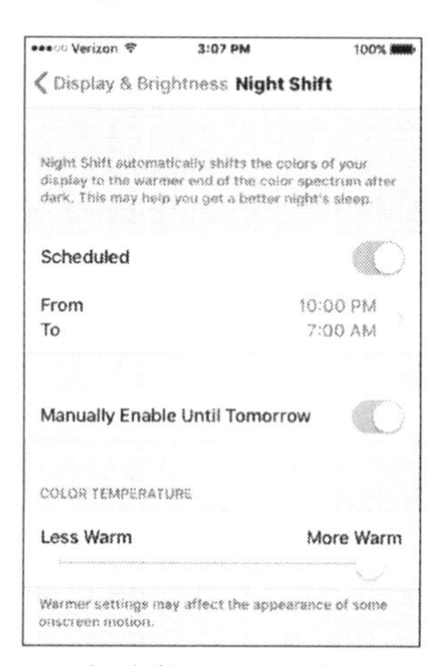

(*top*) f.lux, an app for synchronizing the color spectrum of your computer screen to the sun; (*bottom*) screenshot of NightShift, the built-in iOS app which does the same thing.

Luckily for us all, a computer app called f.lux is available that synchronizes the color spectrum from your computer screen to that of the sun—full spectrum during the day with a shift to the red end of the visual spectrum after sundown. The progressive adjustment towards evening red prevent blue spectrum suppression of melatonin and resulting sleep disruptions. f.lux automatically adjusts to your local time of day, year and location (latitude). Humanity often becomes too smart for its own good, but in this case f.lux can help save us from our own inventiveness.

Find f.lux at: https://justgetflux.com/. The same screen customization is built into all iOS devices (iPhones, iPads, iPods). Simply go to **Settings > Display & Brightness** and turn on the **NightShift** program, which allows you to also easily calibrate the evening warmth of your screen to suit your preference.

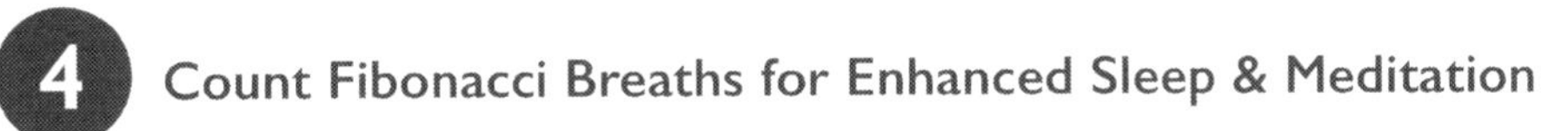

4 Count Fibonacci Breaths for Enhanced Sleep & Meditation

This easy method for easing into deep sleep was adapted by **Bruce Mandelbaum**, a master acupuncturist and massage therapist. You simply pay attention to each breath and count each full inhalation/exhalation to the Fibonacci Sequence: 1 breath (in & out), 1 breath, 2 breaths, 3 breaths, 5 breaths, 8 breaths, 13 breaths, 21 breaths, 34 breaths, 55 breaths...and so on. **The key is to keep each breath deep and full.** As Bruce notes,

You simply cannot be tense and contracted when your breath is full and deep.

You may find that by going to sleep counting your breaths to the Fibonacci Sequence you wake up more refreshed. Bruce has yet to make it past breath 55 before he's sound asleep. If on the other hand, you haven't fallen asleep and are still counting by morning, you will have super-oxygenated your system by having taken 5,760 breaths. This happens to be somewhere between the 19th and 20th Fibonacci numbers (19th: 4,181; 20th: 6,765), assuming that you take an average of 12 breaths per minute.

5 Reload Your Catapult by taking Fibonacci Power Naps

These naps will help reduce any sleep deficits from the night before, as well as "reloading your catapult" for the rest of the day. Naps or siestas recharge your system and elevate your efficiency, information processing and improve emotional health and immune function. The trick is to get just deep enough into the lighter stages of sleep to get some restful and regenerative effects, yet not long enough to awaken feeling groggy (sleep inertia). Numerous authoritative sleep studies show that the ideal length of a nap is from 5 to around 20 minutes. Here are some nap lengths to experiment with in your schedule. These naps are calibrated to Fibonacci numbers that interestingly correspond to practical nap time lengths and are named after some famous successful nappers. You may want to use an alarm to awaken you from your nap so as not to overnap.

Time To BeneFIT 8 Seconds

- Φ **The Einstein ∞: 8–13 minutes**. Einstein is one of the preeminent Golden Ratio geniuses in history. He was also a frequent napper, who clearly benefited from the increased creativity and mental acuity that naps bestow.
- Φ **The Edison : 13–21 minutes**. Inventor of over 1000 different devices including the light bulb, phonograph and moving pictures, Thomas Edison took short naps daily to make up for the fact that he only slept 4-5 hours per night. Naps gave him the ability

to walk a fine line between the worlds of unlimited imagination and waking reality, to bring his great insights back to waking consciousness.

Φ **The Bucky ⚽: 21-34 minutes.** According to *The Economist*, 2/15/07, Golden Ratio Genius Buckminster Fuller advocated taking 30-minute naps every six hours. He is reported to have abandoned the practice only because *"his schedule conflicted with that of his business associates, who insisted on sleeping like other men."*

6 Caffeinate Only Until 2pm for Sounder Nighttime Sleep

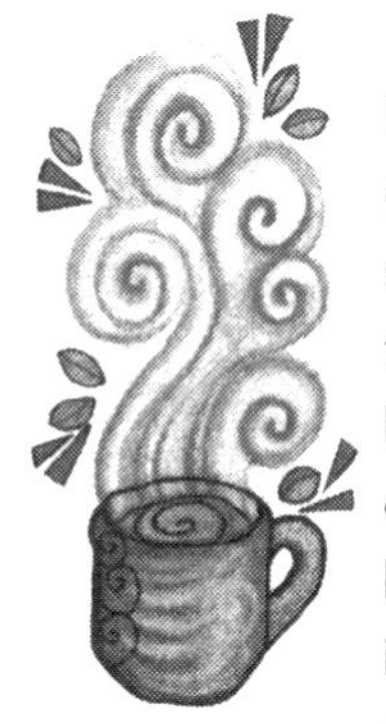

Caffeine and related compounds (methylxanthines) are the active ingredients in coffee, tea, cola, chocolate and many energy drinks and energy bars. Many people don't realize that the caffeine from these sources circulates in your system for many hours after you consume them. Caffeine is metabolized in your liver and has a half-life of around 5 hours. Contraceptive use, pregnancy, liver problems or medication use can extend caffeine's half-life to 24-48 hours or longer. This means that **5 hours after you drink coffee, fully half of the caffeine is still circulating in your system.** In another 5 hours half of the half—or ¼ of the original amount—is still around. So, if you have an afternoon tea or coffee at tea-time, say around 4 pm, you'd still have some stimulant activity in your system at bedtime, lasting through the night. Your ability to drop into deep sleep would be compromised and rejuvenation wouldn't be optimal. So it's best to limit your caffeine consumption to the early and mid parts of the day, so that your liver can metabolize most of it before you retire in the evening. Of course an easy substitute for coffee or black tea is a cup of caffeine-free herb tea, which can be enjoyed anytime.

7 Sleep Apnea/Snoring: Taming a Dangerous Sleep Disrupter

Sleep apnea occurs when breathing stops for 10 seconds or longer on multiple occasions throughout the night. Often happening hundreds of times during the night, it leaves the person feeling totally fatigued the following day. Long-term, there is also an increased risk of cardiovascular disease and stroke. Snoring often accompanies sleep apnea. During the snoring/apneic episodes, oxygen levels in the blood fall and CO_2 levels rise, which then activate an alarm reaction in the brain. The person then usually has a startle reaction, regains their breath and then briefly falls asleep again—until the dangerous cycle repeats itself. In sleep labs, physiologic recordings document the constant disruption of deep restorative sleep phases in this condition.

The most common type of sleep apnea is obstructive, which means that there is a biomechanical problem in the neck or throat, e.g., loose or collapsing pharyngeal tissue that is blocking the airway. Poor sleeping posture or positions—sleeping on your back, face-up, as opposed to on your side with a pillow between your knees—can also predispose you to snoring/sleep apnea. Many patients get relief from Continuous Positive Airway Pressure (CPAP) machines that hold the airways open while breathing. This malady highlights the importance of healthy breathing as the #1 driver of health and longevity. Many times weight loss along with exercise and postural improvement can create more airway space, realign airways and strengthen weak throat muscles, alleviating the problem. An unusual treatment that has shown remarkable improvement in patients with moderate obstructive sleep apnea is didgeridoo playing. The didgeridoo is an Australian Aboriginal wind instrument made from eucalyptus trunks that have been hollowed out by termites and then shaped into resonant instruments by craftsmen. After several months of practice, obstructive apnea patients have been able to tone and strengthen the muscles of their upper airways, resulting in a dramatic improvement in sleep apnea symptoms.

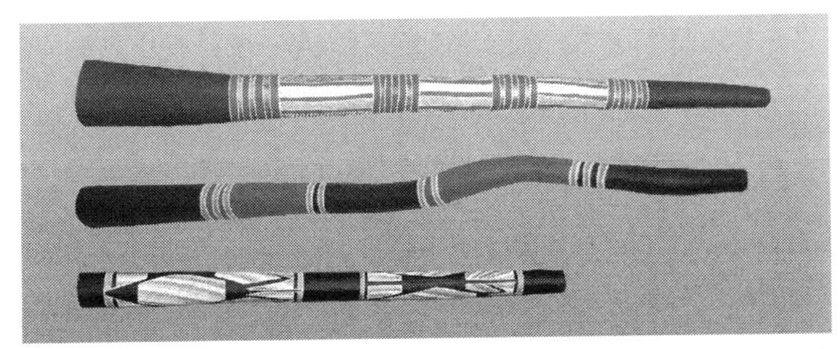

Didjeridoos come in various shapes and sizes and have been discovered to be a very effective therapeutic device for obstructive sleep apnea.

8 The Human Star Technique for Sounder Sleep

This simple exercise takes 5 minutes at bedtime, setting the stage for deep, refreshing sleep. When the 5 "star points" of your body (hands, feet and head) are relaxed, a wave of growing relaxation ripples back to your core. This theory has its roots in the practice of reflexology: your soles, palms and scalp/ears are said to each contain a fractal map of your whole body. When you massage each of these 5 "mini-maps" for a minute or so, you initiate a chain relaxation reaction which leads you easier into sound sleep. **Try it:**

1. Get into bed and turn off lights before beginning.
2. Massage the sole of one foot for a minute. Press firmly, as comfortable. Repeat the above on your other foot for a minute.

3. Spend a minute massaging one of your hands with the other. Repeat on the other hand. Press into your palms.
4. After massaging both hands, move to your head for a minute. Start by gently massaging your temples and scalp with your fingertips for 30 seconds. Spend a few seconds gently massaging your ears, then move to your jaw muscles, Left hand on Left jaw, Right hand on Right jaw. Press into your jaw muscles with your fingers and thumbs firmly, yet comfortably. Lastly, gently massage your third eye (the point between your eyebrows) with one of your middle fingers for a few seconds, to activate your pineal gland's melatonin secretion.
5. Take a few deep, relaxed Golden Breaths: **Inhale to a count of 3; Exhale to a count of 5.** Let yourself go... and sleep well…

> *The genius of things is to make things simple. We are built to be happy, strong and healthy. We just need to go back to Nature, the natural laws within us, and connect again. Very simple.*
>
> **Iceman Wim Hof, on *The Joe Rogan Podcast***

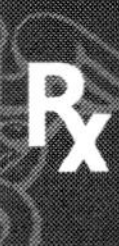

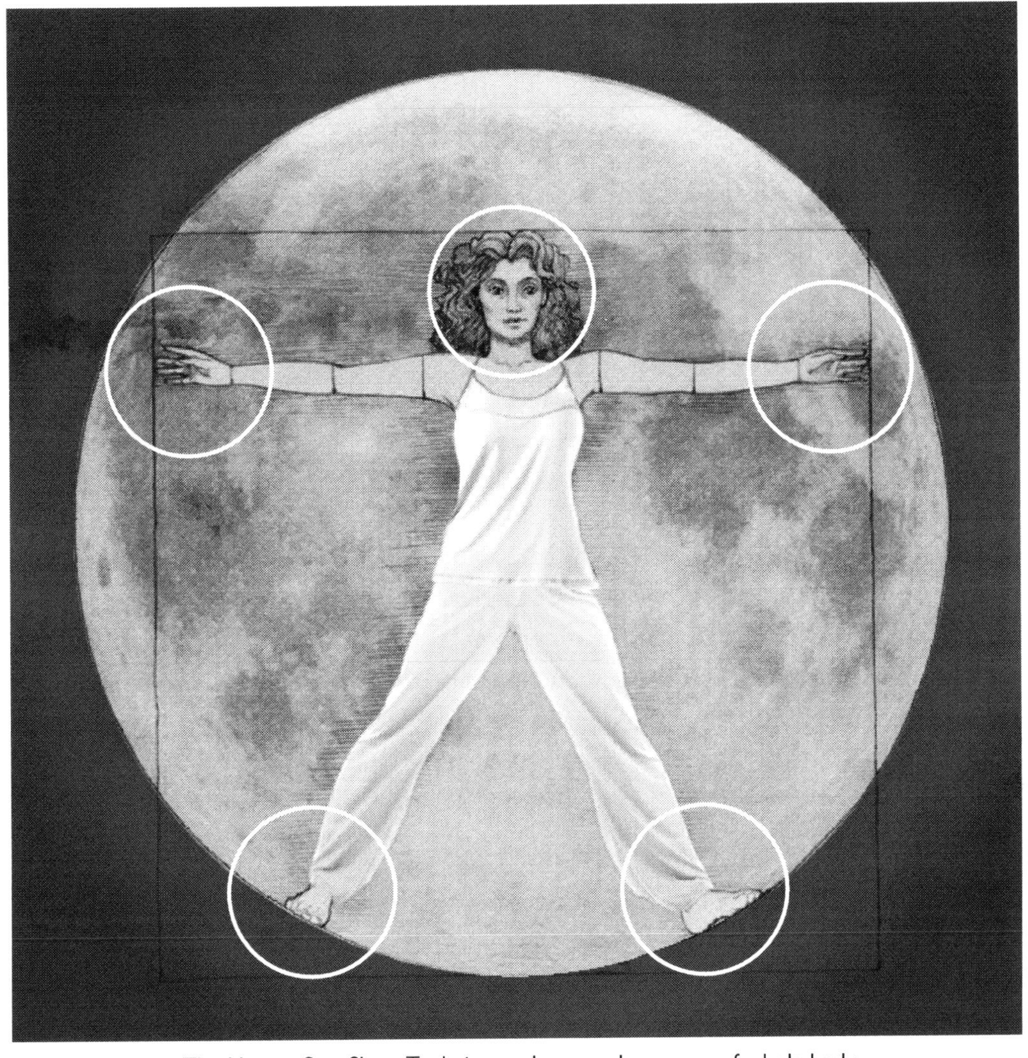

The Human Star Sleep Technique releases a deep wave of whole body relaxation and gently reinforces your natural Golden Star geometry, setting the stage for an uncommonly good night's sleep.

SECTION II: Wake~Sunlight Rx's

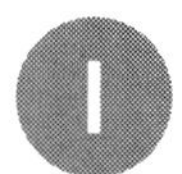

Reset Your Circadian Biorhythms with Morning Sunlight

Morgenstund hat Gold im Mund.
(The Early Morning Hour has Gold in its Mouth).
German proverb; a favorite of Benjamin Franklin

Time To BeneFIT 3 Seconds

3

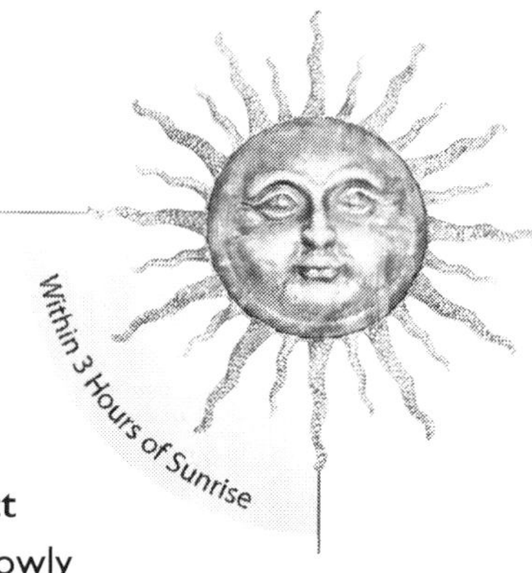

Light is a vital cue that your brain relies on to reset your circadian rhythms each and every day. Here's an easy yet potent method to establish and maintain healthy biorhythms, which directly enhances both waking *and* sleeping states.

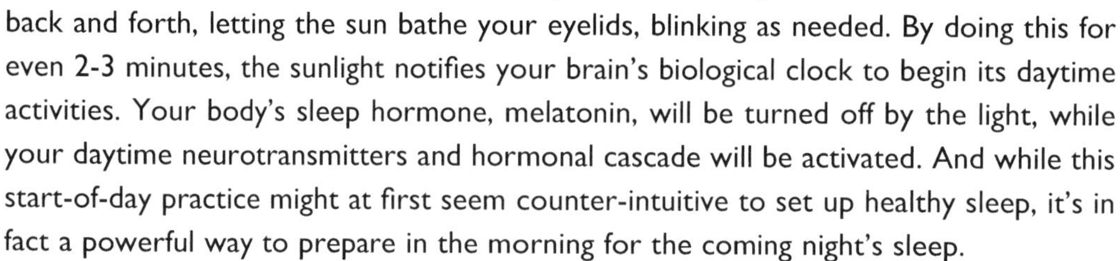

Upon arising, go outside and face the sun, ideally within the first 3 hours after sunrise. You want direct sunlight—no windows or screens. Move your head slowly back and forth, letting the sun bathe your eyelids, blinking as needed. By doing this for even 2-3 minutes, the sunlight notifies your brain's biological clock to begin its daytime activities. Your body's sleep hormone, melatonin, will be turned off by the light, while your daytime neurotransmitters and hormonal cascade will be activated. And while this start-of-day practice might at first seem counter-intuitive to set up healthy sleep, it's in fact a powerful way to prepare in the morning for the coming night's sleep.

If you're up within the first hour after dawn, as the sun crests the horizon and before it's too bright, do the exercise with your eyes open for perhaps 30-60 seconds. Remember not to stare directly at the sun, just be aware of it in the periphery of your visual field, blinking as you move your head from side-to-side. This exercise also works well to help mitigate jet lag. People with Seasonal Affective Disorder (SAD) can also use full-spectrum lights in the winter to modulate melatonin, neurotransmitters and hormones. You may want to get full-spectrum indoor lights if you live in northern latitudes with pronounced seasonal changes or frequent cloud cover. *So let there be light* every morning .

2 The Sunlight Dose Makes the Medicine—Or the Poison

The Goldilocks principle of finding the dose of *Just Right* applies to just about everything, including finding the correct dose of UV Sunlight, vitamin-D and DHA. Too small a dose and there's no beneficial effect; too large a dose produces side effects. Essentially, as we see with all NSN health priority drivers, *The Dose makes the Medicine or the Poison*. There are easy ways to monitor the dose of Sunlight, vitamin-D and DHA:

UV Sunlight: UV exposure can be estimated with a free app called **DMinder**, an iPhone and Android app that monitors UV exposure and estimates the amount of Vitamin-D produced in your skin. This free app calculates the amount of vitamin-D produced by measuring the amount of your UV exposure as determined by your location (latitude and elevation), time of day and year and duration in the sun. This app, used in conjunction with vitamin-D blood testing, is another excellent way to fine-tune the *Just Right* amount of your sun exposure and vitamin-D production to maximize generation of NSN.

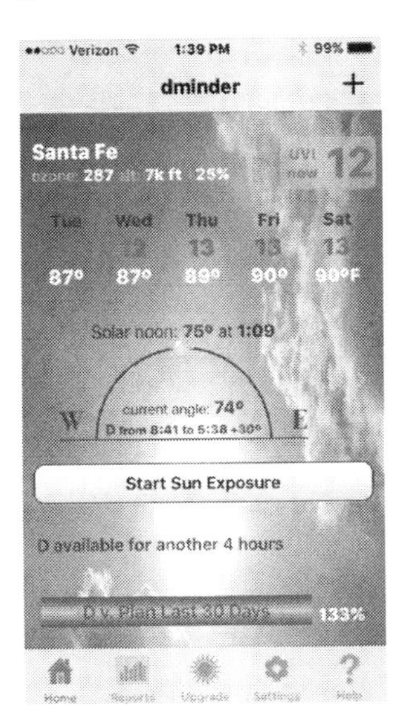

Vitamin-D: 2 25-OH Vitamin-D levels can also be checked with an in-home finger-stick test. Your results can be compared to those in the **Recommended Golden Ratio Vitamin-D Levels** chart below. You ideally want to be in the Golden Ratio range of 38-62ng/ml. As vitamin-D synthesis is dependent on UVB light, this test can also be used as an indirect measure of UVB exposure. If your 25-OH Vitamin-D level is low, you know that you need to increase sun exposure or begin supplementing with oral or intramuscular vitamin-D.

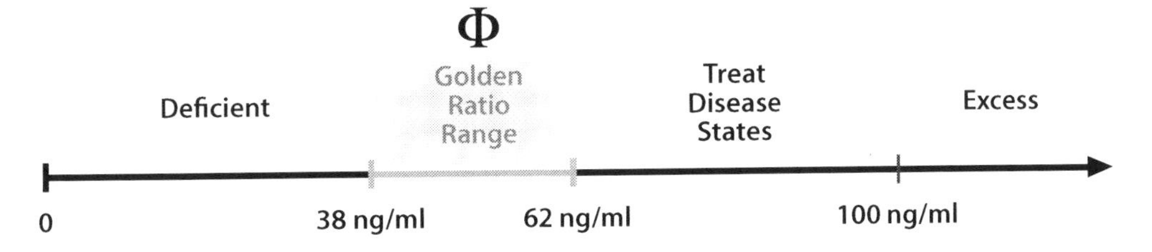

DHA: The Omega Check™ report indicates your levels of both Omega-3 (DHA & EPA) and Omega 6 fatty acids as well as your risk of cardiovascular disease (DHA is required to convert photons from sunlight into body-charging DC electricity).

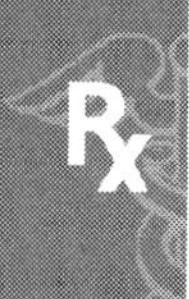

An in-home finger stick finger-stick drop of blood is all that's required. If your DHA level is low, you know that you need to increase DHA intake through either eating more high Omega-3, non-farm-raised seafood or via supplements.

Links to order test kits and app:

Omega Check: http://tinyurl.com/j3duesg
Vitamin D test: http://tinyurl.com/k8gvg5x
DMinder app: http://tinyurl.com/j53km9d

3 The Fibonacci Sunbathing Timer

The Fibonacci Sunbathing Timer is an easy general guide for determining the duration of safe sun exposure. It uses Fibonacci Sequence Numbers as a progressive guide for how much time to stay in the sun without burning, tied to a person's skin type and sun sensitivity. Each person needs to find their own Golden RAYtio amount of sun exposure, where the dose becomes the medicine, but not the poison. The ideal way to get solar benefits while preventing over exposure is to *first sunbathe without sunscreen according to the Fibonacci Sunbathing Timer*. Then, *after* you've had a chance to absorb adequate sunlight, you can apply sunscreen or use other sun blocking methods.

Even as little as 1 to 3 minutes may be the limit for those with light or extremely sensitive skin. Even if you're very sensitive to the sun, it's still possible to increase time in the sun as your skin develops more tolerance. These individuals can begin at the

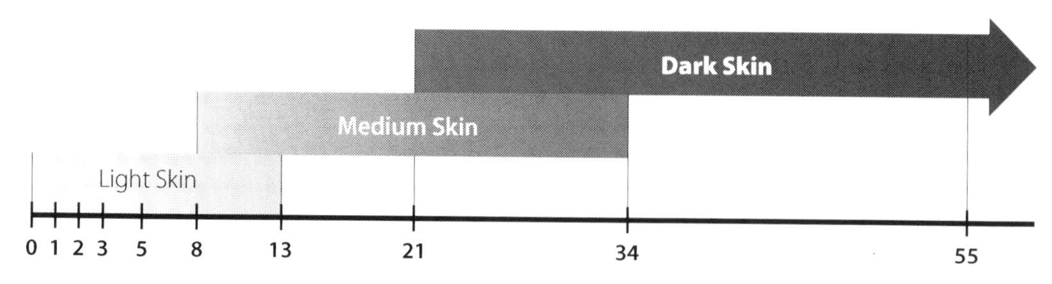

The Fibonacci Sunbathing Timer is an easy general guide for healthy sun exposure duration according to skin type. Each skin type has a range of minutes within which you can safely sunbathe. For example, if you have light or sensitive skin, a beginning range would be from as little as 1-2 minutes, building up as tolerated over time. If you have medium skin, a beginning range would be anywhere between 13 minutes, and so on. However, it's always recommended to start with the lowest number in your skin category to give your skin time to build sun tolerance before moving up. Remember to alternate your front and back, so that the actual time on each side is halved. If you begin at the 13 minute level, you'll have 6½ minutes on front and 6½ minutes on back for a 13 minute session. Note: Depending on the season you'll need to adjust up or down your total daily sun exposure time.

1 minute mark and progress up to 3, 5 or even 8 minutes as their tolerance develops over time. Light-skinned people have less melanin pigment in their skin as an evolutionary adaptation to northern latitudes, where it was advantageous to maximize sun absorption in a low sun environment. Paradoxically, light-skinned people have an advantage over people with more pigmentation in that they don't need as much time in the sun to absorb an adequate amount of UV light.

People with medium skin pigmentation have moderate sun tolerance and have a wider range of sun exposure on Fibonacci's Sunbathing Timer. These individuals can begin at the 13 minute mark and progress up to 21 or even 34 minutes as tolerance develops over time. If any over-exposure occurs, you need to drop down to the next lower Fibonacci Number after your skin recovers and you are ready to begin again. Darker skinned individuals have the most resilient skin with more melanin protection and can easily tolerate intense sun exposure from 34 to 55 minutes or beyond. They need longer sun exposure to generate an equivalent amount of vitamin-D as the lighter skinned person. However, they benefit in not having to be as concerned with over exposure and burning as people with light and medium skin pigmentation. Sunlight has the potential to deliver life-giving medicine without side-effects—if we monitor ourselves with respect to *duration, intensity and frequency*. As with all the NSN health priority drivers, remember the following:

- Start low & go slow.
- As sun intensity ↑, sunbathing time ↓
- Moderation is the Key
- As sun intensity ↓, sunbathing time ↑

Healthy Sun Protection Methods—External & Internal

Golden RAYtio Sunscreen: Determine the amount of sun exposure you can safely tolerate based on your skin type, time of day & year, latitude & location. Aim to get the correct dose of sunshine according to **Fibonacci's Sunbathing Timer** and download the *DMinder* app to estimate UV exposure and vitamin-D production and then you'll have Golden RAYtio sun protection. Remember, *the dose makes the medicine or the poison.*

Φ **Barrier methods:** Hats, clothing, umbrellas, trees, porches or other types of shade. Ultraviolet Protective Factor (UPF) clothing is specifically designed with special fabrics to give increased sun protection.

Φ **Sunscreens:** The Environmental Working Group's (EWG's) 2016 Sunscreen Guide rates the safety and efficacy of more than 750 sunscreens, more than 500 daily moisturizers and 100 lip products with SPF values. Safety assessments are based on ingredients disclosed on product labels. The product's score ranges from 0 to 10 and reflects both the degree of both UVA & UVB protection and the safety of all ingredients on the label. Two-thirds of the overall score is based on a product's UV protection, while one-third of the score reflects the hazard score, based on toxicity concerns of listed ingredients. See EWG.org for more information.

Φ **Internal Sunscreens:** A simple, natural, yet overlooked way to get sun protection is to orally ingest certain foods and supplements which become incorporated into your skin over time. Photo-protective phytonutrients from food or supplements increase in concentration in your skin over time, taking sun protection to the cellular level where it's most effective. This natural approach totally avoids exposure to potentially toxic external sunscreens. The only drawback with this biohack is that you really can't be sure of how much sun protection you're actually getting, in that unmeasured variables include amount and duration of intake as well as cellular penetration. The wisest way may be to combine both external *and* internal protection, using only the safest ingredients. Below are a few of the research documented foods and supplements that can help protect your skin from the inside out. Adequate tissue levels and best results are obtained by eating moderate portions/doses over a period of months or longer.

- **Lycopene**: red fruits & vegetables.
- **Astaxanthin**: red pigment from seafood & algae.
- **Resveratrol**: grapes, wine, supplements.
- **DHA & EPA**: fish, supplements.
- **Green Tea**: tea, supplements.
- **Blueberries**: berries, supplements.
- **Leafy greens & cruciferous vegetables**: kale, romaine, spinach, parsley, cilantro broccoli, leeks, onions, garlic, broccoli, cauliflower, cilantro, celery and parsley.
- Life Extension's **Oral Sun Protection Formula** is a triangulation of fire combination of red orange extract, polypodium leucotomos extract and nicotinamide. The formula is designed to prevent DNA damage and promote DNA repair via decreasing the inflammatory response to radiation exposure.
- **Dark chocolate**: greater than 70%. A 2009 study in the Journal of Cosmetic Dermatology revealed that eating high-flavanol dark chocolate can significantly protect your skin from UV light. This double-blind study tested 15 subjects who ate 20 grams of high-flavanol chocolate daily compared with 15 subjects who ate 20 grams of low-flavanol chocolate daily. After 12 weeks the MED

(MED—Minimal Erythema Dose—is time-to-reddening of the skin) more than doubled in the high-flavanol group. The takeaway is that eating high-flavanol dark chocolate can double the time you can stay in the sun before UV rays cause reddening of your skin. Note: The cacao percentage of your chocolate doesn't necessarily indicate flavanol content, because flavanol content of chocolate is dependent on many factors, including agricultural and manufacturing practices, as well as the cultivar of cocao bean. That being said, it's best to eat chocolate with 70% cacao or higher.

5 Circadian Rhythms du Soleil: Morning Sun Supports Optimal Weight

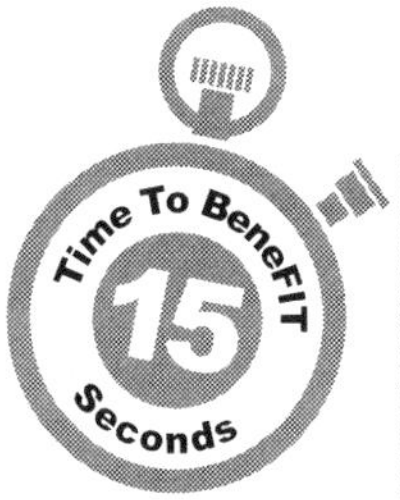

Time To BeneFIT 15 Seconds

All mitochondriac's, at a fundamental level, know that physiologic solar exposure is the most critical part of the equation for fat burning.

Jack Kruse, M.D., neurosurgeon & biophysicist

Sun exposure of specific *timing, intensity and duration* is associated with a decreased BMI (Body Mass Index). BMI is a ratio of weight to height reflecting varying degrees of obesity or leanness. Researchers have determined that when these 3 elements are blended together, a decreased BMI results. Variations or absence in any of the 3 critical factors wouldn't decrease BMI. The specific requirements of the 3 elements are:

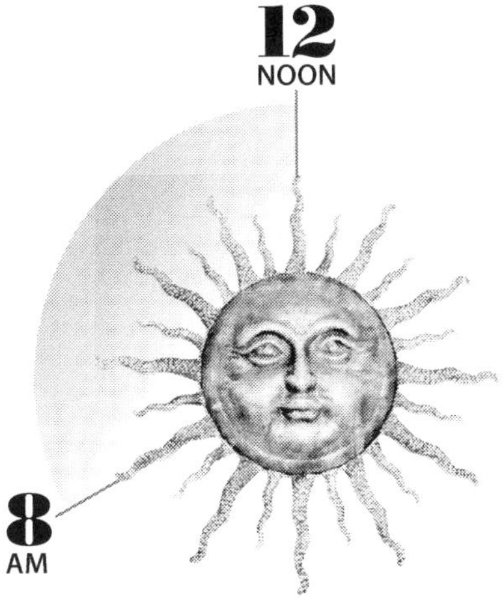

- Φ **Timing:** Morning sun exposure between 8 am and 12 noon
- Φ **Intensity:** Natural outdoor sunlight
- Φ **Duration:** Up to 20 minutes of direct morning exposure daily. Adjust exposure duration up or down depending on season and intensity of sunlight.

12 NOON

8 AM

The best hours for sunning to activate weight reduction are between 8 am and 12 noon.

This solar triangulation of fire practice is a simple, 3-faceted approach to activate and reset your biorhythms and support optimal weight reduction. By realigning with one of Nature's premier essential nutrients—the sun—you can lose weight, lower your BMI and experience improved health and vitality.

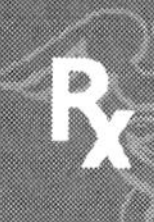

6 Use Full Spectrum Lights to Bring the Sun Inside

Full-spectrum lighting contains many wavelengths found in natural Sunlight and is a suggested upgrade to conventional indoor lighting for use during daylight hours. Full-spectrum lighting relieves eyestrain, reveals more natural colors and is effective in treating Seasonal Affective Disorder (SAD) during winter months in northern climates. Conventional incandescent, fluorescent and LED (light emitting diodes) bulbs project

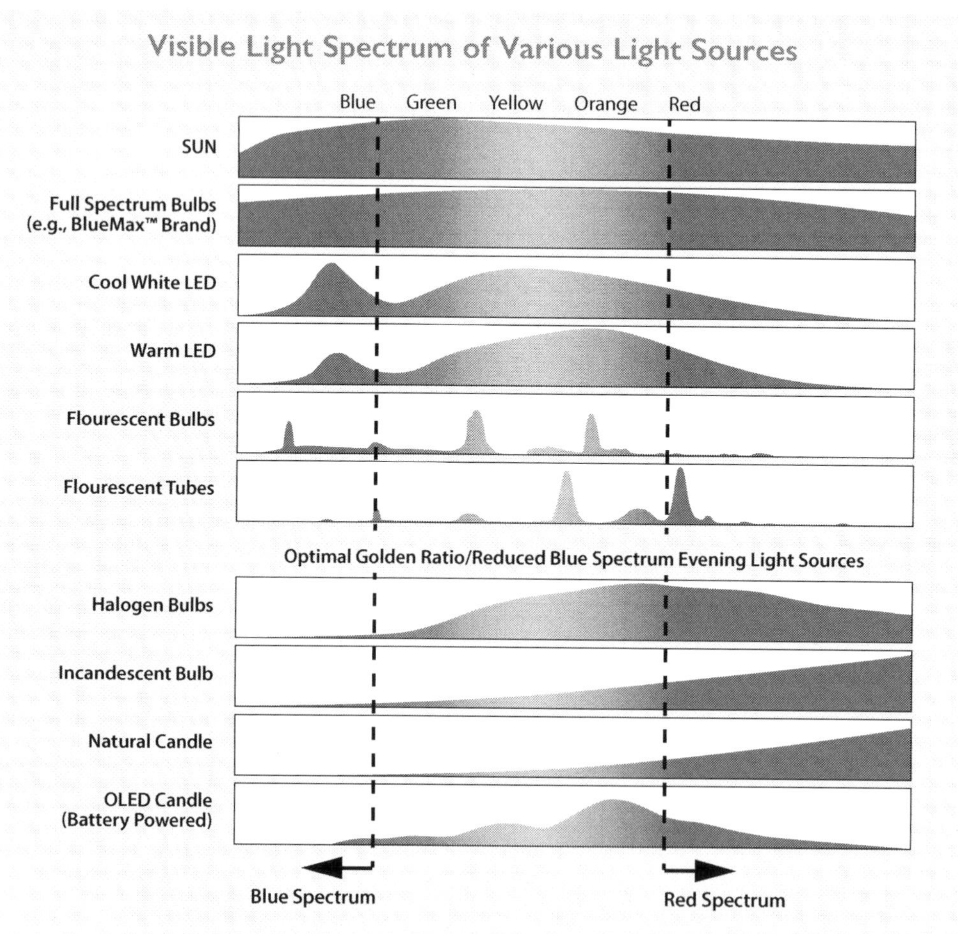

Different types of light bulbs emit different light frequencies, including various amounts of blue light. Although Sunlight has the highest amount of blue light, it of course only shines during daylight hours. **It's the artificial evening blue light that desynchronizes us from our natural circadian rhythms and wreaks havoc with normal hormonal secretions including melatonin, which induces sleep.** Of the common light bulbs compared, incandescent bulbs have the lowest amount of blue frequency emission; their spectral frequencies are shifted towards yellow, orange and red, while CFL and LED bulbs retain a fair amount of blue light emission.

The Visible Light Spectrum

Wavelength (meters)

10^{-14} 10^{-12} 10^{-10} 10^{-8} 10^{-6} 10^{-4} 10^{-2} 1 10^{2} 10^{4}

Gamma Rays | X-Rays | Ultraviolet Rays | Infrared Rays | Radar | FM | TV | Short-wave | AM

Visible Light

ULTRAVIOLET | VIOLET | BLUE | GREEN | YELLOW | RED | INFRARED

380 450 495 570 590 620 750

Wavelength (nanometers)

Visible sunlight is a small band in the electromagnetic spectrum ranging from around 380nm to 750nm. Ultraviolet rays (UVA, UVB and UVC) have shorter wavelengths (100-400 nm) just to the left of visible light and are invisible to the human eye. Infrared rays have longer wavelengths (700 nm-1 mm) and are the invisible warming rays of the sun just to the right of the visible red region. The region of visible blue light is from around 450-495 nanometers. Excessive blue light has the undesirable property of destroying DHA in the retina faster than it can be regenerated, as well as upsetting circadian signaling, hence the reason for avoiding blue light in the evenings from computers, cell phones, TV's, etc. Use blue blocker lenses or apps for more retinal protection from blue frequencies when using digital at night.

an uneven light spectrum which can cause irritability, lethargy and eyestrain. As evening comes, transitioning towards bulbs with more of the green, yellow and red part of the spectrum prevents circadian desynchronization and allows the body to gradually prepare for sleep. Some of the newer incandescent and candle light OLED (organic light emitting diodes) bulbs have eliminated much of the blue light and are a good choice for evening lighting.

7 The Golden Ratio Evening Light bulb

The hypothetical ideal light bulb for evening use would emit light frequencies that are only within the 62% of the spectrum that encompasses *green/yellow/orange/red*. These frequencies avoid the toxic blue light that can disrupt our circadian rhythms if we're

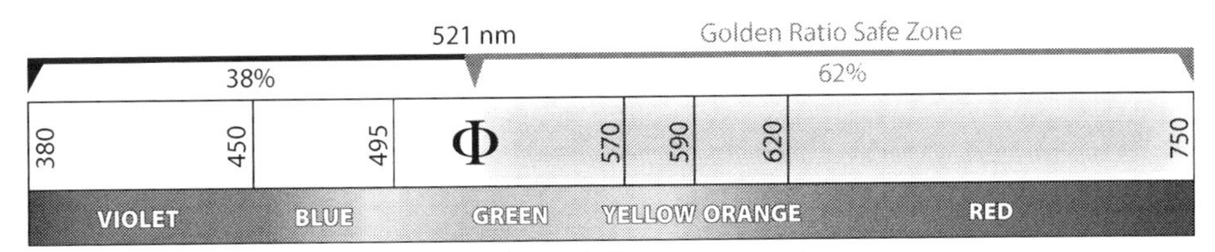

Wavelength (nanometers)

The Golden Ratio division point is at 521nm, in the green part of the spectrum. As the evening progresses, so should your light bulbs move further to the right, towards the red frequencies. Light bulbs in the red range are also advisable for night lights.

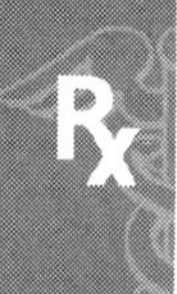

exposed to them after sunset. Natural candle light, candle light-style OLED's, traditional incandescent and halogen bulbs eliminate most of the blue light and thus fit into the Golden Ratio safe zone (the candle options are recommended, due to their softer light).

8 Morning Sunlight + Coffee/Tea for Optimal Circadian Reset

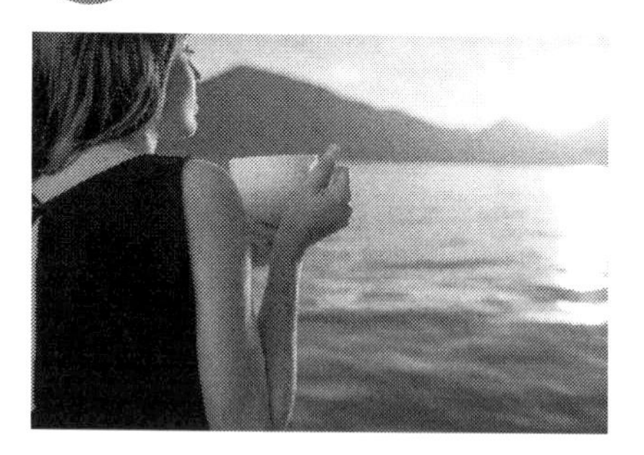

Time To BeneFIT 2 Seconds

As we've seen, daily morning exposure to sunlight for at least 3 minutes is critical for the circadian reset that inactivates the sleep hormone melatonin and turns on and stimulates synthesis of many essential daytime hormones and neurotransmitters. To add to your bright start every day, compliment your morning sun exposure with a cup of sunshine's liquid circadian surrogate—coffee or tea. You'll then get your circadian reset with a double shot of sunshine—in your cup and on your face.

9 Ignite Your Circadian Wake-up With A Fibonaccino

The *Fibonaccino* is a tasty way to get your surrogate circadian wake-up, as well as a morning dose of NSN.

1. Combine 2 shots (2 oz.) of espresso with 3 oz. of either steamed or frothed milk.
2. This gives a total of 5 oz. for a perfect Fibonaccino Ratio of 5 to 3 to 2.
3. To top it off, decorate your milky canvas with a golden spiral, golden rays of sunshine or any design that will brighten your day.

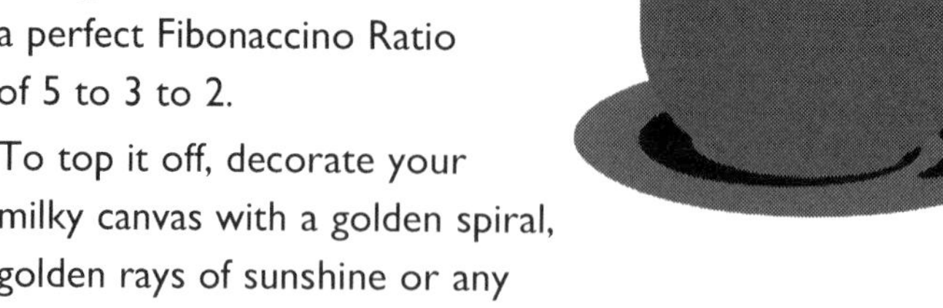

For an innovative gourmet coffee alternative, visit biohacker Dave Asprey's Bulletproof.com and see pages 124 and 409 to learn about Bulletproof Coffee's health and detox benefits.

Quantity, Quality & Timing of Coffee Consumption

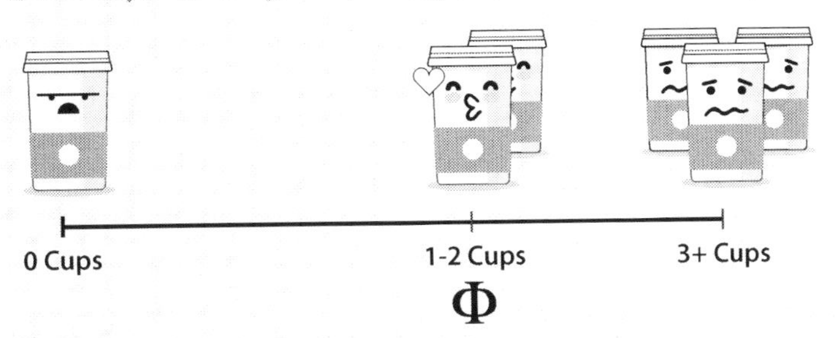

Sunsplashed coffee is the world's most popular beverage and principal source of antioxidants for many people, yet coffee consumption is no exception to the axiom of *All Things In Moderation*. Respect that limit or you'll likely suffer the consequences of anxiety, queasiness or even elevated blood pressure. Find your daily Golden Ratio ***Quantity*** of coffee consumption to get an optimal dose of NSN. Additional benefits from coffee include a lower risk of liver and colon cancer, decreased risk of type 2 diabetes, lowered risk of eyesight degeneration/blindness, improved memory, dementia prevention and delayed onset of Alzheimer's disease. ***Also remember Quality*** and ***Timing. Always go organic, as coffee is one of the heaviest toxic pesticide-sprayed crops on earth***. While the weakness and jitters many feel after drinking coffee may be a result of too much caffeine, it can also just as well be due to the toxic pesticides or mycotoxins (mold toxins) present in non-organic/poor quality coffee. As a general rule, avoid coffee consumption after 2pm, as caffeine has a half-life of 5-6 hours and thus can disrupt sleep for the upcoming night.

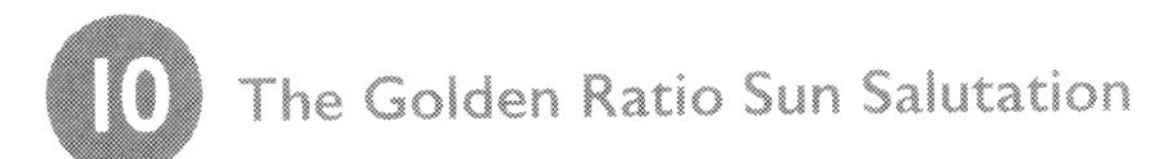

10 The Golden Ratio Sun Salutation

The Sun Salutation is a classic yoga practice to welcome each day and get your solar circadian reset at the same time. Use the featured Golden Spiral flexion/extension demonstration poses as a guide to this exercise. Listen to your body and stretch only as far as you're comfortable. If you're not initially very flexible, just go slow and easy. Increasing flexibility and suppleness comes with consistent practice.

1. **Facing the Sun, stand tall and relaxed.**
   Take 8 deep, Golden Ratio breaths: **Breathe in to 3 and out to 5.**
   With each inhalation move your attention up your spine, gently aligning each vertebra as you focus rises. Reverse direction on each exhalation.

2. **On the next inhalation, gently arch backwards, opening up your spine.**
   Let your hands and arms move back and to the sides as you go.
   Imagine you're a plant stretching to soak up maximum sunlight.
   Hold this fully extended position for 1-2 seconds...

3. **After 1-2 seconds, slowly reverse the position.**
   Continue exhaling as you move into a forward bend, head following last.
   Allow all the solar energy you've just gathered to permeate and
   energize your entire being. Cover your eyes gently with your palms.
   Hold this position for 1-2 seconds. Repeat steps 2 & 3 three to five times.

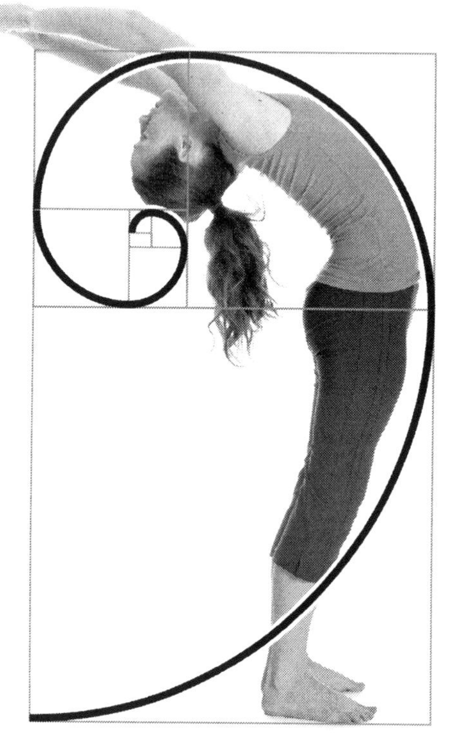

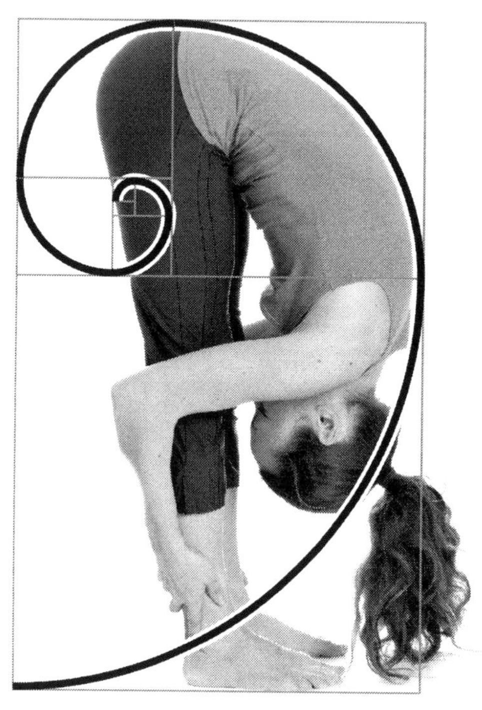

In your morning Golden Ratio Sun Salutation, visualize yourself tracking a Golden Spiral in both spinal extension and flexion.

> *Your body is a Golden Ratio/GR machine... built according to GR specs, running programs designed with GR operating systems and running cleanest and strongest on GR fuel. With that in mind the logical strategy is to consume as much GR as possible—in whatever form—for optimal performance, health and longevity.*
>
> **Robert Friedman, M.D.**

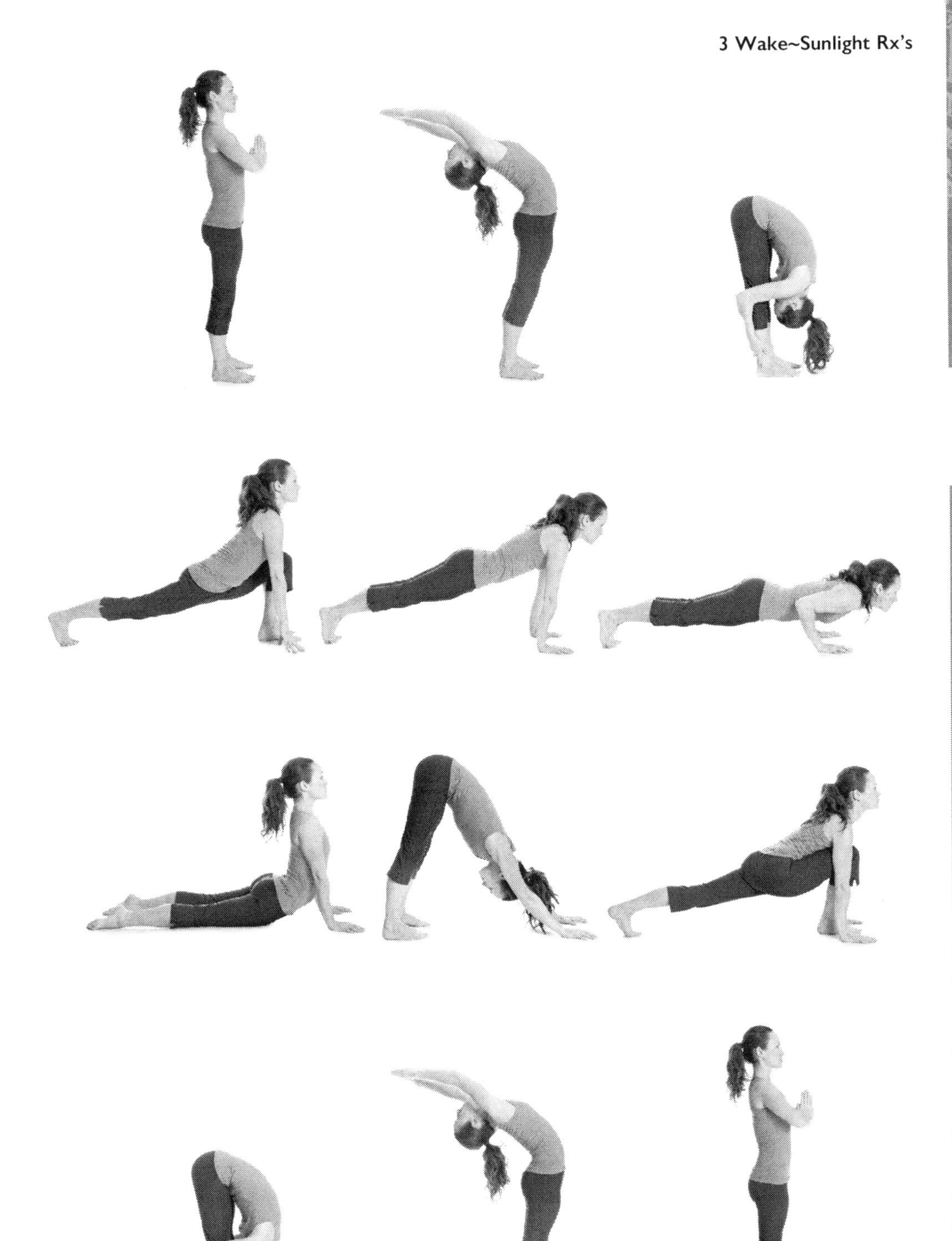

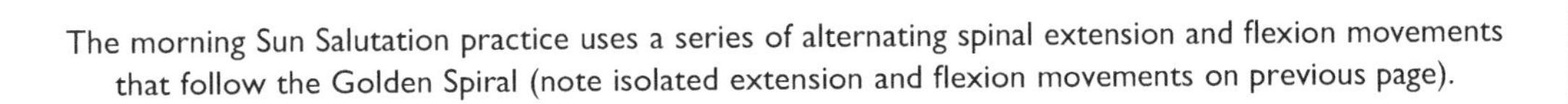

The morning Sun Salutation practice uses a series of alternating spinal extension and flexion movements that follow the Golden Spiral (note isolated extension and flexion movements on previous page).

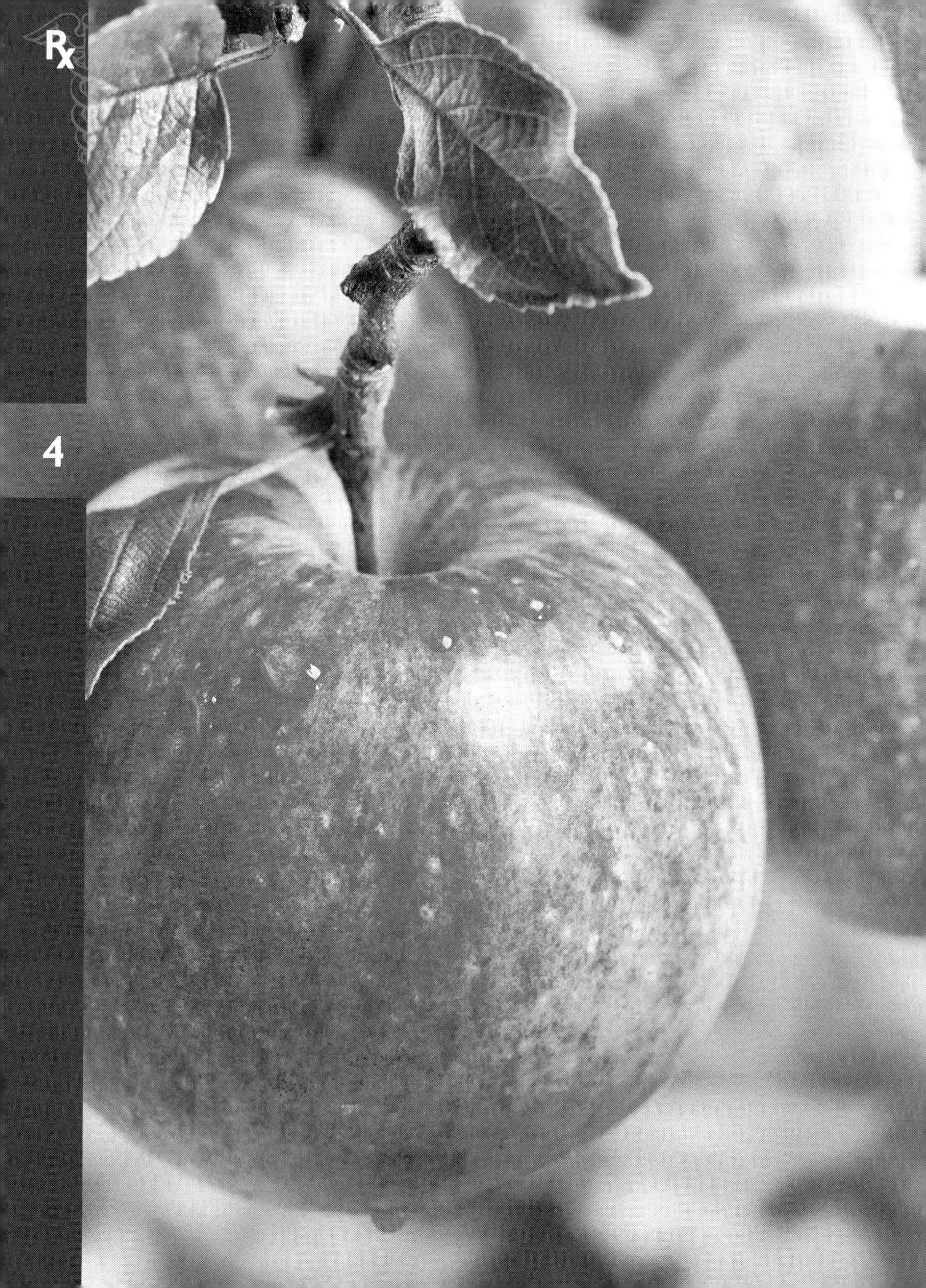

Rx
4

4 Nutrition ℞'s

Pick one or more of the following Rx's to add to your NSN daily health regimen.

1 Optimize the MacroNutrient Balance of Your Food: The 40/30/30 Golden Ratio Zone

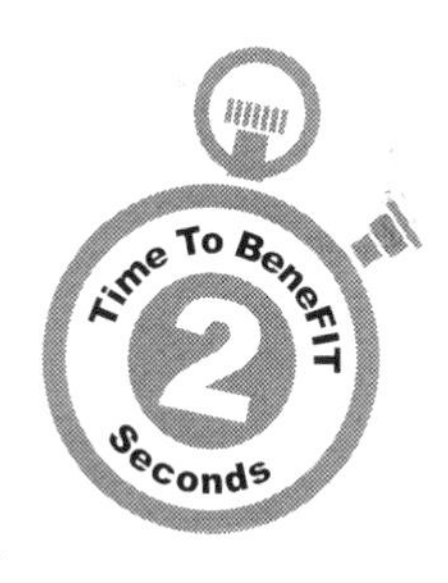

The 40/30/30 Golden Ratio Zone is adapted from the original breakthrough research of **Dr. Barry Sears**, author of *The Zone.* It interprets The Zone by approximating Golden Ratio balance in calories consumed at meals between our 3 key macronutrients of Carbohydrates, Protein and Fat: 40% Carb, 30% Protein and 30% Fat. This special proportion provides huge health and longevity benefits. **You know you're in The Zone when you have that *hum*—that special feeling of satisfied satiation after a meal.** Satisfaction is the signal that you've balanced your nutrients according to the 40/30/30 (40:60 Golden Ratio Zone) and that NSN has been activated. By eating according to the Golden Ratio Zone, you can extract the power of Nature's Secret Nutrient/NSN from your diet and enjoy these powerful cross-reinforcing benefits:

- Steady energy, mental clarity and focus throughout the day
- Reduced obesity and weight control via balanced insulin and metabolic hormones
- Inflammation control—a crucial factor in disease prevention and life extension
- Optimal sustained health, setting the stage for maximum longevity.

Here's an easy, non-mathematical way to approximate a 40/30/30 Golden Ratio of Carb, Protein and Fat at each meal, from Zone Master Dr. Sears:

> *Fill your plate with a Golden Ratio balance of lean protein and colorful, non-starchy vegetables—a little more than 1/3 lean protein & a little less than 2/3 colorful, non starchy vegetables. Add small amounts of monounsaturated fat, e.g., olive oil, avocado, almonds, etc. Whole grains or beans may be added, in small amounts. Smaller meals or snacks will have the same ratios, yet are merely more appetizer-sized portions. It's that simple!*

With the Zone approach the majority of your carbs come from colorful vegetables and fruits, vs. the over-indulgence in grains, white potatoes and processed carbohydrates common in the Standard American Diet (SAD). Here's a concise summary of how the Zone Diet works in Dr. Sears' words:

> *The more white you put on your plate, the more inflammation you create. Its inflammation that makes us fat—and keeps us fat.; it's inflammation that makes us sick; it's inflammation that increases the rate of aging. So if you really want to take control of your life, follow the Zone diet.* ***Again, it's not a weight loss program, it's a blueprint; a [Golden Ratio] blueprint to retake control of your future by retaking control of the expression of your genes.*** *That's a powerful statement. Drugs can't do that; but the Zone diet is more powerful than any drug, because it allows you to basically change the expression of your genes, and by doing so, live that longer and healthier life we all crave for.*

The 40/30/30 Golden Ratio Meal Zone is refreshingly simple and easy to achieve. **See Dr. Sears' *Zone* cookbooks for easy recipes, meal plans and creative ideas.**

2 Healthy Macronutrient Review—Always Go Organic, Non-GMO

All calories are not created equal. Always consume the highest *quality* calories.

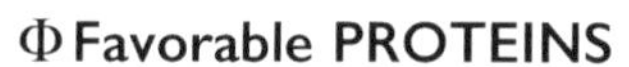

Φ Favorable PROTEINS

- Fish (high in omega-3): Salmon (NON farm-rasied), sardines, mackerel, herring.
- Grass-fed beef, buffalo, lamb
- Free-range chicken, turkey
- Free-range eggs
- Grass-fed goat/sheep dairy—milk, cheese, yogurt, kefir, butter
- Tempeh (versatile cultured/fermented soy/grain cake)
- Organic protein powders, e.g., whey, pumpkin, hemp, pea, rice

Golden Φ Ratio Zone Diet Chart

The 40/30/30 MacroNutrient ratio is based on the work of Zone Nutrition genius Dr. Barry Sears.

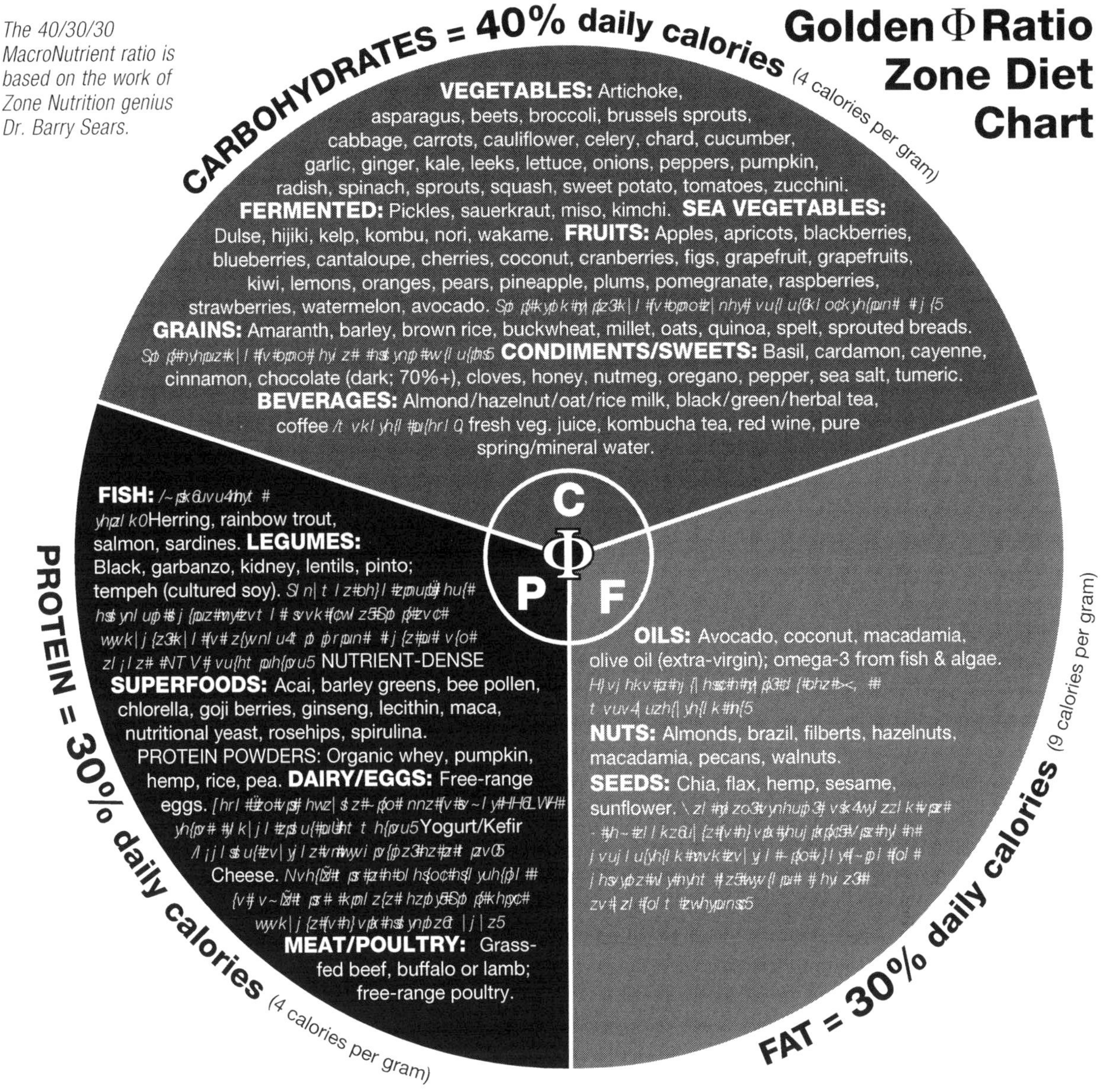

CARBOHYDRATES = 40% daily calories (4 calories per gram)

VEGETABLES: Artichoke, asparagus, beets, broccoli, brussels sprouts, cabbage, carrots, cauliflower, celery, chard, cucumber, garlic, ginger, kale, leeks, lettuce, onions, peppers, pumpkin, radish, spinach, sprouts, squash, sweet potato, tomatoes, zucchini. **FERMENTED:** Pickles, sauerkraut, miso, kimchi. **SEA VEGETABLES:** Dulse, hijiki, kelp, kombu, nori, wakame. **FRUITS:** Apples, apricots, blackberries, blueberries, cantaloupe, cherries, coconut, cranberries, figs, grapefruit, grapefruits, kiwi, lemons, oranges, pears, pineapple, plums, pomegranate, raspberries, strawberries, watermelon, avocado. *Sp µ#kyþk#ny µz3k| l #v#þpmo#z| nhy# vu{l u{6kl ockyh{µun# #j {5*
GRAINS: Amaranth, barley, brown rice, buckwheat, millet, oats, quinoa, spelt, sprouted breads. *Sp µ#nyhµz#k| l #v#þpmo# hy z# #nsyn#w{l u{þs5* **CONDIMENTS/SWEETS:** Basil, cardamon, cayenne, cinnamon, chocolate (dark; 70%+), cloves, honey, nutmeg, oregano, pepper, sea salt, tumeric.
BEVERAGES: Almond/hazelnut/oat/rice milk, black/green/herbal tea, coffee */t vkl yh{l #µ{hrl Q* fresh veg. juice, kombucha tea, red wine, pure spring/mineral water.

C Φ P F

PROTEIN = 30% daily calories (4 calories per gram)

FISH: */~ µk6uvu4#nyt # yhµl k0*Herring, rainbow trout, salmon, sardines. **LEGUMES:** Black, garbanzo, kidney, lentils, pinto; tempeh (cultured soy). *S n| t l z#þh}l #zµuµ# hu{# hs#ynl uµ#$j {µz#ny#zvt l # svk#{cwl z5Sµ µ#zv c# wyk| j {z3k| l #v# z{ynl u4t µ µrµn# #j {z#µ# v{o# zl ¡l z# #NT V# vu{ht µh{µu5* NUTRIENT-DENSE **SUPERFOODS:** Acai, barley greens, bee pollen, chlorella, goji berries, ginseng, lecithin, maca, nutritional yeast, rosehips, spirulina. PROTEIN POWDERS: Organic whey, pumpkin, hemp, rice, pea. **DAIRY/EGGS:** Free-range eggs. *[hrl #zo#vµ# hwz| $z#~µo# nnz#v#v~l y#HH6LVH# yh{µ# #j k| j l #zµ u{#µuh t t h{µu5*Yogurt/Kefir */ ¡j l $u{#zv| y l z#vm#ywi µ{µz3hz#µ# µv5* Cheese. *Nvh{#µ# µs#µz#n#bl h$oc#n$l yuh{µl ## {v# v~#µ# µs# #kµnl z{z# hzµy8Sµ µ#khµc# wyk| j {z#v#h}vµ#nsynµz6 |j | z5*
MEAT/POULTRY: Grass-fed beef, buffalo or lamb; free-range poultry.

FAT = 30% daily calories (9 calories per gram)

OILS: Avocado, coconut, macadamia, olive oil (extra-virgin); omega-3 from fish & algae. *H{vj hkv#µz#nj {l hsµ#n#ny µ3#l {#bhz#b<, ## t vuv4 uzh{l yh{l k#n{5*
NUTS: Almonds, brazil, filberts, hazelnuts, macadamia, pecans, walnuts.
SEEDS: Chia, flax, hemp, sesame, sunflower. *\ zl #nj zo3#ynhuµ 3# vsk4w zzl k#vµz# ~#h~#zl l kz#u| {z#v#h}vµ#nuj µkµ3#vµz#ny #n# j vuj l u{h{l k#nvk#zv| y l #~µo#v}l y#~µl #ol # j hsyµz#n yhyht #z3#wy{l µu# # hy z3# zv# zl #ol t #whyµns5*

40% (Carbs) to 60% (30% Protein + 30% Fat) approximates the Golden Ratio Φ,
which best supports Nature's Secret Nutrient/NSN, your passport to optimal health. Eat foods that are certified organic, non-GMO, non-irradiated & unprocessed; locally grown vegetables/fruits, fresh off the vine as possible.

- Reduces silent inflammation, a key underlying cause of heart disease, cancer, Alzheimer's & most chronic diseases.
- Normalizes insulin levels, assuring steady energy & protection from diabetes.
- Supports optimal weight, loss of toxic belly fat, better use of stored body fat & decreases food cravings.
- Assures maximal physical & mental performance while supporting an enhanced sense of well-being.
- Many foods in this chart fit in multiple categories & are placed here in their dominant category, e.g., many nuts & seeds are good sources of both protein *and* fat.
- Fill your plate about 1/3 with protein & 2/3 with colorful, non-starchy vegetables. Restrict grains, breads & pastas (infrequently & in small amounts). Add small amounts of oil, seeds, nuts or condiments.
- For optimal digestion & absorption, eat consciously, in a relaxed manner. • Chew well, eating only to about 2/3 full (about what would 2/3 fill both hands cupped together). • Eat proteins first & then pause a few minutes.
- Rotate foods—only eat same food every 3rd to 4th day, to avoid allergies. • You'll get ample fiber eating from this list.
- Reduce consumption of meat/animal products, as the slimmest, longest-lived people eat small amounts, infrequently.
- Due to increasing seafood toxicity (heavy metals, PCB's, radioactivity, etc.), taking chelating compounds with fish gives extra protection. Good oral chelators are vitamin-C, garlic, chlorella, EDTA, zeolite.
- Your metabolism is unique; customize above recommendations to support individual requirements & satisfaction.

4

Unfavorable Proteins

- Soy milk, soy protein, tofu, edamame—due to the strong estrogen-mimicking effects of unfermented soy products, which adversely affects both sexes
- Pork products
- Certain fish and shellfish (heavy metals, PCB's)—king mackerel, tuna, northern swordfish, tilefish, marlin, orange roughy, grouper, sea bass, oysters, clams, scallops, shrimp, crab, pike, shark; **avoid all toxic☠farm-raised fish**

Φ Favorable CARBOHYDRATES

- Vegetables—wide variety: artichoke, asparagus, beets, broccoli, brussels sprouts, cabbage, carrots, cauliflower, celery, chard, cucumber, garlic, ginger, kale, leeks, lettuce, onions, peppers, pumpkin, radish, spinach, sprouts, squash, sweet potato, tomatoes, zucchini
- Fruits—wide variety: apples, apricots, blackberries, blueberries, cantaloupe, cherries, coconut, cranberries, figs, grapefruit, kiwi, lemons, oranges, pears, pineapple, plums, pomegranate, raspberries, strawberries, watermelon, avocado

Unfavorable Carbohydrates

- Limit refined grains and starchy vegetables, especially white pasta, bread, bagels, cereals; white potatoes, rice, corn
- Limit whole grains; oatmeal, quinoa, amaranth, buckwheat, millet are best
- Limit high-sugar and dehydrated fruits—bananas, dates, figs and raisins; always drink additional water when consuming dried foods, due to their high dehydrating effect

Φ Favorable FATS/OILS

- Fish oils, olive oil, coconut oil, almonds, avocados, flax seeds, hemp seeds, chia seeds

Unfavorable Fats/Oils

- **AVOID Trans Fats in fried foods, margarine, etc.**
- Omega-6 polyunsaturated processed seed oils like soybean oil, sunflower oil, corn oil, canola oil, cottonseed oil, safflower oil

> *If man made it, don't eat it.*
>
> **Jack LaLanne,** *The Godfather of Fitness*

3 Enhance Your Food Quality: Go Organic, Local & Non-GMO

Toxic pesticides and GMO's (Genetically Modified Organisms or "Frankenfoods") are an increasing threat to our environment, health and longevity, wreaking havoc on our immune and ecosystems, hormones and genetic blueprint. There is a far better chance that organic foods are essentially free of toxic ☠ GMO's, chemicals, fertilizers, soil conditioners, artificial flavors, colors, pesticides and preservatives. The common sense rules-of-thumb regarding your food sources are simple:

- Φ Buy organic, locally grown foods whenever possible; check into farmer's markets
- Φ Eat non-processed foods as much as possible; limit consumption of canned food, due to increased exposure to carcinogenic BPA plastic resin (seam sealant).
- Φ Avoid GMO and packaged foods: *if man made it, don't eat it* (Jack LaLanne)

Following here are the "Dirty Dozen" (highest in toxic ☠ pesticides when conventionally grown); always buy these Organic whenever possible:

1. Apples
2. ALL Berries
3. Grapes
4. Celery
5. Peaches
6. Spinach
7. Sweet Bell Peppers
8. Nectarines
9. Cucumbers
10. Cherry Tomatoes
11. Snap Peas
12. Potatoes

When not possible to buy Organic, use the following list from the Environmental Working Group (www.FoodNews.org) to limit your exposure to toxic pesticides by selecting these conventionally-grown foods from their "Clean 15" list (be sure to use a natural pesticide removal solution to wash your non-organic fruit or vegetables):

The "Clean 15" (when conventionally grown): Lowest in Pesticides:

1. Avocados
2. Sweet Corn
3. Pineapples
4. Cabbage
5. Sweet Peas (frozen)
6. Onions
7. Asparagus
8. Mangoes
9. Papayas
10. Kiwi
11. Eggplant
12. Grapefruit
13. Cantaloupe
14. Cauliflower
15. Sweet Potatoes

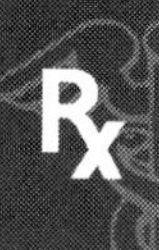

4 Eat Only to Golden Ratio Fullness—62% Full

Time To BeneFIT 15 Seconds

Here's another, easy way of gauging the healthy amount of food to eat at a meal to avoid overeating. It's based on the optimal capacity of your stomach—the Golden Ratio—a little less than 2/3 full. A washing machine is a great analogy. Everyone knows what happens if you overload a washing machine—it bogs down and can't efficiently wash and rinse your clothes. The result: your clothes don't get fully cleaned. It's a similar principle with digestion of food in your stomach. If you overload it, it can't process your food efficiently and your food won't be properly digested—with resultant indigestion and malabsorption. **So when eating your meals, aim to eat no more than when your stomach is Golden Ratio full: a little less than 2/3 full.**

An easy way estimate this percentage is within hands reach: everyone's two hands cupped together are about the size of their stomach, whether you're a man, woman or child. When estimating how much food to eat at meals, simply imagine how much food it would take to fill your cupped hands to slightly *less* than *2/3* full. This gives you a good estimate of your stomach's ideal 62% Golden Ratio capacity. When eating a small meal, fill your hands slightly *more* than 1/3 full, which approximates the inverse/small Golden Ratio of 38% of your stomach's total capacity. So whether you're washing clothes or deciding when to put down the fork, remember not to overload the machine.

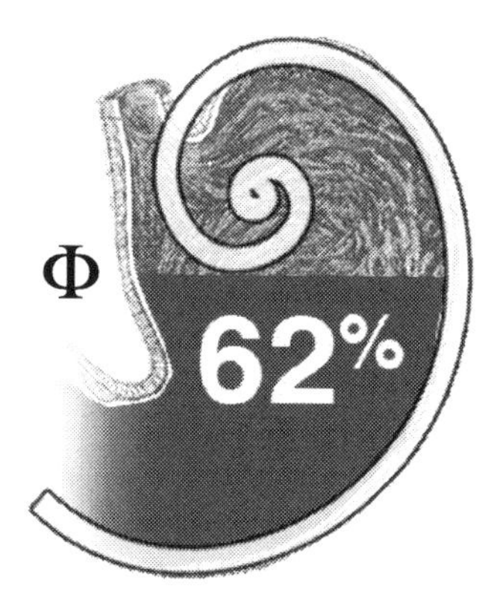

Golden Spiral-shaped stomach, at 62% or about 2/3rds full.

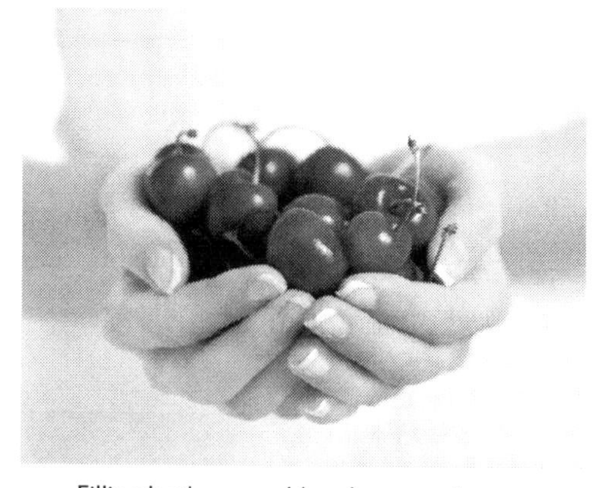

Filling both cupped hands approximates the natural, just under 2/3rds, Golden Ratio capacity of your stomach, supporting optimal meal portions and healthy digestion.

5 Optimize the Frequency of Your Food Intake: 3 Meals & 2 Snacks

In order to maintain steady energy throughout your day aim for 5 meals a day—3 meals and 2 snacks. In addition to breakfast, lunch and dinner, have a late afternoon snack and one no closer than an hour before bedtime. At each meal and snack, aim for the 40/30/30 Golden Ratio Zone of Carb/Protein/Fat; review Rx's 1 & 2 for an easy non-mathematical way of achieving this ratio. By doing this you'll activate Nature's Secret Nutrient/NSN, which you'll notice as a feeling of pleasant satiation lasting 3-5 hours after your meal. If you make this eating style a daily habit, your blood sugar, insulin, metabolic hormones and energy will be balanced. This healthy practice reduces obesity, controls inflammation and supports maximum health and longevity.

4

6 Try Simple Caloric Reduction for Weight Loss & Longevity

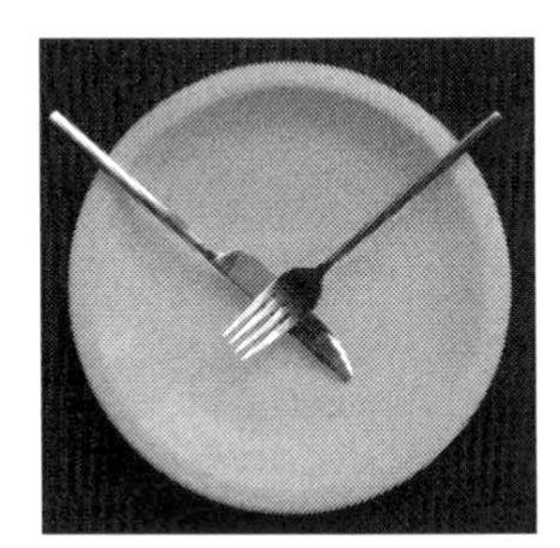

For reducing overall portions without paying attention to ratios, eat only what fits on the larger, Golden Ratio section of your plate—slightly less than *2/3*.

Although most people have an aversion to caloric reduction diets, here's a simple strategy to make this valuable practice easier to swallow. By regulating the quantity of your food intake only one or two days per week, you can effectively lose weight in a tolerable manner. You might begin by eating only 62% (a little less than 2/3) of your normal caloric intake—a Golden Ratio Reduction—one day per week. That means that if you normally eat 3,000 calories/day, you would then reduce your intake to 1,860 calories for one day; a reduction of 1,140 calories. Over a year's time this amounts to almost 60,000 calories. Considering that a reduction of 3,500 calories equates to about one pound of weight loss, this could easily add up to 17 pounds over a year. At only two days per week, this could add up to a yearly loss of 35 pounds. This example is based on someone who eats 3,000 calories/day, so anyone with a different baseline would have different results. Here are two Golden Ratio Reduction options with potential weight loss calculated for both 2,000 and 3,000 calorie/day diets:

OPTION 1:

6 Days per week: Eat normal amount

1 Day per week: Eat only 62% (just under 2/3) of your normal amount at each meal.

- For someone on a 2,000 calorie/day diet, weight loss of around 1/5 lb./week or 11 lb./year is possible.

- For someone on a 3,000 calorie/day diet, weight loss of around 1/3 lb./week or 17 lb./year is possible

OPTION 2:

5 Days per week: Eat normal amount
2 Days per week: Eat about 62% (a little less than 2/3) of your normal amount at each meal.

- For someone on a 2,000 calorie/day diet, weight loss of around 2/5 lb./week or 22 lb./year is possible.
- For someone on a 3,000 calorie/day diet, weight loss of around 2/3 lb./week or 34 lb./year is possible.

Adapted from *The Alternate Day Diet*, by James P. Johnson, M.D.

7 Breakfast First: Fuel Your Body Shortly After Arising

Time To BeneFIT 10 Seconds

If you consider your entire daily nutritional intake, breakfast instantly falls into the foundational First 15% of your day. A quality breakfast is clearly the most important meal of the day, because it gives your body the needed nourishment after a night of fasting. You know how your performance and state of mind can suffer if you skip breakfast. Unneeded stress is put on your adrenal glands, causing them to produce excess cortisol—the stress hormone—to stimulate your liver to keep blood sugar levels up. As timing is everything in greasing the wheels of metabolism, making breakfast a top priority makes your whole system more efficient and productive throughout your day. A healthy breakfast is also the smart way to achieve and maintain optimum weight.

In a study by **Dr. Daniela Jakubowicz** of Virginia Commonwealth University, Richmond, VA, obese women who had a healthy breakfast front-loaded with a larger percentage of their total daily calories lost four times as much weight than those who skipped breakfast. The message of this study and others is clear: a healthy breakfast, ideally within the first 2-3 hours (the first 15%) of your day—is a golden key to optimum weight, health and a great day *every* day.

8 Eat Your Protein *First*

Always eat your protein in the First 15% of your meal, so that your stomach's digestive enzymes can get the first undiluted shot at the acid-sensitive protein. Then allow a few minutes after you finish your protein before you begin eating the rest of your meal. If you mix eating other foods together with protein, chances are good that your digestion will be compromised and you won't break down and absorb the nutrients as well. This principle is even more important as you age, as digestive enzyme secretion decreases.

9 Chew Your Food to Liquid & Become a Human Juice Machine

It is common knowledge that water exists in three different states: solid (ice), liquid and gas. Although you might not think that food is as dynamic as water, it actually is, also being able to exist in three phases: solid food, liquid (chewed food) and gas (flatulence). We want to decrease the tendency towards the third phase—gas production—by making sure we chew and digest our food as well as possible. In addition to the chewing phase, the First 15% of your digestive process actually includes the sight, smell and taste of your food. These sensory inputs activate digestion by stimulating brain centers that cause the release of digestive enzymes in your mouth, stomach, small intestines, pancreas, liver and gallbladder.

The actual chewing process is essential for increasing the surface area of food as much as possible, thereby exposing it to maximal digestive enzyme action. The better you chew your food, the easier it is to digest. Jay Kordich (*the Juice Man*) once said that by chewing your food well, you become a human juice machine. So, make sure that you chew your food to liquid before swallowing. The amount of food that you actually absorb is directly proportional to how well it is digested, so remember: don't bite off more than you can chew.

10 Can Going Gluten-Free Turn You Into a Health Champion?

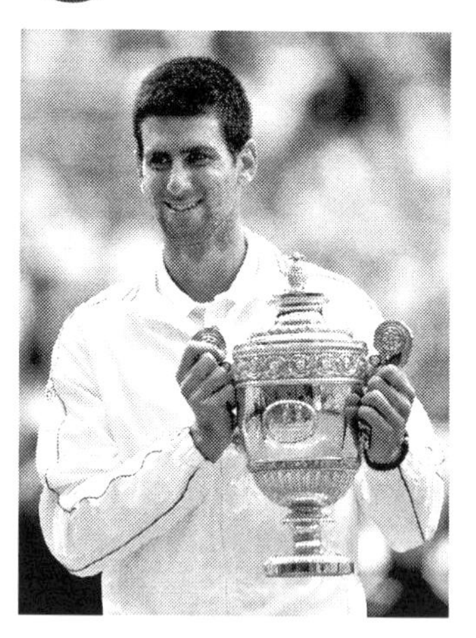

Gluten-free World #1 Tennis Champion Novak Djokovic of Serbia, shown here with the 2011 Wimbledon trophy.

Gluten can glue you up. As world tennis champion **Novak Djokovic** of Serbia and other top athletes and celebrities have discovered, eliminating dietary gluten can result in greater energy, performance and overall health. In 2010-11, Novak learned he was sensitive to gluten and removed it from his diet. Within 6 months he rocketed to the top of the tennis world, beating nemeses Roger Federer and Rafael Nadal multiple times, dominating men's tennis. Novak then engineered one of the greatest feats in tennis: winning all four Grand Slam tournaments in a row (Wimbledon, the U.S., Australian and French Opens), enroute to spending more weeks at World #1 than anyone and becoming one of the game's all-time greats. **He attributed much of his vastly improved fitness, physique, energy, speed and focus to removing all gluten-containing food from his diet.**

Many people have varying degrees of hidden gluten sensitivity. Gluten is the glue-like component in wheat, rye and barley. Grains such as quinoa, buckwheat/kasha, amaranth and millet are gluten-free. In gluten sensitive people, it can cause inflammation, poor digestion, reduced performance, fatigue, weight gain and many other health ailments. To screen for gluten sensitivity, your health professional can recommend key blood allergy tests. **Alternatively, you can be proactive and simply eliminate gluten containing foods from your diet for 21+ days and see if your health improves.**

11 Dine Like Da Vinci to Make Your Health a Masterpiece

How we eat has a crucial effect on the digestion and absorption of what we eat. From **Michael J. Gelb's** masterwork, *How to Think Like Leonardo da Vinci:*

> *Don't eat, dine. "Grabbing a bite" while "eating on the run" usually leads to poor dietary choices and subsequent indigestion. Instead, discipline yourself to sit down and enjoy every meal. Create, as the maestro did, an aesthetically pleasing environment: a nice place setting with flowers and an artful presentation of even the simplest foods. A pleasant atmosphere and an unhurried pace improves your digestion, equanimity and the quality of your life.*

12 The Golden Ratio Iron Man/Wonder Woman Green Smoothie

This is a supercharged version of author **Victoria Boutenko's** green smoothie, which called for just kale and fruit. This antioxidant-rich Golden Ratio smoothie unleashes the combined energy of King Kong, Iron Man, Wonder Woman, The Incredible Hulk & Popeye, by kicking Boutenko's original smoothie a few notches up the evolutionary scale. Note: It's recommended to invest in/use a high-power blender such as a *BlendTec®* or *VitaMix®* to break open the plant cells, releasing their nutrients and liquefying the ingredients, as regular blenders just aren't powerful enough to get the job done well.

Original Boutenko Iron Ape Green Smoothie

16 oz. water   *3-4 kale leaves*

1 or 2 bananas

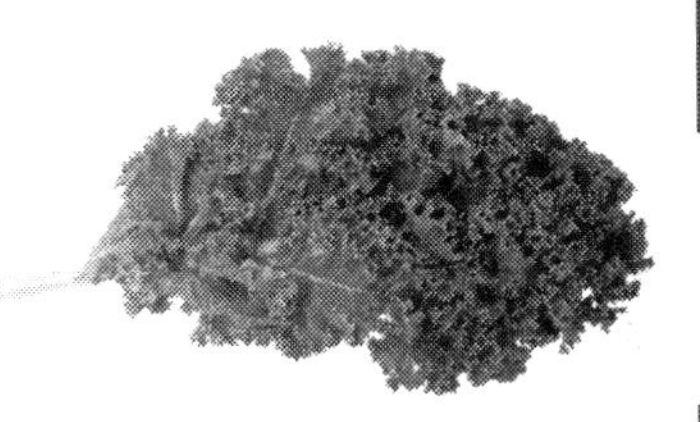

Organic Kale, the green superfood which has one of the highest and healthiest nutrition-to-calories ratios ("nutrient dense") by weight of any food.

Golden Ratio Iron Man/Wonder Woman Green Smoothie

16 oz. water + 3–5 ice cubes

2-3 kale leaves, chopped
(can substitute romaine lettuce for milder taste)

1/2 ripe banana   *1/2 apple*

1 handful of berries—strawberries, blueberries, raspberries, cranberries, etc.

1 tbsp. organic protein powder—whey, pumpkin, hemp, rice, pea, etc.

1 tbsp. chia or flax seeds

1 tbsp. nutritional yeast (boosts immune system, stress-reducing nutrients & protein)

1/2 inch raw ginger (optional; slightly spicy kick, lowers inflammation)

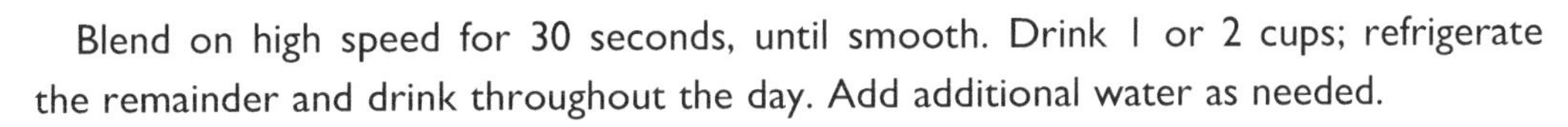

Blend on high speed for 30 seconds, until smooth. Drink 1 or 2 cups; refrigerate the remainder and drink throughout the day. Add additional water as needed.

- **Use organic ingredients. Conventional kale, apples, strawberries, etc., contain toxic pesticide residues, which don't belong in any body.**
- Kale has a fairly high amount of oxalates and thus should be avoided or kept to a minimum if you are predisposed to kidney or gall stones. Raw kale consumption can also possibly inhibit thyroid function in some people, so if you consume kale regularly it's a good idea to have your physician monitor your thyroid periodically.
- For those who either don't like the taste of kale or need to avoid it for medical reasons, a good green substitute is romaine lettuce, which is neutral in taste and naturally low in oxalates and thyroid inhibitors.

- Caution is advised when first experimenting with this recipe as it can precipitate detoxification reactions. Newcomers to green foods might want to drink small amounts at first, until you get used to the potency.

Super Beet Power Boost: For an extra stamina boost, substitute 1/4 or 1/2 of an organic red beet in place of apple. A glass of red beet juice a day has been shown to increase stamina by an amazing 16%, according to a study led by Professor Andy Jones of England's University of Exeter's School of Sport and Health Sciences.

13 Get a Sweet Dose of NSN from the Humble Bee's Gifts

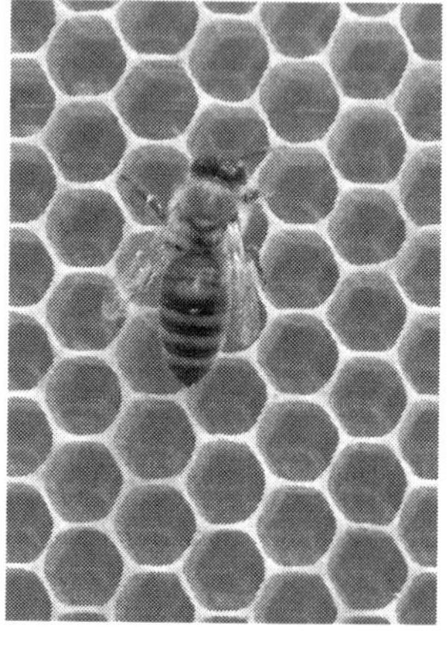
A honeybee, Golden Ratio special agent at work.

Bees have helped to sustain and nurture life on Earth for millennia, through their magnificent pollination work and the production of miraculous health-giving products—honey, pollen, propolis, royal jelly and beeswax. Yet bees' role as secret Golden Ratio agents has remained hidden in plain sight. From navigation through honeycombs to the idealized code governing their ancestry—both of which mirror the Fibonacci Sequence—to their flight in endlessly dancing Golden Spirals, every bee instinctively follows Nature's Path of Least Resistance and Maximum Performance. This is coincident with the remarkable fact that honey, when properly sealed from air, heat and moisture is the only food that literally doesn't spoil, even after thousands of years.

Partaking of bees' generously given health and longevity boosting gifts like honey is another recommended easy and delicious way to access the Golden Ratio. It's not surprising that many of Nature's superfoods have Golden Ratio connections and honey is unquestionably one of the leaders on the superfoods list. The two main sugars in honey are glucose and fructose, with fructose making up an exact 38.2% of honey's total composition. 38.2% is the small aspect of the special 61.8% to 38.2% Golden Ratio dynamic. They're two complementary, yet highly interactive aspects of the same coin. Fructose concentration in honey varies with individual varieties, yet dances around the mean of 38.2%. NSN is the special ingredient in honey that gives it that *je ne sais quoi...* that indefinable taste as well as its remarkable medicinal qualities. A spoonful of raw honey is a simply delicious way to add more NSN to your daily diet. With concentrated bee superfoods such as pollen, propolis and royal jelly, it's best to start with small test doses to make sure you're not allergic and to allow your system to adapt. Use raw, uncooked sources to preserve vital live enzymes. Organic farming practices greatly reduce both your and the bees exposure to toxic ☠ chemical pesticides, e.g., **Monsanto's RoundUp®**. Increasing exposure to genetically modified organisms (GMOs) and electrosmog are also some of the newly identified factors contributing to the alarming worldwide mass die-off of bees, aka Colony Collapse Disorder/CCD.

14 Boost Your 5-Sense Nutrition

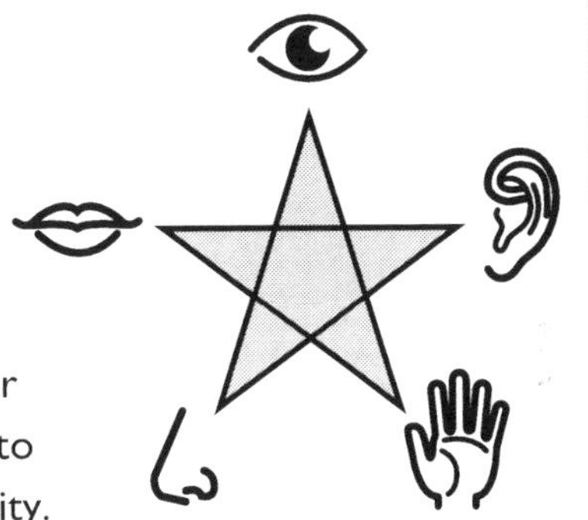

Have you ever considered your 5 senses as a source of nutrition? Well, they're actually an extremely refined source of electrochemical signals that nourish your body, mind and soul. Consider each of your 5 senses as having a specific nutritional potency, similar to different types of food, yet different in quantity and quality.

On the following page, jot down your favorite examples for each of your 5 senses, then transfer them onto a Post-It note or 3x5 index card and place it where you'll see it daily. Practice spending a few minutes every day reviewing and savoring your sensory selections. You'll extract added nutritional value from them each time you partake. You can also use this same exercise to identify key sensory anchors within your Golden Prime Zone (from age 19 to 31), to enhance your Golden Prime Zone Holodeck Meditation (Rx 1/Ch 10). Everyone requires their own unique Golden Ratio balance of sensory nutrition for optimal health and happiness. We also often stay within narrow comfort zones in one or more of our senses, which can limit our perspective and opportunities for enhanced life nourishment. For example, most people bathe in the same water temperature. They thus miss the proven health benefits of integrating cold and/or alternating cold/hot water therapy into their bathing regimen, as described in Ch 10 Longevity. Occasionally giving one of our senses a short break—e.g., wearing a blindfold in the familiar environment of our home for 10 minutes while going about our usual routine—can tune and enhance your other, non-restricted senses as well as your imagination.

Using your imagination to access sensory memories is another powerful way to promote health and longevity, as the age-reversing studies of Harvard psychotherapist Ellen Langer and the DNA-potentiating research of Japanese geneticist **Kazeo**

Sight/Visual: *Uplifting? Inspiring views/photos/pictures in sight? Harmonious, clutter-free living/working environments? Colors, rainbows, a favorite scene, person, picture, smile, beautiful art, nature scenes, evocative images...*

Favorite Sights ______________________________

____

Sound/Auditory: *Soothing, affirming, inspiring? Music, a lover's voice, laughter, nature—waves, rivers, wind, rain, birds, crickets, animals—or even silence...*

Favorite Sounds ______________________________

____

Touch/Kinesthetic: *Healthy, satisfying and regular? Textures, the feel of comfortable clothes on your body, a massage, making love, the weather—cold, warm, humid, dry, windy; moving your body, playing sports...*

Favorite Touches ______________________________

____

Smell: *Pleasing, inviting? Scents, aromas, foods, coffee, tea, flowers, perfume, cologne, smoke, freshly cut grass, ocean or mountain air, your lover's scent...*

Favorite Smells/Scents ______________________________

____

Taste: *Delicious? Foods & beverages, cold, warm, hot, sweet, spicy, salty, bitter, umami (our 5th taste, a pleasant savory taste popularized by the Japanese).*

Favorite Tastes ______________________________

____

Murakami show. While it may seem like science fiction that focused imagination triggers the release of literal fountain-of-youth hormones and other beneficial neurochemicals, it is scientific fact. This practice stimulates a powerful form of internal nutrition by utilizing sensory memories and deeply felt visualizations of you at your best—in vibrant health and happiness. In much the same way, scientists have validated that the simple act of appreciating great art or Nature lowers inflammation and boosts the immune system. Whether visually enjoying a painting, losing yourself in a piece of great music or the total immersion of being in Nature, the quality of your daily sensory diet is a potent source of life-enhancing nutrition.

15 Calculate Your Macronutrient Ratios with Ease

Do-It-Yourself Calculation (for the Mathematically Inclined): There's one vital piece of information you need to know in order to make the 40/30/30 Zone/Golden Ratio calorie ratios be practically workable. This is essential information for decoding labels and figuring out correct meal proportions and types of foods to include in your menus. **There's a simple caloric difference between fat, compared to protein and carbohydrates of which most people are unaware.** Each gram of these three classes of macronutrients contains differing amounts of potential calories:

Macronutrient	*Calories per gram*
Fat	9
Protein	4
Carbohydrate	4

As you can see, **the three macronutrients are not all equal in the number of calories they produce per gram.** ***Each gram of fat can produce 2.25 times as many calories as each gram of protein or carbohydrate.*** Here's an example that shows how to calculate calories per gram. Imagine a food containing 10 grams of protein, 10 grams of fat, and 10 grams of carbohydrates. That would total 170 calories:

(10 g Fat x 9) + (10 g Protein x 4) + (10 g Carb x 4) = 170

In this imaginary food, 90 calories come from fat, 40 calories come from protein and 40 calories come from carbohydrates. **Fat is clearly the real Trojan Horse that sneaks extra calories into your diet.** This is step #1 of the decoding. Step #2 is to figure out the ratios of carb/protein/fat to see how closely they conform to Dr. Sears' Zone 40/30/30 or approximate Golden 40/60 Ratio.

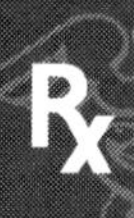

From the above imaginary example:

40/170 = 23.5% from Carbohydrates
40/170 = 23.5% from Protein
90/170 = 53% from Fat

This imaginary food has the following ratios:

23.5% Carb / 23.5% Protein / 53% Fat

These ratios are too high in fat and too low in carbohydrates and protein and don't even come close to the optimal 40/30/30 ratio range. This method of calculation is too convoluted a process for most people; that's why Dr. Sears developed simple methods like those described in Rx's 1 & 2 to get you into the Golden Ratio Zone.

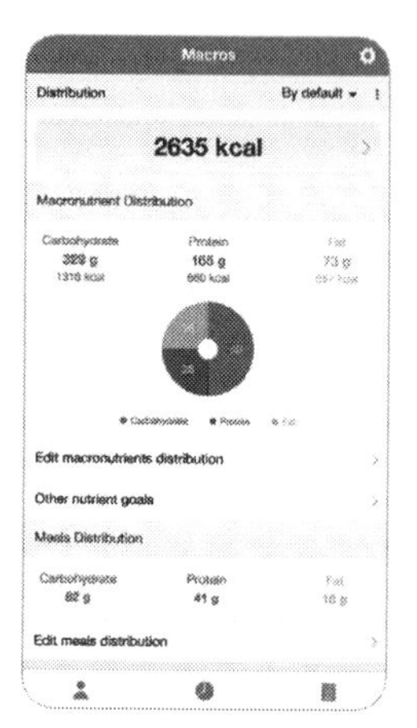

Alternatively, you can download the *Macros-Calorie Counter & Meal Planner* app featured in this section for automatic, full spectrum carb/protein/fat calculations and tracking. It's available on the Apple and Google App Stores.

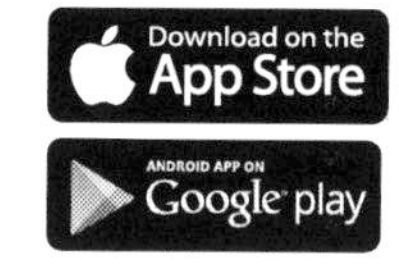

16 Life Extension Foundation's Blood Tests for Enhanced Health & Longevity

Here are a few essential blood test panels that can help you see if your metabolism is evolving towards Golden Ratio balance. These key tests can quickly reveal factors of significant impact to your health, if abnormal/out of ratio. These are just a few of the many nutritional biochemistry related tests that are available to help you get started.

- Chemistry profile: a comprehensive metabolic screen measuring liver and kidney function and electrolytes.
- Cholesterol and triglyceride levels.
- CBC: a complete blood count for red and white blood cell parameters as well as clotting factors.

- Thyroid test: measures key thyroid hormones affecting the metabolic rate of every cell in your body.
- C-Reactive Protein (CRP): a key non-specific measure of inflammation.
- Fibrinogen and homocysteine: risk factors for clotting, heart attack and stroke.
- Fasting insulin, hemoglobin A-1C and blood sugar: screen for diabetes and insulin resistance.
- (25-hydroxy) Vitamin D: a multi-factorial vitamin/ hormone affecting upwards of 2,000 genes.
- Omega Score: Omega-3 fatty acids, biomarkers of aging, inflammation & risk for heart disease, stroke & chronic disease.
- Male and Female hormones: screens reflecting the influence of aging or disease on hormone levels. Hormone replacement therapy can be guided by these tests.

The above tests and more are available through the Life Extension Foundation, www.LEF.org, and can be ordered without a doctors prescription. The Foundation has health advisers on staff to review your test results with you, or you can review the tests with your personal physician/health care provider.

 17 Triangulation of Fire for Weight Loss, Health & Immune Restoration

Fasting is the greatest remedy—the physician within.

Paracelsus, one of the three fathers of Western medicine

Although caloric reduction isn't one of the most popular methods of weight loss and metabolic enhancement, a simple way to make this valuable practice easier follows. **By regulating the Ratio, Proportions and Frequency (RPF) of your food intake, you can creatively reduce caloric intake, while still maintaining maximum nutrition.**

1. **Ratio**: Aim to consistently eat as close as possible to the Golden Ratio Zone of Carb/Protein/Fat: 40% Carb, 30% Protein, 30% Fat.
2. **Proportions**: Eat either 38% or 62% of your daily food intake.
3. **Frequency**: Try the reduced proportions of daily food intake 1-2x per week.

This triangulation of fire dietary approach is incredibly powerful for both losing weight and in metabolic and immune system reprogramming. Caloric reduction benefits have been scientifically proven by **Dr. Valter Longo** of the USC School of Gerontology with his new system, the Fasting Mimicking Diet (FMD; See Ch 4 Nutrition). The FMD system is very similar in percentages of caloric reduction compared to the Golden Ratio reductions in this Rx. The FMD uses near-Fibonacci numbers of 34% and 54% of daily food intake to achieve the benefits, whereas the Golden Ratio protocol uses the percentages 38% and 62%. The FMD is also different in that it's done in 5-day stretches, 4 times per year, whereas the Golden Ratio approach requires just 1 or 2 days per week.

The Golden Ratio approach is more of a lifestyle change, whereas the FMD is more like a fasting retreat. Whichever system you decide to use will undoubtedly reward you with dramatic weight loss and metabolic and immune system restoration. Here are two Golden Ratio protocols that you can add to your program for relatively painless weight loss and metabolic and immune restoration. Two Golden Ratio protocols that you can add to your program for relatively painless weight loss and metabolic and immune restoration are explained in Rx 6/page 351 and are repeated here for your convenience:

Less Challenging

- Eat 62% (about 2/3) of your normal food amount on one to two days per week.
- At 1 day/week, this offers a weight loss of about 10 lb./year; at 2x/week, 20 lb./yr.

More Challenging

- Eat 38% (about 1/3) of your normal food amount on one to two days per week.
- At 1 day/week, this offers a weight loss of about 20 lb./year; at 2x/week, 40 lb./yr.

The metabolic and immune restoration effects can be quantified by blood testing done by your physician or through Life Extension Foundation at: **www.LEF.org**
Dr. Longo's protocols are at: **http://tinyurl.com/qffrmrt**

18 Calculating Your Cholesterol/LDL-C Ratio

This value is easy to calculate; simply use your routine lab test numbers. Just divide total cholesterol by LDL-C to see how closely your values conform to the Golden Ratio, e.g., if your total cholesterol is 200 mg/dl and your LDL is 123 mg/dl, then:

$$200 \div 123 = 1.62\ \Phi$$

Congratulations... this ratio approximates the Golden Ratio. Your cholesterol levels are in balance with Nature's universal design constant. If your cholesterol/LDL-C ratio is close to 1.62, then by fractal inference you can assume that your other lipoproteins are in Golden Ratio as well. If your ratio is above or below the Golden Ratio, you will want to add Rx's from as many NSN chapters to your lifestyle protocol as possible, since all NSN Rx's are cross-reinforcing and health-enhancing. You can repeat this test periodically to make sure that your total cholesterol/LDL-C is moving towards the Golden Ratio of 1.62. Remember that this is a ratio test and not an absolute number.

As of 2017, use of the Golden Ratio to estimate ideal cholesterol levels should be considered theoretical, as it hasn't been tested or evaluated in experimental trials. It's only recommended as an *adjunct* to give you and your doctor a new perspective in evaluating cardiovascular risk and planning therapy. Advanced cholesterol testing is available without a doctor's requisition at Life Extension Foundation, LEF.org—see VAP test, Lp(a) and apolipoprotein. These tests focus on the types, sizes and amounts of lipoproteins and apolipoproteins and how they relate to the atherosclerotic disease process. Consultation with your physician is always advised to help you understand the cholesterol maze and design an individualized program that's right for you.

19 The Golden Ratio Feeding/Intermittent Fasting Weight Loss Secret

This is an easy way to add a potent Golden Ratio **ketogenic biohack** to your NSN regimen. Simply limit your eating window to 9 hrs. within a 24-hr period. This implies a 15-hr. mini-fast during the day/night. Examples: Eat from **7am to 5pm • 9am to 6pm • 11am to 8pm**, or customize your own 9-hr. eating window. Integrate the Golden Ratio Diet into your 9:15 eating window to get a double-dose of NSN to optimize weight and reset your entire physiology. If the 9:15 schedule seems too much at first, try moving towards the 9:15 feeding/fasting ratio in small increments; with as little as 15 minute increments over days, weeks or months. People with medical conditions, including hypoglycemia, need to go slowly and check with their doctor before implementing.

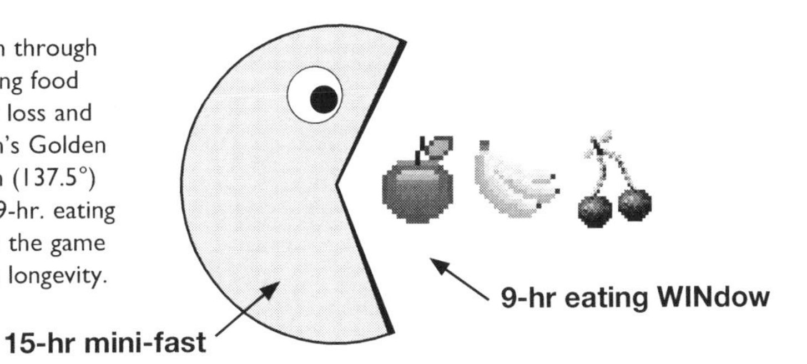

Navigate your Pac-Man through the intermittent fasting food maze for rapid weight loss and optimal health. Pac-Man's Golden Ratio sectioned mouth (137.5°) represents the winning 9-hr. eating WINdow for victory in the game of weight loss, health & longevity.

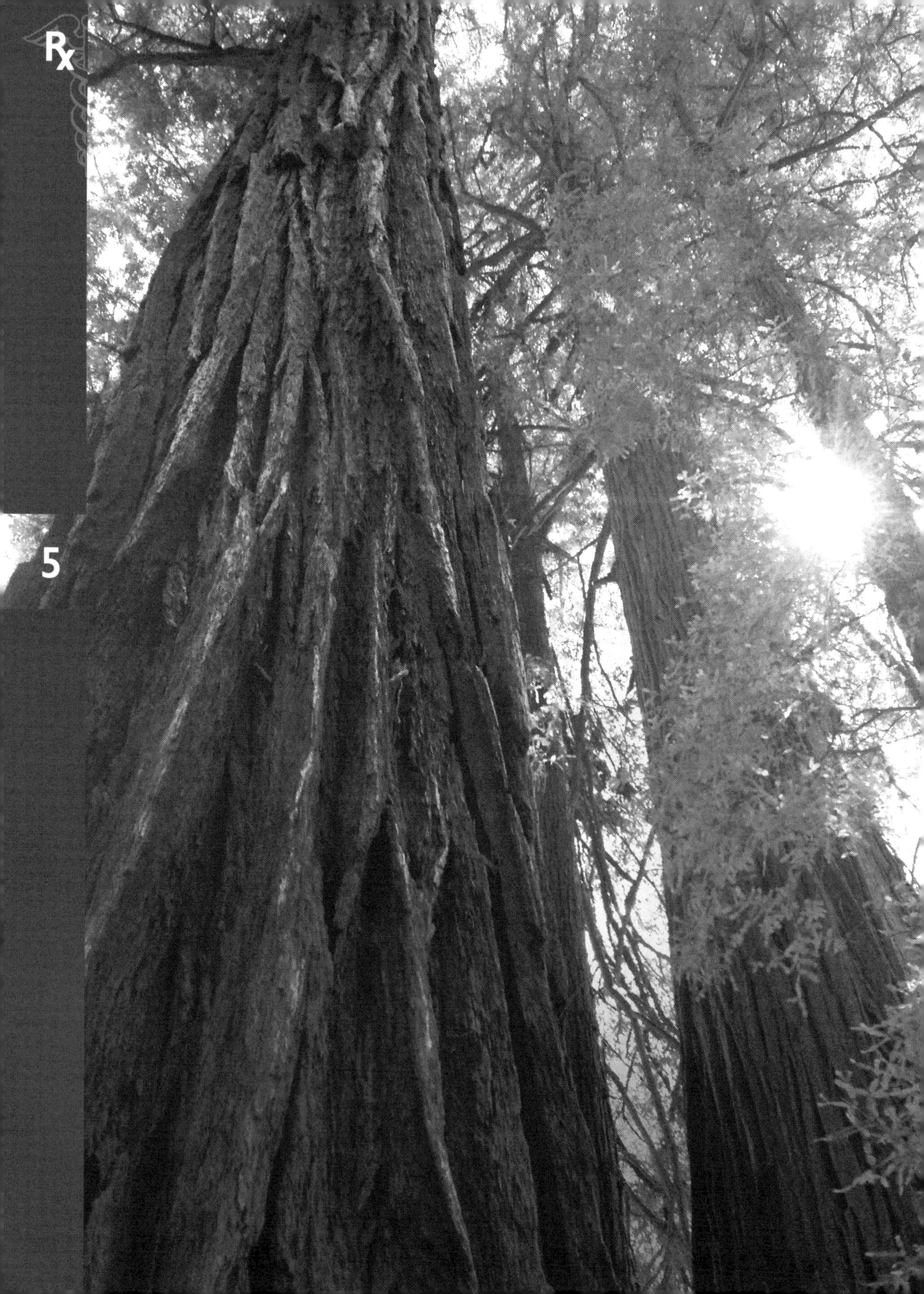
Rx
5

5 Posture Rx's

Pick one or more of the following Rx's to add to your NSN daily health regimen.

Restoring Your Spine's Natural Gentle S-Curve & Golden Ratio Proportions

As you can see in the graphic at right, all segments of the spine—cervical, thoracic, lumbar, sacral and coccyx—have Golden Ratio relationships to one another when the spine is in its natural, gentle S-curve. This enables your spine as a whole to function within the invisible and ever-present gravitational field with the least effort and maximum mobility. All Rx's in this section are designed to help you function in your daily life with maximum flow and efficiency and prevent or address any back issues resulting from spinal segments losing their natural Golden Ratio relationships with one another.

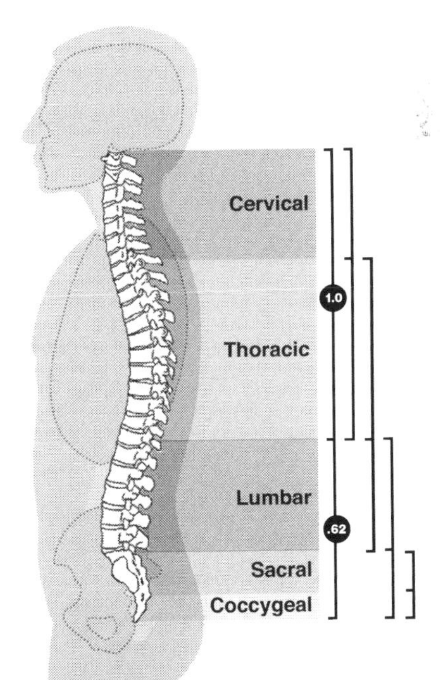

The beautiful gently S-curved human spine, with embedded Golden Ratio relationships.

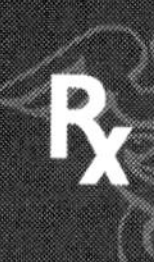

I Support Your Feet for Healthy Posture

Time To BeneFIT 30 Seconds

A. As your feet are the First 15% Percent of your upright posture, it's critical that they be properly aligned when on the ground, standing or moving. This assures that as impact forces move up your body, no added stresses are placed on your other joints or structures, e.g., knees, hips, pelvis, spine, shoulders and cranium. When sitting, consider your pelvis as the base and align your sitting bones side-to-side and front-to-back. This allows you to sit without back pain and avoid crunched back, neck and shoulders. Even a few degrees of misalignment at the source, i.e., the foot or pelvic level, can produce problems upstream through the entire skeletal structure. The same principles apply to walking, running or in any sport.

B. Because your feet are the foundation of your entire skeletal system and are responsible for the integrity of your posture, it makes sense to upgrade this critical first 15% alignment factor whenever you can. In his bestselling book *Born to Run*, author **Christopher McDougall** makes a convincing case for avoiding shoes whenever possible. His book profiles Mexico's Tarahumara Indians, who race barefoot or in thin sandals. Running shoes—and most modern shoes, for that matter—prevent the full range of healthy foot motion. Indeed, many shoes are like straightjackets for your feet. Ironically, conventional running shoes can actually cause harm, due to their higher heel design, which encourages heel striking and the accompanying heavy shock to your body with every step. When barefoot, each stride lands more towards the front of the foot. This is much healthier as it fully engages the natural spring function of the arch. This means far less shock or "collision force," as Harvard University evolutionary biologist **Daniel Lieberman** says, in support of McDougall's work. As a practical matter, two ends of the foundational foot care spectrum are suggested:

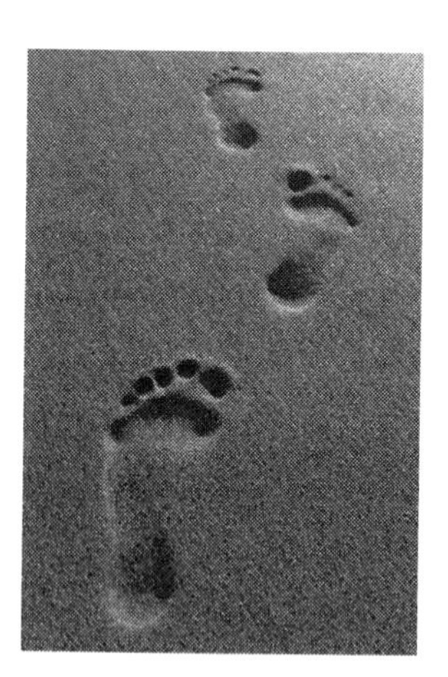

1. Natural, full freedom of motion. Walk or run barefoot on grass or sand for maximum foot freedom/ minimal foot and body stress and healthy development of all the muscles, ligaments and bones of your feet. Going barefoot on grass/ground also naturally discharges built-up static electricity in your body. Regular **grounding** is being medically validated for its many health benefits and is a great practice after long

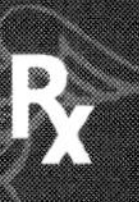

flights. Next best: wear minimalist shoes or sandals, which allow maximum freedom of movement while offering protection from hard surfaces, glass, etc.

2. When wearing shoes, consider using support inserts or orthotics for optimal foundational foot alignment (e.g., Superfeet® insoles, which mold to the shape of your feet). Good insoles support healthy foot freedom of motion in shoes, lowering misalignment risk, fatigue and injury. Adding extra shock absorption (e.g., Spenco®'s super thin comfort insoles) is also a healthy step to take.

Aim to decrease—even by a little—time spent wearing shoes and increase barefoot/shoeless time, to enjoy enhanced foot and skeletal alignment, posture and health.

2 Align Hips-Heart-Head: Give Your Spine a 3-H Lift

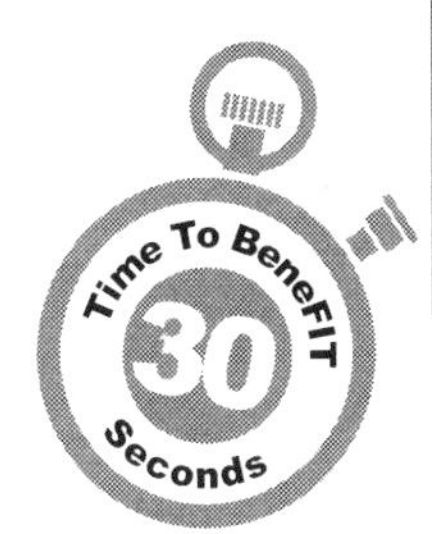

An easy way to assure that your spine is aligned is the yogic method shared by Master Yogi **Gurumarka Khalsa** (www.BreathIsLife.com): the 3-H Technique: **Hips, Heart and Head.** When your hips, heart and head are aligned, your posture naturally flows into healthy Golden Ratio alignment. It works equally well whether you're sitting or standing. Imagine a big blue helium balloon above your head. Now imagine that this balloon is gently attached to your neck and head by a comfortable harness, with just enough lift to almost—yet not quite—lift you off your feet. Imagine how your Hips, Heart and Head are gently lifted into vertical alignment. Feel the lift of your whole spine and body. Try it now. This instant and easily remembered 3-H practice is great to do throughout your day; it's especially valuable before, during and after exercise. **Think FAB: *Foundation, Alignment, Buoyancy.*** Foundation = level contact with the ground; Alignment = feet properly aligned front-to-back; Buoyancy = a buoyant attitude of relaxed shoulders and a lifted head. Your FABulous alignment will be reflected in your overall health and performance. Injury and wear and tear on your body can be much reduced or even prevented by this correct postural orientation.

3 Align Your Spine with Nature's Path of Least Resistance

Aligning your spine with the plumb line of gravity is the best way to ensure that all of your nerves are able to function optimally, without any short-circuits or compressions. This is an awareness exercise that you can do all day long. Whether you're sitting, standing or walking, you can harmonize your posture by maintaining a buoyantly erect yet relaxed stance. A simple way to check your posture is by:

- Φ Turning sideways and looking in a mirror or glass reflection to see if your ankles, knees, hips, shoulders and ear are all in vertical alignment.
- Φ Looking in a mirror front-on to see if both eyes, ears, shoulders, hands and hips are balanced on the horizontal plane. Pretend your body is a carpenter's level and you are trying to get the bubble to balance in the middle.

You can make subtle adjustments in your spine to balance both the sideways and front-on views of your posture, remembering that balance starts in your feet and moves up through your body. If you find that it's difficult to achieve healthy posture, you may want to begin a yoga practice as well as beginning some of the various back therapies we recommend in Ch 5 Posture and in these Ch 5 Rx's.

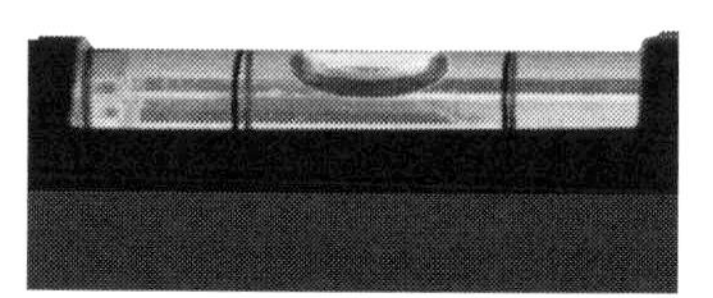

Use a mirror for a *front view* posture check. Use the analogy of a carpenter's level to balance your eyes and ears, shoulders and hips on the horizontal level.

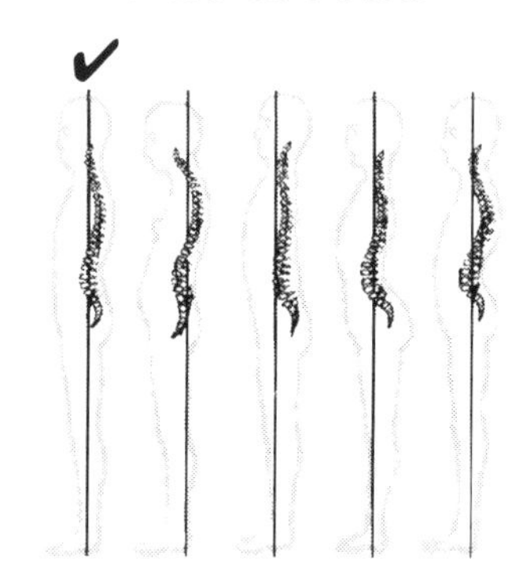

Side view posture check: Your spine is naturally meant to form a gentle S-curve. Sit and stand tall, lifted and relaxed, with ankles, knees, hips, shoulders and ears aligned like the example on the left ✔.

5

4 Go Palms-UP for Healthy Golden Ratio Posture

Maintaining healthy posture is a must to support the Golden Ratio relationships in your spine and throughout your body. Portland, Oregon-based acupuncturist **Sara Calabro** learned a powerful yet easy method for posture improvement from renowned Boston, Massachusetts area acupuncturist **Kiiko Matsumoto**, summarized here from AcuTakeHealth.com, where Calabro is founding editor:

Turn up your palms. That's it. Whenever you're doing something that doesn't require use of your hands, turn one or both of them so that they're palm-side up. You can also do it while standing or walking, leaving your arms down at your sides and turning your palms so that they face outward in the direction you're facing… In less than two weeks, I saw a marked improvement in my posture. I also noticed a general feeling of more openness in my chest. It felt easier to breathe.

Easier to breathe—**remember that the quality and quantity of your breath is Driver #1 for health, performance and longevity.** This simple palms-up action gently opens up your chest, rolls your shoulders down and back and lifts your spine. It helps to counteract your likely predominantly more hunched, palms-down attitude (typing, texting, driving, sitting, etc.). Calabro theorizes that an added benefit to the Palms-Up method is also acupuncture related. It turns out that the main acupuncture meridians running along the inside of your arms, from your chest/underarm to your palms, are the Heart, Pericardium and Lung. When you open your posture by practicing Palms-Up, you also open the energy that flows through these meridians, improving organ function and efficiency. Try it now. Go Palms-Up throughout your day and feel the difference.

5 Tools & Techniques to Bring Your Spine Back Into Golden Ratio

Time To BeneFIT 30 Seconds

There are many effective methods and tools to strengthen your core spinal muscles, regain and maintain spinal flexibility and restore your natural Golden Ratio postural proportions. Some favorites include:

- **Two tennis balls** tied tightly together in a sock makes a great low-tech, high-value spinal therapy tool. Lie down on a soft surface and place the tennis balls on either side of your spine. Start at either the base or top of your spine. Feel the tension in your back melt away as you breathe. Move the balls a few inches along the spine, continuing to breathe until you reach the end, then reverse direction. Also a great travel tool.
- Exercising on & stretching over a **Swiss Exercise Ball** is a simple, effective method for gently stretching & restoring your spine's Golden Ratio Proportions.
- Limit spinal disc compression: **Avoid heavy backpacks/shoulder bags**. Even moderately weighted bags can compress discs and throw off healthy posture (children's spines are especially adversely affected by overloaded backpacks).
- **Yoga, Chiropractic, Rolfing, Pilates, Alexander Technique, Feldenkrais Method, Massage** are all great body alignment & structural integration systems.
- **Floating** in a flotation tank filled with buoyant epsom salt water is an excellent way to gently support and restore healthy spinal alignment and posture, while

simultaneously promoting deep body relaxation and regeneration. An increasingly popular practice, float spa centers can be found in many cities worldwide.

- Lying on a **Foam Roller** is an easy, effective way to lengthen & relax your spine.
- The **Body Bridge** is a semicircular shaped apparatus on which you lie to decompress your spine. Lying supine (face-up) on the Body Bridge for even 3 minutes allows your spine to gently relax and lengthen. www.BodyBridge.com
- The **Elaine Petrone Miracle Ball Method**™ uses two soft, 4" air-filled balls to roll on and decompress your back. The balls are easy and fun to use and are a proven system for relieving back pain and stress. www.ElainePetrone.com
- The **MA Roller**: A rolling pin-like back self-massage tool. It stimulates acupressure points as you roll on it and lengthens your spine; helps restore your spine's Golden Ratio proportions. It has a comfortable spinal contour and can quickly relieve tight spots in your back. www.TheMaRoller.com
- The **MedX Core Spinal Fitness System**™ is a breakthrough spinal rehabilitation system that delivers the four factors essential to spinal health: strength, stability, flexibility and endurance. The workout is delivered via five biomechanically designed machines which isolate and strengthen the low back, neck and torso muscles. Designed by Nautilus®/Golden Ratio inventor Arthur Jones, it's used by doctors and chiropractors worldwide. Profound benefits are reported from sessions lasting just 20 minutes, once or twice a month. MedxOnline.com
  If near NYC, **Mike Arteaga's Health & Fitness Centers in Poughkeepsie, NY** is one of the country's premier MedX facilities, with a highly trained staff.
- **Spinal inversion therapy** is an excellent practice for the spine; see Rx 7 ahead.

Remember to breathe slowly & deeply while engaging any of the above practices/tools and consult your physician/health care provider prior to trying any of these therapies.

6 Avoid Sitting Death Syndrome: *Get Up & Move!*

Sit less, live longer; sit more, live less. A vast 13-year study of over 123,216 healthy men and women by the American Cancer Society (ACS) revealed sobering details about a regular practice most people do in excess without thinking. As reported by CNN reporter William Hudson (6/24/11):

Φ Hours of excessive sitting each day does significant, lasting damage to human health—*which cannot be undone by exercising.*

- Φ Women who sat more than 6 hrs./day compared to women who sat less than 3 hrs./day were 37% more likely to die during the 13 year study. Likewise, men sitting more than 6 hrs./day were 18% more likely to die during the study than those sitting less than 3 hrs./day.
- Φ **Even when people do significant and regular exercise, they still increase their risks of serious illness from hours of physical inactivity.**

Hudson also points out that:

> *...these findings are also consistent with lifestyles in so-called "Blue Zones," longevity hot spots places such as Okinawa, Japan, and Sardinia, Italy, where people live much longer on average than the rest of the developed world [see Ch 10 Longevity for more on Blue Zones]. In addition to plant-based diets and strong communities, near-constant yet moderate physical activity is the norm in these areas. More Americans are adapting modern work environments to suit these physiological needs better by installing standing and adjustable desks that allow for switching between sitting and standing positions, and treadmill desks, which operate at low walking speeds.*

Some suggested new habits to address the dangers of sitting for too long:

- Sit less—get out of your chair every hour or so, even for a short walk to get some fresh air, stretch and get your blood circulating. Standing, stretching and walking is especially important on planes, to reduce the risk of potentially deadly blood clots forming (ample hydration is also key; see page 72/Ch 2 Hydration).
- In addition to sitting tall and buoyantly with good posture, gently rock or spiral from time to time. Even a little movement is a good thing while sitting.
- Vary your sitting position from time to time. Experiment sitting cross-legged on the floor if possible, using a cushion to raise your pelvis, thereby relieving low-back strain. Interestingly, much of the world's population does not sit in chairs and are healthier for it.
- Alternating standing and sitting at your desk is a healthy alternative to just always sitting. A good adjustable desk makes this an easy upgrade, e.g., at Ikea.
- **As with breathing, the important thing is to sit consciously.** Don't sit on autopilot—until your autopilot is trained to maintain healthy posture.

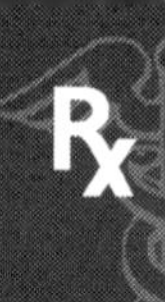

7 Go Upside Down, Lengthen Your Spine & Gain New Perspective

Dan Brown, bestselling author of *The Da Vinci Code*, further expands his perspective and creativity when writing by hanging upside down every hour for a few minutes, as a part of his hourly writing breaks. Should you decide to turn your world upside-down, we recommend the **Teeter Hang Ups/DEX II** Spinal Decompression/Extension/Inversion System, one of the most comfortable and supportive do-it-yourself gravity traction devices available. By safely supporting you from your pelvis—vs. from your ankles as in other devices—your spine slowly lengthens as it's gently tractioned by gravity. The Teeter/DEX II is one of the quickest ways to give your spine a Golden Ratio tune-up. Recommended hang time is anywhere from 30 seconds up to 5 minutes. ***NOTE:*** *Inversion therapy is NOT for everyone, as there are certain contradictions; ALWAYS check with your physician before using inversion therapy.* Available at: www.EnergyCenter.com

8 Activate Your Superhuman Posture Via Golden Ratio PowerPosing

Time To BeneFIT 2 Seconds

With something as easy as changing your physical posture you can send strong subconscious signals to yourself, resulting in increased confidence and performance. *Power Posing* is a valuable technique for any upcoming situations requiring enhanced self-assurance, including public speaking, interviews, competitions or any situations where a Superhero-like presence would result in a favorable outcome.

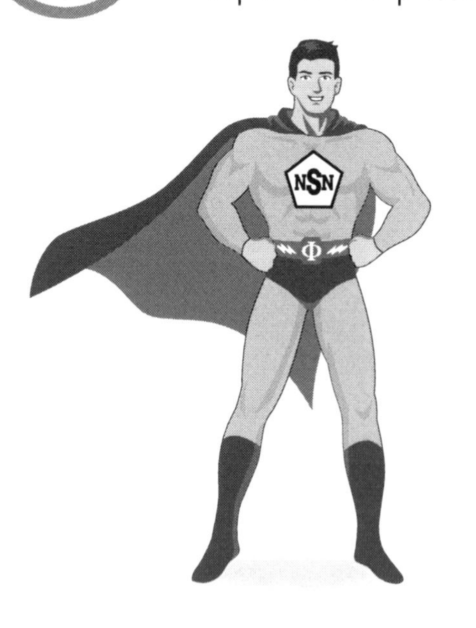

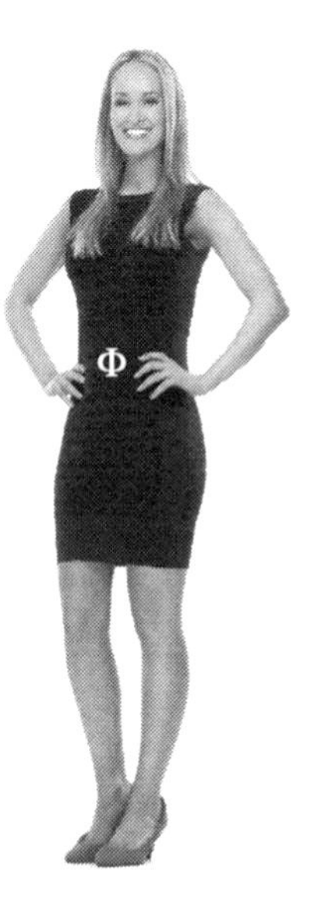

NSN Man and Super Business Woman have the classical "hands-on-hips" pose. A Golden Ratio secret of standing in Power Poses is that your hands are resting at and pointing directly to your navel region/core, which is the main Golden Φ Ratio division or Power Point of your whole body.

Dr. Amy Cuddy has researched the science of Power Posing, where expansive, confident postures are held for 1-3 minutes, such as those modeled by Superheroes like Wonder Woman, Batman and Superman and also with hands held high in the "V for Victory" pose. She discovered that there were positive downstream effects of such poses in subjects' cognitive, emotional and behavioral areas, especially in vastly increased self-confidence. The physiological effects were also impressive: power poses resulted in *increased* testosterone (power/confidence hormone) saliva levels of up to 20% and *decreased* cortisol (stress/anxiety hormone) levels of up to 25%; yoga power poses such as the Cobra revealed similar results. You can emulate the power poses shown here to get a quick hit of natural testosterone to amp up your personal power and self-confidence. At the same time, you'll be lowering your cortisol to remain calm, cool and collected. Featured here are two essential power pose options, namely NSN Man/Super Business Woman "hands-on-hips" pose, which is at the root of Dr. Cuddy's research and the Vitruvian Man/Woman arms-high "starfish" variation. By practicing either of these poses, **you're affirming, amplifying and broadcasting your own hidden-in-plain-sight Golden Ratio power to yourself *and* to the world.** So what are you waiting for? The next time you need to amp up your self-confidence, personal power and equanimity before an important meeting, presentation or competition:

1. **Center your mind. Tune into your breath.**
2. **Imagine your favorite Superhero, or Vitruvian Man/Woman, standing tall and proud. Smile and breathe deeply and confidently.**
3. **For 1 to 2 minutes...** ***Strike a Pose!***

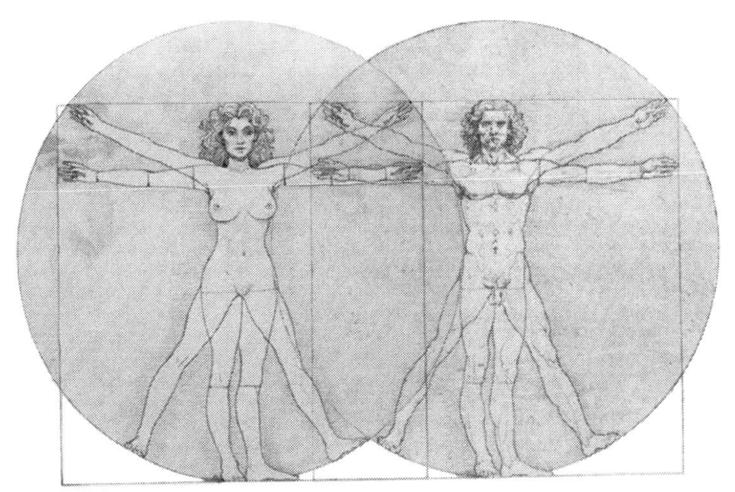

An alternative to the Superhero's and Super Business Woman's Power Pose is demonstrated by Vitruvian Man/Woman. In this 500 year-old pose, they demonstrate how to "Square the Circle" and access the energies of both Heaven and Earth. No doubt even the great Leonardo da Vinci himself used this Power Pose before soliciting grant money from the Borgia Pope :)

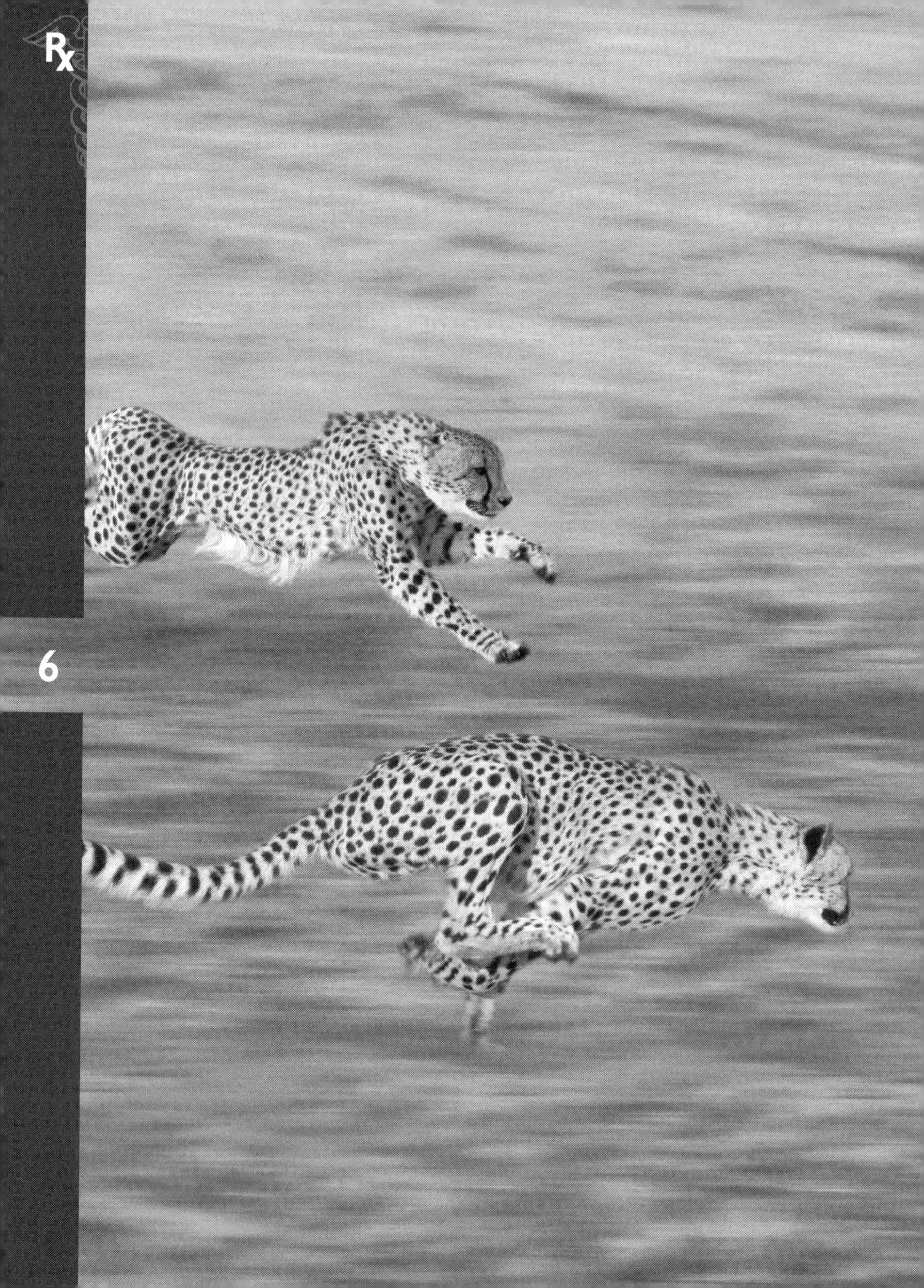
Rx
6

6
Exercise Rx's

Note: *Consult your health professional before trying this or any new exercise regimen. If you're a beginner, out-of-shape or have a medical condition, get evaluated by your physician with a maximal cardiac stress test. We also recommend that you establish an endurance baseline with a personal trainer before beginning any Fibonacci-based FIT workouts.*

General Exercise Recommendations to Maximize NSN

Maximally beneficial exercise for health, heart and longevity exhibits the following facets and forms our recommendations. Rx's addressing these points and more follow:

- Exercise should be a *good stress*—a fun and invigorating way to achieve natural health, peak performance and longevity—never a burden or source of negative stress.
- Always spend 8-13 minutes warming-up & cooling-down before and after exercise.
- Integrate Golden Ratio Breathing into your workouts for an added dose of NSN.
- Always hydrate before, during & after exercise to maximize performance & recovery.
- For recreational athletes and fitness exercisers, keep each non-stop aerobic workout session to 55 minutes or less.
- Strengthen your Golden Ratio Core Zone (navel area), foundation for total health.
- Vary the intensity and duration within ***individual*** workout sessions, e.g., by integrating FIT intervals, to support healthy Heart Rate Variability (HRV).

- Vary the intensity & duration between ***day-to-day*** workouts, always taking days off as needed in order to recover & *catapult load* before the next exercise session.
- Use Fibonacci Sequence Numbers (1,1,2,3,5,8,13,21,34,55,89...) and Golden Ratio Numbers (38,62,100) for number of reps, sets and interval duration.
- Make regular, low intensity Blue Zone movement as much a part of your natural lifestyle as possible: walking/biking for transportation, gardening, outdoor games, etc.
- For optimal fitness use the 40/30/30 Golden Olympic Training (GOT) Ratio to maximize your Endurance, Strength and Flexibility/Balance/Coordination (FBC).
- Use the FIT Short, Medium & Long Wave Workouts to integrate NSN into your workouts over varying time scales—second, minutes and hours. Adjust Intensity, Frequency & Duration of workouts to 50/30/20 Fibonacci ratios

Pick one or more of the following Rx's to add to your NSN daily health regimen.

1 Workout with the Fibonacci Fitness Code

Walk or jog 5 minutes, then rest and stretch for 3. Repeat three times. Increase the intensity as endurance and desire allow, or experiment with other Fibonacci Ratios—3:2, 8:5, 13:8. These Fibonacci workout/recovery ratios are an easy, fun way to tap NSN's power in your workouts and give your body ample time to clear lactic acid and recharge. Another easy way to integrate the Golden Ratio into your exercise routine is to modify the number of repetitions per set of any exercise.

By using adjacent Fibonacci numbers for the number of repetitions per set, you automatically add the power of the Golden Ratio to your workout. It may seem a little odd at first, doing for example 8 pushups followed by 13, rather than 10 followed by 10. Yet this simple change in your reps counting method can switch your body into reactivation of your latent Golden Ratio performance capabilities. Here are some example adjacent Fibonacci number pairs with which you can structure the number of repetitions in sequential sets:

3:5 5:3 5:8 8:5 8:13 13:8 13:21 21:13 21:34 34:21 34:55 55:34

When your exercise intervals correspond to Fibonacci Sequence numbers (and thus Golden Ratios), you send a powerful message to your nervous system to synchronize with the Golden Ratio and extract NSN for greater performance and endurance.

Lighten Your Load with Golden Ratio Weight Lifting

The next time you're lifting weights, using exercise resistance bands or using a Nautilus,® Bowflex,® or other machine, try synchronizing your repetitions with Golden Ratio Breathing. Begin with a light weight or easy resistance until you get accustomed to the Ratio. As you lift the weight or move against the resistance, breathe out to a count of 5. As you release the weight or resistance, breathe in to a count of 3. Your motions should be slow and synchronized with your breath. For variability, experiment with different ratios, such as 2:3, 3:2, 3:5, 5:3 or 5:8. Different ratios give different results. When you're working out with the Golden Ratio, you can make amazing gains in a short amount of time.

Golden Ratio Exercise Breathing

Since your entire respiratory system is designed around the Golden Ratio, it makes perfect sense to tune your breathing during exercise to the ratio for optimal benefits. For example, while walking or running try inhaling to the count of 3 and exhaling to the count of 5. If you need more air, try a 2:3 ratio of inhalations to exhalations. Find the ratio that feels right for you. This way of breathing offers a valuable alternative to the standard 1:1 inhalation to exhalation ratio. You may keep up the breathing ratio through 3, 5 or 8 breathing cycles, and then let the practice go and breathe in and out without consciously thinking about the ratio for a while. Then try it again, perhaps with a different set of Fibonacci numbers and ratios. If you're strenuously exercising, you may not be able to keep up with Golden Ratio breathing because your system may try to revert to your habitual inhalation to exhalation ratio of 1:1, 2:2 or 3:3 to keep up with maximal oxygen and CO_2 demands. However, when you slow down or stop, you can resume Golden Ratio breathing. When Golden Ratio breathing is continued for at least 3 minutes it will relax you, lower your blood pressure and calm you down. These breathing exercises can be done anytime, anywhere: driving, lying in bed, at work or exercising. What makes these breathing exercises so effective? They simply yet powerfully rebalance and repattern your autonomic nervous system in accordance with the Golden Ratio. This opens the door for more of Nature's Secret Nutrient to enhance your health and restore overall wellbeing.

2 Split Workouts For Better Results & Easy Weight Loss

Split your daily workout into two sessions in Golden Ratio to obtain greater benefits for less effort. This simple practice optimizes the ratio of your exercise and recovery cycles. For example, workout for 13 minutes in the morning and 21 minutes in the afternoon. For longer workouts, try ratios such as 21:34 or 34:55. For shorter workouts, try an 8:13 ratio. Splitting your daily workout amplifies the benefits of your workout and saves overall time invested.

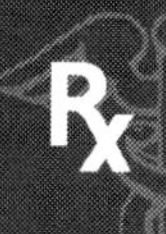

3 Strengthen Your Golden Ratio Core Zone for Total Body Upgrade

The modern focus on **core training** reflects both the Golden Ratio and the First 15% principle. The Golden Ratio division point of your body—the navel region—is a most powerful First 15% starting point for building optimal fitness, posture, balance and strength. It's no accident that oriental medicine and the martial arts place such emphasis on this region known as the Hara/Dantian, slightly below and behind the navel. In addition, the solar plexus, the 2nd largest nerve center in the body (aka the "second brain") is slightly above the navel. This core postural/nerve/gravitational matrix that surrounds your navel—above, below, sides and back—also strengthens your balance, poise and focus. **This translates to strengthening the same qualities in your mind, emotions and spirit as well.** A few simple, effective methods for strengthening your Golden Ratio Core Zone include:

- Φ Yoga, Jumping Rope, Pull-ups, Hula-Hoop, Pilates.
- Φ Sit-ups: knees bent & variations, e.g., diagonal sit-ups, enhanced core workouts.
- Φ Golden Breathing: Full Buddha-belly, expanding up into your chest on inhale; then letting the breath out fully, navel pulled towards the spine on exhale. Strengthens your diaphragm and core muscles simultaneously. See Breathing Rx's, Rx Ch 1.

The Golden Ratio Core Zone is composed of three distinct parts—Solar Plexus, Navel and Hara/Dantian. The Navel is at the center of the Golden Ratio Core Zone and is also the Golden Ratio dividing point of the body, from head to toe.

- The Solar Plexus is the major abdominal nerve plexus.
- The navel marks the primary *vertical* Golden Ratio division point of the body.
- The Hara/Dantian is the body's primary internal energy center in oriental medicine and the martial arts.

Strengthening your Golden Ratio Core Zone is crucial for building and maintaining healthy Flexibility/Balance/Coordination (FBC).

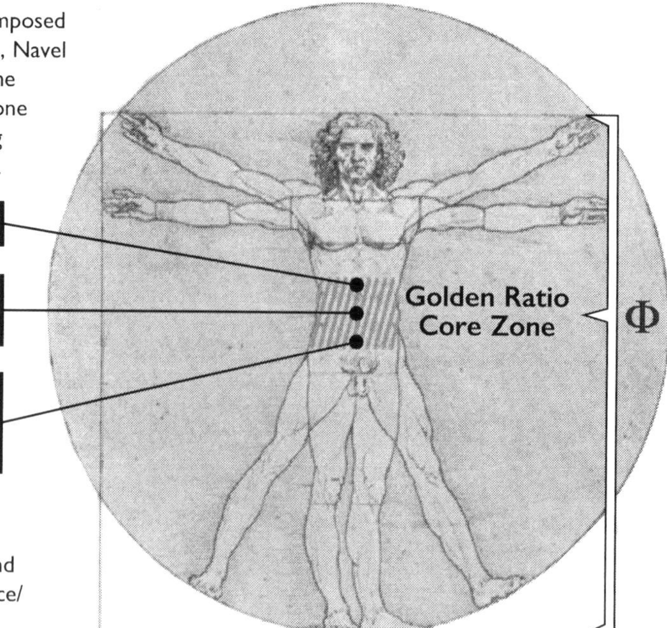

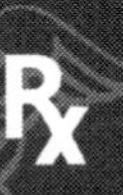

- Φ Wobble Board: Stand and balance on one for a few minutes daily; activates & strengthens your core. **BETTER BALANCE = GREATER CORE STRENGTH.**
- Φ Medicine Balls: www.Spri.com
- Φ Kettlebell workout: www.PowerByPavel.com
- Φ *ABCore Medicine Ball Workout* video, by co-author Matthew K. Cross; coming soon to: www.NSNpower.com

As with all suggested exercises in this book, always consult a health professional before any new exercise regimen, go at your own pace and listen to your body.

4 Treat Your Body Like a Finely-Tuned Race Car

The benefits of interval training are being incorporated into virtually every aerobic/cardio exercise, including running, biking, skiing, swimming, rowing and various gym aerobics. In these sessions, intervals of various lengths and intensity are mixed in during the course of a workout to build in more dynamism and Heart Rate Variability (HRV). A good metaphor for the variability factor interval training offers is to imagine that you're shifting through the gears in a finely-tuned race car. For maximum performance, fuel efficiency and minimum wear, you upshift or downshift as appropriate, sometimes paying attention to your RPM/tachometer so as not to red-line or over-rev your engine. In the same manner it's a good idea to take a similar approach during your exercise by shifting or varying your gears/speed during exercise sessions. This both enhances your performance and endurance and minimizes the effects if you happen to redline your system. Remember to include adequate pit/refueling stops as necessary and pay special attention to sufficient rest and rehydration in support of your workouts.

5 Remember to Warm-Up & Cool-Down Properly

Time To BeneFIT 8 Seconds

Just as you would warm-up your car on a cold day before driving, so should you warm-up your muscles, tendons, ligaments and whole body before exercising to reduce the chances of injury and poor performance. Like every serious athlete, always begin your exercise sessions with an adequate warm-up before shifting into higher intensity workout phases. Your warm-up should be long enough that you break a light sweat, usually after about 8-13 minutes. This signals that your body has reached a safe "green zone" operating temperature which allows you to get the most from your workout. Reversing this process at the end of your workout over 5-8 minutes completes any optimum exercise cycle; this is the easy "runner's victory lap" after the race is over. By decreasing exercise intensity with adequate cool-down time, your body can properly process excess adrenaline and neutralize accumulated lactic acid in your muscles. So always warm-up before your workouts and allow an ample cool-down period by gradually decreasing activity afterwards.

6 The FIT Wave Workouts: Short, Medium & Long

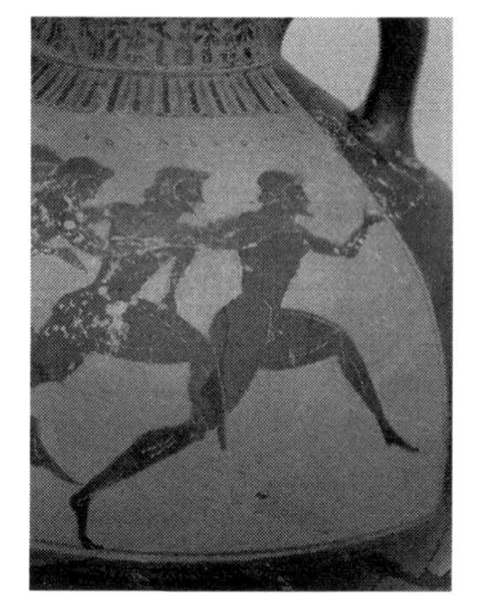

Rx 6 has 3 parts—a, b & c—that comprise the breakthrough exercise protocols of the FIT Wave Workout System. **All FIT Wave Workouts are tuned to the Golden Ratio via Fibonacci Sequence numbers and follow the classic Elliot Wave pattern of 5 total waves up to 3 total waves down.** This supports your body's natural production of Nature's Secret Nutrient/NSN—the secret ingredient for building and sustaining great health and peak performance. **Each workout is scaled to its own fractal time segment and can be used by itself or in conjunction with the others to create a super-synergy**. While a watch or stopwatch can be used to keep track of Fibonacci Numbers for medium and long wave workout intervals, the low-tech method of simply counting off the numbers to yourself during intervals works well for short wave workouts. Once the Fibonacci Sequence numbers are in your mind, keeping track is easy. At the end of each interval, you transition into the rest/recovery phase with a jog or a relaxed walk (the **DOWN waves**). Every rest/recovery cycle is a natural catapult-loading phase for your next exercise cycle (**the UP waves**). When you've recovered your breath and sense of well-being, or when your heart rate has come down if using a heart rate monitor, you're ready for your next interval/up wave.

The 3 FIT Waves for Rx 6 are:

Rx 6a—The FIT SHORT Wave, uses Fibonacci Numbers on a scale of *seconds*, with 3 workout options: 55, 89 & 144 seconds.

Rx 6b—The FIT MEDIUM Wave, uses Fibonacci Numbers on a scale of *minutes*, with 3 workout options: 13, 21 & 34 minutes.

Rx 6c—The FIT LONG Wave, uses Fibonacci Numbers on a scale of *minutes & hours*, with 3 workout options: 55 minutes (~1 hr.), 89 minutes (~1½ hrs.) and 144 minutes (~2½ hrs).

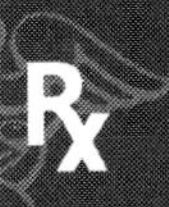

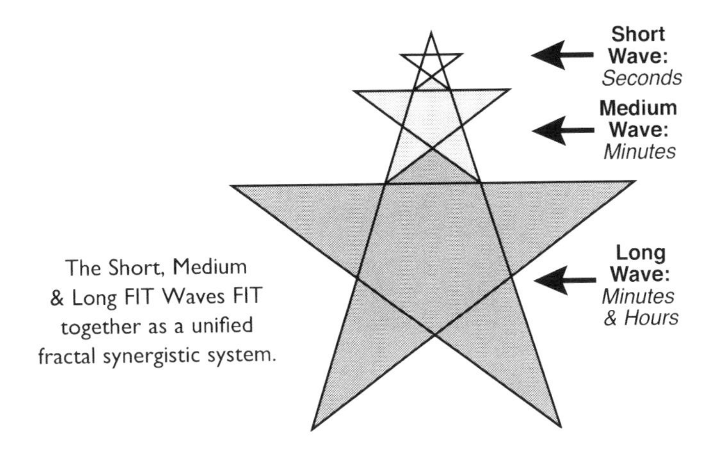

The Short, Medium & Long FIT Waves FIT together as a unified fractal synergistic system.

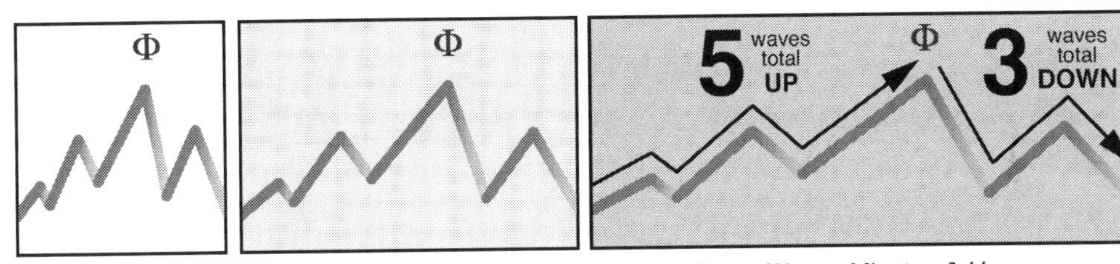

Short Wave: *Seconds* **Medium Wave:** *Minutes* **Long Wave:** *Minutes & Hours*

The 3 FIT Workout Waves: Short (seconds), Medium (minutes) and Long (minutes & hours). As the Golden Ratio-based star allows for fractal embeddings of self-similar, smaller stars, so do the 3 FIT Fibonacci-based training waves embed within one another for super-synergy fitness and performance. **NOTE HOW ALL FIT WAVES exhibit the classic Elliott Wave pattern of 5 total waves UP to 3 total waves DOWN.**

Fine-tuning Your FIT Wave Rx's

Keep in mind that the real benefits of exercise are obtained in the days and nights after your workout. This is the time during which your body regenerates, especially during sleep. While exercise naturally provides us with great feelings of achievement, freedom and even transcendence, intense exercise—especially when rigorous and/or too frequent—is actually physically damaging to the body. In addition to causing micro muscle tears and increased wear, it also generates excessive free-radical activity, due to the higher oxidation rates generated during exercise. This is why it's vitally important to allow ample rest/recovery periods in any exercise regimen, to honor your body's need to properly heal, recover and come back even stronger. **The secret to effective FIT Wave Workouts is the *quality* of your exercise cycles vs. their *quantity*.** By tuning your FIT workouts to the Golden Ratio via Fibonacci Sequence numbers, you support your body's natural production and concentration of Nature's Secret Nutrient/NSN—the secret ingredient for building great heath and peak performance. At the end of each interval, transition slowly into the rest/recovery phase—come out of your exercise into a fast walk, followed by a slower, relaxed walk. Every rest/recovery cycle is a natural catapult-loading phase for your next exercise cycle (no need for perfection in timing your exercise cycles. While a watch/stopwatch can be handy, the low-tech/high-ease method of counting off the numbers to yourself during your exercise cycles works very well). Once the Fibonacci Sequence numbers are in your mind, it's easy.

Key FIT Wave Workout Points

- The FIT Wave workout system is applicable to exercise enthusiasts from all sports.
- Over a period of weeks, aim to build up to your subjective sense of safe maximum intensity. Alternatively, your safe maximum pulse rate would be around 85% of your maximum heart rate. A ballpark formula for calculating 85% of your maximum heart rate is: **(220 - age) x .85 = 85%.**
- If FIT Wave workouts are done with high intensity, limit them to twice/week; if done at low to moderate intensity, they can be done 3-5 days/week.
- Although the exercise phases are structured according to Fibonacci Numbers, the intensity of each interval is variable and is totally up to you.
- Start easy and respect your body's natural feedback signals. On some days you may need longer rest/recovery cycles; on others, less. The same goes for the intensity of your exercise cycles; vary as needed.
- Experiment with longer or shorter exercise intervals by selecting the next higher or lower Fibonacci number to define your exercise upwave cycles.
- If a longer total workout is desired, just repeat a workout or add in one or more of the other workouts, i.e., easy, moderate or competitive.
- An easy way to make sure you're not overtraining is to take your resting pulse in the morning before arising. If your pulse is 10 beats or more higher than normal, you need to back off training until your body recovers.
- To more accurately assess overtraining and optimize your total fitness, track your Heart Rate Variability (HRV) with the HRV app (Rx #9, this chapter). FIT workouts naturally enhance HRV and dynamism, as your heart rate repeatedly rises and falls in sync with the FIT Wave Fibonacci-based intervals.
- The alternating upwaves and downwaves build in key rest/recovery cycles throughout your whole workout. The downward rest/recovery waves have a catapult-like effect, giving your cells vital time to reboot and recharge before your next upwave surge.
- Although not as accurate as heart rate monitors, you can sense where you're at in your intensity zone by subjective sensations—sweating, breathing rate, burning muscles, or just feeling good when you get your second wind. A caveat: since competitive athletes train with a higher % of max heart rate, they will want to use a heart rate monitor for more precision. Heart rate monitors can be valuable

for any level athlete, since it's often difficult to accurately gauge where your target heart rate is in both exertion and recovery phases.

- Moving from aerobic through anaerobic levels exercises your endocrine, nervous, cardiovascular and musculoskeletal systems' full range of intensity.
- The FIT Workout Waves comprise an exceptional system combining Fibonacci Sequence numbers and Golden Ratios **to generate the secret weapon of optimal exercise: NSN.** Enjoy riding the FIT Waves to greater fitness and performance!

6a FIT Short Wave: 3 Interval Workouts of 55, 89 or 144 Seconds

To use the FIT System for short interval sessions, try any of the following FIT Short Wave workouts as a starting point. Always begin workouts with an easy 8–13 minute warm up. When fully warmed-up, as indicated by a light sweat, you're ready to begin your workout. All FIT workouts are divided into alternating exercise and rest/recovery phases. The exercise phase can be done anywhere from low to high intensity, depending on your goals and energy levels on any given day. For recreational or fitness exercisers, you don't need to do high intensity intervals to reap the benefits, as many of the benefits come from the NSN-generated from the Golden Ratios between intervals. Competitive athletes will get a super-boost of NSN because of the additional high-intensity effort put into the workouts. **Your rest/recovery downwave cycle length is up to you; enough**

FIT SHORT Wave Workouts in SECONDS

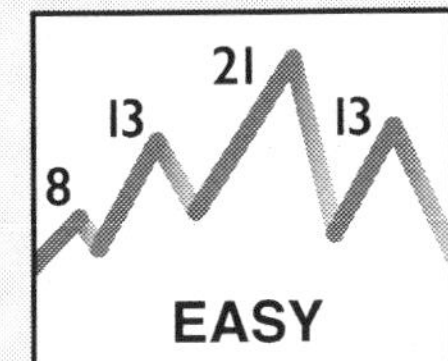

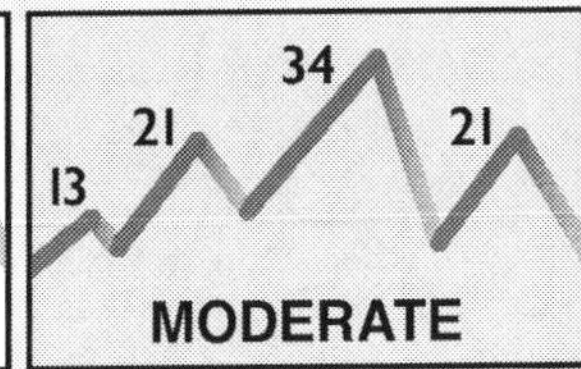

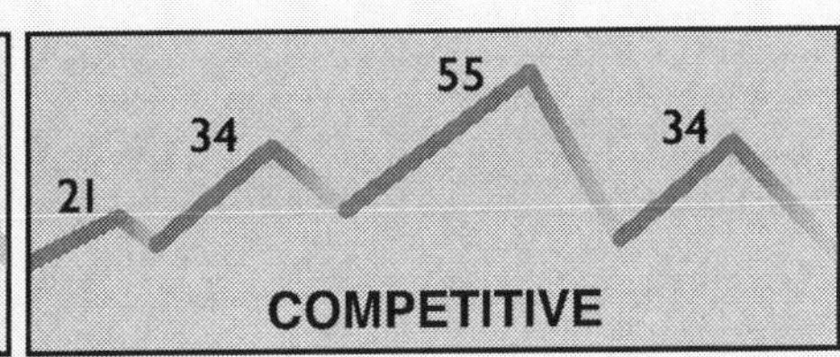

1. EASY: Actual exercise time = 55 seconds.

2. MODERATE: Actual exercise time = 89 seconds.

3. COMPETITIVE: Actual exercise time = 144 seconds.

These super-efficient FIT Short Wave Workouts range from 55 to 144 seconds of actual exercise time. All wave intervals are in Golden Ratio proportion to one another via their Fibonacci Sequence Numbers structure, the key to producing NSN. Upwaves are exercise phases and downwaves are rest/recovery phases. Downwaves load the catapult for the next up wave. If a longer total workout is desired, simply repeat the workout or add in one or more of the other Short Wave Workouts—easy, moderate or competitive.

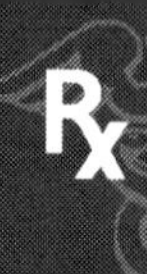

time to get your breath back, lower your pulse from its former high and load your catapult for your next upwave burst with renewed energy.

Choose the workout that feels right for you. If you're just starting out, start with the FIT Short Wave 55 second workout and move up to the 89 or 144 second workout as your endurance improves over time. The workouts sound much easier than they actually are. For example, the 55 second workout is composed of 4 exercise upwave sprints of 8, 13, 21 and 13 seconds. Although the intervals are short, the intensity factor can make them challenging, especially if you repeat the entire cycle several times. For longer workouts, feel free to move up to the 89 or 144 second workouts and repeat them as many times as you require to satisfy your workout appetite and goals. *Note: workout lengths don't include your critical warm-up and cool-down periods of at least 8-13 minutes each.*

FIT Medium Wave: 3 Interval Workouts of 13, 21 or 34 *Minutes*

The FIT Medium Wave is an easy way to incorporate the Golden Ratio into moderate length workouts for powerful performance enhancement and injury protection benefits. You have the choice of three workout options of either 13, 21 or 34 minutes. Each workout is tuned to the Golden Ratio by using alternating Fibonacci Sequence numbers

FIT MEDIUM Wave Workouts in MINUTES

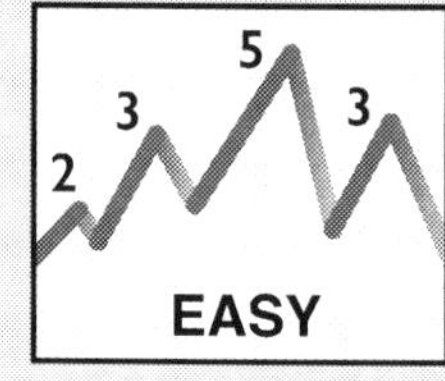

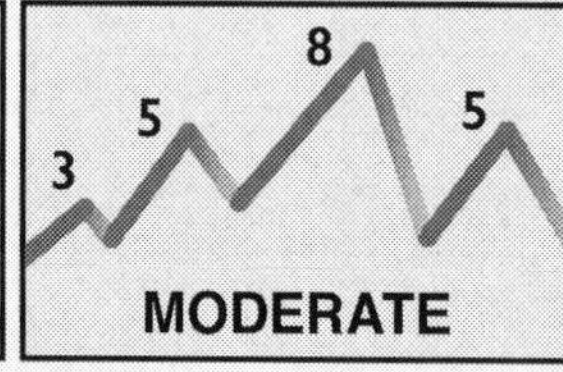

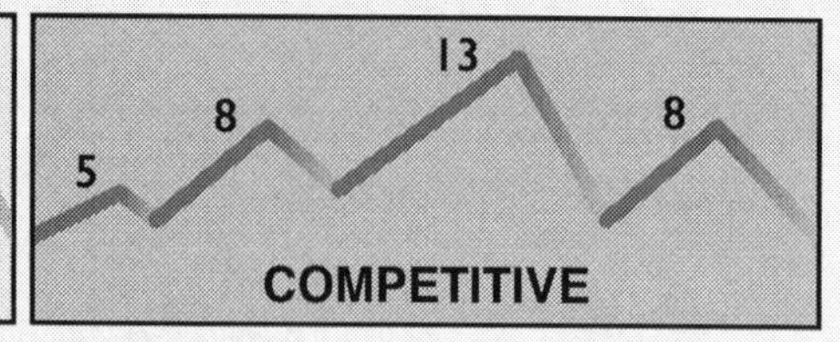

1. EASY: Actual exercise time = 13 minutes.

2. MODERATE: Actual exercise time = 21 minutes.

3. COMPETITIVE: Actual exercise time = 34 minutes.

The FIT Medium Wave Workout intervals are delineated by Fibonacci Sequence numbers, forming Golden Ratios between intervals. All downwaves are recovery phases, loading the catapult for the next upwave. You determine the length of each downwave recovery phase, based on your heart rate combined with your subjective sense of readiness/recovery for the next sprint. Rest/recovery times aren't included in total number of minutes for each workout (13, 21, 34), since all rest/recovery periods vary by being left up to you.

between intervals. Since the FIT Medium and Long Wave workouts are more aerobic in nature than the FIT Short Wave sprint workouts, they can be done 3-5 times per week.

The FIT Medium Wave charts show the 3 different workouts, with total times of 13, 21 or 34 minutes. Each exercise upwave uses Fibonacci Sequence numbers (listed at bottom of chart) to generate Golden Ratios between intervals and maximize NSN. The length of your rest/recovery downwaves between exercise intervals is up to you. Choose the workout that feels right for you. If you're just starting out, start with the 13 minute workout and move up to longer workouts (21 or 34 minutes) as your endurance improves over time. Remember that both intensity level and length of rest/recovery periods are up to you.

6c FIT Long Wave: 3 Interval Workouts: 55 minutes (~1 *Hour*), 89 minutes (~1½ *Hours*) & 144 minutes (~2½ *Hours*)

The FIT Long Wave applies the same NSN generating principles as the FIT Short & Medium Waves, yet over longer periods. We know from the research of cardiologist **Dr. James O'Keefe** that **nonstop exercise of around one hour is a safe limit, past which the risks of overtraining begin to exceed the positive benefits of exercise.** Many sports/games routinely exceed one hour in duration, yet due to the nature of the sports they have natural built-in breaks that give the heart time to recover. This avoids the nonstop stress on the heart that is seen for example in long-distance runners who

FIT LONG Wave Workouts in Minutes/HOURS

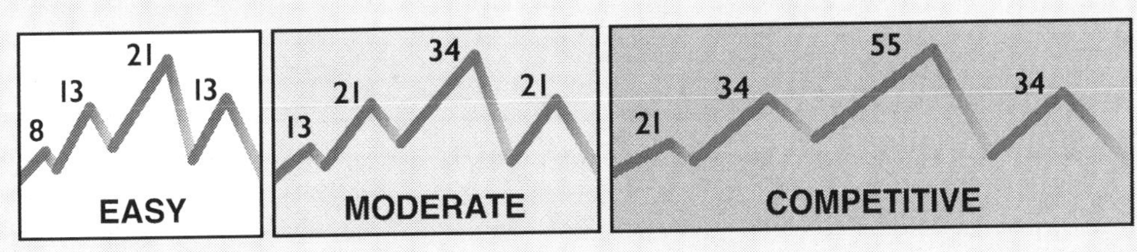

1. EASY: Actual exercise time = 55 minutes.

2. MODERATE: Actual exercise time = 89 minutes.

3. COMPETITIVE: Actual exercise time = 144 minutes.

The 3 FIT Long Wave workouts have the same general structure, differing only in the Fibonacci Numbers used for each upwave. The duration of the downwaves, i.e., rest/recovery periods, is left up to you and is dependent on your ability to catch your breath and regain your sense of well-being and readiness for the next wave.

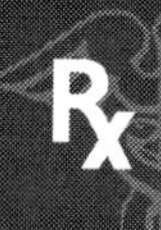

routinely train with runs of over an hour. Sports/games where frequent rest/recovery breaks can be used to natural advantage to safely exercise over an hour include hiking, cycling, swimming, tennis, basketball, soccer, skiing, etc. For the average recreational or fitness exerciser this isn't a consideration, as most people's workouts are usually around an hour or less. However, for competitive or professional athletes, longer exercise sessions can be done safely by simply incorporating the FIT Long Wave and its strategic rest breaks into their workouts. Three FIT Long Wave options for safe, extended workouts are featured in the graphs on the previous pages.

7 Nature's Energy Wave / N•E•W™: Optimizing Workouts & Rest/Recovery Periods Over Days, Weeks & Months

Nature's Energy Wave / N•E•W™ is based on the work of Golden Ratio performance pioneer Dr. Ron Sandler. It is simply the world's most effective and rewarding training system, where both fitness enthusiasts and serious athletes can access the NSN winning edge on demand. By optimizing training and rest cycles with the Golden Ratio, athletes at any level can insure healthy and Predictable Peak Performance on Demand™ *and* optimal fitness. To perform at your best for any race or competition, you simply select a target date on the calendar when you need to experience peak performance. **You then schedule *backwards* from that date to the present day,** setting in motion a building wave that will set you up for peak performance on your chosen day. The four N•E•W training cycles with exact training & rest periods are on the opposite page:

- **3-month (97-day):** More major/longer events; embeds all 3 next cycles.
- **5-week (35-day):** Mid-length events; 1-week cycle is embedded at end.
- **3-week (26-day):** Shorter events; 1-week cycle is embedded at end.
- **1-week (6-day):** Good in a pinch; ideally the final catapult effect in the above cycles.

The 3 shorter cycles especially assume you already have an initial training/ fitness base. Use the longest cycle possible before your event for optimal results, e.g., all 4 cycles are embedded in the 3-month (97-day) cycle for maximum power. N•E•W reduces/eliminates injury and supports peak performance for competitive athletes, fitness exercisers and performers on and off the field. It also adds a dose of fun, unique structure to your training regimen. With Nature as your master coach, you'll be at your best when you need it most.

See Dr. Sandler's & the author's comprehensive book *50 Pages to Peak Performance* for more detail, including interactive training calendars.

Nature's Energy Wave™ [N•E•W]: Peak Performance & Fitness on Demand

Nature's fundamental wave motion, mirrored by the Golden Ratio Spiral & Fibonacci Sequence, can be harnessed to schedule Peak Performances on exact days, weeks or months ahead. **N•E•W** puts the wind at your back to be your best when you need it most, while building in the vital rest/recovery catapult loading periods optimal performance requires. All athletes & fitness enthusiasts can use the Wave to safely maximize health & fitness, keep workouts fresh and optimize sports performance and enjoyment over a lifetime. Whether on the field or in the classroom, boardroom or stage, anyone wanting to perform their best in any arena can use Nature's Energy Wave as their secret success weapon.

- **NATURE'S ENERGY WAVE [N•E•W]** tapers you **up** for 2 days prior to your event vs. tapering **down** as in conventional systems. *A predictable peak occurs on the 3rd day back after a rest/recovery period.*
- **TO SET YOUR PEAK PERFORMANCE** count backwards from your event/race date, using the 1-wk (6-day), 3-wk (26-day), 5-wk (35-day) or 3-month (97-day) cycles. All 4 cycles can be superimposed for maximum synergy.
- **N•E•W REST & RECOVERY** down-waves are essential to load the Fibonacci catapult effect: 3 steps back/5 steps forward, or 5 steps back/8 steps forward.

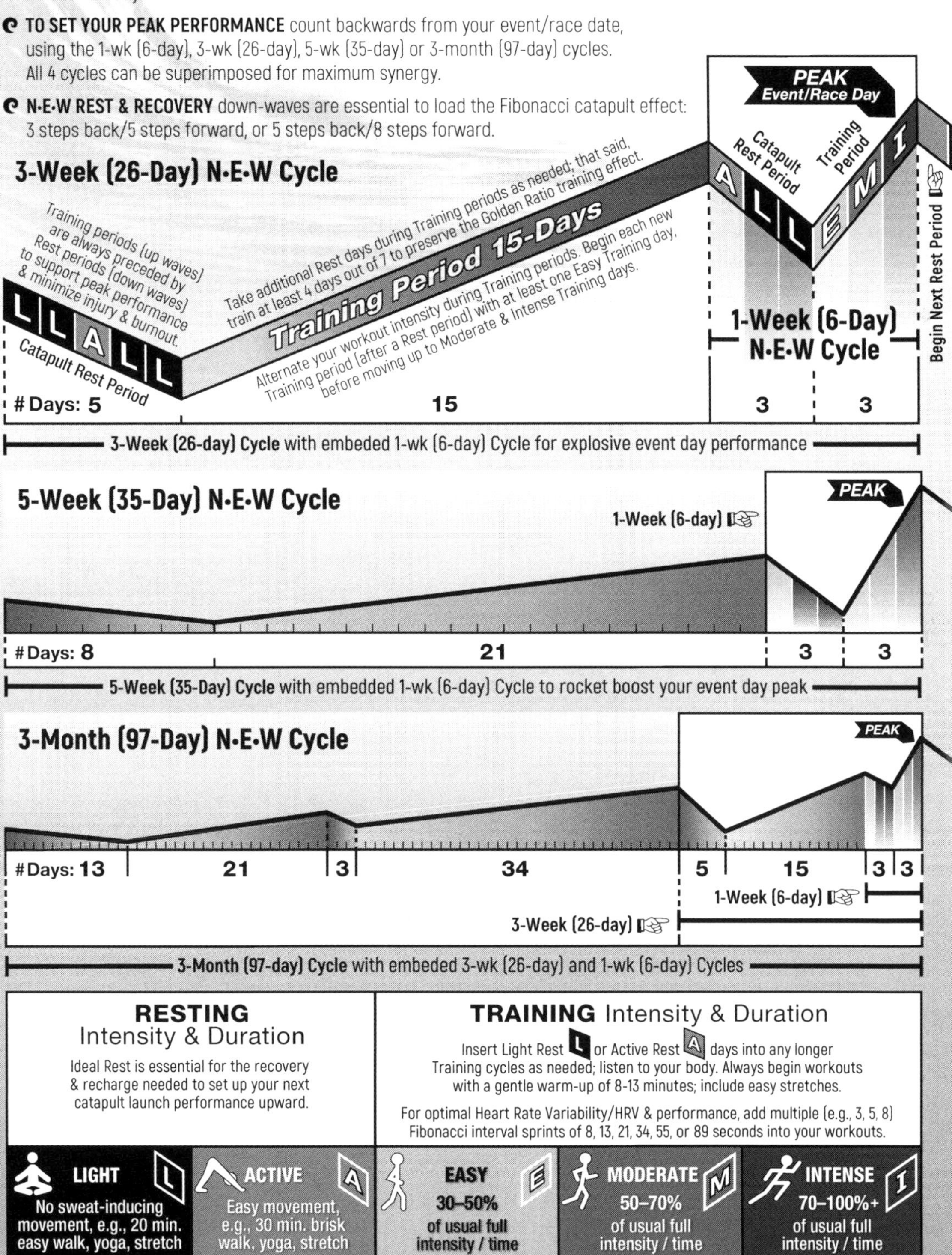

3-Week (26-Day) N•E•W Cycle
PEAK
Event/Race Day
Training periods (up waves) are always preceded by Rest periods (down waves) to support peak performance & minimize injury & burnout.
Take additional Rest days during Training periods as needed; that said, train at least 4 days out of 7 to preserve the Golden Ratio training effect.
Training Period 15-Days
Alternate your workout intensity during Training periods. Begin each new Training period (after a Rest period) with at least one Easy Training day, before moving up to Moderate & Intense Training days.
Catapult Rest Period
Catapult Rest Period
Training Period
L L A L L
A L L E M I
1-Week (6-Day) N•E•W Cycle
Begin Next Rest Period
Days: 5
15
3
3
3-Week (26-day) Cycle with embeded 1-wk (6-day) Cycle for explosive event day performance
5-Week (35-Day) N•E•W Cycle
PEAK
1-Week (6-day)
Days: 8
21
3
3
5-Week (35-Day) Cycle with embedded 1-wk (6-day) Cycle to rocket boost your event day peak
3-Month (97-Day) N•E•W Cycle
PEAK
Days: 13
21
3
34
5
15
3
3
1-Week (6-day)
3-Week (26-day)
3-Month (97-day) Cycle with embeded 3-wk (26-day) and 1-wk (6-day) Cycles
RESTING
Intensity & Duration
Ideal Rest is essential for the recovery & recharge needed to set up your next catapult launch performance upward.
TRAINING Intensity & Duration
Insert Light Rest L or Active Rest A days into any longer Training cycles as needed; listen to your body. Always begin workouts with a gentle warm-up of 8-13 minutes; include easy stretches.
For optimal Heart Rate Variability/HRV & performance, add multiple (e.g., 3, 5, 8) Fibonacci interval sprints of 8, 13, 21, 34, 55, or 89 seconds into your workouts.
LIGHT L
No sweat-inducing movement, e.g., 20 min. easy walk, yoga, stretch
ACTIVE A
Easy movement, e.g., 30 min. brisk walk, yoga, stretch
EASY E
30–50% of usual full intensity / time
MODERATE M
50–70% of usual full intensity / time
INTENSE I
70–100%+ of usual full intensity / time

Everyone's body has natural cycles of ups and downs. If you don't believe it, keep your own workout records for several weeks/months. Each day, note how you feel about your physical stamina and strength. For example, rate your day's workout on a scale from 1 to 10, where 10 is a great day; 5 is average and 1 is a day when you drag or barely get through your workout. When you review your workout data, you'll recognize the rising and falling performance cycles which reflect the natural Golden Ratio wave fluctuations occurring in your body. Performance is revealed to move in predictable waves, where your exercise UP waves are in Golden Ratio to your rest/recovery DOWN waves. This means that each complete cycle ends with your performance at a higher baseline than when you began, and that your next exercise cycle will start from that higher level. In Fibonacci and Elliott Wave terms, this illustrates a **5-steps up to 3-steps down progressive improvement wave**, which builds a regenerative catapult effect into your workouts and total fitness regimen over time.

These Golden Ratio-based waves are all part of your natural physiologic cycles and biorhythms. Learning to ride these waves so that you maintain high energy and drive—and peak when needed if you're competitive—is what Nature's Energy Wave / N•E•W offers. *For the average exerciser, this means you don't need to force yourself to exercise when overly tired, because you know you'll gain more from resting and allowing your body to recharge.* On rest days you could take a short, easy walk to keep your body loose—yet not a fast one that would create an aerobic or anaerobic training effect. For competitive athletes, you can actually predict and schedule in advance when your peak day will be—weeks and even months ahead of your event. The predictive health and performance power of this universal principle at the heart of N•E•W applies to ALL sports at ALL levels, from fitness exercisers to competitive and world-class athletes.

8 The Golden Olympic Training Ratio: Endurance, Strength, Flexibility/Balance/Coordination (FBC)

Finding your personal **G**olden **O**lympic **T**raining (**GOT**) Ratio is a golden key to increasing the efficiency, enjoyment and safety of your sport or exercise regimen. Here's how to structure your workouts to keep your body in a more balanced state. Use the easy 40/30/30 form of the Golden Ratio to allocate workout time in the areas of Endurance—Strength—Flexibility/Balance/Coordination (FBC). Each of these components cross-reinforces with the others, giving your workouts a dynamic synergy. You'll achieve a stronger, healthier and better proportioned body than if you focus on only one discipline. Here are 3 easy ways to divide single workouts into the GOT Ratio;

of course, this doesn't mean you need to fit all three categories into every workout; ideally, your weekly training totals will reflect the 40/30/30 ratio. The number of minutes used in these examples are chosen so that they divide into easy-to-remember numbers; however, if you want a different length workout, use a calculator to customize the 40/30/30 divisions (multiply total minutes of workout by 0.4, 0.3 & 0.3). **Examples use Endurance as the larger 40% division; customize the larger proportion for your desired focus area, whether Endurance, Strength or Flexibility/Balance/Coordination (FBC).**

20 min. workout: 8 min. Endurance—6 min. Strength—6 min. FBC
35 min. workout: 15 min. Endurance—10 min. Strength—10 min. FBC
65 min. workout: 25 min. Endurance—20 min. Strength—20 min. FBC

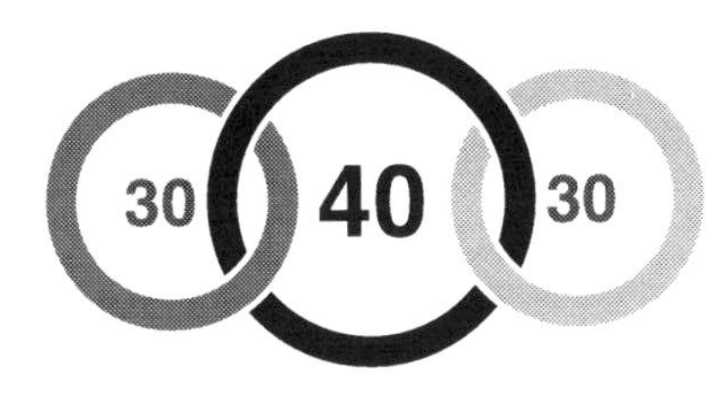

Example of Endurance-weighted **G**olden **O**lympic **T**raining Ratio of Endurance, Strength and Flexibility/Balance/Coordination (FBC). The larger/40% segment is always weighted towards your chosen sport's focus, to optimize your results in that arena. Maintaining a healthy balance of these 3 training segments is a cornerstone of optimal fitness, performance and longevity.

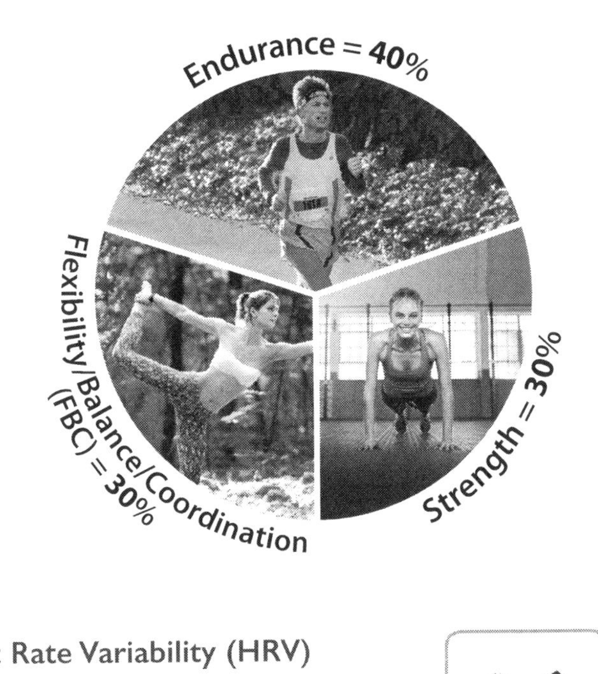

9 Measuring Your Heart Rate Variability (HRV)

HRV4 Logo

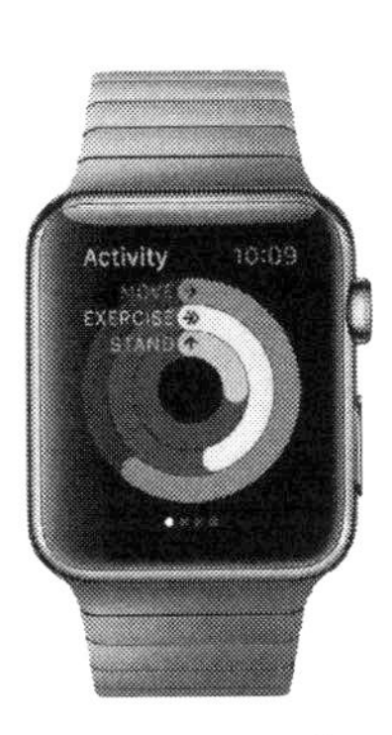

Apple Watch®

Knowing and optimizing your Heart Rate Variability (HRV) on a regular basis is a secret health, performance and longevity weapon you can't afford to be without. The great news is that measuring your HRV is now very simple, as the technology has become easily and cheaply available on smartphones and other devices, such as the Apple Watch. The most convenient way is via the app HRV4TRAINING, available at: www.hrv4training.com This easy-to-use app, which also measures your Heart Rate, works by simply placing your fingertip over your smartphone's camera lens.

10 Easy Golden Spiral Movement & Sitting Upgrade

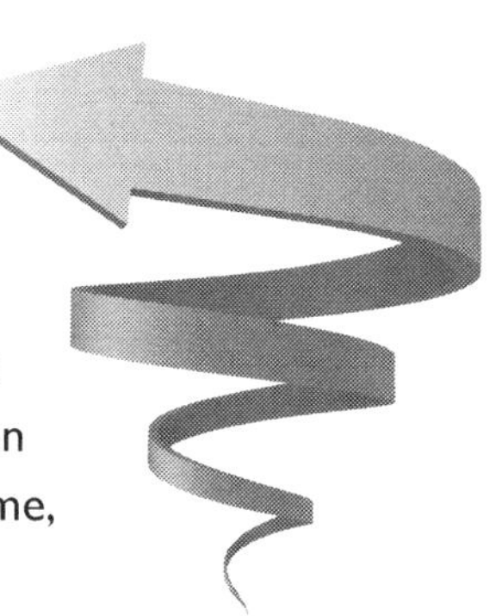

Try following a gentle Golden Spiral the next time you get out of bed, rise from a chair, get out of a bathtub or exit a car. With your spine relaxed, allow your body to gently *spiral up* as you rise. You'll feel less effort and put less stress on your back when you follow Nature's spiral path of least resistance. Modifying movements by incorporating the Golden Spiral also enhances your balance and breathing; at the same time, stiffness and rigidity in both body and mind is gently released.

For a healthy movement break when sitting, try this: with your spine erect and weight equally balanced on your sitz bones (your derriere's bony part), begin moving your pelvis in a gentle spiraling motion, starting in the center of an imaginary spiral and unwinding 3 times, tracing an expanding Golden Spiral. Then spiral back to the center by reversing direction. These spirals can be traced in both clockwise and counterclockwise directions. Note that the Golden Spiral moves up through the spine and entire body, even though it's initiated in your pelvis. As you spiral back to center, the center of the spiral may feel like a gentle still point. Pause for a few moments and enjoy the feeling.

11 Upgrade Your Body-Mind Integration

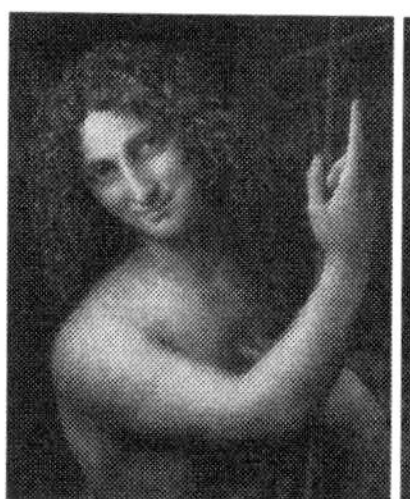
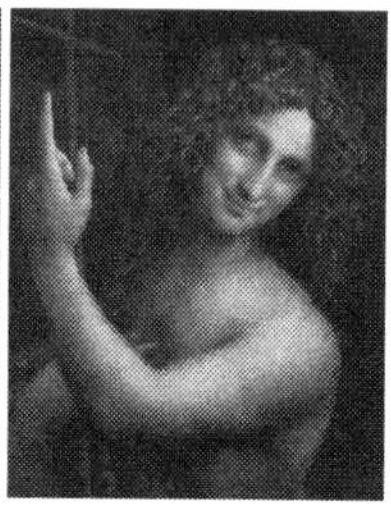

Leonardo da Vinci's *St. John the Baptist*, aka *St. John the Ambidextrous*.

One of the fascinating talents of Golden Ratio genius Leonardo da Vinci was his ability to use both his left and right hands with near-equal skill. Yet most people are 100% right or left dominant and never question it; we've come to accept without question the notion that one side does all and fits all. This is like using only a portion of your whole potential. Ambidexterity is not just a freak talent reserved for the lucky few. In fact, not cultivating your non-dominant hand/side wastes a huge opportunity to upgrade your brain synchronization, creativity and health. So invite your non-dominant side to the table and get your whole brain and body more in the game. Take some baby steps to move from a 100:0 ratio of Right or Left side dominance towards a more Golden 62:38 Ratio. At first it may be challenging, yet like learning any valuable skill, the rewards are vast.

Benefits

- More integrated, whole-brain function and synergy
- Enhanced creativity, innovation and problem solving
- Better body-balance, symmetry, proportion and movement
- Increased ability to adapt to physical and mental challenges

Exercises—Practice switching to your non-dominant side while

- Brushing your teeth, combing hair
- Holding a fork, knife or glass
- Practicing sports, e.g., tennis, ping-pong, baseball, basketball, archery
- Opening doors, flipping switches
- Dialing your phone or entering data
- Using your mouse or trackpad
- Writing, signing your name, drawing, painting

> *Balance the body, balance the brain.*
> *The future lies with the ambidextrous human!*
> **Professor Raymond Dart, Australian anatomist & anthropologist**

A dramatic increase in your ambidexterity is "at hand." By practicing these simple exercises with your non-dominant hand/side, you'll soon be surprised by your improved balance, coordination and creativity. It's never too late to start enjoying a more synchronized and integrated body-mind-spirit.

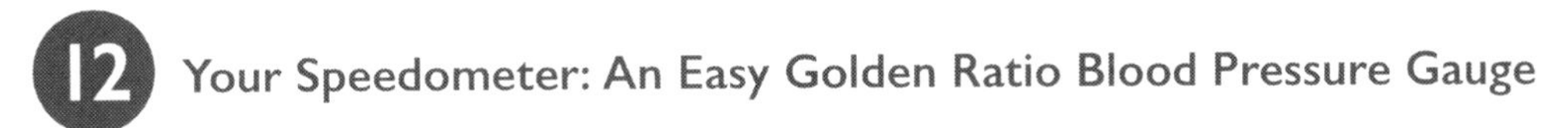

12 Your Speedometer: An Easy Golden Ratio Blood Pressure Gauge

With a simple conversion scale, you can quickly plot your blood pressure readings to see how close they are to the Golden Ratio. This scale is derived from a speedometer, which shows miles per hour (mph) alongside kilometers per hour (km/h). This scale also reveals an intriguing fact: the ratio of mph to km/h is very close to the Golden Ratio—and can also be used to evaluate blood pressure readings. Look at your speedometer and you'll see the following Golden Ratio readings, which resemble various possible blood pressure readings:

100 km/h = 60 mph
120 km/h = 75 mph
160 km/h = 100 mph
} **Φ 1.6 Golden Ratio**

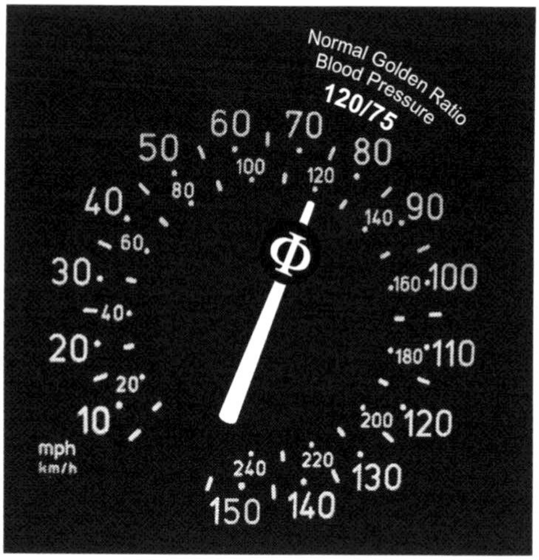

Golden Ratio Blood Pressure

Your speedometer is really a *Golden Ratio Blood Pressure Gauge*. Kilometers per hour (km/h) to miles per hour (mph) gives the full spectrum of Golden Ratio blood pressure possibilities.

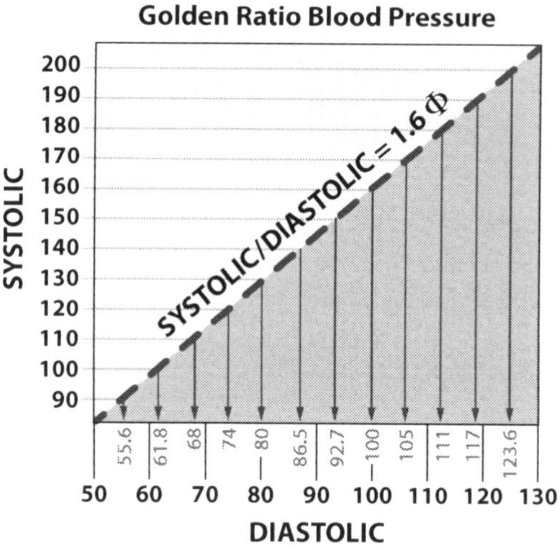

This graph shows Golden Ratio blood pressure readings across a wide range.

To see if your blood pressure readings are in Golden Ratio range, you'll need a recent blood pressure reading (home arm blood pressure monitors which offer quite accurate, near-instant readings can be purchased online). Next, find your systolic reading (the higher of your two blood pressure numbers) on the speedometer's km/h line. Then look directly across at the mph line and plot your diastolic reading (the lower of your two blood pressure numbers) in mph. **If your systolic reading is directly across from your diastolic reading, then they are in Golden Ratio. Golden Ratio blood pressure evaluations always look at quality *and* quantity; whether or not the systolic and diastolic readings are in Golden Ratio determines the *quality* of the reading.**

How high or low the readings are determines the *quantity*. In the speedometer examples above, 100/60 is considered borderline low blood pressure, yet still maintains a Golden Ratio. 120/75 is in the normal range and is also in Golden Ratio. 160/100 is considered high blood pressure, yet still maintains the Golden Ratio. Even if a blood pressure reading is too high or too low—quantity—there is still a presumed physiologic advantage if it's in Golden Ratio—quality.

If your blood pressure readings are either too high or too low and/or aren't right across from one another on your speedometer, start incorporating the Nature's Secret Nutrient recommendations into your life, in addition to consulting with your physician or health care professional.

13 Check & Track Your Morning Heart Rate

One of the quickest and easiest ways to get a broad spectrum reading on the status of your body's overall operating system is to monitor your morning heart rate. This simple bit of information will let you know if your body is sufficiently rested to let you perform at your best in the upcoming day. There are both low-tech and high-tech methods to check your heart rate. **Make sure you do your pulse measurement *before you get out of bed in the morning,* as you always want to use your lowest morning heart rate to establish an accurate baseline.** Any elevation above your baseline average heart rate gives you a basic reading of the tone of your autonomic nervous system and can alert you to the possibility of general stress, overtraining syndrome, inadequate sleep or even an increased mortality risk. A Golden Ratio resting heart rate of 62 beats/min is a good ballpark figure to be at or below in order to help keep overall mortality risk low and life expectancy high; see the section on Golden Ratio Heart Rate & Longevity near the end of Ch 6 Exercise to review the heart rate and mortality risk link.

Low-tech heart rate check method:

Take your carotid artery pulse for 15 seconds and multiply by 4 to get your heart rate in beats per minute. Using your index and middle fingers, press gently to feel the pulsation in your neck, just to the side of your trachea (wind pipe). Check either left or right carotid pulses, whichever is easier. Use a watch or stopwatch to count your pulse for 15 seconds and multiply by 4, or for greater accuracy, measure for a full minute.

High-tech heart rate check methods:

1. Use the free Azumio Instant **Heart Rate Monitor app** (other free apps are available). It's a simple way to check your AM heart rate. Just place your finger over your smartphone's camera flash for 10 seconds… *and that's it.* The app automatically calculates your heart without any counting or using a watch or stopwatch.
2. The finger clip-on, laser-activated **Pulse Oximeter** is another quick and easy way to check your AM heart rate as well as monitor the oxygen saturation of your blood. Readings can be taken multiple times per day to help you correlate bodily sensations of rest or exertion with actual data points. Low oxygen saturation is an instant reminder to take a series of Golden Breaths to recharge your blood with life-giving oxygen. Various models are available online for under $20.

Heart rate monitors are of great value for checking not only AM resting heart rate before you get out of bed, they can also be used during exercise to help fine-tune your workouts. Everyone has a differing resting heart rate depending on age, gender,

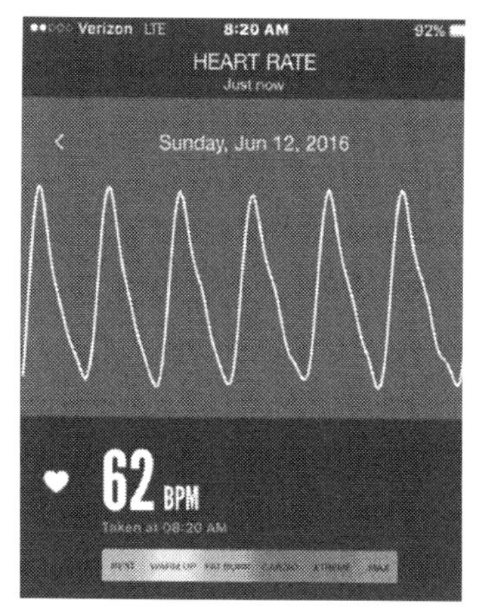

Screen shot from Azumio's free Instant Heart Rate Monitor app. In 10 seconds it measures your heart rate by use of your smartphone's camera flash.

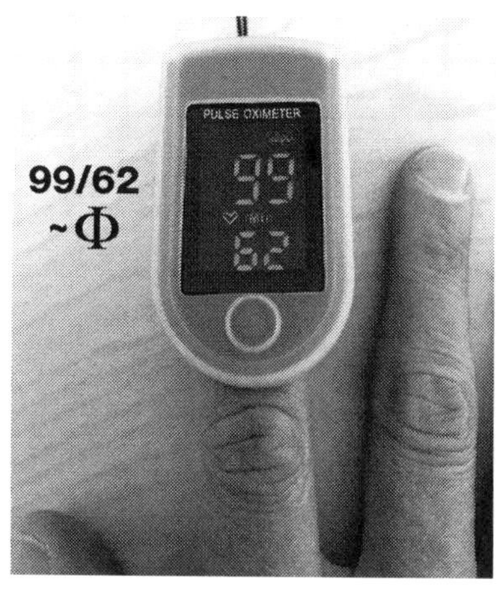

The pocket laser-activated Pulse Oximeter fits like a gentle clothespin on the end of your finger. In 10 seconds, it shows both the oxygen saturation % of your blood (top number) and heart rate (beats per minute; bottom number).

medical conditions, overall athletic conditioning and activity level. You have to establish baseline readings over a week or so to then be able to decide if your heart rate is in a healthy range for you. This one measurement can change over time and gives a great amount of information, considering the time it takes to do it. If you want to glean more detailed information about your heart rate, see Rx #9, Heart Rate Variability (HRV). Consultation with your physician or athletic trainer is advised, since every person has variable considerations and goals. Be sure to log your AM heart rate—before you get out of bed in the morning—in the Priority Coach app or in the paper version at the back of the book to monitor and learn from your resting heart rate over time.

14 Yoga & the Golden Ratio are both Unified Fields

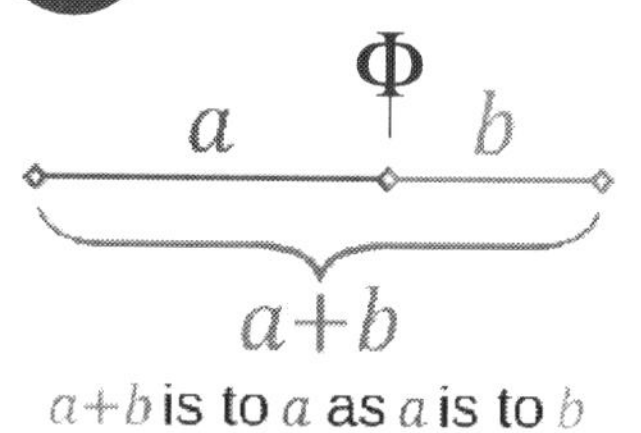

Yoga, the ancient Sanskrit word for Union, is the oldest mind-body-spirit exercise system in recorded history, with myriad variations existent around the world. Like the ancient science of acupuncture, Yoga's origins are lost in the mists of time. At its root is an integrated system for working with and tuning the body to support optimal posture, muscle tone, organ function, blood and energy flow and overall health, performance, happiness and longevity. Both Yoga and the NSN system are premier examples of *biohacking*, or integrating multiple,

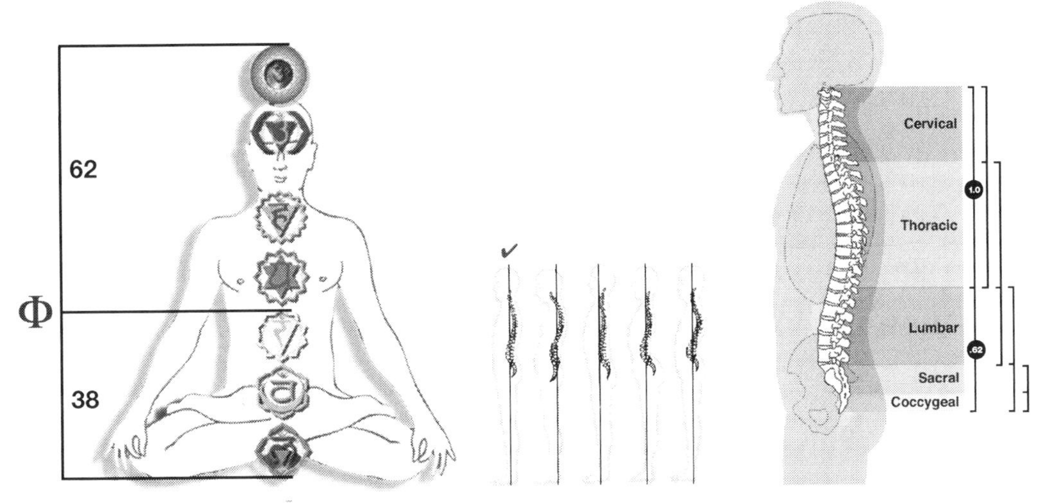

(L) Emotional equilibrium occurs when upper chakras (humanistic & transcendent functions) are in balance with lower chakras (primitive survival functions). (R) Perfect spinal alignment occurs when vertebrae are in Golden Ratio relationship to one another.

cross-reinforcing practices simultaneously in order to generate megadoses of life energy (prana) or NSN. Interestingly, the Golden Ratio is humanity's foremost geometrical expression of Union, Unity or the Unified Field. The most basic example of the Golden Ratio as a Unity phenomenon is the classic line diagram, where two lines of specific lengths (a & b) are combined such that **a + b is to a, as a is to b**. Essentially, the whole becomes greater than the sum of its parts, which is the very definition of *synergy*. In addition, its parts are fractalized, so that each is self-similar to the others.

This geometrical Unity function has its corollary in the Yogic system of health and spirituality. When our body, mind and spirit are harmonized and fractalized not only within ourselves, but with society and the world at large, we experience the Union that is Yoga—and the Unified Field that is the Golden Ratio. Our physical structure has its own potential for Unity as well. Regarding spinal alignment, we can practice refining and perfecting our integration with the gravitational field until we have a zero-stress body that promotes vibrant health, wellbeing and longevity. Yogic spinal Union is exemplified in the diagram above, where we see that in ideal posture, each group of vertebrae is in Golden Ratio relationship with the others. When spinal balance and dynamic integration is achieved, optimal energy flow up and down the spine (kundalini) promotes a state of profound health and vitality in body, mind and spirit. On an energetic level, the resulting equilibrium in all of the body's primary energy centers (chakras) is often experienced as peace, bliss and union.

The Human Spine follows the Golden Spiral

One of the many amazing capacities of the human spine is that it has the inherent flexibility to move in fluid Golden Spirals. The following images artfully demonstrate how we have the ability for spinal flexion and extension that reflect two aspects of the Golden Spiral, infolding and outfolding. These Yin and Yang complementary movements are the foundation that gives us the flexibility and adaptability to carry out the wide-ranging movements necessary for both surviving and thriving in the physical world. As such, they're also the core movements around which yoga is structured. Add rotation, inversion, breathing and meditation variations and you've got the essence of all yoga practices.

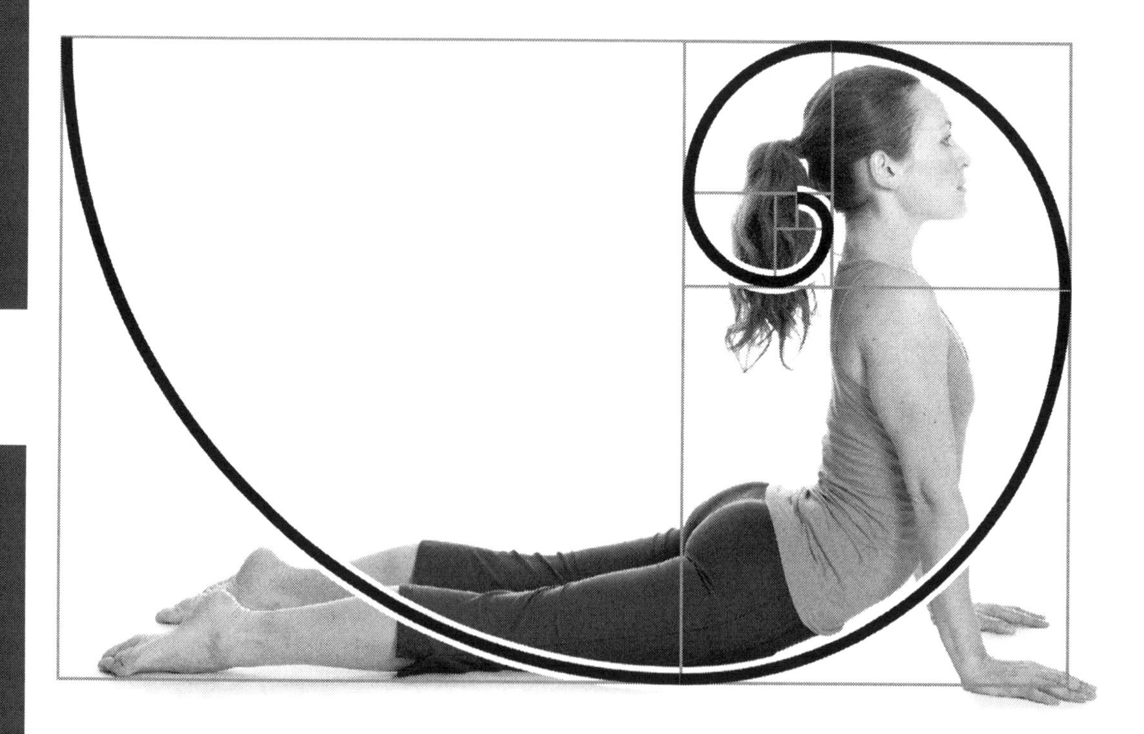

The human spine naturally tracks a Golden Ratio Spiral in both extension and flexion. In addition to being a super posture reset, Harvard Professor Amy Cuddy points out that just 2-3 minutes in Cobra pose (above) has been shown to simultaneously increase testosterone/power & confidence hormone by approx. 16%. and reduce cortisol/stress & anxiety hormone by approx. 10%. This +16%, -10% ratio is the Golden Ratio in dynamic action.

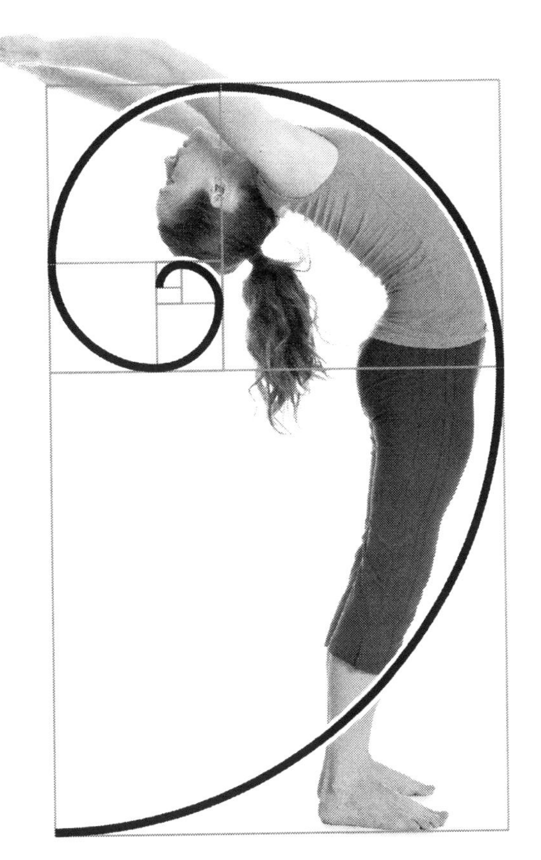

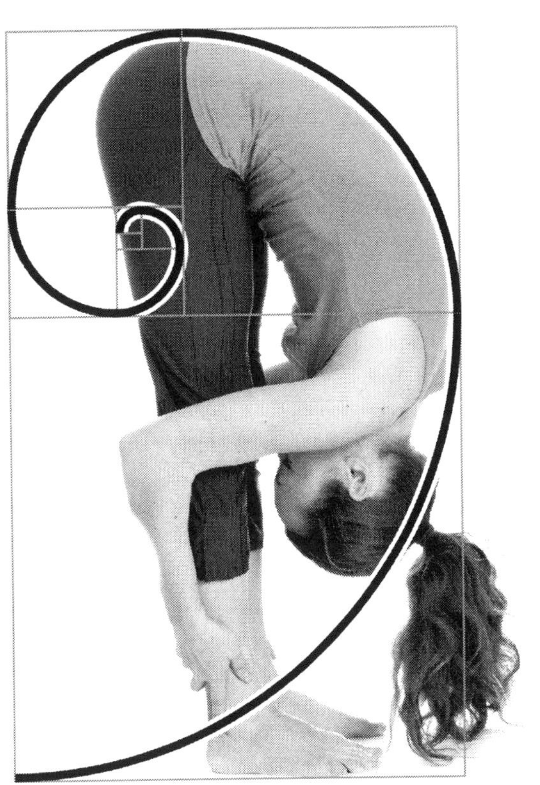

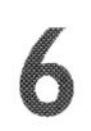

Health is the First Secret of Success.

Charles Atlas, American health & bodybuilding pioneer

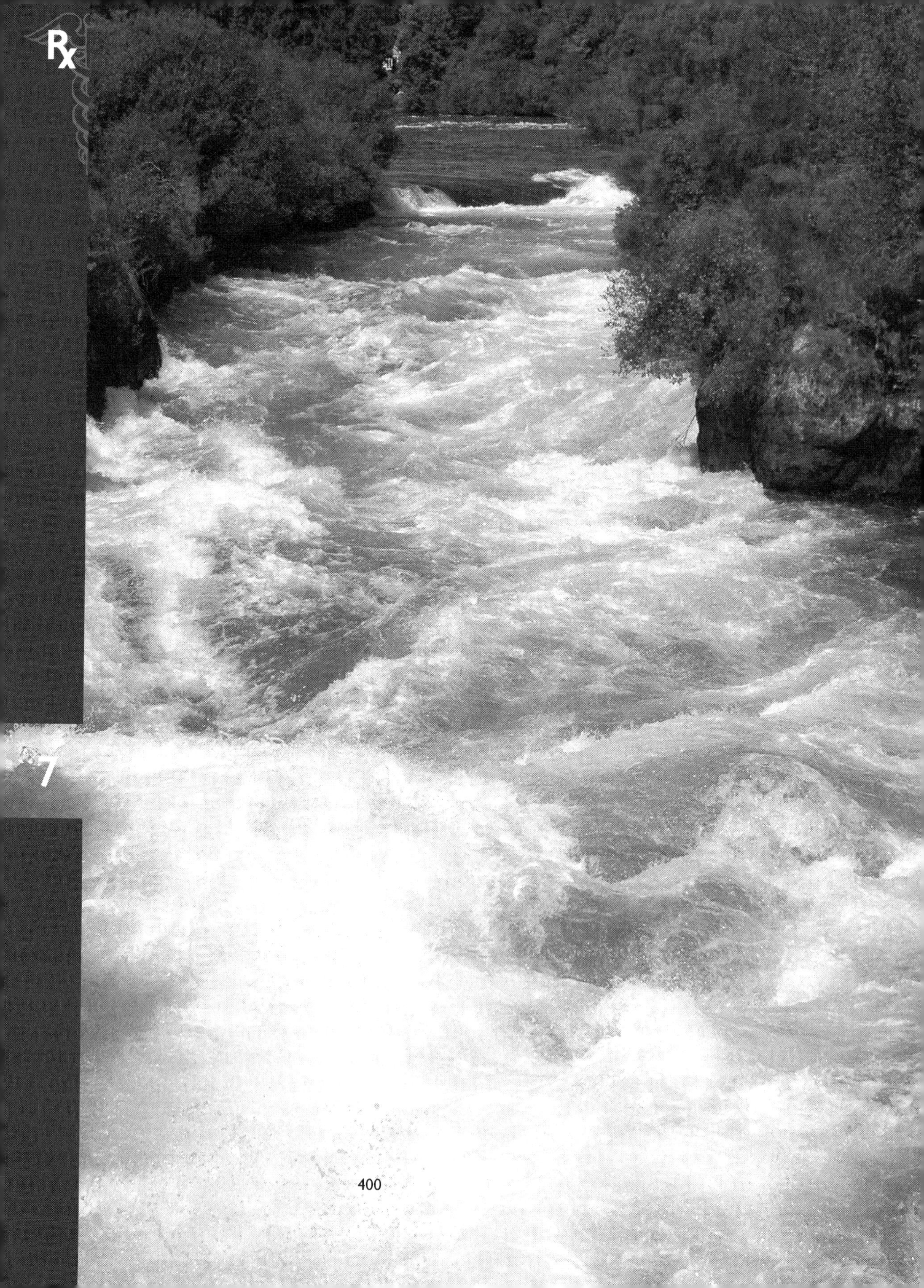
Rx
7

7

Detox Rx's

Pick one or more of the following Rx's to add to your NSN daily health regimen.

1 Activate Your AM BM: Morning Bowel Movement

As we saw in Ch 3 Sun/Light, light is a potent cue for daily resetting and synchronizing our circadian rhythms. Regular morning bowel movements can also be used to reset and maintain our biorhythms. We need a way to tune our internal clocks to ensure bowel movements happen in the AM, as morning bowel movements are essential to detoxify and remove waste products collected from the previous day and night. Here are several helpful ways to assist and cleanse a sluggish colon.

- Drink one or two glasses of pure water with lemon upon arising.
- Activate your colon by doing 30 seconds of stomach pumps: after a deep exhalation, roll your stomach muscles up and down 5-8 times. Rest and repeat 2-3 times. This motion activates your colonic reflex.
- Increase the fiber in your diet, easily done via adding one to two tablespoons of fresh ground flax or chia seeds to your meals, e.g., mixed into oatmeal, sprinkled over salads or mixed into any dish. Or, soak a tablespoon of chia or flax seeds in 1/4 cup of water overnight to hydrate them for easier digestion. Eating more raw foods is also advised; experiment with increasing your intake. Go slow; it can take your

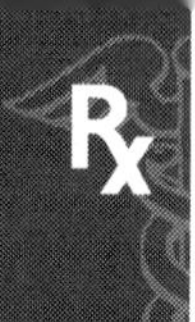

digestive system a few weeks to adjust to an increase of raw foods.

- Colon cleansing can be advantageous. You may benefit from some gentle herbal colon cleansing formulas which also provide laxative and bulking assistance. Excellent intestinal fiber/cleansing products are **Dr. Richard Schulze's** Intestinal Formulas #1, #2 and #3 and can be found at www.HerbDoc.com.
- Add fermented/cultured foods to your diet, such as yogurt, kefir, kombucha tea, sauerkraut, pickles, miso, kimchi or powdered or encapsulated probiotics.
- If your colon is particularly sluggish, you may want to get a series of colonic irrigations to help jump-start the detoxification process and reestablish regularity.
- Take Vitamin C (1-2 grams) and Magnesium (200-400mg.) before bedtime.
- Enjoy a cup of coffee or tea: caffeine often triggers AM bowel movements.

2 Practice Hot & Cold Water Therapy Detox

Cold water stimulates and hot water relaxes! Together, they are like a hydrostatic pump that makes blood flow! Circulation produces cures! Herbs cannot cure, if the blood cannot circulate! Hot & Cold Water Therapy can bring about better circulation, because the hot water stimulates blood flow to the surface of the body, while the cold water stimulates blood flow to the core of the body, thus bringing fresh blood to the organs and glands and all parts of the body! In other words, OXYGEN & NUTRIENTS IN + TOXINS & PATHOGENS OUT! Dr. Richard Schulze

Time To BeneFIT 3 Seconds

Hot and cold water therapy is a great way to harness water's unique healing abilities, via its amazing capacity to absorb and transfer heat through your body, as well as being the solvent for transporting nutrients to your cells and getting toxins out through perspiration. We've incorporated Fibonacci numbers and ratios into this practice in order make it more fun and easy to remember, as well as to activate NSN.

1. At the end of your warm/hot shower, go full cold for 13–21 seconds. Start the cold water on hands and feet first, then your front, back and lastly, your head.
2. At the end of your 13–21 second cold water treatment, switch back to warm/hot water for the next higher Fibonacci number of seconds, e.g., **13 cold/to 21 warm -or- 21 cold/to 34 warm**
3. Do 3 to 5 repetitions. Always end with *cold* water, which restores blood and energy to your core/vital organs.
4. For optimal detoxification, do the showers 1-2 times per day.
5. Drink a glass of pure water before and after to facilitate your detox.

3 Try the Triangulation of Fire Detox Strategy

Since many environmental toxins are stored in fat tissue, the only way to eliminate them is through a strategy that we call Triangulation of Fire. This 3-pronged approach attacks the challenge from 3 different angles, greatly amplifying the efficacy when combined into one strategy. These 3 angles are: **Exercising, Hydration & Sweating.** Once fats are mobilized by aerobic exercise, toxins are released into general circulation. Only at that point will they be able to come out in sweat. So, if you walk, jog, swim or bike for 20 minutes before going into a sauna or steam bath, you'll be able to get rid of fat-soluble toxins which are normally hard to detox. Sweat glands and sebaceous glands are a great pathway for the exit of many fat-soluble toxins. Be sure to drink adequate water while exercising to replace fluid losses. You can add electrolytes such as Emergen-C to your water in order to maintain mineral balance as well as take advantage of Vitamin C's ability to bind toxins in the gut and kidneys. This can help prevent possible reabsorption of toxins from the blood and gut back into your body. *NOTE: If you have a medical condition or don't have sauna or steam bath experience, check with your physician first before trying this detox method.*

Here's a summary of the process:

- Ample fluid replacement before, during and after exercise and sauna; add electrolytes, such as a packet of Emergen-C, to a LARGE glass of water.
- Aerobic exercise for 13-21 minutes.
- Sauna or steam sweating. Alternate going in and out of the sauna or steam room as tolerated. Take a cold shower during sauna breaks for 13, 21 or 34+ seconds for a great thermal pump boost. Remember not to overdo it. Use Fibonacci numbers for your sauna in-and-out and cold shower times to avoid monotony.

Example of possible sauna or steam bath and cold shower ratio:

5 mins. in, then 21 sec. cold shower, then 3 min. out; repeat or try new ratios.

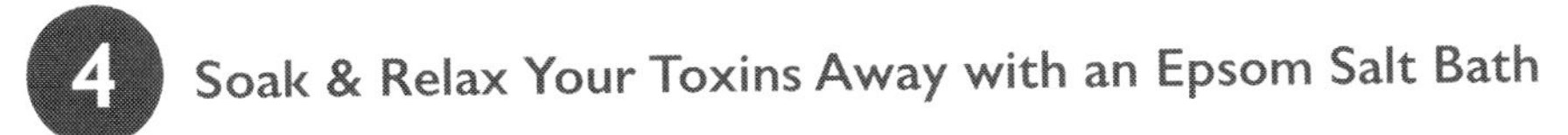

4 Soak & Relax Your Toxins Away with an Epsom Salt Bath

Another easy and enjoyable way to detox is by taking a warm Epsom salt (magnesium sulfate) bath. Epsom salt has many beneficial properties, including relaxation and detoxification. The magnesium helps with muscle relaxation and the sulfate is important for detoxification. Skin becomes more permeable in warm water, so absorption of magnesium and sulfate can occur, as well as passage of toxins out of the body. Epsom salt soothes tired, overused muscles and induces a deep feeling of calm. It's also great for travelers and as a post-workout soak for athletes. **To prepare your soak: run a warm/hot bath and add 1 to 3 cups+ of Epsom salt, available at drug stores and many food stores.** Soak 13-21 minutes; longer as desired. To enhance your soak, add a few drops of essential oil into the running water as your tub fills; eucalyptus oil is a common favorite. Before and after your bath, make sure you have a large glass of water to replenish fluid lost through sweating. If your bath is in the evening, notice the quality of your sleep and how you feel upon arising the next morning.

5 The NSN Parasite Eradication Program (PEP)

IF, in the last few years, you've...

- Dined in a restaurant • Eaten organic or unwashed produce
- Eaten raw sushi, shellfish or rare/under-cooked fish or meat
- Travelled to any country with questionable sanitation or water standards

...THEN you're very likely to be one of the many people who has undiagnosed intestinal parasites that are living off of your vital life force. These parasites not only steal your nutrients, they deposit their toxic waste products in your intestines and other vital organs. This constant internal poisoning disrupts your entire microbiome—microorganisms that make up your intestinal environment—wreaking havoc with your immune system's ability to regulate and protect your health. Yet most people are oblivious to the fact that their mysterious nagging symptoms and even serious health challenges may be directly related to parasites. Of course, parasites also interfere with your body's ability to extract maximum nourishment and NSN from your diet. Therefore, identifying and eradicating parasites is a *critical* starting point in restoring, maintaining and enhancing your health.

A highly effective approach is offered by **Ann Louise Gittleman**, M.S., CNS., who popularized parasite testing with her best-selling book, *Guess What Came to Dinner.* She uses the Parasite Flexi-Test to screen for many types of abnormal bacteria, fungi, protozoans and helminths (flukes and worms). In the privacy of your home, 3 stool samples and 2 saliva samples are collected and sent to the lab. Results go directly to Dr. Gittleman's office; you then receive a personalized letter of treatment recommendations to rid yourself of any discovered parasites. In the majority of cases, you'll be able to totally eradicate the parasites with herbal therapy. If, after several rounds of treatment you're not improving, you may need to repeat the test and see if the sensitivity testing indicates that drug therapy may be a desirable next-step option.

In the end, eradicating your parasites is worth the effort it requires as long as you're being monitored by your doctor for any side effects. The self-led Parasite Eradication Program (PEP) addresses the fact that many parasites have a little-known protective biofilm mucus layer that effectively shields them from any therapy meant to eradicate them; you must first disrupt the biofilm in order to expose them to the treatment. A Triangulation of Fire approach seems to be helpful in side-stepping the parasite's evasive strategy. This 3-pronged approach includes the following elements with varying protocols lasting from 5, 8, 13 or more days:

1. Colon cleansing to break down the parasites biofilm.
2. Herbal remedies to kill the parasites. Repeat treatment protocol 2–3 times, due to any dormant ova/eggs hatching after the initial treatment phase has finished.
3. Reflorastation of your microbiome with a mix of different natural probiotics, including yogurt, kefir, sauerkraut, miso, kimchi, or alternating on a weekly basis several different strains/formulations of over-the-counter encapsulated probiotics.

Recommended protocols and products can be purchased at the following websites:

1. Colon Cleansing: Dr. Schulze's Intestinal Formula's #1, #2 & #3; HerbDoc.com
2. Parasite Treatment Protocols: a. Ann Louise Gittleman's Colon Cleanse for Parasite Elimination: www.unikeyhealth.com/my-colon-cleansing-kit. b. Dr. Hulda Clark's Herbal Parasite Removal 13-day program: www.DrClarkStore.com
3. Probiotic Reflorastation: Garden of Life Raw Probiotics and Prescript-Assist Probiotics; both available online. 4. Biokleen Produce Wash: available online.

In the future, avoid all raw or under-cooked fish/meat and make sure all produce eaten is washed well. Biokleen Produce Wash removes chemical sprays and utilizes grapefruit seed and orange peel extract to kill any critters; also use it to clean kitchen prep areas as well. Repeat the PEP cleanse treatment on a seasonal basis (4 times/year) to maintain intestinal health and be proactive against reinfestation. Add this Rx to your NSN Priority Coach app and note how you feel before, during and after your treatment.

Additional Parasite Removal & Life Cleansing Practices

The parasite dynamic plays out in other areas of our lives in addition to internal parasites. From bed bugs to dust mites to funguses to parasitic/draining people, we are surrounded by often overlooked yet easily addressed drains on our vital life force. These drains pull us out of life alignment, fragment our focus and rob us of energy. To reduce the parasitic drag of these factors on your health and happiness, consider integrating any/all of the following strategies which may not already be a part of your lifestyle:

1. Wash your bedding weekly in hot, perfume-free, soapy water.

2. Vacuum and clean your house weekly, as dust traps and holds toxic chemicals, e.g., flame retardants, building materials, etc. (HEPA filter vacuums are best).
3. Do a deep house cleaning and clutter removal seasonally.
4. Irrigate your sinuses with a Neti Pot 2-3 times/week; use skin temperature water with a pinch of sea salt or 3-5 drops of colloidal silver.
5. Address any athletes foot or nail fungus issues.
6. Optimize good oral hygiene with regular dental cleaning. Add a few drops of colloidal silver to your teeth brushing regimen.
7. Stop exposure to emotionally parasitic/draining people, places, situations, thoughts.

6 Periodically Detox Your Body's Main Detox Organ

Your liver is your largest and heaviest internal organ (about 1/40 of total body weight), weighing an average of 2.9 lbs. (1.3 kilograms) in women and 3.5 lbs. (1.6 kilograms) in men. **Everything you eat or drink** passes through your liver to be metabolized for assimilation or detoxified and prepared for removal from your body. Toxins are made water-soluble by the liver and secreted into bile and then into the stool. Water-soluble toxins may also be cleared through the kidneys. As the liver is your main organ of detoxification, it can become overworked, sluggish and occasionally even clogged, leading to numerous health challenges, including fatigue, nausea, loss of appetite, brain fog and immune dysregulation. One effective way to both maintain and restore healthy liver function is to do a liver detox. **We recommend Dr. Richard Schulze's Liver Detox system, available at: www.HerbDoc.com.**

7 Go Smoke Free in 21 Days

The Golden Ratio principle exhibits equally powerful expansive and contractive action. As a unique method to go smoke-free, the following pattern of accelerated reduction follows the *Fibonacci Sequence in reverse,* down a 21-Day reduction spiral to zero cigarettes. The Fibonacci Sequence is used for determining both the number of cigarettes smoked, and the days on which you reduce that number. To start, pick the nearest Fibonacci number below the number of cigarettes you currently smoke per day. For example, if you currently smoke a pack a day (20 cigarettes in USA packs), then 13 is the closest lower Fibonacci number, so you'd smoke 13 cigarettes for the first

8 days. Then you'd drop to 8 cigarettes for the next 5 days. Continuing your Fibonacci deceleration cycle, you'd drop to 5 cigarettes for the next 3 days, and so on until you've gotten to zero cigarettes.

Number of Cigarettes	13	8	5	3	2	1...
Number of Days	8	5	3	2	1	1...

If you're smoking significantly more or less than in the above example, you'll want to create a custom deceleration cycle, e.g., beginning with the higher Fibonacci numbers 34 to 55 for more, or extending the days of smoking less cigarettes, to allow for modifications of the standard 21-Day new habit cycle.

8 NSN Nicotine Withdrawal Therapy

If you're using a nicotine patch to control smoking withdrawal symptoms, consider experimenting with decreasing dosages, sequenced to Fibonacci days. A friend of the authors chose nicotine patches to help stop smoking. He changed the strength of his patches every 8 days, which kept him aware that he was achieving his habit change in tune with Nature's Path of Least Resistance. Nicoderm® nicotine patches (21mg–14mg–7mg) are the closest of the smoking reduction patches that approximate Fibonacci Sequence Numbers of 21–13–8. Nicotine is a unique drug in that it exhibits homeostatic (balancing) properties. It acts as a mental, emotional and physical body balancer. So, if you're tired a cigarette gives you a lift; conversely, if you're nervous or anxious, it calms you down. As nicotine and smoking's addictive, negative health impacts are well-known, we need to find a healthful alternative—a new habit to take its place. As you've learned, *you can never fully erase a negative habit; you can only replace or "overwrite" it with a new, healthy, more ingrained behavior.* **We suggest replacing smoking with Golden Ratio Breathing**—inhaling to 3, exhaling to 5—a natural, healthful way to regain balance in your autonomic nervous system. During the 21-Day smoking deceleration cycle, the carbon monoxide that has been blocking your body's oxygenation processes will rapidly be replaced with healthy oxygen, supporting detoxification without throwing your body into physiologic withdrawal. Doing Golden Ratio Breathing throughout the day supports a smoother transition to a healthier, smoke-free life.

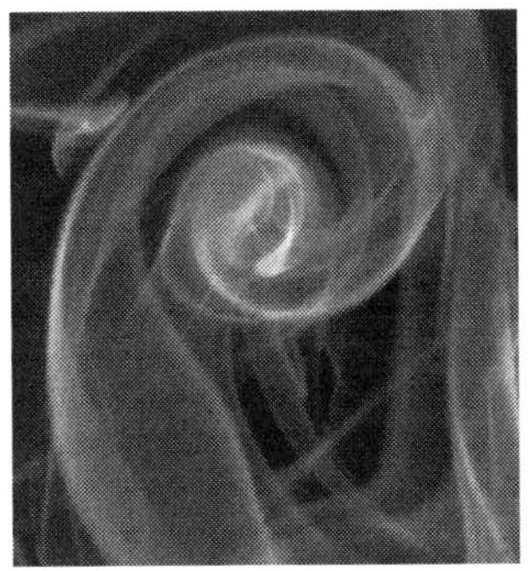

Even smoke follows Nature's Path of Least Resistance—the Golden Spiral.

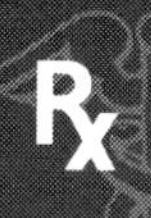

9 Fibonacci's Critical Electromagnetic Fields (EMF) Detox

Reducing exposure to modern life's omnipresent, toxic ElectroMagnetic Fields (EMF's) from cell phones, WiFi, power lines, household wiring, electric appliances, "Smart" meters, etc., is a required practice if optimal health and longevity is a serious goal.

Expanding the range of what is normally thought of as toxic pollution, we must now include exposure to man-made EMF's (ElectroMagnetic Fields) as an environmental poison. This silent yet intensifying toxicity source includes EMF's emanating from:

Cellphones, cordless phones, computers, routers, WiFi, television, "smart" power meters, power lines, electric outlets, cords & appliances, e.g., clock radios.

Note: see standard radiation detoxification protocols on pages 228-9.

While man-made EMF radiation may be invisible to the naked eye, its proven ability to disrupt a wide range of biomolecules (in cell membranes, mitochondria and DNA) and biorhythms is cause for immediate remedial action (numerous references corroborate this finding: search on the web under "EMF/DNA damage"). **Man-made EMF's interfere with the natural earth, sun and moon EMF's to which we synchronize all of our biologic activities.** The most basic biorhythm is our light/dark regulated wake/sleep cycle. As this most basic biorhythm is being disrupted by man-made, unnatural EMF's, we are surely experiencing negative health-impairing consequences. The risk to your health and longevity over time is a very real and one that must be reduced as much as possible. Compounding the problem is that this source of technological toxicity has become an addiction in modern times. We just can't seem to do without being plugged in to the EMF Matrix 24/7. In this technological age, it's seemingly impossible to live without a generally high degree of connectivity to "the grid." Rather than reducing exposure by going cold turkey, you can strive to cut down your exposure by a meaningful amount, yet not so much as to throw yourself into withdrawal, e.g., a reasonable amount of decrease would be to reduce by the Golden Ratio amount of 38%.

Using Fibonacci numbers is the quickest and easiest way to hit this 38% marker and easily figure out how many hours of exposure to cut. For example, if your combined daily cellphone/computer/tablet time is 13 hours, then move to the next lower Fibonacci number to see how many hours would be your new high limit. In this case, you would limit usage to 8 hours. Just moving down one interval on the

Fibonacci ladder can have a dramatic improvement on the way you feel and in your overall health. This decreased EMF exposure time will also force you to be more focused and efficient in accomplishing what you really need to. Junk surfing and random gossiping will be eliminated, leaving you with an upgraded plugged-in experience. **A very simple yet effective way you can address the constant EMF bombardment experienced in the modern world is to simply turn off the WiFi transmitter (and ideally the electricity in your sleeping area) in your home when you sleep.** As sleep is the critical time when your body does most of its healing and regeneration, it's especially important to reduce/remove toxic EMF interference while sleeping. This one practice assures that your body is protected from EMF's during at least the smaller Golden Ratio portion of each day as you rest and regenerate. Be sure to reduce other silent sources of EMF exposure as mentioned previously, to give your system even more relief from this all-consuming yet invisible 21st century toxin. If you're a city dweller and have a chronic health challenge, you'd be wise to experiment with moving out of the light polluted, toxic EMF city environment and into the countryside, to let your system readjust to a more healthy natural light, EMF-free environment that only Dr. Mother Nature can provide.

10 Bulletproof® Coffee Detox to the Rescue

When ingenious entrepreneur and Bulletproof Executive **Dave Asprey** took an age old Tibetan recipe calling for combining yak butter with tea and adapted it to coffee-loving Westerners, an innovative new morning biohack was created. Dave intended his new creation, Bulletproof® Coffee (BPC) to be consumed as a slow, fat-burning and long-lasting morning energy beverage that would hold physical and mental energy levels steady anywhere from 4-6 hours. In addition to BPC's growing popularity in this arena, Dave perhaps unknowingly also discovered a convenient and enjoyable way for people to detox their bodies. Since consumption of both coffee and fat independently cause a strong bile-secreting and toxin-releasing action in both the liver and gallbladder, BPC can act as a daily mini-liver/gallbladder flush and colon stimulant. Asprey's BPC innovation accomplishes so much so easily that it could become known as the *6th Tibetan Rite*. Meanwhile, we'll use BPC as a unique cleansing and energizing biohack to compliment the other powerful NSN Detox Rx's. Visit www.BulletProof.com for the BPC recipe and more information on Dave's trailblazing human performance work.

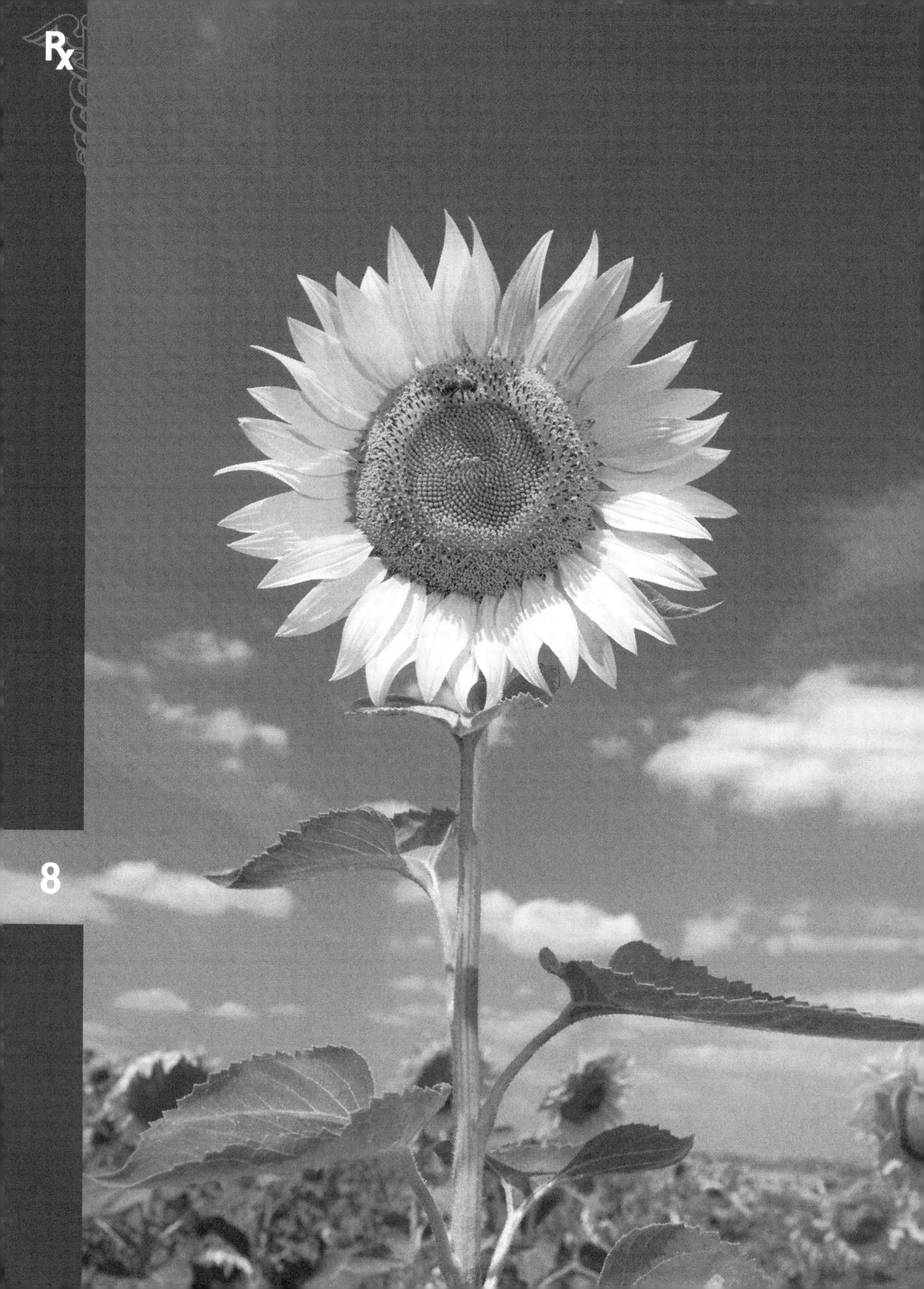

Rx
8

8

Happiness Rx's

Pick one or more of the following Rx's to add to your NSN daily health regimen.

1 Honor the Golden Doors of Your Day

Time To BeneFIT 5 Seconds

When you awaken each morning you are presented with the golden gift of another day. At the end of your day when you lay down to sleep, you are preparing to relax deeply and recharge for the next day. Sleep is the great mystery we all share and require and through which these golden doors are linked. Taking up around 1/3 of every day, sleep is foundational to your health, performance and longevity. It is similar in a sense to a scuba diver taking a long deep dive every night and then emerging every morning. Yet many of us fail to properly honor and prepare for both our descent into sleep and our reemergence from it. We hurry to bed, all too often staying glued to a screen right up until we close our eyes. Upon awaking we rocket out of bed and into our day. We know that if a diver surfaces too rapidly decompression sickness is very possible and the results can be serious, even deadly. Similarly, rushing through the Golden Doors of each day is deleterious to your health, performance and fulfillment. How can you honor and strengthen the twin Golden Doors each day presents? Following is an easy, powerful 5-minute Golden Door practice. Try it for 21 days and

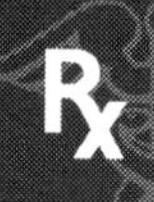

see the difference for yourself. This exercise has the added benefit of *clustering* several optimal health and happiness habits into *one* easy practice. Result? A growing sense of accomplishment, as well as effective habit upgrade and transformation.

Golden Doors Practice

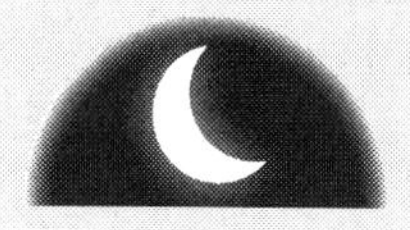

PM

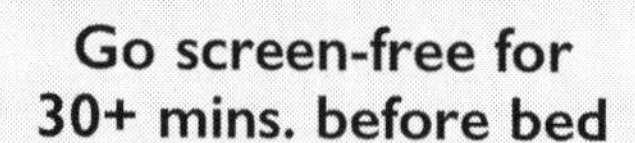

Go screen-free for 30+ mins. before bed

Sit tall or lie down. Go ***Palms Up*** *for good posture and breathing. Close your eyes and take...*

Φ **3 Golden Breaths**
inhale deeply to 3, exhale to 5

Φ **3 Gratitudes**
Imagine 3 things you're grateful for, e.g., your health, family, life

Φ **Set Your Intention**
e.g., *I will sleep wonderfully*

Φ Imagine your body filling with **Blue Light**. Let the light flood you with healing, love and wisdom

Ease into deep, relaxing sleep...

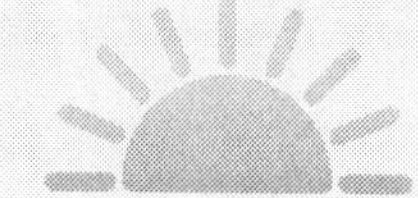

AM

Return to bed or sit after waking; set alarm for 5 mins.

Drink a tall glass of water. Then go ***Palms Up*** *for good posture and breathing. Close your eyes and take...*

Φ **3 Golden Breaths**
inhale deeply to 3, exhale to 5

Φ **3 Gratitudes**
Imagine 3 things you're grateful for, e.g., your health, family, life

Φ **Set Your Intention**
e.g., *I will have an amazing day*

Φ Imagine your body filling with **Golden Light**. Let the light flood you with healing, love and wisdom

Open your eyes, start your day...

2 Elevate Your Happiness with Gratitude & Appreciation

As 1964 Olympic 10K Gold Medal winner **Billy Mills** points out, ***your subconscious mind cannot tell the difference between reality or imagination.*** Said another way: *Whatever you APPRECIATE (regularly focus your heart and mind on, value) APPRECIATES (grows, like assets in a bank).* Mills rehearsed his historic victory in his mind daily for four years, leading to his achieving one of the greatest upsets in Olympic history. There is enormous hidden power in using your imagination to focus on what you most want to create and grow in your life. Focused appreciation, gratitude and expectancy are like super magnets—they attract their counterparts. When you focus on both what you want and are most grateful for in life, you attract more of it. Focusing on happiness attracts more of the same. Then, appreciate—focus with feeling—on as many appreciation points as you wish with eyes closed for a few moments. Remember to sit tall and breathe deeply. Let your mind flow over your Appreciation Points. Feel them as if they are real, *now*. Then, open your eyes and release those good feelings into your day. Whenever you need a boost, repeat. As **Oprah Winfrey** said,

> *The more you praise and celebrate your life, the more there is in life to celebrate.*

Gratitude & Appreciation List

Φ **I am most Grateful for** *(aim for 2–3 items)*:

____

____

Φ **My Greatest Strengths:**

____

____

Φ **Inspiring Activities** *(things I LOVE to do)*:

____

____

Φ **Inspiring People** *(past or present)*:

____

____

Φ **Inspiring Places** *(places where I feel GREAT)*:

____

____

Φ I am Happiest when I:

____

____

Φ My Wild Dreams *(e.g., travel around the world, climb Everest, write a book)*:

____

____

Φ My Unique or Hidden Talents:

____

____

Φ My Greatest Life Triumphs:

____

____

3 Reactivate Your DNA with the NSN Mandala Meditation

Time To BeneFIT 5 Seconds

The use of mandalas is an ancient and powerful method to de-stress, ground and center. This mandala exercise helps you communicate with one of the most microscopic, archetypal parts of yourself—your Golden Ratio-based DNA. Gazing at this DNA cross-sectional image drops you into a relaxed state of meditative reflection.

Softly gaze at the DNA image on the following page, as you breathe slowly and deeply for 3 minutes in a cadence of 3 seconds in to 5 seconds out. Then close your eyes and continue to see this beautiful Golden Ratio latticework in your mind's eye. When it fades, slowly open your eyes. You'll feel deeply relaxed and more in sync with the Golden Ratio, the underlying blueprint of life.

> *There is ALWAYS something to celebrate, so long as life is being lived.*
> *Seeing your cup as at least* [62%] *full is the key to enduring happiness.*
> **Neale Donald Walsch, author of *Conversations With God***
> [with a slight modification—from *half* to **62%** full—by the authors]

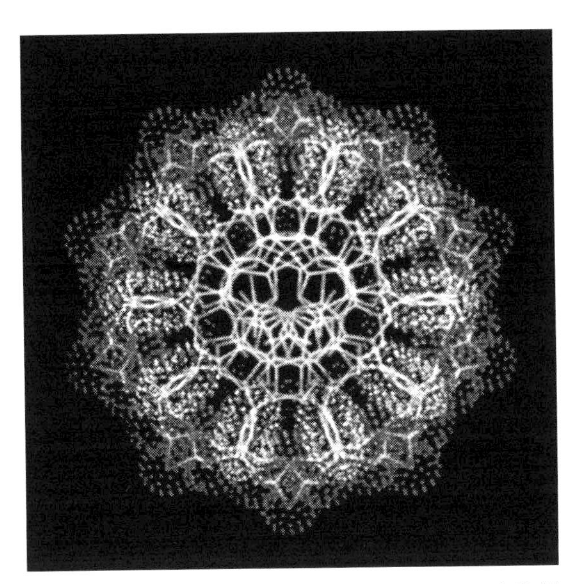

Cross section of DNA. Note multi-petalled decagonal Golden Ratio geometry. As a decagon is basically two pentagons overlaid, we're all living reflections of the Golden Ratio, right down to our DNA core.

4 Upgrade Your Working/Personal Time Ratio

Consider the amount of time you work in relation to your personal time. Is the proportion healthy and fulfilling? The easiest way to get a sense of this is to simply record the actual hours you spend on work and commuting time in any given week in your daily planner. Then, simply divide your total time spent working vs. your total non-working or personal time. If you feel that your working time is out of ratio and is stressing you out, try these small steps to restore a healthier balance:

Small Steps for Continuous Improvement (Kaizen)
Consider ONE of your current top challenges for a moment. Next, surface ONE small meaningful yet manageable step that would move you forward regarding your challenge or aim. Next, take the step! Then, ID another small step and schedule it. Read Dr. Robert Maurer's book *One Small Step Can Change Your Life: The Kaizen Way* to gain more insight into this powerful principle.

The 80/20 Pareto Principle (or the 62/38 Golden Ratio Pareto Principle)
Start thinking 80/20 by taking targeted small steps to enhance the 20% causes or actions which lead to the 80% desired outcomes/results. For example:

- 20% of activities or work deliver 80% of happiness:
  ACTION: ID & expand the key 20% to increase happiness or fulfillment.

- 20% of customers generate 80% of business:
  ACTION: ID & focus more on the 20% to grow your business.
- 20% of people known generate 80% of fulfillment.
  ACTION: Clarify the 20% group & increase meaningful time spent with them.

Combining 80/20 focus with small steps sets the stage for breakthrough results. Read Richard Koch's book *The 80/20 Principle* and Tim Ferriss' *The 4-Hour Workweek.*

5 The Easy NSN Inner Peace Meditation

Time To BeneFIT 5 Seconds

Meditation is one of the oldest methods known to regain and maintain inner peace. Its benefits are profound and scientifically proven to also enhance health and performance. There are many meditation practices to choose from, e.g., Benson Relaxation Response, Transcendental/TM, Vipassana, Zazen, etc. A few minutes of breathing to a 3 seconds IN to 5 seconds OUT cadence infuses your meditation with the Golden Ratio, enhancing the benefits of meditation with a relaxing dose of NSN. Try this easy version for 5–8+ minutes a day to reap the many rewards of meditation, including reduced stress, enhanced health, focus, presence and performance.

- To start, choose a place and time where you won't be disturbed.
- Sit relaxed yet buoyantly on a cushion on the floor or in a comfortable chair.
- With eyes closed, begin to deepen and slow your breath. Experiment with Golden Ratio Breathing: breathe in deeply into your belly to the count of 3; breathe out fully to the count of 5. Let the count go whenever you like.
- Gently focus on your breath. If thoughts come into your mind, simply return to focusing on your breath. Variations include focusing on one word, image, sound or feeling along with your breath. Find what works for you.
- When the time feels right to finish, raise your hands and bring them up a few inches in front of your eyes, palms facing your face. Slowly open your eyes, allowing them to acclimate first to your palms; after a few seconds, lower your hands.
- Allow yourself a few minutes to return to your activities, refreshed and calm. Jot down any insights you may have had while they're fresh.
- Certain music can enhance your meditation experience. One of the author's favorites is *Becoming Creation* from the ***Chakra Sound System*** program, by Golden Ratio therapeutic sound master David Ison.

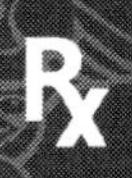

6 Practice the Vitruvian Happiness Exercise

Study Da Vinci's *Vitruvian Man* and Hedden's *Vitruvian Woman*. Then, mirror either image, standing with your feet slightly wider than shoulder-width apart and your arms extended from your sides, so that your silhouette forms a five-pointed star—a classic symbol of the Golden Ratio. Close your eyes for a moment; breathe deeply. Feel your idealized five-fold symmetry. Know that your entire being is reflecting the Golden Ratio, which links you with everything in creation, from the tiniest atoms to the great spiraling galaxies in the heavens. Allow feelings of love, gratitude, happiness and inner peace to spiral out from your heart, spreading into a vibrant connection with all creation.

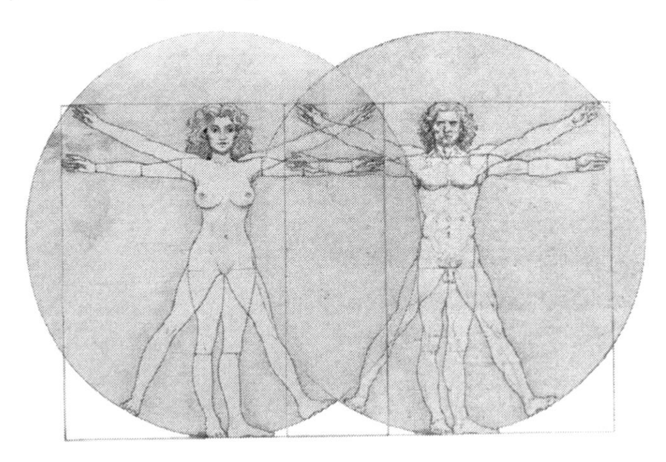

007 James Bond's Suave Φ Formula for Inner Peace

An enjoyable way to achieve a state of inner peace is to occasionally follow James Bond's advice and drink a martini *stirred, not shaken*... or would that be *shaken, not stirred?* In the Bond books, author Ian Fleming originally wrote ***stirred, not shaken***, yet in the film adaptations the order was reversed to ***shaken, not stirred***. In terms of psychological equanimity, James Bond had numerous encounters with villains where his peace of mind was challenged to the core.

Due to the intensity of the situation, his composure could be externally shaken, but he appeared to not be stirred at his core. On the flip side, encounters with beautiful yet deadly vixens were especially unnerving, leaving him visibly stirred on the outside, yet inwardly unshaken. What was Bond's secret that allowed him to handle beauties and beasts alike, yet still retain his suave poise? Perhaps James Bond's imperturbable nature had something to do with his frequent martini consumption...those martinis that were *stirred, not shaken*—or was it *shaken, not stirred?* In any event, here's a Golden Ratio adaptation of the classic Bond martini, guaranteed to calm your soul and leave you happy for no reason... we'll leave the mixing ratio to you.

The Golden Ratio ASTON MARTINi Formula

A delicious NSN twist on the Bond martini, utilizing juice from the preeminent Golden Ratio fruit, the apple:

For Drier: *40% Vodka (e.g., Grey Goose), 30% each: Sour Apple Schnapps (e.g., DeKuyper) & Apple Juice, preferably organic & fresh pressed.*
Note that 40/30/30 is the same as 40/60, approximating the Golden Ratio.

For More Tart or Sour: *40% Sour Apple Schnapps, 30% each Vodka & Apple Juice.*

For Sweeter: *40% Apple Juice, 30% each Vodka & Sour Apple Schnapps.*

Finish with a dash of Vermouth and garnish with a thin slice of fresh apple, cut horizontally to show the Golden "Star of Knowledge" at the heart of every apple. To easily achieve the above Golden Ratio mixes, measure 1¼ jigger for the 40% portion and 1 jigger for the 30% portions. Experiment with Golden Ratios in your favorite drink. When you mix drink components according to the unifying Golden Ratio, they will tend to blend in a more harmonious and delicious way.

Note: A word of sensible caution—not everyone tolerates or should drink alcohol. Some people are very sensitive to alcohol or additives from processing. Remember that alcohol is also very dehydrating, so honor NSN factor #2 and **drink at least twice as much water as alcohol consumed.** Many people may have a low threshold to alcohol's effects or are susceptible to the addictive nature of alcohol. Some people may also have other adverse effects that impede social interaction as well as the well-known risk of driving while intoxicated. *Avoid alcohol consumption if any these warnings apply to you and substitute one of the many other Rx's in this book as a source of NSN.*

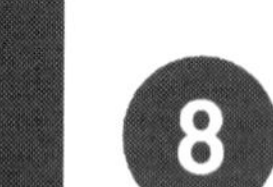 The Art & Science of Order From Chaos

Take the following small step to begin upgrading your workspace to the *Cockpit Office*, point #1 from **Liz Davenport's** brilliant ***Order From Chaos*** book and system:

1. Clear your desk of all items currently within both hands and arms reach.
2. Mindfully replace all items, papers or files you access *daily* within Hands Reach.

3. Place all items, papers or files you access *several times a week* within Arms Reach (beyond the Hands Reach zone).
4. Items you access monthly can stay in your workspace—just away from your desk. *All other items go out of your workspace.*

Picture
Vase
Monitor
Hot File
Phone
Keyboard
Work Space
Chair
Work Space

The Order From Chaos system upgrades working space to enhance productivity. Positioning key desk items using a Golden Ratio grid can provide an added boost.

9 Access the Power of Mona Lisa's Smile

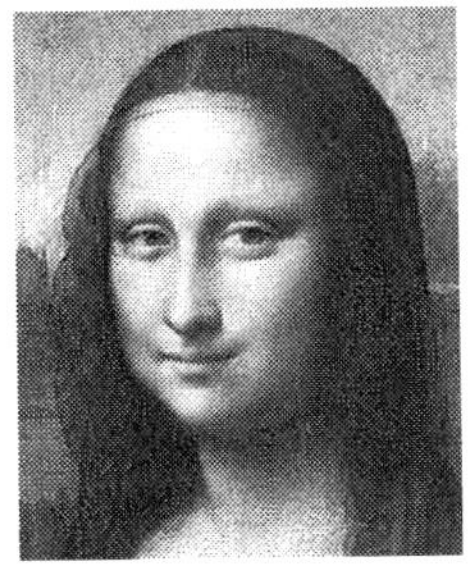

Mona Lisa's Divinely-Coded smile.

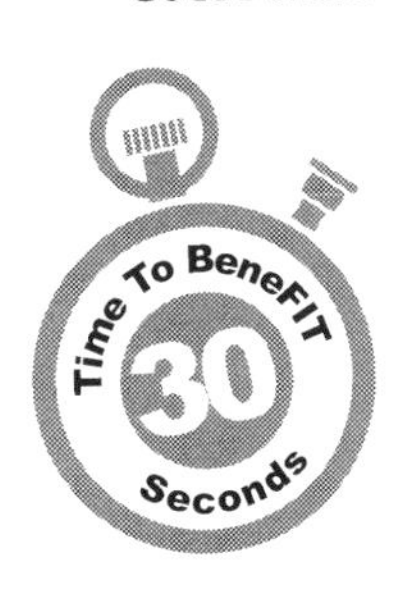

Look at Mona Lisa's smile. For a few moments, try to mirror her subtle smile—about 62% happy. See if you can find that Golden Ratio balance point. Try it first without a mirror and then with one. This is a playful way to raise and balance your emotions throughout your day. How does it feel when you smile like *Mona Lisa*? You may want to get a small picture of *Mona Lisa* to keep on your desk so you can fine-tune your inner state of mind whenever you like. Of course, if you feel the the need to expand your range or balance a smile-less day, you can always take Mona Lisa Smile star Julia Roberts' cue and unleash your best megawatt superstar smile!

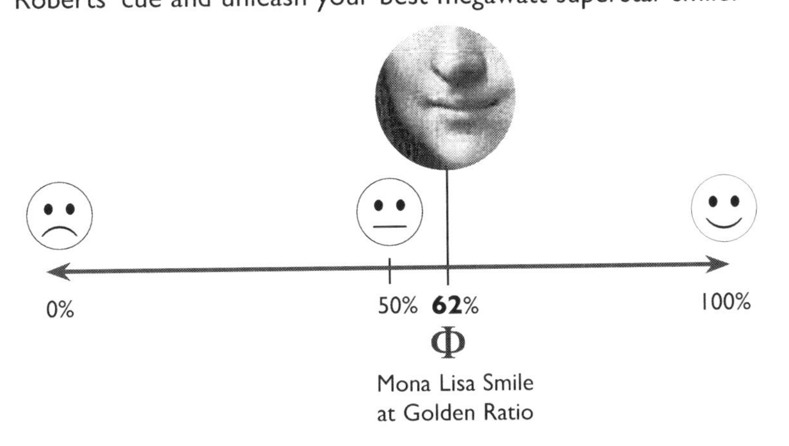

10 Strengthen Your Inner Peace & Focus with Candle Gazing

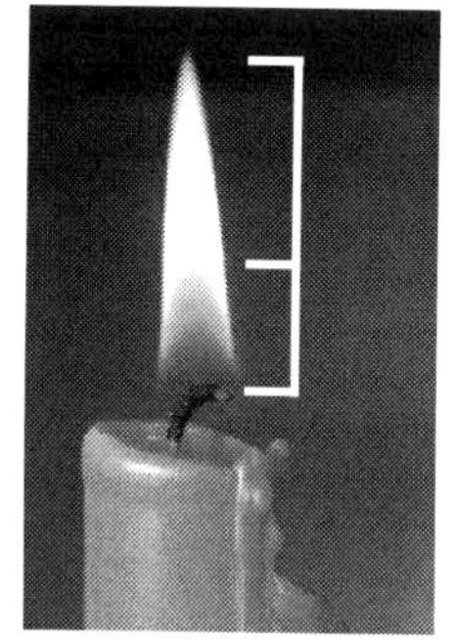

This is a simple and relaxing method for both calming and focusing your mind, adapted from mindfulness master **Dr. Phil Nuernberger's** *Strong and Fearless*:

1. Practice in a dark, quiet room with an even-burning dinner candle placed about arms length before you. If the wick of your candle is the right length, the flame will divide itself into Golden Ratio by natural color and temperature gradients, allowing you to tune into your sense of Divine Proportion.
2. Sit with tall, relaxed posture. Close your eyes and breathe slowly and deeply.
3. Open your eyes and gaze steadily at the flame. Focus on just the flame. Ignore any other thoughts or feelings; should they arise, let them simply float away.
4. Let the exercise be effortless and relaxed. After 5 minutes or so, close your eyes and visualize the flame in your mind's eye for as long as comfortable. The smaller and clearer the image of the flame, the better the training for meditation. Don't worry if the flame's image is undefined or vague at first. With practice, the flame's image will become clearer and more defined. By visualizing the flame in your mind's eye, you upgrade the exercise from external to internal orientation. Begin by gazing at the flame for 5 minutes with eyes open, then visualize for 3 minutes with eyes closed. For best benefit, practice twice a week. Your new powers of concentration and relaxation will transfer to enhanced concentration and creativity in your work and life in general.

Note: Do the candle gazing exercise in a room that has some ventilation, yet not so much that your flame overly flickers. To avoid excess smoke and perfume smell use clean burning/fragrance-free candles, e.g., beeswax. Make sure your candle is in a stable candle holder and that there is nothing near or above the candle that could catch fire.

11 Fibonacci's Reverse Psychology Secret for Happiness & Inner Peace

This exercise is an easy, powerful way to reclaim your natural state of happiness and inner peace in minutes. By using the Fibonacci Sequence to balance your emotional state before going to sleep or upon awakening, subtle stresses on your nervous system are released. Many of us have people who, at one time or another, caused us a bit of grief. It may be one person or many with whom we were at odds. The perceived injustice to us might be real or maybe some projection was involved, yet the effect on your nervous system is real and affects your health, happiness and peace of mind. The good news is there's a unique way to short-circuit such unhealthy states. **By reversing Fibonacci's Sequence and using it to release *your* projections and reactive feelings, you can clear your nervous system of needless psychological stress and grief.**

NSN Stress Reduction Technique

21————13———8——5—3—2-1-1-0

Enemy–Negative Charge–Problem
Disharmony

Friend–Neutral Charge–Resolution
Peace

Time To BeneFIT 5 Seconds

The Process: Imagine that your feelings towards a particular person with whom you are/were at odds with are at their most intense—we'll call this **Level 21.** With a deep breath in, feel that intensity for about 5 seconds and then, as you exhale, feel the intensity drop down to a 13. *Whew!* That feels much better. Take another deep breath and as you exhale, feel the intensity drop down to an 8. Now that the intensity is lessening, feel a deep relief and relaxation emerging in your nervous system. With another deep inhalation and exhalation, feel the intensity drop down to Level 5. The negative emotional pattern is really weakening now, especially as you take another deep breath and move down to 3. Those invisible knots in your nervous system are totally unraveling, as you continue breathing and drop to Level 2. Now it's just one more gentle breath and you can let go down to 1...and breathing through 1 another time... and one last deep breath in and out, and the intensity is all the way down to Level 0. Now, just breathe gently 3 more times, letting those feelings of renewed happiness and inner peace resonate through your body... *Ahhhhhh...* You've just harnessed the power of Fibonacci's Reverse Psychology Method to dissolve a negative emotional charge, which was potentially damaging your health and transmuted it to a state of enhanced inner peace. Now you can *act without reacting* the next time you interact with your friend. Repeat the process as often as desired if you feel any residual charge or recurrence. This exercise was inspired by renowned psychospiritual freedom fighter Lester Levenson.

12 Journey to the World's Sacred Sites for Inner Peace & Wisdom

What do the Great Pyramid, Stonehenge, the Pyramid of the Sun, the Parthenon and Chaco Canyon all have in common? In addition to being places of profound peace and

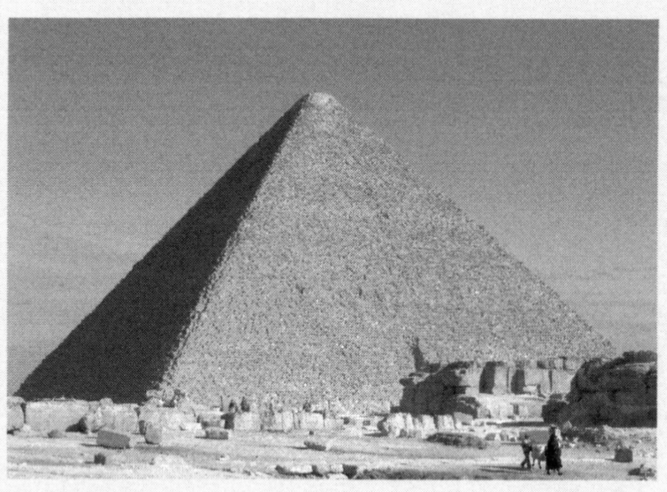

Egypt's Great Pyramid, as well as many other pyramids and ancient structures found across the world, contains precise Golden Ratio design elements. To this day, no one knows for sure who built it, when it was built—or why.

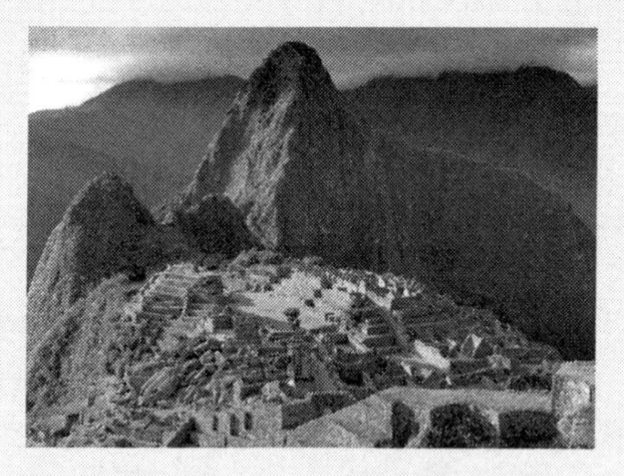

Machu Picchu, lost city of the Incas in Peru.

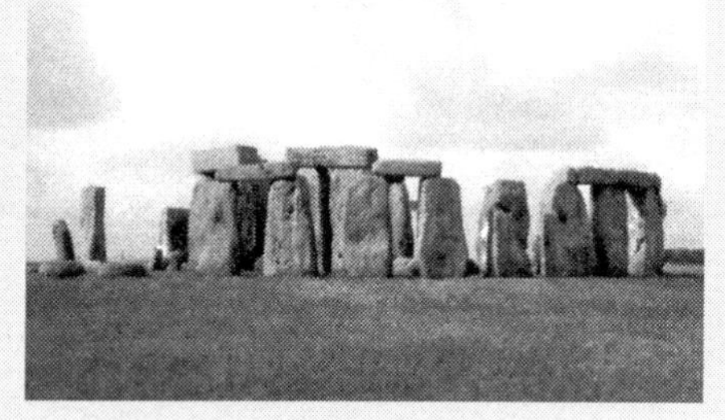

Stonehenge in England is loaded with Golden Ratio layout elements.

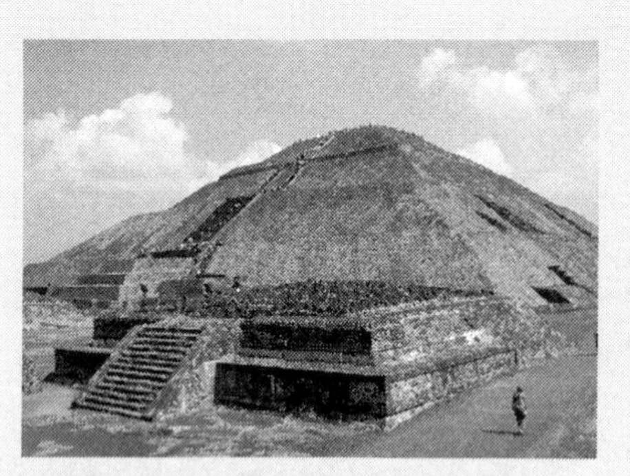

Pyramid of the Sun, Mexico. Its footprint exceeds that of Egypt's Great Pyramid.

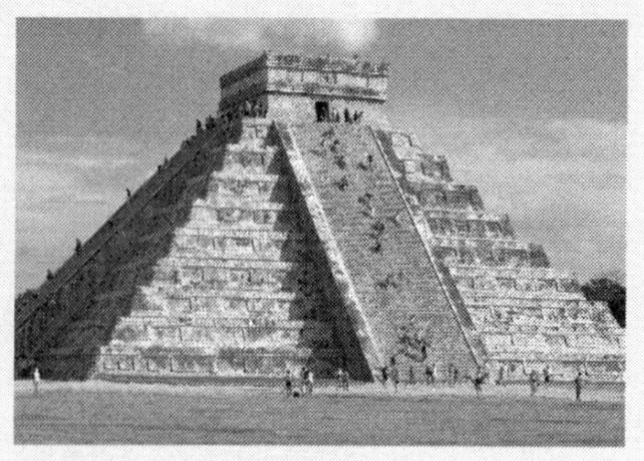

Pyramid at Chichen Itza, Yucatan, Mexico.

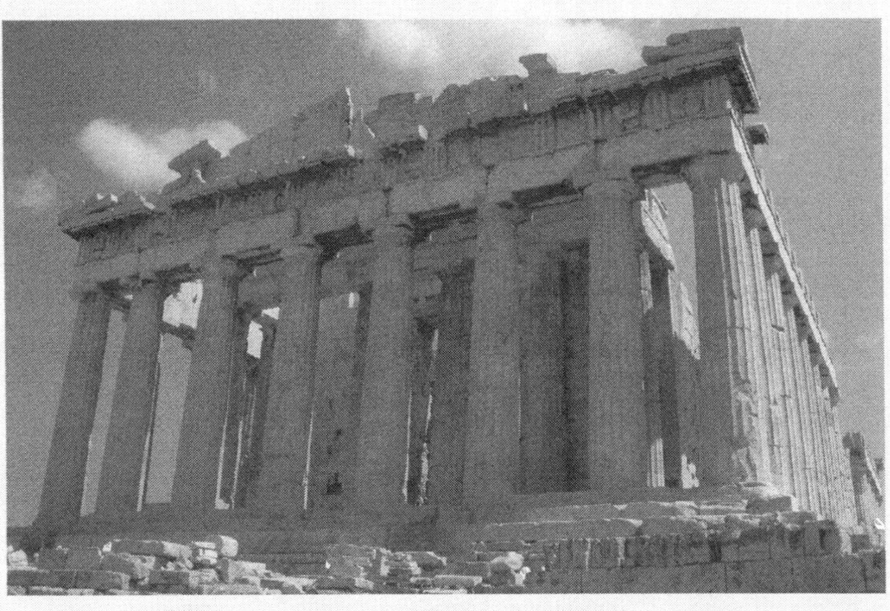

The Parthenon in Greece, whose front façade fits neatly within a Golden Rectangle.

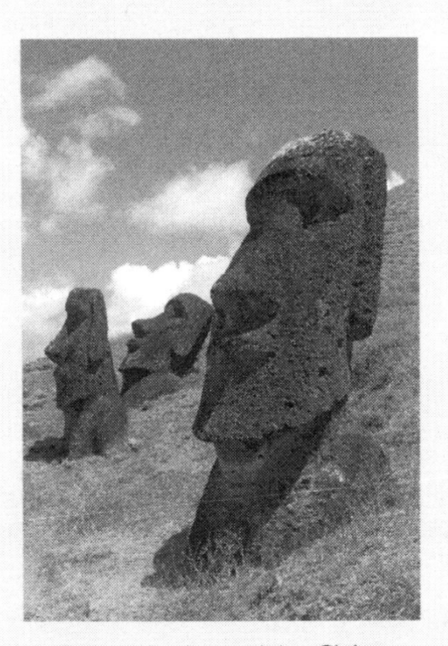

Easter Island monoliths, Chile.

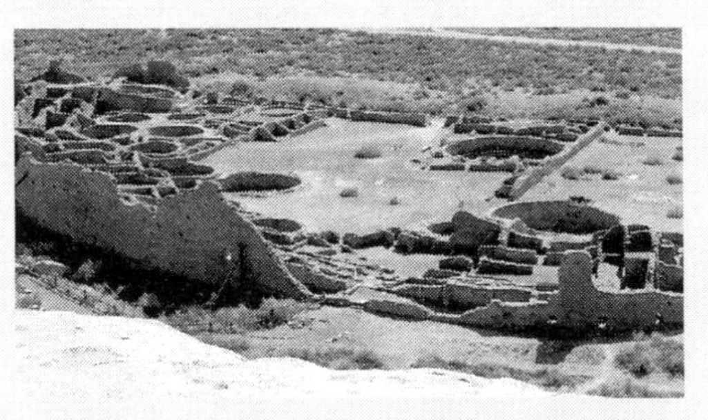

Pueblo Bonito ruins, Chaco Canyon, NM, USA.

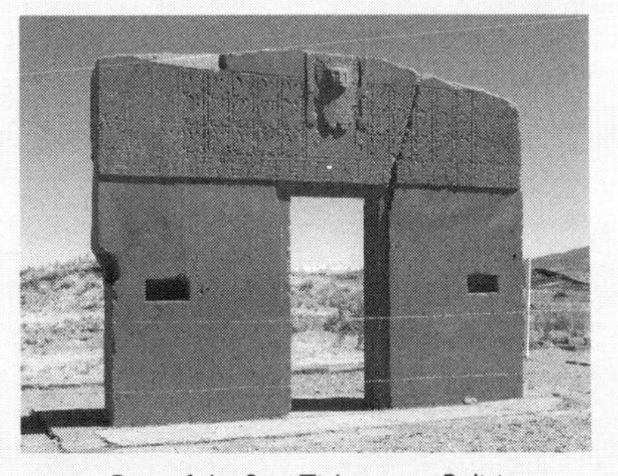

Gate of the Sun, Tiahuanaco, Bolivia.

majesty, these ancient sacred sites integrate the Golden Ratio in their design and/or layout (see ***The Divine Code of Da Vinci, Fibonacci, Einstein & YOU*** for deeper analysis). Sacred sites are often visited as a way to connect with their visible and energetic link to the advanced wisdom encoded in their geometry, along with their mysterious, awe-inspiring beauty (read the brilliant ***Fingerprints of the Gods*** and ***Magicians of the Gods*** by Graham Hancock and ***The New View Over Atlantis*** by **John Michell** for explorations into the deeper meaning of the world's ancient sacred sites). Select the site that appeals to you on the preceding 2 pages and examine it for a few moments. Then, close your eyes, picture the site in your minds eye and gently explore it, being aware of any sensations or meaning that surfaces. Let your inner peace and joy be strengthened by your mind's journey to your chosen sacred site. Recommended picture books for more images are *Heaven's Mirror* by **Graham Hancock & Santha Faiia**, *The Sacred Earth* by **Courtney Milne** and *Sacred Earth: Places of Peace and Power* by **Martin Gray**. Each features magnificent photographs of sacred sites the world over to further fire your imagination.

13 Rediscover Your Essential Childlike Nature *on the* Yellow Brick Road

Some childlike qualities that many adults seem to have lost along the journey of life include an innocence, the effortless ability to dwell in a state of joy in the present moment and a deep curiosity for Nature. A child's beginning is much like that of a newly sprouted fern, innately following the magical unfurling path of a Golden Spiral. With the arrival of adulthood—after many years of heavily regimented schooling, largely removed from Nature—numerous physical, mental and emotional capabilities develop, yet sadly many of our amazing childlike qualities retreat into deep hibernation. The challenge for most every adult is how to regain that childhood innocence, curiosity about Nature and effortless happiness and present-mindedness? The answer must be a simple one if so many children the world over naturally embody these principles. A well known, rarely heeded bible verse offers some profound guidance: ***Truly I tell you, unless you change and become like little children, you will never enter the Kingdom of Heaven.*** Perhaps a closer look at the Golden Spiral can provide insight into how to reaccess the essence of our native childlike state. When most people look at a Golden Spiral they usually envision the spiral unfurling from the center outward. After all, isn't that how spiraling galaxies appear in the sky and how humans develop—from a small outwardly spiraling fetus into a mature adult? Yet if we retrace the spiral in the *opposite* direction, from expanded galaxy to black hole and from adulthood back to our conception, we gain subtle yet valuable insights. At the very center of the Golden Spiral is the creation or "still" point, which could also be called the Kingdom of Heaven. That's the target, so by metaphorically going back to our origin and regaining a child's perspective, our natural childlike qualities can more effortlessly reemerge.

Life is too precious and beautiful to take too seriously. Over-seriousness is often a sign of unhealthy, out-of-ratio stress—which weakens the immune system, shortens telomeres and lowers life quality and length. As in the classic film *The Wizard of Oz,* the secret is to metaphorically **follow the Yellow Brick Road** (which auspiciously begins as a Golden Spiral below) back to your more innocent, joyful, childlike state and dwell in the **Now**—the only place where inner peace and true happiness live. Go outside in Nature and look for the Golden Ratio in the world around you. Meet the face of the nearest flower or animal and see the child in you staring back. Since children are closer to the Golden Spiral origin point in their lives and are less stressed, they more frequently dwell in the present moment and in the realm of imagination. They also have a curious and innocent appreciation for Nature and all life, often drawn to express their connection via the stars, spirals, geometric shapes and Nature in their art. A simple practice to reconnect with your childlike nature is to draw a Golden Spiral on a piece of paper, or use the one here, and track the spiral with your finger or a pen back to its center, reminding yourself to *play, have fun and laugh, be curious and be like a child more often...*

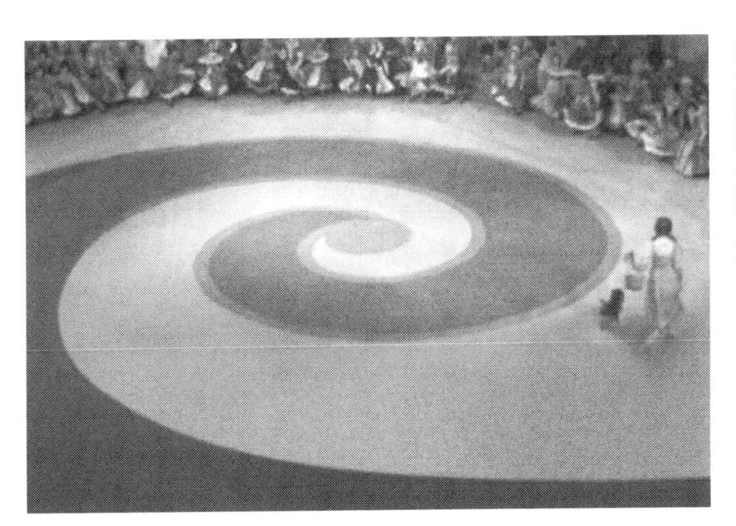

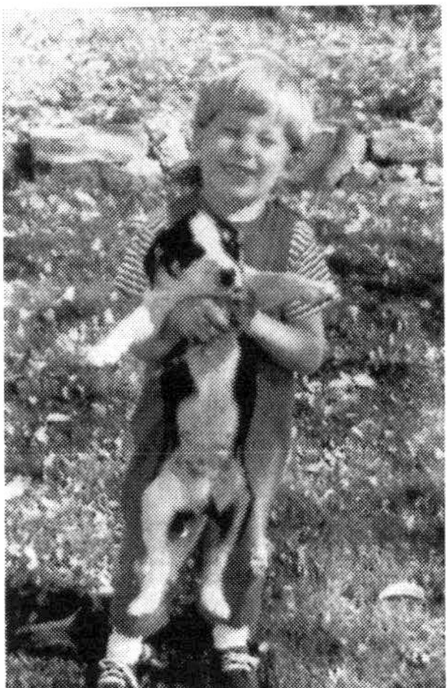

> *When we are no longer children, we are already dead. I consider that what makes us live the most is the feeling of a permanent childhood in our life.*
>
> **Constantin Brancusi, master Romanian sculptor**

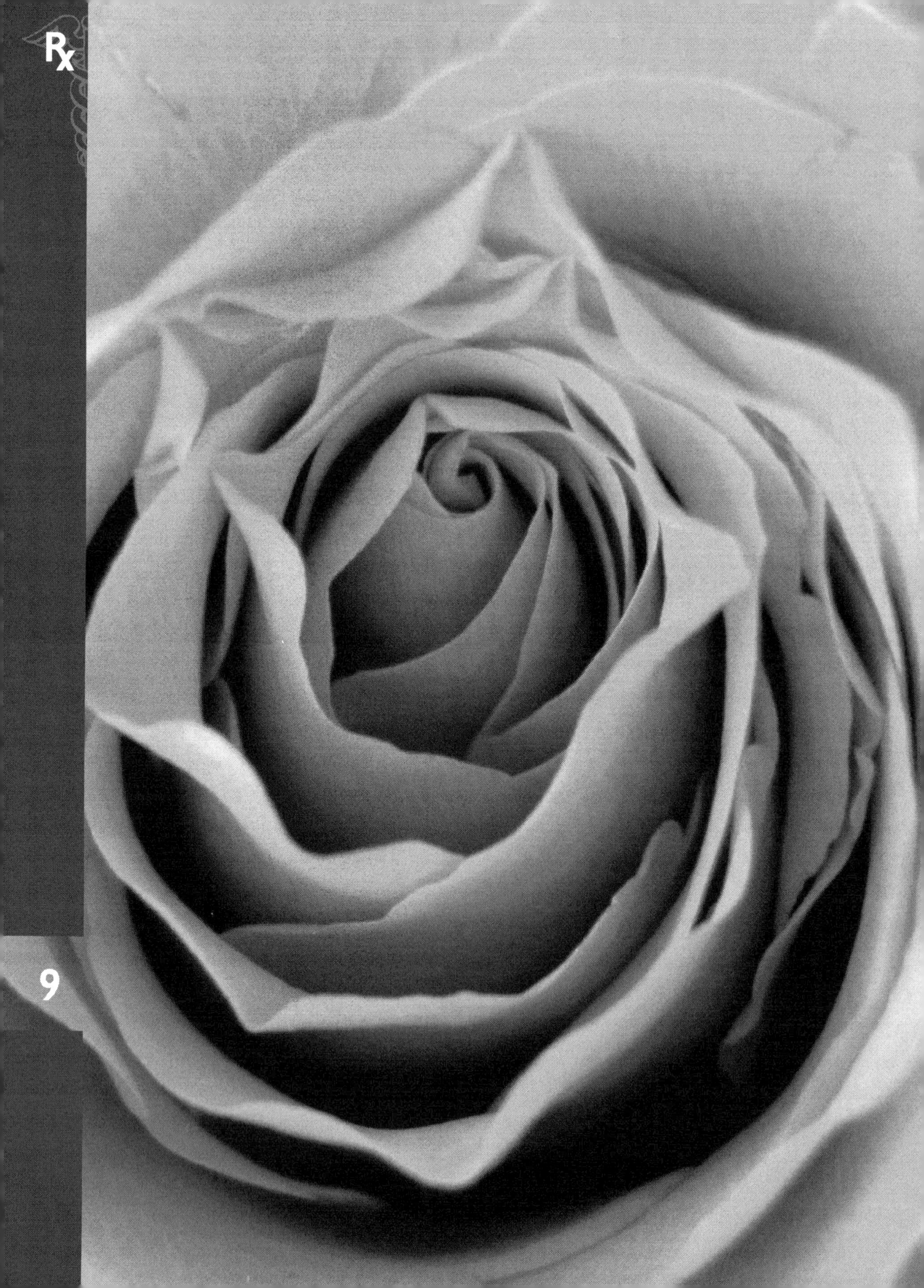
Rx
9

Beauty/Relationships Rx's

Pick one or more of the following Rx's to add to your NSN daily health regimen.

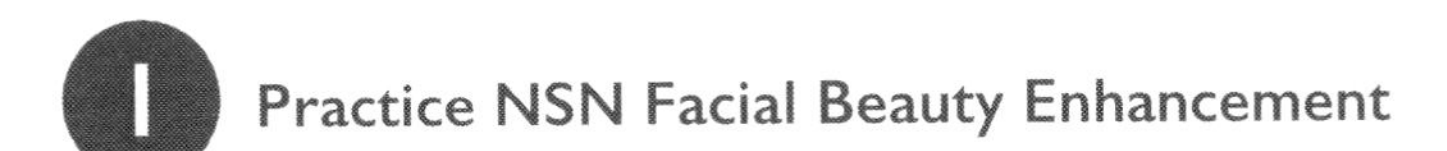

1 Practice NSN Facial Beauty Enhancement

Time To BeneFIT 3 Seconds

Your face is the primary point of focus and interaction with others. While everyone is gifted with their own unique facial features, most faces can benefit from some extra TLC. Let's look at a few simple things you can do to enhance your natural Golden Ratio attributes. **These easy techniques will make a meaningful difference in how you feel about yourself—*and how others perceive you.*** Remember, it's not only the quantity of actions taken, it's their quality and consistency. Try adding one of the following to your regimen for 21 days and observe how it makes you look and feel, inside and out.

- **Facial Hydration:** Hydration is the #2 NSN health priority driver and facial hydration is an important subset of that. Proper daily facial hydration is essential for keeping your face glowing and youthful as well as strengthening your skin's role as a resilient barrier against dehydration and environmental toxins. Select a high quality facial moisturizer without toxic ingredients, as creams and lotions are absorbed through your skin directly into your bloodstream. Many toxic ingredients are easily identified by being multi-syllabic, hard-to-pronounce and/or have CAPITALS or numbers in their names, e.g., PEG-13. Visit the Skin Deep website: www.cosmeticsdatabase.com to evaluate most cosmetic or personal care products and ingredients to check their safety. **Ideally, your moisturizer**—*indeed, anything you put on your skin*—**should be pure enough to eat; if not, it doesn't belong on your face. Organic coconut, almond or olive oils make excellent natural facial moisturizers.**

- **Exercise your facial muscles:** It's fun and easy—just make as many different faces as you can in front of a mirror for 1 minute. Try it daily for a week and see, feel and delight in the increase in your facial tone and flexibility.

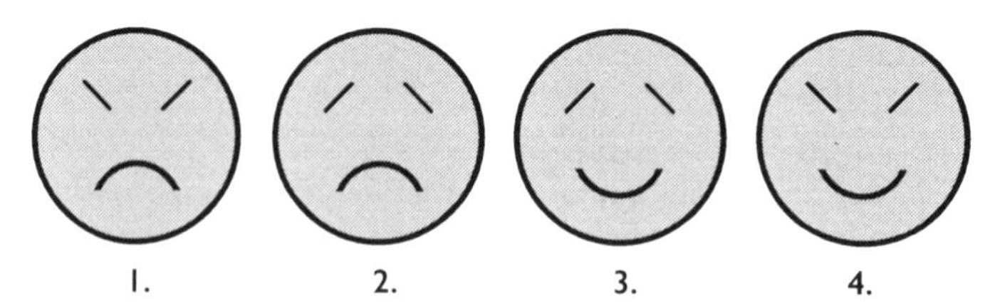

As a starting point, here are four *emoticons* that you can imitate to guide your facial muscles through the range of archetypal human emotional temperaments: **1.** Choleric (angry, irritated), **2.** Melancholic (gentle sadness, pensive), **3.** Phlegmatic (not easily disturbed), and **4.** Sanguine (happy, cheerful). Note: you might want to spend just 38% of your time exercising the left two examples (1-2) and 62% on the right two (3-4).

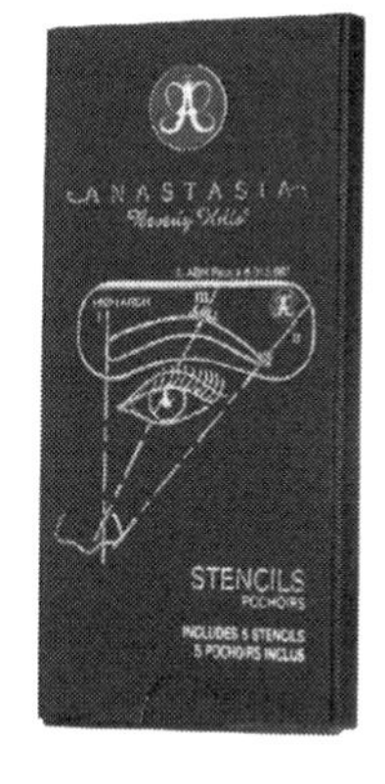

- **Anastasia Beverly Hills Golden Ratio Eyebrow Stencil Kit:** Patented Golden Ratio eyebrow stencil kit makes it fun and simple to sculpt your eyebrows to enhance the natural beauty of your face. Kits feature an assortment of custom stencils to accommodate all faces and eyebrows, giving anyone the ability to be their own Golden Ratio facial beauty and magnetism master. Available at Nordstroms and Sephora or: www.AnastasiaBeverlyHills.com
- **The Natural Facelift At Your Fingertips:** *The Empress's Secret* describes the remarkable restorative program of facial massage used by classic Chinese empresses. In this book, Robert Klein, Ph.D., presents an easy-to-learn method for facial rejuvenation and beautification, through gentle massage of facial acupressure points. The original *Bionic Woman*, actress Lindsey Wagner, along with Robert Klein, Ph.D., were early pioneers of this method, as shared in their superb book and video *The Accupressure Facelift*.

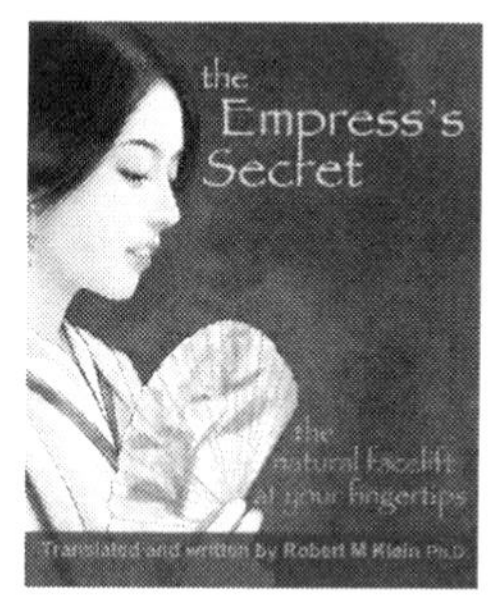

- **Sleep!** Honoring NSN health priority driver #3: Sleep is one of the huge hidden factors in maintaining a healthy, vibrant face. Many people continually compromise this key health, longevity and beauty driver. Don't be one of them.
- **Eat Anti-Oxidant-Rich Foods:** Eating super-charged antioxidant-rich spices such as cloves, cinnamon, turmeric, curry, nutmeg, etc., and berries such as cranberries, blueberries, raspberries, acai berries, goji berries, etc., can result in dramatic improvements in your skin's (and body's) health.

2 Activate Your Natural Beauty & Attractiveness

How can you best support and maximize your innate Golden Ratio symmetry and magnetism? Simply by following the cornerstones of the NSN system, the presence and power of the Ratio will begin flowing naturally. Natural Beauty and Attractiveness is available to anyone at anytime by moving towards the Golden Ratio range in each of the 10 primary health drivers. Remember to be especially mindful of your breathing, posture and movement. A few easy methods that support these factors include:

- Φ Golden Ratio breathing: inhale fully to a count of 3, exhale to a count of 5. A sense of relaxation and inner balance will naturally follow after 8 breathing cycles.
- Φ Stand with your feet firmly grounded—ideally barefoot on *real* ground—and allow your spine to rise to its full, natural length. You'll find that your neck and head are in a relaxed position and that your chest and heart are more open. This will tend to support and enhance the natural Divine Proportions in your body. As an added bonus, when you work on improving your static posture, it will automatically enhance your dynamic, moving posture.
- Φ Move with grace, e.g., when dancing, allow your movements to unfold in *flow-motion*. Gentle circular, ellipse or spiraling movements allow your body to move with more fluid and attractive grace.

3 The Power of the Golden 62/38 Communication Ratio

Based on the work of UCLA Professor Emeritus **Albert Mehrabian**, the strength and impact of your primary channels of communication reflect the Golden Ratio: approximately 55% of your communication power is in your body language, e.g., eye contact, facial expression, hands, posture; 38% is in your voice tone, and only the remaining 7% is in the actual words you use. This is a Golden Ratio distribution, as:

$$55 + 7 = \boxed{62} + 38 = \boxed{100} \qquad 100/62 = \Phi$$

Since the top two categories equal the vast majority—93%—of your communication power, this ought to inspire you to prioritize your communication enhancement efforts towards improving your non-verbal, body language and voice tone skills. All of these subtle communication upgrades will be perceived as enhancing your overall expression of beauty, inner attractiveness and connection.

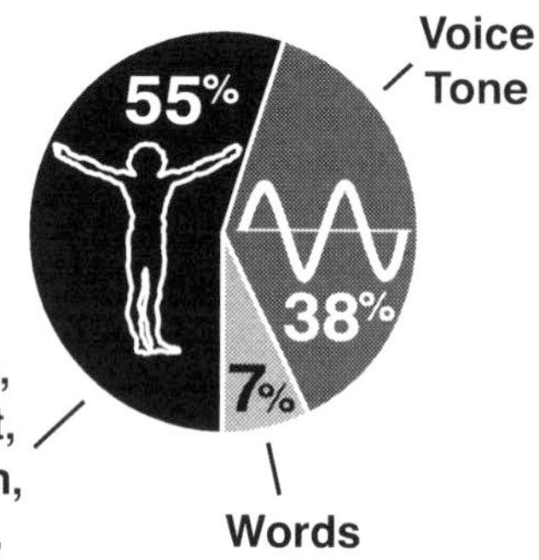

The 3 primary channels of communication are in Golden Ratio: 55+7=**62** + **38**=100, therefore **62**:**38**=Φ. They're optimized by the energy, intention and heart of the communicator.

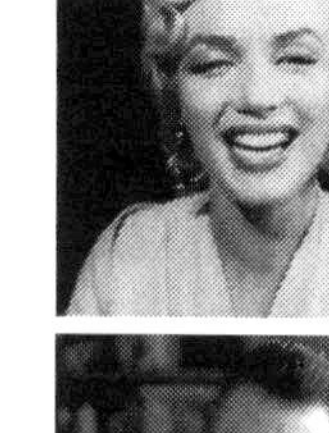

A GIF is Worth More Than a Thousand Words. GIFs are very popular because they're 1-2 second nonverbal mini-movies conveying a huge amount of information in a compact format. See Monroe & De Niro in GIFY action at https://gfycat.com/

4 Activate the Divine Rose Spiral

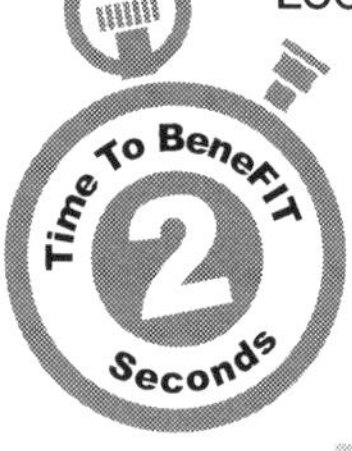

Look at the multiple Golden Spirals in this picture of a rose. Notice how the petals gracefully trace the spiral leading into and coming out of the heart of the rose. Close your eyes for a moment. Take a deep, full Golden breath, inhaling to 3, exhaling to 5. On your exhale, send this Golden Spiraling love energy to the heart of your beloved. Repeat 3 times.

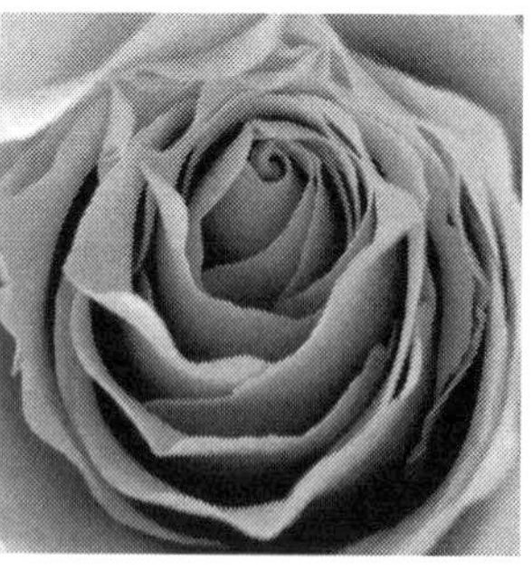

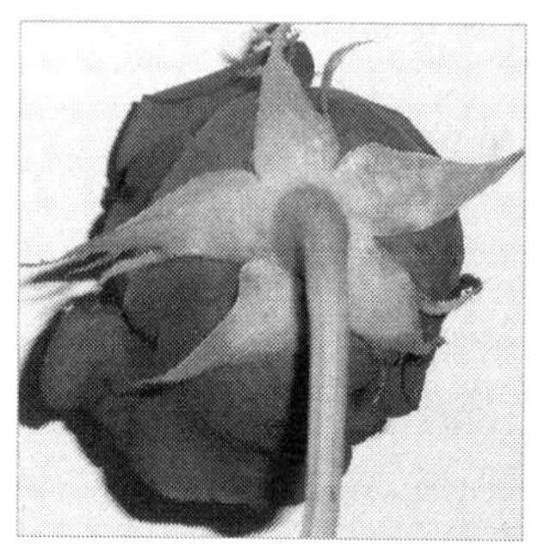

The rose sends a double imprint of the Golden Ratio: petals unfolding in Golden Spirals on the face and a five-pointed Golden Star on the back.

5 The 60/40 Power of Sight, Sound & Feeling to Enhance Your Communication Effectiveness

60%
20%
20%

In *How To Make People Like You in 90 Seconds or Less,* author **Nicholas Boothman** explores how to optimize your ability to more rapidly and meaningfully connect with people. It turns out that the three primary modalities we use to connect and communicate approximate the Golden Ratio. They are: Visual (images), Auditory (sounds) and Kinesthetic (sensation of position & movement in space). **These three modalities are how we communicate with *ourselves* internally—and with others externally. Yet each individual prefers to communicate predominantly via *one* of the three.**

It turns out that approximately 60% of people are visually dominant, with the remaining 40% being nearly evenly split between auditory and kinesthetic dominance: 60/40, approximating the Golden Ratio. This is another example of how human as well as universal structure and function align with the Golden Ratio. In order to know yourself better and communicate with greater grace and effectiveness with others, become more aware of your communication preference and strength. How do you prefer communicating (sending and receiving) with others? Via images, sounds or hands-on? How do those close to you prefer to receive communication? How can you create strong bridges of understanding and value with others? The answers to these questions are golden keys which unlock life success skill #1: building meaningful communication and relationships with others. Enhanced communication skills will help you more fully express your natural personal magnetism.

6 The Magic of Golden Ratio Relationships: Time-Sharing & More

- Φ Become more aware of how much time you and your mate are spending together and apart, on a daily, weekly and monthly basis. Where do your time ratios fall with respect to the 38/62 or 62/38 Golden Ratio? If it feels right now, simply continue what you're doing. Otherwise, to mix it up/keep it fresh, experiment by shifting the time ratio one way or the other to reflect Divine Proportion in your relationship.
- Φ Experiment with the many ratios in your relationship, such as decision making ratios, giving vs. receiving, listening vs. talking (often a big one), action vs. rest, etc. If any of these ratios are unfulfillingly out of proportion, experiment with shifting the balance one way or the other toward the unifying Golden Ratio: 38/62 or 62/38.

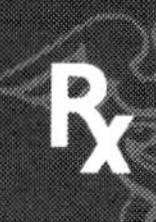

Golden Lovemaking Ratio for Enhanced Beauty & Longevity

In his book *Secrets of the Superyoung*, Scotland's **Dr. David Weeks** revealed the age-reversing and beautifying power of intimacy. This was arrived at through impartial ratings of the study subject's pictures. He discovered that those who were enjoying satisfying intimacy with the same partner about 4 times a week were perceived by others to be 4 to 7 years younger than their actual age. According to Dr. Weeks,

The key ingredients for ***looking younger*** *are staying active...and maintaining a good sex life.*

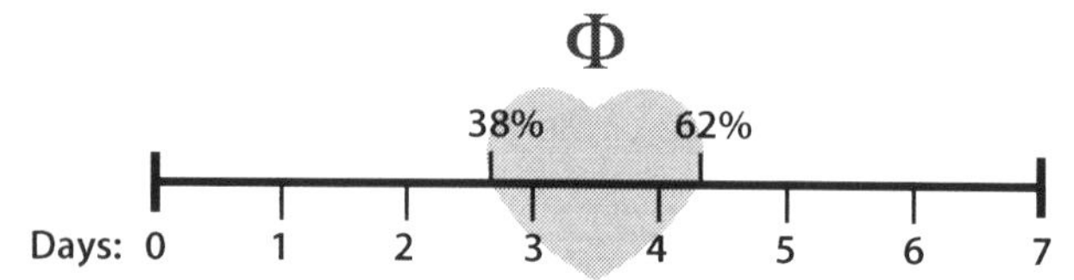

The 4 times per-week lovemaking frequency found in *Superyoung* people falls within the Golden Lovemaking Ratio range of 2.6 to 4.3 times a week, which frames the 38% to 62% range within a 7-day week.

Try and establish your own Golden Ratio Lovemaking range based on desire, state of health, physical conditioning and of course, your partner. The above research highlights the potential benefit regular intimacy holds for beauty and longevity. In light of this, you might consider adding intimacy as a tracking category to your 21-Day Priority Coach.

Play with Fibonacci's Foreplay

What would it be like to enjoy infinite foreplay? Impossible you say? The inspiration for this playful practice in extended foreplay is courtesy of **Zeno** and his famous paradox (Greece, 5th century, B.C.) The exercise also echoes the infinite nature of the Golden Ratio, which forever approaches, yet never actually arrives at the infinite number 1.618033... Leonardo Fibonacci might have explained it as follows:

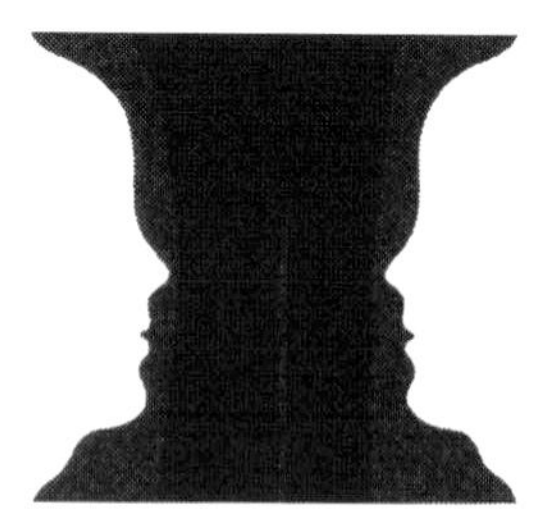
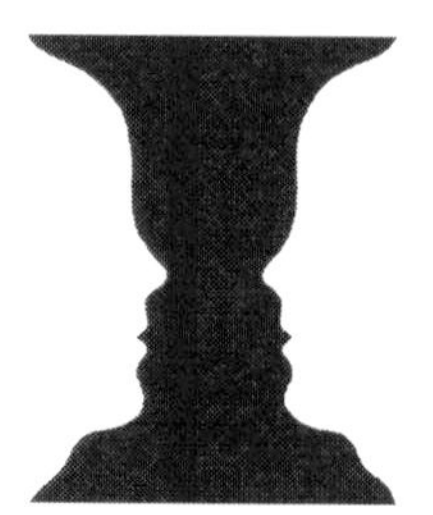
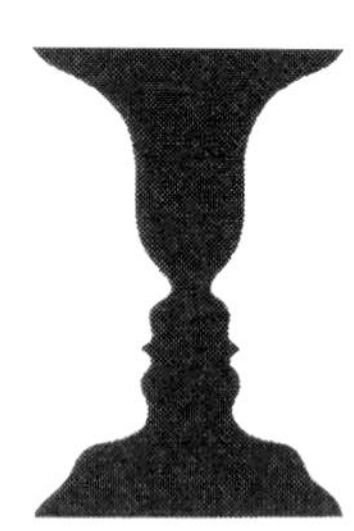

The illusory Fibonacci Foreplay or Zeno's Kiss. Look closely: what else do you see besides three shrinking candle holders?

You are 10 inches away from your mate and you want to kiss them. In order to meet the lips of your love, you will need to progressively reduce the distance between you. However, by continually moving towards him or her in approximate Golden Ratio reductions, you will get infinitely closer… without actually touching. How is this so? You'd first move from 10 inches to 6.2 inches…then to 3.8 inches… 2.3 inches… 1.5 inches… infinitum frustratum... continually approaching each other, yet in theory never actually touching.

9 Give & Receive a Golden Ratio Foot Reflexology Massage

Time To BeneFIT 10 Seconds

Buddhist artisans obviously had knowledge of the Golden Ratio when they placed the Dharmachakra (Golden Flower design) and the Three Jewels design at the precise locations on the Buddha's footprint that correspond to Golden Ratio points. Armed with this knowledge, you can now treat your partner, friend or even yourself to a Golden Ratio foot massage. Be especially mindful to massage the charged points indicated on the Buddha's footprint. It's said that a good way to reach—and lift—a person's soul is through their soles.

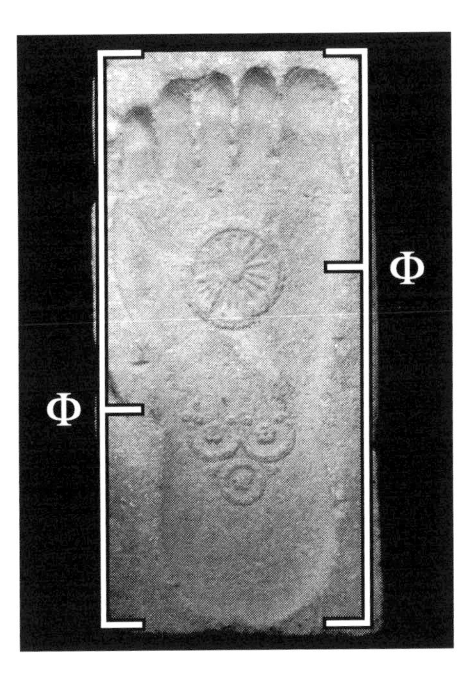

Buddha's Footprint: Dharmachakra and Three Jewels are at Golden Ratio points of the foot. Imprint from the Gandhara, ZenYouMitsu Temple, Tokyo; 1st century.

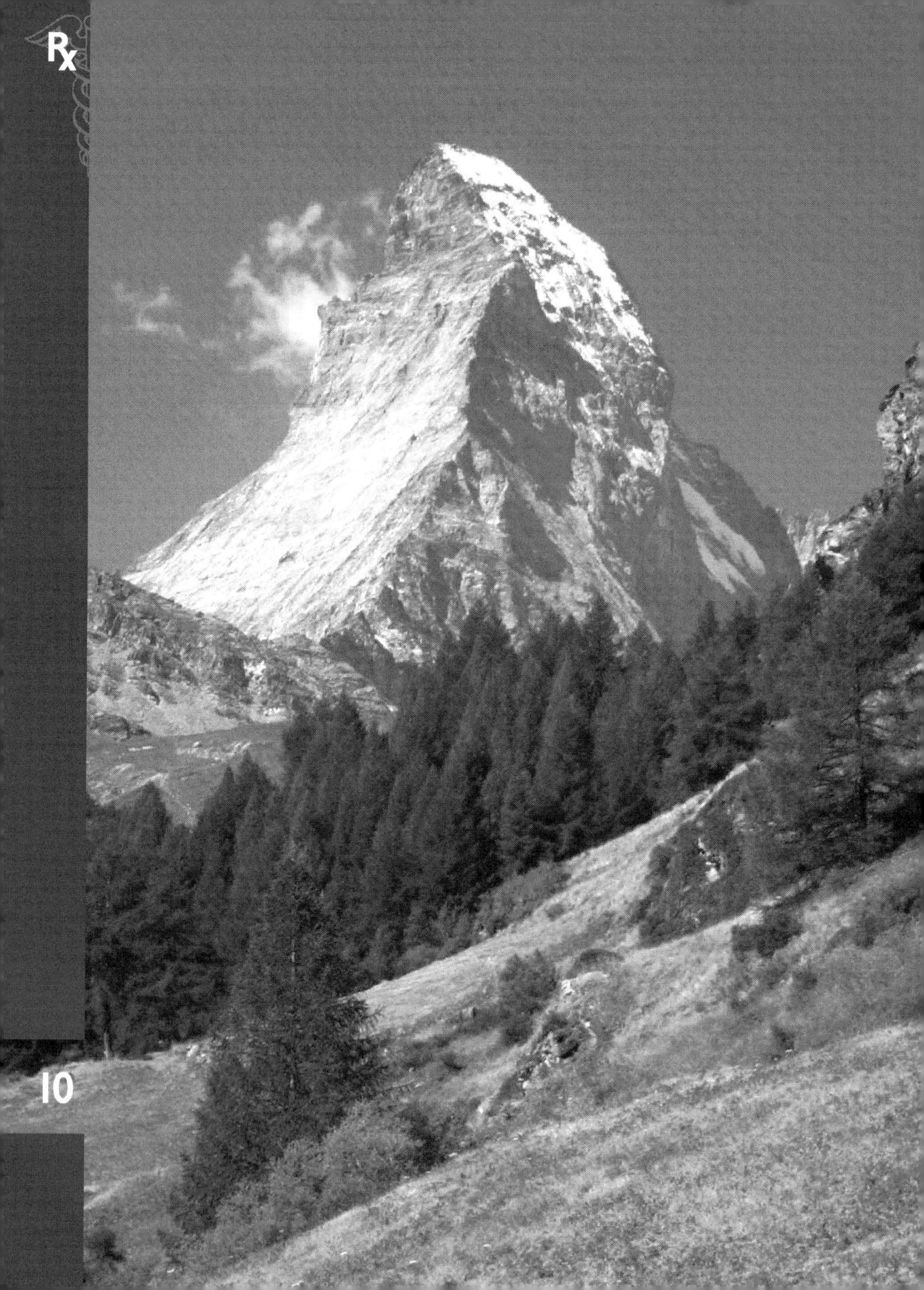
Rx

How old would you be if you didn't know how old you are?

Satchel Paige, American baseball legend

10 Longevity Rx's

Pick one or more of the following Rx's to add to your NSN daily health regimen.

1 Power Up Your Golden Prime Zone Age-Reversing Holodeck

Time To BeneFIT 13 Seconds

In Ch 9, we identified the ages 19 to 31 range as the Golden Prime Zone. Recall that 19 and 31 are both prime numbers and 31 divided by 19 equals the Golden Ratio of 1.6. **This is the prime time range when your life force is especially vibrant.** All of your hormones are at their peak, including growth and sexual hormones. If you're in your 19–31 Golden Ratio Prime Zone now, you can bask in the prime of life and skip this Rx. However, if those years have passed and you'd like to revisit them to revitalize today, we've designed the following Rx in the spirit of **Dr. Ellen Langer's** landmark Counterclockwise study. In this Rx you'll revisit and reactivate the vitality of your 19–31 years and enjoy for a second time a glowing period of maximal health and potency. An easy, imaginative process for reactivating your Golden Prime Zone consists of creating and periodically visiting your own virtual *Holodeck* (a virtual reality simulator popularized in *Star Trek*, where a person can select and visit any chosen reality/timeframe and experience it as if it were real). Turn the page to set up your personal Golden Prime Zone Holodeck.

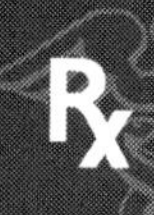

To create your Golden Prime Zone Holodeck, set your:

1. **TIME TARGET** Circle the years on the spiral TimeMap™ (opposite page) when you were ages 19 and 31. Those years and the years in between delineate your personal *Golden Prime Zone.*
2. **PEAK MEMORIES** Jot down *3–5 Peak Memories* from within your age 19–31 Golden Prime Zone on the spiral TimeMap.™ Mark the year they occurred, along with people, places or events.
3. **ONE PEAK MEMORY** Select one *Peak Memory* from your 3-5 and write it down at the top of a 3x5 index card, your **Peak Memory Card** (or on a large Post-It note).
4. **LOCATION TARGET** *Add the Location* of your One Peak Memory to your Peak Memory Card.
5. **SENSORY ACTIVATION CUES** Add a few *Sensory Activation Cues* from the 5-senses list below to your Peak Memory Card:

Visual Favorite scene, person, picture, smile; any evocative images.

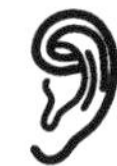
Auditory Favorite song, a lover's voice, cheering crowds, city sounds, laughter, nature sounds: ocean, wind, rain, crickets; or even silence.

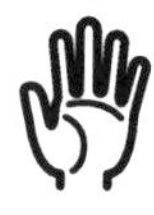
Kinesthetic What you were wearing, the weather, sun, warmth, cold, or how you were moving your body. Put yourself *in* your memory and ***pay special attention to how you're feeling in your Peak Memory.***

Taste A particularly wonderful meal or drink and how it tasted: how delicious was it? sweet, spicy, sour, cold, warm or hot?

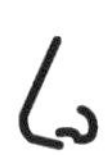
Smell Any scents or aromas associated with the scene—food, coffee, a cocktail, flowers, perfume or cologne, smoke, freshly cut grass, ocean or mountain air. Your sense of smell is deeply connected with emotional memory in your brain's limbic system. Scent thus plays a very powerful role in both encoding and recalling memories. Now complete your Peak Memory Card.

You're now ready to start your Holodeck time travel journey...

1. **PLAN** 13+ minutes when you can be undisturbed, focused and relaxed.
2. **SIT** relaxed, or lie down. Breath deeply, in to 3, out to 5. Release any tension.
3. **REVIEW** your Peak Memory Card for a moment. When ready, close your eyes.
4. **IN YOUR MIND,** step into your chosen Peak Memory. Begin to experience and enjoy it as if it were happening **Now**. Let it unfold *(continues on p. 438)*...

The TimeMap™ Graph: Blueprint for Activating Your Inner Fountain Of Youth™

Circle the years when you were ages 19 to 31. This 13-year range is your personal Golden Ratio Prime Zone.

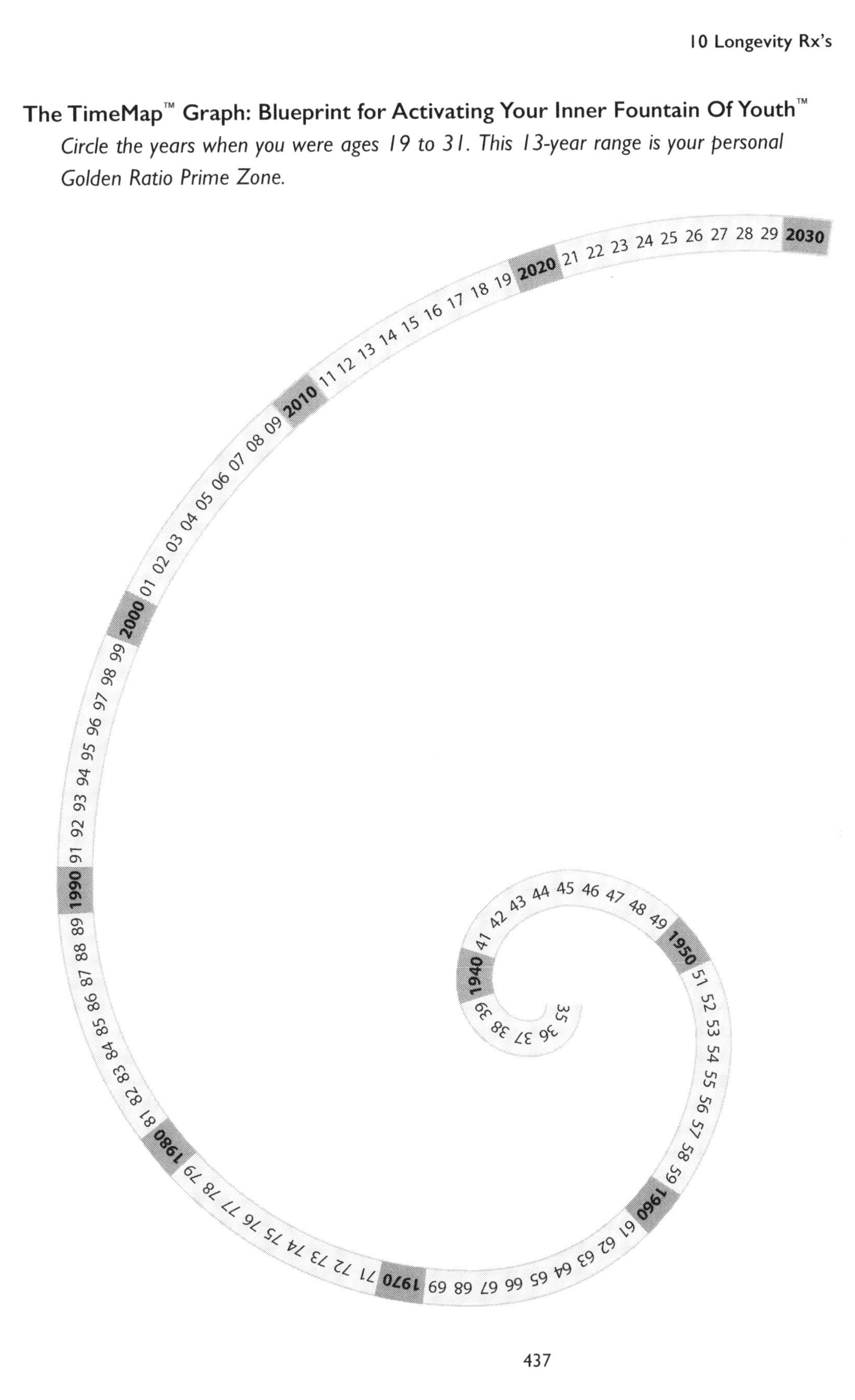

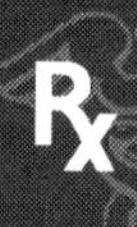

5. **SURF** the sensory waves of your Peak Memory. Savor any particularly wonderful scenes, with your physical, mental and emotional energies at their PEAK (know that you're fully protected and safe in your Holodeck as you enjoy your Peak Memory). Let the positive feelings permeate your body and soul. If there are any areas of your body today that aren't feeling their best, welcome the great feelings of healthy times past into those areas. **Feel these rejuvenating sensations as if they are real again NOW. Dwell on *all* of your senses from this memory: sights, sounds, touch, tastes and scents.** This further amplifies your memories into feelings, deepening the impact of your Holodeck journey.

When ready, prepare to return to the present. *Slowly* open your eyes. Jot down any insights on a 3x5 index card or Post-It to inspire you during your week ahead. **Your Golden Prime Zone Holodeck meditation need not be long—as little as 8–13 minutes can reactivate your age-reversing neurotransmitters and hormones.** Practice the Golden Prime Zone Meditation at least weekly for maximum benefits. In the weeks ahead, you might be surprised at who's looking back at you in the mirror.

To further amplify your Holodeck experience, review the prior 5-Sense checklist with your age 19–31 Peak Memory timeframe in mind and gather any/all of these items from that time:

- Φ A picture (of you between 19–31) or a newspaper or magazine from that time.
- Φ A favorite song from that time; see Rx #6 ahead in this chapter for more here.
- Φ Something to hold or touch from that time: any favorite item or knick-knack, e.g., a baseball or tennis racket or sentimental item from that 19–31 time range.
- Φ A specific favorite taste item and/or an affiliated scent.

These will be the sensory memory trigger items to review prior to your Holodeck meditation, along with your Peak Memory Card. Once you've secured any/all of these items, keep them handy in a special place or container, ready for future Holodeck journeys into your Golden Prime Zone. This practice allows you to hack into your core Golden Ratio DNA and access and activate your latent, vast capacity for super health, happiness & longevity.

2 Cold & Hot Therapy for Life-Extending NSN

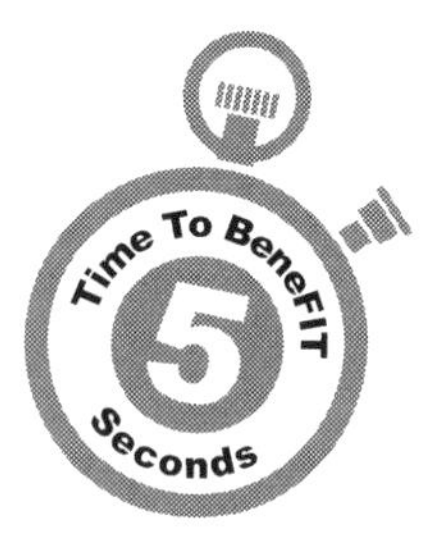

A. The easiest way to shift your metabolism into a higher metabolic gear and reclaim your natural fat burning ability is to start embracing the cold by wearing less clothing and turning down the thermostat. This new habit sends a subtle signal to your

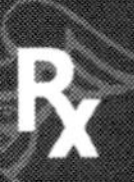

nervous system to throw more fuel on your metabolic fire and crank up your internal thermostat. This simple adjustment can result in increased fat burning and weight loss over weeks to months, not to mention boosting your immune system.

B. As you progress in your tolerance to colder air, you can slowly introduce yourself to cold-water therapy by alternating cold and hot water in the shower. Begin by alternating hot and cold water in Fibonacci Ratios—start with 8 seconds hot, 5 seconds cold and progress to higher Fibonacci Ratios as desired, e.g., **13:8, 21:13, 34:21. Try 3-5 sets of alternating hot and cold.** Utilizing Fibonacci Ratios gives your nervous system a thermal dose of Nature's Secret Nutrient and adds some fun structure to the process. Hot water brings blood to your muscles and skin, which is great for soothing aches and pains as well as for releasing toxins. When you switch back to cold, you activate a thermal pump—blood is shunted back to your core, and your internal organs get bathed in oxygen and nutrient-rich blood.

While not as rigorous as **Katherine Hepburn's, Jack Kruse's, Iceman Wim Hof's** or co-author **Matthew Cross**' Biostack (see Rx #7, this chapter) strictly cold methods, alternating hot and cold has its own unique benefits in balancing your immune, nervous and endocrine systems. The added advantage of alternating hot and cold-water therapy is that Nature's Secret Nutrient becomes available, since you're aiming for a dynamic balance of hot and cold by using Fibonacci Ratios in the process (as your tolerance builds, try spending the larger Fibonacci number in the cold water). ***Note: If you can't tolerate cold air or water, have your doctor check your thyroid for proper functioning. Avoid cold water therapy if you have heart problems.***

3 Partake of the Longevity Food of the Gods: Chocolate!

Time To BeneFIT 3 Seconds

Chocolate in various forms has enjoyed high esteem and popularity for thousands of years. Believed by the Maya to have been discovered by the Gods (its scientific name, *Theobroma*, means "Food of the Gods"), chocolate has been used as an endurance booster, aphrodisiac and even as a form of currency. Itzamna, legendary Mayan Sky God, founder of Mayan culture and early champion of chocolate, is said to have taught his people to grow maize and cacao, as well as writing, calendars and medicine. The ancient Maya created a cacao concoction called *Kukuha*, which they flavored with chili and black pepper, spices and honey. It was consumed hot or cold by the Maya to boost strength. Due to chocolate's potent mix of nutrients and divine flavor, it certainly fits the profile of a super health and longevity food of the gods—and humans. If we look deeper into the structure of cacao pods we find, to no surprise, that they exhibit Golden Ratio design geometry: 5 cacao beans per pod, distributed in a Golden Ratio pentagonal array. Every cacao pod, and thus chocolate the world over, carries a distinct Golden Ratio imprint. Key chocolate's benefits include:

- Darker, raw chocolate or cocoa (ideally as raw cocoa nibs) means a higher concentration of polyphenols and flavanols, which make it 2-3 times more potent than red wine or green tea. These factors decrease the "stickiness" of blood, improve circulation and lower blood pressure.
- Chocolate contains phenylethylamine, anandamide, tryptophan and theobromine—all natural neuroactive compounds—which enhance mood, induce relaxation and have aphrodisiac-like qualities. Also, the comforting fragrance and taste of cocoa is thought to enhance theta brain waves, leading to a more relaxed state of mind.
- Consuming chocolate as cocoa in a hot drink makes its antioxidants more bioavailable. Sweeten to taste with raw organic honey, agave, coconut sugar or xylitol.

Chocolate shopping can be daunting, with a burgeoning number of companies and chocolate products to choose from. Aim for the darkest, most unprocessed organic cocoa in bar, nib or powder form you can find. Obviously, taste is a critical factor as well, so you may want to sample various new products on the market to find one that suits your taste. A great review of various chocolate bars with percentages of cacao can be found at: http://healthyeater.com/dark-chocolate-best-and-worst Enjoy a guilt-free daily portion of chocolate and savor the blessings of this Divine Food of the Gods.

Itzamna's Golden Ratio Hot Cocoa Recipe; Serves 3-5 People
Aphrodisiac, Mood Booster & Super-Energizer, All Rolled Into One

3 cups milk (substitute water, almond, rice, oat or hazelnut milk as desired)

5 rounded tsp. organic darkest cocoa powder

1-3 tsp. agave nectar, honey, xylitol or organic sugar—sweeten to taste

1 vanilla bean (split into pieces), or a few drops of organic vanilla extract

1 or 2 cinnamon sticks (can substitute ground cinnamon, ½ tsp.)

½ tsp. nutmeg. To invoke the power of the Mayan Gods,
try adding a pinch of cayenne pepper or chili powder.

In a saucepan on medium heat, add milk, cinnamon, nutmeg and vanilla (and cayenne pepper or chili powder as desired). Gently heat until warm, then reduce heat and add cocoa powder and sweetener, stirring ingredients until smooth. Pour into cups; if desired, garnish with a Golden Spiral of whipped cream. Makes 3-4 cups. Note Fibonacci number usage and attendant Golden Ratios in this recipe which activates cocoa's inherent NSN.

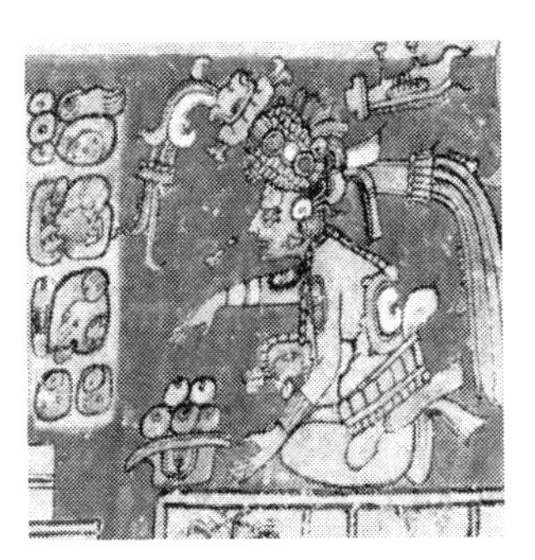

Mayan God Itzamna, early champion of chocolate's divine powers.

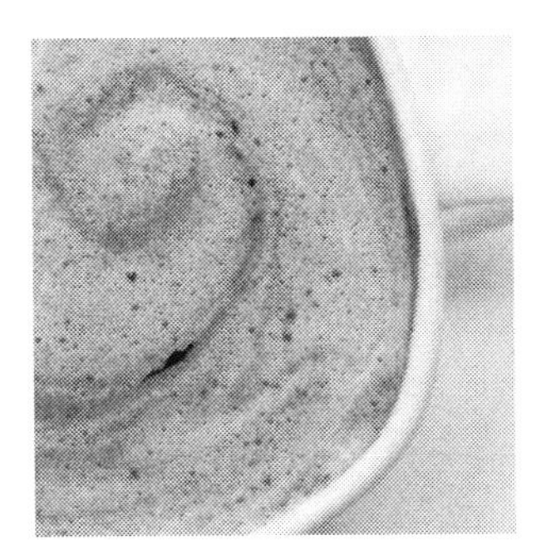

Sharing hot chocolate is a great way to bring people together (note subtle Golden Spiral in foam).

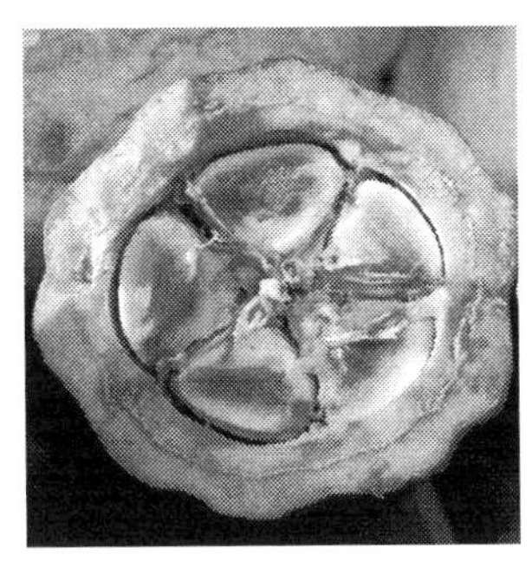

A Golden Ratio Star frames the cacao beans in all cacao pods.

4 Cacao Butter: Nature's True Golden Ratio Food

It's like striking gold whenever we find a food that has exact Golden Ratio proportions of its constituents—and cacao butter is one of those foods. Nature offers us a free dose of NSN just for the tasting. In touting cacao's benefits, most "experts" focus only on the mood altering components like anandamide (bliss chemical) and phenylethylamine (PEA, love chemical). Yet the hidden NSN jewels are in cacao's fatty acid components. In the Nutrition Data Facts label for cacao butter, we can see that:

- Total Fat to Saturated Fat ratio is 1.67 (218 / 130 = 1.67); this approximates the Golden Ratio of 1.62.

Nutrition Facts
Serving Size 1 cup 218g (218 g)

Amount Per Serving	
Calories 1927	Calories from Fat 1927
	% Daily Value*
Total Fat 218g	335%
Saturated Fat 130g	651%
Trans Fat	
Cholesterol 0mg	0%
Sodium 0mg	0%
Total Carbohydrate 0g	0%
Dietary Fiber 0g	0%
Sugars 0g	
Protein 0g	
Vitamin A 0% • Vitamin C	0%
Calcium 0% • Iron	0%

*Percent Daily Values are based on a 2,000 calorie diet. Your daily values may be higher or lower depending on your calorie needs.

©www.NutritionData.com

Nutrition Facts label for Cacao Butter.

So, whenever you need a quick dose of NSN, just take a healthy bite of organic, dark chocolate and saturate yourself with bliss and love.

Red Wine in Moderation: Ancient Elixir for Health & Longevity

To reap wine's full benefits, be sure to sip it slowly. Swish it around in your mouth for 8-13 seconds before swallowing. This allows the polyphenols to absorb directly through the mucous membranes in your mouth into your blood stream, giving you maximum benefits. Up to 100 times more resveratrol—one of red wine's key health-bestowing polyphenols—can be absorbed by this method, compared to just swallowing the wine. If you immediately swallow your wine, it goes into your stomach and then directly to your liver where the beneficial nutrients are inactivated before your body can extract their full nutritional value. Wine connoisseurs will swish their wine before swallowing to be able to discriminate the nuances of various flavors. However, they also unknowingly benefit from increased absorption of the longevity-promoting polyphenols by this practice. **So, in addition to enjoying the taste of your wine, be sure to get more of the life-extending benefits as well by swallowing no wine before its time.**

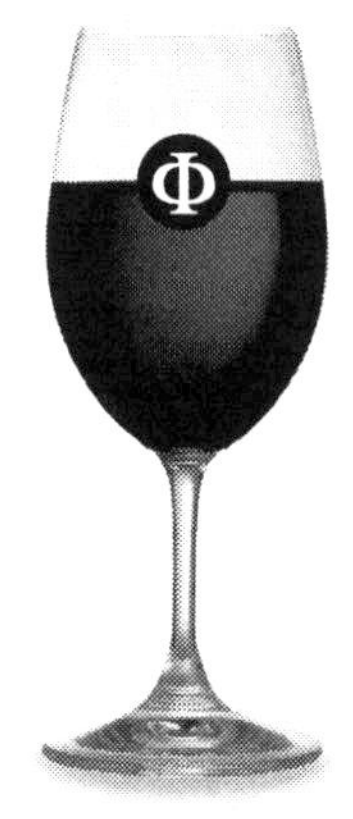

Fill your wine glass to slightly less that 2/3rds full, to visually represent the 62% Golden Ratio.

To ensure that you drink a Golden Ratio "pour," practice filling your glass to slightly less than 2/3 full. This approximates the 62% Golden Ratio volume of your glass. In general and depending on weight, a woman's ratio would be around 1 Golden Ratio glass and a man's average ratio would be 1–2 Golden Ratio glasses. Filling wine glasses to an approximate Golden Ratio amount helps your brain integrate this classic proportion into memory, so you can recall it for use in other areas of your life as desired. By practicing moderation—in wine consumption *and* as a metaphor for moderation in all aspects of life—you'll be well on your way to becoming a centenarian—or if you're of an especially good vintage, perhaps even a supercentenarian. As a doctor of the future, one of the most potent elixirs you can prescribe yourself, in addition to an occasional glass of Sardinian red (such as **Cannonau**) or other high polyphenol wine, would be to heed the advice in the inscription over the ancient Greek temple of Apollo at Delphi,

Meden Agan—Nothing in Excess

If you make this timeless wisdom a part of your life, then Nature's Secret Nutrient will be yours for the drinking. A toast: ***To Your Healthy, Happy and Long Life!***

Note: A word of sensible caution—not everyone tolerates alcohol. Some people are very sensitive to alcohol or allergic to various components of wine or additives from processing. For those choosing wine as one of their NSN Longevity Rx's, drink organic wine only to minimize side effects/toxic reactions from additives. Remember that alcohol is very dehydrating, so honor NSN driver #2, Hydration: ***drink at least twice as much water as the alcohol you consume.*** Many people may have a low threshold to alcohol's effects or are susceptible to alcohol's addictive

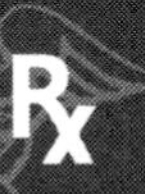

potential; some people may have other adverse effects that impede social interaction as well as the well-known risk of driving while intoxicated. Avoid alcohol consumption if *any* of these warnings apply to you and substitute one of the many other Rx's in this book as a source of NSN. If you do decide to make wine a part of your NSN longevity protocol, aim to limit your consumption to just 3-4 days out of 7. This Golden Ratio range embeds another layer of NSN synergy and moderation into your life.

6 Turn Back Time & Restore Your Youth with Golden Ratio Oldies

Get your smartphone or iPod and download your favorite Golden Ratio "Oldies" that were your favorite songs during your Golden Prime Zone years, those years from 19 to 31. These songs will reactivate key memories imprinted in your subconscious mind and emotions during those especially vibrant years. Music from other non-Prime Zone eras in your life is also enhancing, yet there's a uniquely deep imprint from your Golden Prime Zone years that's particularly strong (as we saw in the miraculous *Alive Inside* music and memory story, pgs. 288-9). **Your goal is simple: to reactivate and resonate with that Prime Time Zone when your life force/élan vital was at its most potent.** As you deploy this simple strategy, note how you feel, look and function. Don't be surprised if soon you start catching glimpses in the mirror of that robust, super-healthy 19 to 31 year old version of yourself! Listen to your selected songs over the next 21 days and watch what happens. You may be amazed in your physical, mental and emotional rejuvenation simply from the power of music to reactivate the latent, youthful areas of your brain. Pop Culture Maestro **Bob Borst** has meticulously compiled a great resource you can use to create your own custom Golden Prime Zone Playlist: 2-minute fractal audio samples of the Top 25 songs for every year from 1946–present at: **www.bobborst.com/popculture/top-100-songs-of-the-year** • *Fun Fact: Jazz legend John Coltrane's masterpiece album Giant Steps was created with the Golden Ratio & Fibonacci Sequence.*

7 The Blizzard Runner: Biostacking Your Rx's to MAXIMIZE NSN

Combining or *Biostacking* multiple Action Rx's at the same time is the ultimate way to generate megadoses of health and longevity-enhancing NSN. In the January 2016 biggest-ever New York City blizzard, co-author **Matthew Cross** seized the perfect opportunity to Biostack *all 10* NSN health Priority Drivers—and tip his hat to Iceman **Wim Hof** in the process. Running in just shorts, sneakers, hat and light gloves for 35 minutes in the extreme snow and blowing cold, he integrated all 10 drivers into a simultaneous *triangulation of fire* for maximum NSN impact, as seen on the next page...

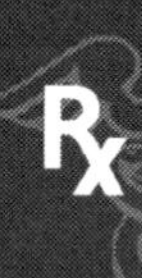

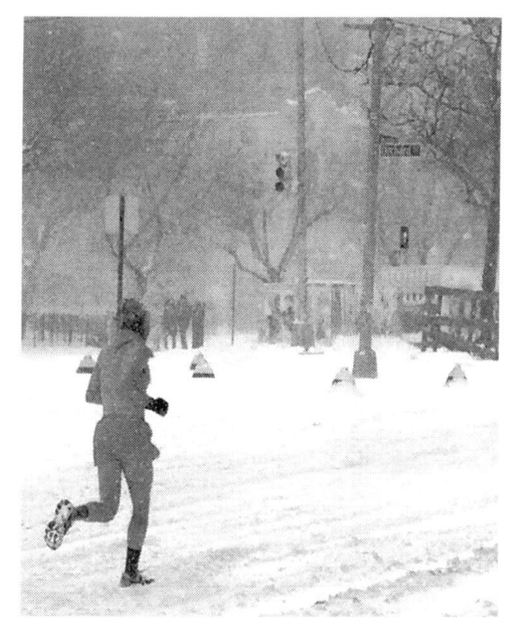

Co-author Matthew Cross, aka *The Blizzard Runner*, running shirtless in shorts at the height of the Jan. 2016 biggest-ever blizzard in New York City. In this radical workout, Matthew *Biostacked* all 10 NSN health priority drivers to extract a megadose of Nature's Secret Nutrient/NSN. Can you spot the hidden Φ? *Picture credit: Raquel Garcia.*

Here's how the 10 drivers Biostacked up:

1. ***Breathing.*** Mindfully took deep, Fibonacci Breaths of snow-purified air.
2. ***Hydration.*** Drank ample pure water before and after his run.
3. ***Sleep/Night~Wake/Sunlight.*** Had Golden Ratio amount of restful sleep the night before; got a solid dose of natural light during his run.
4. ***Nutrition.*** Ate a Golden Ratio Zone balanced breakfast before running.
5. ***Posture.*** Set Golden Ratio spinal posture by stretching before and after the run; he also ran tall and relaxed.
6. ***Exercise.*** In Blue Zone fashion, he kept the run to under 1 hour. The cold wind & snow activated his cold thermogenesis (heat production). Along with Fibonacci Interval Training (FIT) sprints added to the run, this kept him warm and toasty.
7. ***Detox.*** The below-freezing, blizzard conditions initially directed blood flow to his core. A hot shower post-run brought blood and toxins to the surface, dilating skin pores so he could sweat out toxins—activating the cold/hot thermal pump detoxifying effect (a sauna would have been great post-run as well).
8. ***Happiness.*** Running through the snow, he experienced a sense of childlike play, along with feelings of freedom, self-empowerment and joy. After the run, mind, body and spirit-elevating endorphins filled his being, as did a sense of invincibility.
9. ***Beauty/Relationships.*** By the end of the run, the cold wind and snow brought blood and vital force to his skin, giving it a vibrant, ruddy glow.
10. ***Longevity.*** Tapped the adaptogenic and longevity-enhancing power of cold therapy. Post-run, he drank a polyphenol rich, adaptogenic mug of hot cocoa. To cap off his mega-Biostack, he treated himself to a rejuvenating and longevity-enhancing deep-tissue sports massage later that day—and a good night's sleep.

Key Takeaway: Combine or Biostack *two or more* health priority Action Rx's to create a synergistic, Biomimicry-amplified effect—and generate more NSN.

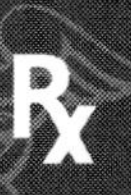

 Implementing NSN Rx Actions & Tracking Your Results

By now you likely have a good grasp on how Nature's Secret Nutrient/NSN can be accessed through implementation of the key health priority drivers, shown here for review in their sequenced FAR (Foundation > Action > Results) order:

Foundation	Actions	Results
1. Breathing **2**. Hydration **3**. Sleep/Sunlight **4**. Nutrition	**5**. Posture **6**. Exercise **7**. Detox	**8**. Happiness **9**. Beauty/Relationships **10**. Vibrant Health & Longevity

NSN's Hoshin North Star FAR (Foundation >Actions >Results) sequence for optimal health and longevity. Note: there is always overlap and cross-reinforcing integration between priority drivers.

All you need now is a motivational tracking system, one that encourages and guides you to implement your chosen NSN Action Rx's. This system—the **Priority Coach**—helps you track and tweak your NSN Action Rx's for lasting lifestyle upgrade. You'll also see how your daily health, performance and happiness—your *Emotional Altitude*—rises by following through on your Action Rx's. A sample pre-loaded **Priority Coach** page is in the next section, addressing each of the key NSN health priority drivers. You can also create your own list of custom Rx's as you get familiar with the multiple Rx choices. The complete NSN system is Nature's ultimate biohack for Vibrant Health, Performance & Longevity. As you begin your journey, may you be inspired and blessed by the timeless salutation of the famous Greek Golden Ratio Genius, Pythagoras:

Great Health To You!

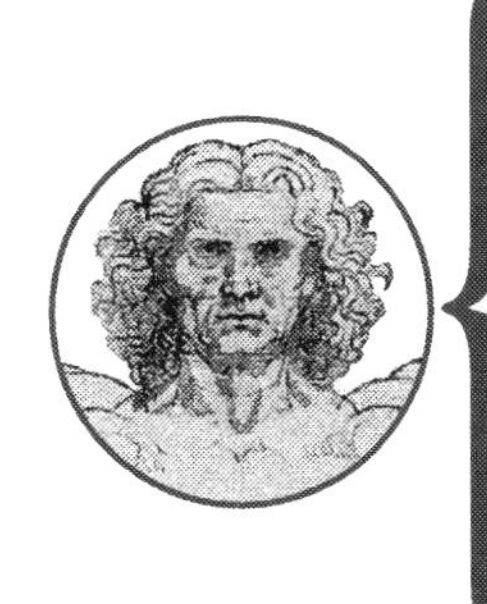

Remember, you're only as ***HEALTHY & ENERGIZED*** *as the degree to which you understand & implement the 3 cornerstones of the NSN system, so:* **1.** Understand how the Golden Ratio is the key to generating NSN. **2.** Learn how the Hoshin North Star prioritized & sequenced the Peak Health, Performance & Longevity drivers of NSN. **3.** Implement the NSN Action Rx's & Priority Coach System to activate & embed the NSN principles & prescriptions into your daily life.

NSN 101: MegaNutrient Health Priorities **Quick Review**

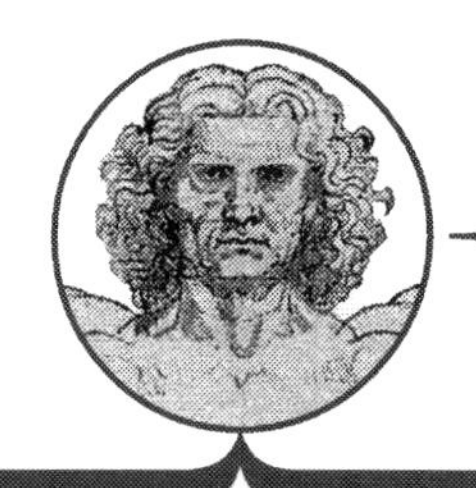

Remember, you're only as...

1

...well Oxygenated as your last ***BREATH****.* So breathe consciously, in Golden Ratio: Inhale to 3... Exhale to 5..... Practice NSN Lung Yoga daily: inhale a few extra sips of air at the top of a full in-breath & exhale a few extra puffs of air at the end of a full out-breath. Feel the powerful surge of life-giving oxygen/prana as it circulates through your entire body.

2

*...****HYDRATED*** *as your last drink of pure* ***Water****.* So pay regular attention to what doctors and nurses call your I's & O's: Inputs & Outputs. Drink before you're thirsty and monitor the color of your urine to keep it in the clear-to-light Chardonnay range.

3a

...Rested and recharged as last night's ***SLEEP****.* So honor the quality and quantity of your sleep by aiming to get a Golden Ratio of 8–9 hours of sleep/rest at least 3 to 4 nights per week. Sleep in a dark, cool, relaxing space with no EMF's.

3b

...Charged Up as your last healthy ***SUN*** *exposure.* So be sure to get your 3-minute morning sun circadian reset as well as a regular dose of UV solar nutrition between 10am–3pm; this activates your vitamin D, neurotransmitter & hormone production, while supercharging your entire system.

4

*...****NOURISHED*** *as your last healthy* ***Meal****.* So eat in the Golden Ratio Zone: 40% carbs, 30% protein and 30% fats. Use organic, fresh, unprocessed, non-GMO food and integrate nutrient-dense SuperFoods into your diet to boost total nutrition. Eat only to a little less than 2/3 full: a Golden Ratio ProPORTION. Prepare and enjoy your food with presence, relaxation and gratitude.

5

...well Aligned as your ***POSTURE*** *is right now.* So sit and stand tall, relaxed and poised to support and maintain Golden Ratio skeletal alignment within the gravitational field. Strengthen your Golden Ratio Core Zone to enhance spinal health and posture. Sit less. Practice yoga and use Power Poses to further boost total body alignment and confidence.

Remember, you're only as...

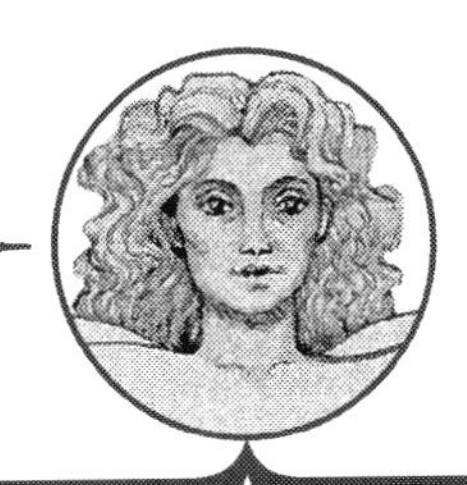

...Fit as your last **EXERCISE**. So be sure to get Golden Ratio exercise at least 3-4 times/wk. Add FIT intervals 1-2 times/wk to release Human Growth Hormone (HGH). Use the 40/30/30 Golden Olympic Training (GOT) ratio for Endurance, Strength & Flexibility & tune Intensity, Duration & Frequency (IDF) of workouts to the 50/30/20 ratio. Strengthen your Golden Ratio Core Zone as a key priority. And last yet not least, one of the best mood elevators bar none is—Exercise!

6

*...**Clean** internally as your last* **DETOX**. So be sure to establish daily bowel movements in the Golden Ratio range of at least 1.6 x/day. Increase fiber intake, e.g., ground flax & chia seeds, exercise your Golden Ratio Core Zone to support healthy elimination. Improve detoxification with deeper breathing, increased hydration and sweating; do periodic colon and liver cleanses. Avoid all radiation exposure.

7

*...**HAPPY** as you feel in any moment.* If you're feeling blue, activate your latent Golden Ratio-blueprinted Happiness genes by practicing gratitude & giving & doing more of whatever makes you happy & strengthening intimate connections and social networks. Last yet not least, turn on your Mona Lisa Smile and take time to meditate daily for even 5–8 minutes, until you're *Happy For No Reason.*

8

*...**BEAUTIFUL** as you feel.* So use all of the Golden Ratio beauty enhancements you desire, yet know that true beauty starts from within. Cultivate your Golden Ratio sense of beauty and passion within and without. Learn to appreciate the uniqueness and special nuances that only your face reflects. Remember that seeing beauty in others enlivens *your* inner feeling of beauty & your relationships as well.

9

*...**YOUTHFUL** as you feel right now.* So if you don't feel as vibrant as you did in your Golden Ratio Prime Zone (ages 19–31), revisit & reignite the energy of those years via the Golden Prime Zone Age-Reversing Holodeck Rx. When used with the other NSN Rx's in this book, you can reactivate your internal Fountain of Youth and kickstart the revitalizing hormonal cascade to regenerate & rejuvenate your mind, body, spirit, and life!

10

The Priority Coach App

Check out the Priority Coach iOS app for the iPhone & iPad

Makes your new commitment & follow-through visible & actionable

Invite a coaching alliance to support your momentum

Powerful features support new habits & lifestyle upgrades

Upgrade your health, performance & life!

Select, track & share your NSN Action Rx's in an easy & fun format

It's *far* easier to upgrade what you can *see*: In Sight = Insight

Chart your daily, weekly & monthly progress.

Download your Priority Coach app at: ***www.NSNpower.com***

Part III: Your 21-Day Priority Coach™

Habit is overcome by Habit.

Desiderius Erasmus

Tapping the Golden Habit Upgrade Principle

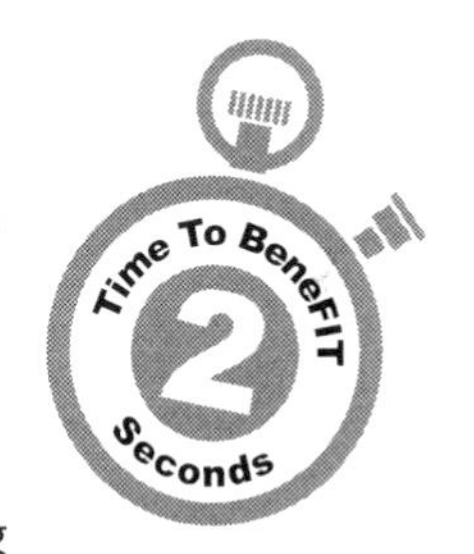

The principles behind the Nature's Secret Nutrient/NSN System are profound yet simple. Yet as with any new practice, incorporating them into your lifestyle requires a behavioral upgrade to new habits. In computerspeak, we first need to install the NSN program and then open the program to use it. This takes us from merely understanding intellectual concepts into the consistent action arena. The "bad" news: upgrading can sometimes be challenging—what may hold us back from making the leap are years of outdated brain software with "bugs," e.g., procrastination, comfort zones, resistance, self-sabotage, etc. **The great news:** The Priority Coach System provides solid support—in just 2 minutes a day—to upgrade old habits and replace them with healthy new ones.

The NSN System provides a solid knowledge base and Action Rx's for health, peak performance and longevity, along with a breakthrough means for activating and habituating them: the Priority Coach System, introduced here. Psychologists specializing in habit upgrade agree that it takes about 3 weeks or 21 days—both Fibonacci numbers—to begin to set a new habit pattern (deeper habit embedding occurs around 55 days, another Fibonacci number). Not surprisingly, the very code guiding our neurophysiology operates according to Fibonacci/Golden Ratio dynamics. It's important to note that forming a new habit pattern doesn't "erase" an old/unwanted one. Evidently our bio-computer doesn't actually "uninstall" unwanted programs of familiar yet maladaptive behavior. Habits, both old and new, are stored throughout our holographic brain. The good news is that as a desired new habit is learned, the old habit is simply deactivated or overwritten—much like a country road becomes overgrown if unused. To no surprise, you can tap Golden Ratio dynamics to support your new habit formation. For example, dietary research reveals that many people stop new diets around Day 13. Yet if they can make it through Day 13 to Day 21, they'll usually succeed in losing

weight and begin embedding the new habit patterns that allowed them to drop the weight. Day 13 is a key threshold—it's as if around that day the old habit reasserts itself to sabotage the new. Armed in advance with this knowledge, you can strengthen your new habit practice on days 12-13-14, escape Day 13's clutches and breeze through those final 8 days until your new habit is better anchored. Propelling yourself through Day 13 is similar to what NASA engineers call *escape velocity:* the tiny percent of added thrust required to break free from the Earth's gravitational field and soar into space.

Priority Coach Launch: A 21-Day Life Upgrade Journey

Priority Coach was designed by co-author Matthew Cross and has been time-tested with thousands of people in Fortune 100 companies and is a dynamic component of the interactive NSN MasterClass system on page 484. It's a powerful yet simple tool for setting new habits to upgrade health, performance and life quality. It takes just 2 minutes a day over the initial 21-day launch phase and integrates the magic of the *Kaizen* small-steps-to-success approach. The theory behind Priority Coach is simple: **You must be able to see and track your progress to stay on target.** When you begin to see the direct correlation between new habits and their impact on the quality of your life, it ignites greater commitment and follow through. It's simple: Out of sight, out of mind—and therefore out of action. On the flip side, **IN–sight** (visible; kept in sight) **= INSIGHT, action, follow through and RESULTS!**

Following is your Priority Coach practice in 5 easy steps. Once you've got it, it takes about 2 minutes a day to track your progress. Review filled-in example on pages 452-3 for guidance. **To set the stage, review the 10 pre-filled Action Rx's on pages 454-5,** which show suggested sample Rx's from each of the 10 Rx chapters. Feel free to modify the list, add other Rx's or fill in your own selected Rx's on the extra blank Daily Tracking pages. **You don't need to fill in all Rx lines—think quality over quantity. Starting with just 3–5 Action Rx's is fine to get going.** *Fill in the month & dates along the graph top and you're ready to begin daily tracking:*

1. **END OF DAY QUALITY RATING.** Start every daily tracking session by quickly Rating the Quality of Your Day (Section 1), in the top shaded row with a 1/Low to 10/High ranking. At the end of each day, assign a "dot" in the shaded 1-10 row across the top of the graph. **This is a quick self-rating of the day just finished,** a visual indication of your day's overall quality or ***Emotional Altitude***. As the days unfold, you connect the dots to form an insightful running graph pattern.

2. **Rx TRACKING.** AFTER assigning your 1-10 Day Quality Rating "dot" in the top shaded area, check off each of your Rx Actions, correlating to today's date. For most Rx's, use a "check mark" to show *I did it.* For others you might fill in a number, e.g., number of hours of sleep/rest for that day (see example). If you missed doing an Rx that day, leave that box blank (no "0's")—you'll want to see the patterns of both blank and checked boxes. These patterns provide valuable course-correcting insight. Patterns are a powerful means to understand the impact of your actions or lack of action. Seeing the correlation between your actions and your day's overall quality rating is especially strong self-motivational medicine.

   Don't judge yourself if you miss doing or tracking an Rx, or miss a day. **Remember, you're simply collecting data in order to upgrade and instill new habits.** *Life Happens*—there will be days when you're derailed and on such days, you may miss doing one or even all of your Rx's. No problem. Let it go. Simply recommit and get back in the game. **Remember, it's not how many times you get knocked down that counts—*it's how many times you get back up.*** So get back up!

3. **WEEKLY PROGRESS NOTES** (section 3; optional). At the end of each week, consider jotting down any insights around your progress.

4. **ACCOUNTABILITY COACH** check-in. Ask a supportive person (spouse, partner, good friend) to be your Accountability Coach. Walk them through the big picture of your Peak Health mission and selected Rx's. Check in with them weekly for 5+ minutes, share your progress—challenges, victories, insights—and consider integrating any course-correcting input that your Accountability Coach offers.

5. **ON DAY 21**, do something to **celebrate** reaching this NSN habit anchoring milestone. Review your progress over the past 21 days; look for patterns or correlations. Commit to closing any gaps where you may have missed the mark; keep following through on what's worked. Consider setting your course to reach Day 55, either by continuing the cycles on paper in this book or in the Priority Coach app. Feel free to modify, add or delete any Rx's as desired going forward. *Remember, the trinity of peak health, performance and longevity is both a journey and a daily destination.*

NSNpower.com also has printable
Priority Coach templates as seen on next pages.

We are what we repeatedly DO.
Excellence, then, is not an act, but a HABIT.
Aristotle

21-day Priority Coach™ System

with Author's recommended Daily Action Rx's for your first 21 days.

1 How was your Day?

Day Quality Rating

At day's end, assign a 1 (low) to 10 (high) rank with a dot ●, signifying the overall quality of that day.

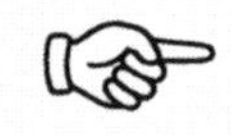

2 How was your follow through on your Daily Action Rx's?

At day's end, check-off (✓) or fill-in data (e.g., **7.5** for hrs. slept/rest or time exercised, etc.) for each action. Important: leave any *missed* actions BLANK.

	My Daily Action Rx Standards	My Target Frequency
1	*GR Breathing: inhale to 3, exhale to 5*	*3x/day, for 1 min.*
2	*Big glass pure Water upon arising*	*Daily*
3	*Sleep/Rest 8-9 hrs.*	*3-4x a wk; track total daily hrs.*
4	*Quality Breakfast; can be power smoothie*	*Daily*
5	*Palms Up or Posture Power Pose*	*Daily*
6	*Golden Core or FIT Wave exercise*	*3-5x/wk, for at least 15 min.*
7	*A.M. BM: morning bowel movement*	*Daily*
8	*NSN meditation or gratitude exercise*	*Daily*
9	*Golden Doors of Your Day practice*	*Daily*
10	*Record pulse rate before getting out of bed*	*Daily*
11		
12		
13	*Coaching alliance check-in*	

3 How was your Week?

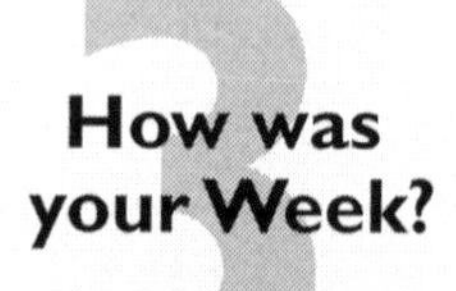

Weekly Journal & Review

At the end of each week, jot down any insights, victories or challenges.

Note any correlations between Actions (hit or missed) and Day Quality Rankings.

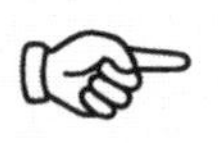

Enter Month: ______________________

Enter Date:	Week 1							Week 2							Week 3						
	M	T	W	T	F	S	Su	M	T	W	T	F	S	Su	M	T	W	T	F	S	Su
10																					
9																					
8																					
7																					
Φ																					
6																					
5																					
4																					
3																					
2																					
1																					

Past week 1-10 rank: ________ Past week 1-10 rank: ________ Past week 1-10 rank: ________

21-day Priority Coach™ System

with Author's recommended Daily Action Rx's for your first 21 days.

1 How was your Day?	**Day Quality Rating** At day's end, assign a 1 (low) to 10 (high) rank with a dot ●, signifying the overall quality of that day.

		My Daily Action Rx Standards	My Target Frequency
How was your follow through on your Daily Action Rx's? **2** At day's end, check-off (✓) or fill-in data (e.g., **7.5** for hrs. slept/rest or time exercised, etc.) for each action. Important: leave any *missed* actions BLANK.	1	*GR Breathing: inhale to 3, exhale to 5*	*3x/day, for 1 min.*
	2	*Big glass pure Water upon arising*	*Daily*
	3	*Sleep/Rest 8-9 hrs.*	*3-4x a wk; track total daily hrs.*
	4	*Quality Breakfast; can be power smoothie*	*Daily*
	5	*Palms Up or Posture Power Pose*	*Daily*
	6	*Golden Core or FIT Wave exercise*	*3-5x/wk, for at least 15 min.*
	7	*A.M. BM: morning bowel movement*	*Daily*
	8	*NSN meditation or gratitude exercise*	*Daily*
	9	*Golden Doors of Your Day practice*	*Daily*
	10	*Record pulse rate before getting out of bed*	*Daily*
	11		
	12		
	13	*Coaching alliance check-in*	

Filled-In Example Page

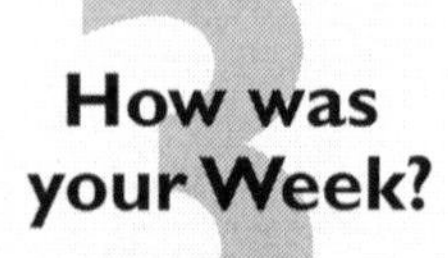

How was your Week?	**Weekly Journal & Review** At the end of each week, jot down any insights, victories or challenges. Note any correlations between Actions (hit or missed) and Day Quality Rankings.

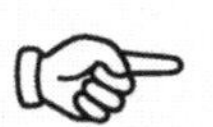

Enter Month: JULY

Enter Date:	7	8	9	10	11	12	13	14	15	16	17	18	19	20	21	22	23	24	25	26	27
	M	T	W	T	F	S	Su	M	T	W	T	F	S	Su	M	T	W	T	F	S	Su

10
9
8
7
Φ
6
5
4
3
2
1

BEST DAY IN MONTHS!

	✓	✓	✓		✓	✓	✓	✓		✓	✓	✓			✓	✓	✓	✓	✓	✓	✓
	✓	✓	✓		✓	✓	✓			✓		✓		✓	✓	✓	✓	✓	✓	✓	✓
	7	8	6.5	6	7.5	8	8.5	7	5.5	6.5	7	8		7	6.5	7.5	8	8	9	8	7.5
		✓	✓		✓	✓	✓	✓		✓	✓	✓		✓		✓	✓	✓	✓	✓	✓
		✓	✓	✓	✓	✓	✓		✓	✓	✓	✓		✓	✓	✓	✓	✓	✓	✓	✓
		✓			✓	✓	✓				✓	✓		✓			✓	✓	✓	✓	✓
	✓	✓		✓		✓		✓			✓	✓			✓		✓		✓	✓	✓
		✓			✓	✓	✓			✓		✓		✓		✓	✓	✓	✓	✓	✓
		✓			✓	✓	✓			✓	✓	✓				✓	✓	✓	✓	✓	✓
						✓								✓							✓

GOT OFF TO A GREAT START, THEN FELL OFF A BIT MID-WEEK FROM OVERNIGHT TRIP/LESS SLEEP... HIGHLIGHT WAS CELEBRATING MAKING IT TO 7 DAYS OF TRACKING ON SUNDAY W/ NICE GLASS OF RED ON THE WATER W/ J.

Past week 1-10 rank: 7

CRAZY WEEK; A BIT ALL OVER THE MAP — AMPLE SLEEP IS A MUST. SAT. WAS A ZOO, SO GAVE SELF PERMISSION TO SKIP TRACKING THAT DAY. GREAT NEWS IS, I'M STILL IN THE GAME! JUMPING INTO NEXT WEEK W/ MUCHO GUSTO!!!

Past week 1-10 rank: 8

ON THE WHOLE A GREAT WEEK! BIG LESSONS:

- ENOUGH SLEEP - HUGE!
- BREAKFAST SMOOTHIES ARE A GREAT LIFT FACTOR IN FEELING FOCUSED + ENERGY
- WEEKLY CHECK-INS W/ ALEX REALLY HELPED.
- PROGRESS FEELS SUPER; PUMPED TO KEEP IT GOING

Past week 1-10 rank: 9+

21-day Priority Coach™ System

Add up to 12 self-selected Action Rx's on lines 1-12 below.

1 How was your Day?	**Day Quality Rating** At day's end, assign a 1 (low) to 10 (high) rank with a dot ●, signifying the overall quality of that day. **My Daily Action Rx Standards**	**My Target Frequency**
How was your follow through on your Daily Action Rx's? **2** At day's end, check-off (✓) or fill-in data (e.g., **7.5** for hrs. slept/rest or time exercised, etc.) for each action. Important: leave any *missed* actions BLANK.	**1**	
	2	
	3	
	4	
	5	
	6	
	7	
	8	
	9	
	10	
	11	
	12	
	13 *Coaching alliance check-in*	
3 How was your Week?	**Weekly Journal & Review** At the end of each week, jot down any insights, victories or challenges. Note any correlations between Actions (hit or missed) and Day Quality Rankings.	

Enter Month: ____________________

Enter Date:	Week 1							Week 2							Week 3						
	M	T	W	T	F	S	Su	M	T	W	T	F	S	Su	M	T	W	T	F	S	Su
10																					
9																					
8																					
7																					
Φ																					
6																					
5																					
4																					
3																					
2																					
1																					

Past week 1-10 rank: ________ Past week 1-10 rank: ________ Past week 1-10 rank: ________

2-minute NSN Self-Test (post)

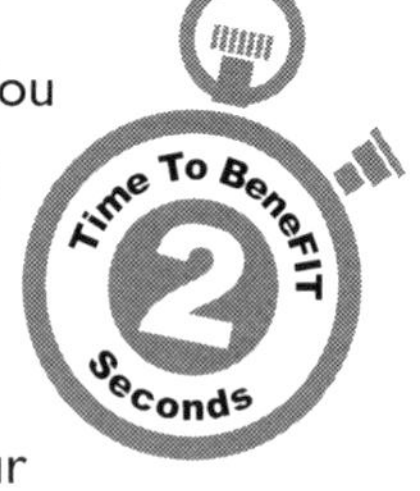

Take this post-test after having completed your first 21-day run through. You can repeat it at various intervals to see where you stand. Continue upgrading your protocol to gain more NSN along your journey for maximum health, performance and longevity.

1. Rate yourself on the 0–4 frequency scale (top of opposite page) on your frequency **today** living the key NSN health and longevity practices. Keep the Golden Ratio, NSN & Biomimicry in mind as you answer these questions.
2. Be honest and non-judgmental rating yourself. Remember, **you're just collecting data to clarify your current position.**
3. When done, tally your score. Give lowest scored items a "*".
   Great News! *The lower your total score, the more you can improve in the coming weeks,* as you practice key elements of the NSN system.

Now that you've completed your 21-Day Priority Coach, compare the results from your first Self-Test on page 47. You'll undoubtedly see positive progress between your *before* and *after* scores. Celebrate your wins! *Note any remaining low scores and commit to elevating them by even 1 point higher in the weeks ahead.* **Challenge yourself!** In this game you're guaranteed to come out the winner. By learning and applying the Golden Ratio Biomimicry principles by which Nature operates, you'll further ignite the power of the NSN Rx's to transform your health, happiness, performance and longevity.

Decode Your Results

85+:	**GREAT**	You're doing really well. Aim for the top by closing any gaps to peak health, happiness, performance and longevity.
71–84:	**GOOD**	You're on track—yet why not kick it up a notch? Are you ready to feel your best *and* live long and strong?
56–70:	**FAIR**	You're hanging in there… yet why just hang? Step up to the plate, select the vital 1-3 biggest gaps to close and *go for it.*
41–55:	**RISKY**	This is your Life Wake Up Call. Will you answer the call?
40 or less:	**HELP!**	You *do* want to *keep* enjoying the miracle of THIS life, don't you? If so, it's time to get serious—**Now.**

Deploy the *Triangulation Of Fire* principle: circle 3 of your lower scored items to focus on for the next 21 days. Select the appropriate Rx(s) from the NSN Action Rx section to lift your 3 chosen lower scored items. Re-test and compare your before and after scores in 21 days.

Self-Score	← LESS	FREQUENCY		MORE →	
	0	1	2	3	4

On a DAILY basis I: *Ch.*

Self-Score		Ch.
1. ______	Breathe with awareness, taking deep breaths throughout my day.	1
2. ______	Drink at least 1 large glass of pure water upon arising.	2
3. ______	Use filtered pure water for drinking.	2
4. ______	Keep my urine in the pale yellow to clear range—no darker than Chardonnay.	2
5. ______	Get between 7.5–9 hours quality sleep at least 4 nights a week.	3a
6. ______	Take a relaxation break or short nap to recharge & reset once a day.	3a
7. ______	Get outdoor sunlight on my face for a few minutes soon after arising.	3b
8. ______	Have a healthy breakfast within 3 hours of arising (a quality smoothie counts).	4
9. ______	Eat only about two-thirds full at meals.	4
10. ______	Include SuperFoods in my diet, e.g., greens, berries, chia seeds, ginger, turmeric, kelp, green tea, dark chocolate, red wine, fish oil, nutritional yeast, spirulina, probiotics, etc.	4
11. ______	Maintain a trim abdomen (a vital health & longevity indicator).	4
12. ______	Am mindful of my posture during the day, keeping my spine relaxed & tall.	5
13. ______	Exercise 3–4+ times a week.	6
14. ______	Include strength, endurance & flexibility training in my regular exercise regimen.	6
15. ______	Have a well-formed, easy bowel movement at least once daily.	7
16. ______	Do regular detox, e.g., deep breathing, exercise, sauna sweating, colon/liver cleansing.	7
17. ______	Experience joy, happiness and satisfaction as my predominant emotions.	8
18. ______	Practice daily meditation, centering, presence, prayer and/or mindfulness.	8
19. ______	Consistently enjoy my work.	8
20. ______	Am happy with my ratio of work to free time.	8
21. ______	Express gratitude daily (e.g., for my body, my life & the good people & things in it).	8
22. ______	Use only non-toxic/organic cleansers & moisturizers on my face & skin.	9
23. ______	Am happy with my romantic life.	9
24. ______	Connect regularly with positive people I care about who care about me.	10
25. ______	Have an inspiring, energizing purpose in my life.	10

Total

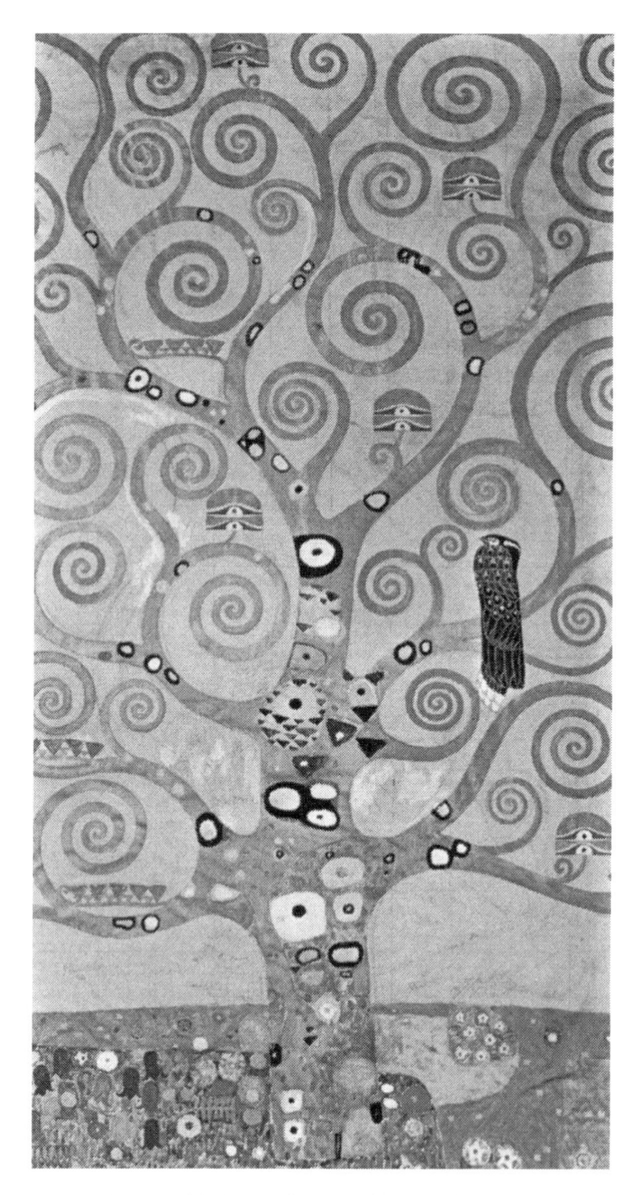

Tree of Life, by Gustav Klimt, 1909.

> *Every living being is an engine geared to the wheel-work of the universe . . . Our entire biological system, the brain and the earth itself, work on the same [Golden Ratio] frequencies.*
>
> **Nikola Tesla, legendary inventor & futurist**

Glossary

21-Day New Habit Cycle: It takes about 3 weeks or 21 days—both Fibonacci numbers—to begin to successfully instill a new habit (about 55 days to really set it in place). Affirming the Fibonacci days within the 21-Day new habit-forming cycle—1, 2, 3, 5, 8, 13, 21—during new repatterning efforts consciously reinforces your desired new habit(s).

21-Day Priority Coach: Kaizen-based, small steps daily journaling system/app for habit and life upgrade. Customized for this book to facilitate charting and implementation of key NSN health and longevity priority Rx's. *Designed by co-author Matthew Cross.*

3-H (Longevity): Mnemonic for Humor/Happiness/Hot-blooded, longevity corollary to Head/Heart/Hips.

3-H (Posture): Mnemonic for Head/Heart/Hips, a simple alignment technique for postural awareness and correction.

40:30:30 (60:40) Zone/Golden Ratio Nutrition: 40:30:30 refers to the ratio of carbohydrates/protein/fat recommended by Dr. Barry Sears, pioneering bestselling author of ***The Zone*** nutrition book series. The 40:30:30 ratio can be reformatted as a 60:40 ratio that closely approximates the more precise 62/38 Golden Ratio.

5-Sense Nutrition: Our combined 5 primary sensory nutrient sources: Visual, Auditory, Kinesthetic (touch), Smell and Taste. *Coined by co-author Matthew K. Cross.*

80/20 or Pareto Principle: A predominant tendency of uneven distribution of causes/effects, actions/results throughout the Universe, commonly expressed as 80% of effects/results come from just 20% of causes/actions. First elucidated by Italian economist Vilfredo Pareto in 1906, the principle was later popularized by quality genius Dr. Joseph Juran. It was subsequently found to have valuable and ubiquitous application to all cause/effect, action/result relationships. It supports the identification of and focusing on the ***vital few*** factors vs. the ***trivial many.*** Not locked to the 80/20 ratio, it can be expressed as *any* uneven ratio, e.g., from 51/49 to 99/1 to 62/38 (the Golden Ratio).

Aquaporins: Molecular water channels on cell membranes that act as microscopic fountains of youth.

Active Isolated Stretching (AIS): Aaron Mattes' stretching technique used by many professional and Olympic athletes. Mattes discovered that muscles can stretch 1.6 times (the Golden Ratio) their resting length before tearing.

AM BM: Morning Bowel Movement.

ANDI Scale: Acronym for ***Aggregate Nutrient Density Index***, developed by Dr. Joel Fuhrman, author of *Eat Right America*; rates the relative healthy nutrient density of foods.

Biohack: A super-effective health and life quality catalyst, providing a transformative physiologic advantage in support of achieving and sustaining optimum performance and longevity. Biohacks can take many forms, e.g., cutting-edge nutritional, medicinal, technological, exercise, mind-body-spirit practices, etc. While associated with the term hacking, *biohacking* has a distinctly *positive* focus, opposite from the common conception of hacking as a malevolent IT practice. Instead, biohacking represents the "white hat" hacker ethic, e.g., free universal access to information, self-determination, quality of life enhancement and ingenious work-around solutions.

Biomimicry/Biomimetics: The art and science of mirroring (and honoring) Nature's eons of experimentation & adaptation to solve current human/ecological challenges. Biomimicry looks to Nature's genius for creative, innovative & sustainable solutions for humanity & the entire ecosystem. Numerous Biomimicry solutions use the Golden Ratio/Spiral for maximum efficiency & performance, e.g., Biomimicry pioneer Jay Harman's Lily Impeller. This beautiful design mirrors a Calla Lily and is used as an ultra-efficient, low-electricity water purification device. Prominent Biomimicry inspirations from Nature include: Bird➔Airplane, Human Brain➔Computer, Eye➔Camera, Whale➔Submarine, Thistle➔Velcro, Plants➔Drugs (as Jay Harman points out, the word *Drug* comes from *Droog*—Dutch for *Dried Plant*). *Imitation is the sincerest form of flattery.* ~ Charles Caleb Colton, 1780-1832.

Biomimicry Medicine™: An innovative bio-engineering and self-healing system that harnesses the Golden Ratio to distill Nature's power into Nature's Secret Nutrient/NSN. Inspired by traditional Biomimicry, Biomimicry Medicine focuses on a wide spectrum of innovations for healthy living and technological advancements in harmony with Nature. Over eons Nature's evolutionary processes have selected the Golden Ratio as the preeminent biological design template for life to grow, survive and thrive. This time-tested principle can now be applied for health optimization and sustainable high performance over a lifetime. Biomimicry Medicine allows anyone to become their own doctor by simply synchronizing their daily lifestyle activities and metabolic processes with Nature's healing rhythms and patterns.

Biostack: Derivative/takeoff of ***Biohacking** (see above)*; ***Stacking*** is a word often used by bodybuilders denoting the combined use of multiple drugs/nutrients for amplified effect. In the NSN context, Biostacking means to combine two or more Action Rx's into the same activity to boost your dose of NSN, e.g., Golden Ratio Breathing + Hydration + Exercise.

Calipers (Golden Ratio): A custom compass for Golden Ratio measuring and designing.

Caloric Reduction: This term is used in contrast to the more draconian phrase Caloric Restriction. In the more user-friendly yet effective practice of Caloric Reduction, overall caloric intake is reduced in varying degrees. Caloric Reduction results in significant activation of the "Skinny Gene" (SIRT-1), resulting in weight loss and normalization of many metabolic processes, including the aging process.

Chaos Theory: A theory for describing and understanding the often-invisible "higher order" that exists in seemingly random patterns, states or occurrences.

Chardonnay: Color standard used to measure urine water concentration. To assure daily water intake is adequate and metabolic wastes are being properly filtered, urine color should be similar to or lighter than the color of a pale Chardonnay wine.

Circadian Reset: Daily biorhythmic resynchronization with Nature's master pacemaker—the Sun—which is easily accomplished with early AM sun gazing.

Circadian Surrogate: A modern stand-in for the morning sun's neurohormonal activating and biorhythmic synchronizing effects. In our modern era the caffeine in sun-drenched coffee has become the sun's circadian surrogate.

Dark Night: Optimal sleeping conditions of maximum darkness, necessary for optimal regeneration and rejuvenation.

Day & Night: Entablatures of the twin maidens Day and Night framing the four clocks which once adorned New York City's magnificent original Penn Station (1910-1963). Created by master sculptor Adolph Alexander Weinman, ***Day and Night*** beautifully represents the true holistic meaning of Diet: *Everything we do in our Day and Night.*

DC (Direct Current) Electricity: An electric current flowing in one direction only, as in a battery or solar cell. When photons from direct sunlight hit the eye's retinas (biological solar cells), electrons are released from DHA molecules present in the retinas, initiating DC electricity which moves through the optic nerve into the brain, supercharging the whole body.

Diet: Holistic, accurate concept of total daily living, represented by the classic sun/moon icon. The word Diet actually means ***everything*** we do in a day—breathing, hydration, sleeping, eating, exercise, relationships, working, etc. *Lifestyle* is really the most accurate definition of the word *Diet.*

Divine: A word most commonly associated with its spiritual connotation, as in ***Divine Guidance***. Lesser known is its equally powerful additional meaning: *To foretell through the art of divination; to know or presage by inspiration, intuition, or reflection.* Thus, ***To Divine*** means to foretell or predict future outcomes. In this context, the Nature's Secret Nutrient System is a powerful way to *divine* optimal health and longevity, at any stage of your life.

Divine or Golden Ratio Code: A term coined by the authors to describe the 5 combined primary, visual manifestations of the Golden Ratio: **1.** The Golden Ratio 1.618:1, or more simply 1.62:1 or 62:38; **2.** The Golden Rectangle, whose sides are in 1.62:1 ratio; **3.** The Golden Spiral, which grows 1.62 larger each complete turn; **4.** The Golden Star, whose every line bisects the other at their precise Golden Ratio points; **5.** The Fibonacci Sequence 0, 1, 1, 2, 3, 5, 8, 13, 21... which showcases the Golden Ratio in the progressive ratios between its successive terms.

Divine Proportion: see Golden Ratio.

Driver(s): Sequenced priorities of lifestyle, health and longevity factors in the Nature's Secret Nutrient, as revealed through the Hoshin North Star™ process.

Elliott Wave Principle: Graphical wave representation of the cyclic growth/ retrenchment patterns in Nature, which are based on Fibonacci numbers, ratios and retracements. First described by R.N. Elliott in 1934 in relation to the stock market; championed in modern times by Robert Prechter, Jr., author and founder of Elliott Wave International, who advanced the principle further with his ***Socionomics*** concept. This principle can also be powerfully applied to health, lifestyle and diet.

FAB: Mnemonic for Foundation, Alignment, Buoyancy; for foot-to-head posture improvement towards healthier Divine Proportion. *Coined by co-author Matthew Cross.*

FAR Principle: The essence of the Hoshin North Star™ prioritization sequence is contained in the eponym FAR: Foundation>Actions>Results. The FAR sequence was used to determine the priorities of the core success drivers in the Nature's Secret Nutrient System. *Coined by co-author Matthew Cross.*

Fatruvian Man/Homo Fatruvius: A play on words on Leonardo da Vinci's famous drawing ***The Vitruvian Man.*** This concept juxtaposes an image of the prototypical modern obese person, ***Fatruvian Man,*** with the ideal body mass representation of mankind as seen in the ***The Vitruvian Man.***

Fibonacci Sequence: The infinite Sequence of numbers created such that each successive number in the series is the sum of the previous two, starting with zero: 0, 1, 1, 2, 3, 5, 8, 13, 21, 34... As the numbers in the sequence get larger, the ratio between them gets ever closer to the Golden Ratio of 1.6180399... *Named after Leonardo Fibonacci of Pisa, (c. 1170-1250), one of the greatest yet forgotten mathematicians in history.*

Fibonacci Sunbathing Timer: A general guide for healthy sun exposure duration according to skin type. Each skin type has a range of minutes, determined by sequential Fibonacci numbers, delineating the ideal amount of time to safely sunbathe.

Fibonacci Trinity: Leonardo Fibonacci's (c. 1170-1250) history-shaping trinity, which he introduced to the West in the 13th century. *Coined by the authors:*

1. Hindu/Arabic numbers (1, 2, 3, 4, 5, 6, 7, 8, 9)
2. Concept of Zero **0**
3. Use of the decimal point

First 15% Principle: Quality pioneer Dr. W. Edwards Deming's principle that 85% of the results in any given endeavor are in the First 15% (the front end) of the process or journey. Used in conjunction with the 21-Day Successful New Habit Cycle.

FIT (Fibonacci Interval Training™): A powerful Golden Ratio enhancement and upgrade of the HIT (High Intensity Training) workout system. By utilizing alternating numbers from the Fibonacci Sequence to demarcate workout/sprint periods over days and weeks and also within single total high intensity workouts, you can tap NSN and greatly augment the impact and results of your exercise. *Coined by the authors.*

Fractal: Any part that reflects the shape or pattern of a whole, e.g., a stalk of broccoli is similar to the larger bunch of broccoli from which it was taken. Fractal geometry, like the Golden Ratio, is present everywhere, at all scales in man, Nature and the Universe. Fractals convey essentially the same principle as the hologram. The Golden Ratio is a master fractal, operating at all scales throughout the Universe.

Fractal Cognition™: The theory of Accelerated Quantum Learning (AQL), which posits that the brain has the ability to rapidly recreate a whole concept or body of knowledge on a larger scale from any similar yet smaller pattern or piece of information. Fractal Cognition is similar to the fact that any piece of a hologram always reflects the whole from which it came. *Coined by co-author Matthew K. Cross.*

Generation PHI™: A new generation of centenarians and supercentenarians that reach their longevity potential through the application of the Nature's Secret Nutrient. *Coined by co-author Robert D. Friedman, M.D.*

Gluten: A sticky, glue-like component of the protein found in grains such as wheat, rye and barley and thus in many common foods (grains such as quinoa, buckwheat, amaranth and millet are gluten-free). In gluten sensitive people, it can contribute to inflammation, poor digestion, fatigue, weight gain and many health ailments.

Golden Ratio/Golden Mean/Golden Cut/Sacred Cut/Phi: The ratio of a small part to a large part or vice-versa which equals 0.618:1 or 1.618:1 respectively. The ratio appears between adjacent numbers in the Fibonacci Sequence, which ever more closely approximates 1.618:1 or 0.618:1 as one moves up or down the Sequence.

Golden Olympic Training (GOT) Ratio: A balanced approach to working out followed by many Olympians and elite athletes which splits workouts into Golden Ratio training percentages, e.g., 40% endurance, 30% strength, 30% flexibility. The larger training segment (40%) is tuned to one's chosen sport.

Golden Ratio Biohack: An integrated system of innovative, simple lifestyle practices and formulas that activate and amplify the Golden Ratio (the universal optimal form and function principle encoded in your DNA) within your body and life. By upgrading and aligning your body's physiologic and behavioral systems and patterns to the Golden Ratio, you can tap the vast health, performance and longevity power of the heretofore unrecognized Über vitality factor known as Nature's Secret Nutrient/NSN.

Golden Rectangle: Any rectangle whose length-to-width ratio equals 1.618:1, the Golden Ratio. Commonly seen in the shape of playing cards, index cards, debit/credit cards, Apple's classic iPod®, etc.

Goldene Schnitt: Der Goldene "Schnitt" is German for the Golden Cut or Golden Ratio. It also just happens to rhyme with the English word *Sh-t*. The phrase is used to denote ideal, healthy bowel movements of about 1.6 times per day.

Golden Spiral: A logarithmic spiral, as seen in a spiral sea shell or galaxy spiral, where each consecutive full turn of the spiral is in 1.618:1 ratio to the previous.

Golden Star: Any equiangular five-pointed star or pentagram, which reflects the Golden Ratio in its design, in that each line bisects the other at its Golden Ratio points.

Goldilocks Principle: The concept of *just rightness* is from the timeless Goldilocks fairy tale and can be reinterpreted through the lens of the Golden Ratio. The point of dynamic balance dividing a line into segments that are not too long and not too short, but just right, isn't at the 50% division point of the line, but at the Golden Ratio or 62% *just right of center* point.

High Intensity Training (HIT): Maximal bursts of exertion with minimal repetition, followed by longer than usual recuperation periods. Pioneered by Nautilus exercise equipment designer Arthur Jones. When the exertion/recovery segments are tuned to the Fibonacci Sequence, we get the FIT system (Fibonacci Interval Training).

Homo Fatruvius: see ***Fatruvian Man***.

Homo Vitruvius: The Golden Ratio's evolutionarily ideal evolved human being, inspired by Da Vinci's ***Vitruvian Man****. Coined by co-author Robert D. Friedman, M.D.*

Hoshin North Star™: The master Japanese strategic planning–prioritization–action system guiding the world's greatest companies. Used to reveal the relative Foundation–Action–Result (FAR) priorities of the health and longevity success drivers in this book. Coined by and from the book *The Hoshin North Star Process,* by co-author Matthew K. Cross.

Human Photovoltaic Charging System: Special ability of the eyes and skin to transmute solar energy into DC electricity that can be used to drive and enhance cellular processes.

Inflammation: A non-specific immune response to injury or irritation with the hallmarks of pain, swelling, redness and heat. Inflammation can also be chronic, low-grade and silent and is suspected of being at the root of many diseases.

Iron Man Green Smoothie: A raw green power drink, inspired from Victoria Boutenko's research into the chimpanzee's Golden Ratio based diet. This Golden Ratio antioxidant-rich blend augments energy and normalizes bowel function.

Kaizen: Japanese for *Continuous Improvement*, especially the practice of consistent, small and manageable steps of improvement. Inspired by the teachings of American quality genius Dr. W. Edwards Deming and his legendary contributions to Japanese/world quality leadership. Kaizen is a close relative of and integrates both the First 15% principle and the Hoshin North Star process. When applied to habit change, Kaizen's small, easy steps approach supports sustainable progress towards successful new habit adoption.

Ketones: Energetically favorable fuel generated during long-duration exercise and fasting, beneficial for the brain, heart and other organs. Ketones are generated from fatty acids in the liver and are an evolutionary survival adaptation developed by our ancestors during times of starvation as an alternate fuel source. The ketogenic diet is an emerging protocol with therapeutic applications for many diseases as well as for performance benefits for athletes.

Markov Chain: A mathematical system that describes transitions from one state to another (from a finite or countable number of possible states) in a chain-like manner. It is a random process characterized as memoryless, i.e. exhibiting the Markov property: ***the next state depends only on the current state and not on the entire past.*** Markov Chains have many applications as statistical models of real-world processes. *After Russian mathematician Andrey Markov.*

Maslow's Hierarchy of Human Needs: A pyramidal ladder representation of human needs, ranging from physiological at the bottom to self-actualization at the capstone. Nature's Secret Nutrient has a similarly themed pyramidal hierarchy, with Air at bottom and optimal Health/Longevity at top. *After humanistic psychologist Abraham Maslow.*

Meden Agan: One of the inscriptions over the ancient Greek temple of Apollo at Delphi, meaning *Nothing In Excess*. This life-guiding axiom is reflected in the Golden Ratio's challenge to live life in moderation in order to foster optimal health, peak performance and longevity.

MicroNutrients are essential metabolic cofactors that are required in very small amounts, such as vitamins and minerals.

MacroNutrients provide the fuel needed to power the body's energetic needs. These are our dietary Carbohydrates, Proteins and Fats which are required in moderate amounts.

MegaNutrients: Potent lifestyle factors unappreciated for their full nutritional value, yet required in far larger amounts than either micro or macro nutrients. They include: *Oxygen, Water, Sleep, Sunlight, Nutrition, Posture, Exercise, Detoxification, Happiness, Inner Peace, Beauty, Relationships & Longevity.* Aligning all 3 nutrient categories—Micro, Macro & MEGA—with the Golden Ratio+Hoshin North Star process results in NSN: master catalyst for Vibrant Health, Performance & Longevity.

Millionaire's MAP™: An interactive book and game for exercising your imagination and preparing your heart and mind to receive greater wealth and abundance. The game involves journaling the daily spending of increasing amounts of money on paper, according to the Fibonacci Sequence. *Coined by and from the book by co-author Matthew K. Cross.*

Nature's Energy Wave / N•E•W™: The incredible Golden Ratio/Fibonacci Sequence-based training system for predictable peak performance and injury avoidance. Developed by Dr. Ronald Sandler and inspired by the Elliott Wave Theory, this breakthrough system tunes and times your training and resting cycles to the Fibonacci sequence, providing direct access to what Dr. Sandler calls *Nature's Path of Least Resistance and Maximum Efficiency and Performance*. Name coined by the authors in honor of Dr. Sandler's genius work and system.

Nature's Secret Nutrient™/NSN: An infinitely self-replenishing, Golden Ratio-based MetaNutrient/nutritional supplement/turbo-charger, obtained simply by learning and applying the Golden Ratio principles to enhancing your MegaNutrients, total health regimen and lifestyle. Nature's Secret Nutrient has no mass, no calories, is tasteless, has no expiration date, never spoils—*and is free for life! Coined by co-author Robert D. Friedman, M.D.*

NSN MasterClass: An custom online course with the authors. Fast-tracks your learning and practice of the Nature's Secret Nutrient system in an engagingly fun way. See page 484.

Nature's SSRI's—Solar Skin & Retina Invigorators: The most natural way to alleviate depression is through sun exposure, since serotonin production pathways exist in both the skin and the retinas. This method can help avoid the use of pharmaceutical antidepressant SSRI's (Selective Serotonin Reuptake Inhibitors) such as Prozac, Zoloft and Paxil.

Order From Chaos: A 6-step system for personal and professional organization, created by author Liz Davenport; from her bestselling book. The system's key sequenced steps are: **1.** The Cockpit Office; **2.** Air Traffic Control System; **3.** Pending File; **4.** Decide NOW; **5.** Prioritize Ongoingly; **6.** OPEN your day, CLOSE your day, CLEAN OFF YOUR DESK at the end of your day. The system greatly increases order and productivity, simultaneously reducing waste, frustration and stress.

Pandiculation: A deep, natural yawn and stretch reflex that automatically resets your oxygen and CO_2 levels, equalizes ear pressure, lengthens muscles, relieves stiffness and increases blood and lymphatic circulation. This Golden Ratio reset is the most primal form of yoga stretching (asana) and breathing (pranayama).

Paradigm: A model used to describe a particular set of assumptions about reality; our mind-set, mental map or theory that shapes how we see and interpret our world.

Pattern Recognition: The ability to see and create meaningful new understandings and insights from seemingly unrelated pieces of data or information. A key skill for higher intelligence; also a component of the ***Fractal Cognition System.***

Peak Performance On Demand™: The ability to schedule in advance peak performances with high predictability using the Nature's Energy Wave / N•E•W™ training system developed by Dr. Ronald Sandler. *Coined by co-author Matthew K. Cross.*

PHI Φ: The 21st letter of the Greek alphabet and another popular term for the Golden Ratio 1.618 : 1.0. Coined by American mathematician Mark Barr, after the first Greek letter in the name of Phidias, the Greek sculptor who lived around 450 BC.

Phyllotaxis: Phyllotaxis or phyllotaxy refers to the arrangement of leaves, stems and seeds on plants. The basic patterns are alternate, opposite, whorled or spiral. They invariably mirror the Golden Spiral/Angle and/or the Fibonacci Sequence/Ratio. Phylotaxis with one "L" is the name of the living Golden Ratio-based artwork by Jonathan Harris.

Priority Coach (process/app): A 21-Day tracking system, designed by co-author Matthew Cross, as a process for implementing daily NSN Rx's. Taking just 2 minutes a day, the system allows you to see direct correlations between new habits and their impact on the performance and quality of your life. *Progress made visible* ignites a chain reaction of commitment and follow through. *Coined by and from the system by co-author Matthew K. Cross.*

Quantum ElectroDynamics (QED): The field of study dealing with interactions of light and matter and also interactions of charged particles with one another. Dr. Jack Kruse is one of the pioneers using QED to explain how quantum physics interfaces with biological processes.

Triangulation Of Fire (TOF): The practice of deploying two or more different yet complimentary, reinforcing angles of approach or action, focused on the same target. TOF exponentially improves the odds of achieving your objective, while reducing complexity and overwhelm. *Definition for this context coined by co-author Matthew Cross.*

Resveratrol: A supernutrient found in grapes, red wine, berries and Japanese knotweed that can slow the aging process by the same genetic mechanism as caloric reduction, via activation of the SIRT-1 "skinny" gene.

℞: A symbol originally used by Leonardo Fibonacci to designate square roots; later used worldwide as the universal medical/healing symbol for prescriptions.

SENS: Strategies for Engineered Negligible Senescence. A tissue repair strategy for human rejuvenation, prevention of age-related decline and extended lifespan. *Coined by maverick English longevity researcher Aubrey de Grey.*

Socionomics: The Golden Ratio-based Elliott Wave Principle as applied to the human moods that underlie all social, cultural and political phenomena. *Concept developed by Elliott Wave International founder Robert Prechter, Jr.*

SuperFoods: Nutrient-dense foods rich in healthy Macro and MicroNutrients, e.g., greens, berries, chia seeds, ginger, turmeric, green tea, dark chocolate, red wine, fish oil, nutritional yeast, spirulina, kelp, probiotics, beets, etc. In addition to tuning your carb/protein/fat MacroNutrient intake towards the 40/30/30 Golden Ratio Zone, it's a great practice to integrate/rotate multiple SuperFoods in your daily diet as well, to supercharge total nutrition.

Synergy: Describes the desirable state where two or more single elements come together to form a *greater whole* which exceeds the sum of the parts. Example: Nature's Secret Nutrient optimizes and focuses the key MegaNutrient priority health drivers to come together to form a breakthrough system for optimum health and longevity. *Coined by Golden Ratio genius R. Buckminster Fuller.*

Telomeres: DNA-protein caps at the ends of your chromosomes, which protect them from deterioration with age. With each cell division telomeres continually shorten, until the DNA in the chromosome isn't protected anymore and begins to unravel, like a frayed shoelace whose plastic tip or aglet has deteriorated. This eventually leads to dysfunction, premature aging and disease. The NSN system is a powerful antidote for telomere shortening.

Unity Principle: A function of Reality that brings together apparent diversity into a harmonious whole. A prime function of the Golden Ratio.

Vesica Piscis: Latin for "Vessel of the Fish," it is the most basic and important construction in sacred geometry, with multiple profound spiritual connections. It is formed when the circumference of two identical circles each pass through the center of the other and is variously linked with Christ, astrological symbolism and the scared canon of ancient wisdom. The design template for the authors' *Vitruvian Man+Woman.*

Vital Capacity (VC): The total amount of air that can be breathed out, after a maximal inbreath. This one lung function is the #1 predictor of longevity; that is, the higher your Vital Capacity, the greater your projected longevity. Deep breaths = long life!

***Vitruvian Human*:** The idealized human being, exhibiting optimal health and vitality, great life meaning and fulfillment and maximum lifespan. Inspired by Leonardo da Vinci's masterwork *Vitruvian Man. Coined by co-author Matthew K. Cross.*

***Vitruvian Man*:** Leonardo da Vinci's masterpiece drawing synthesizing art and science by depicting an idealized human in two simultaneous poses, both inscribed in a circle and square. The drawing is replete with Golden Ratio symmetry and as such serves as a prime icon for Nature's Secret Nutrient/NSN.

***Vitruvian Woman*:** The commissioned-by-the-author's counterpart of *The Vitruvian Man,* by contemporary artist Chloe Hedden. When *Vitruvian Woman* is positioned side-by-side with *Vitruvian Man,* the dynamic balance necessary for the creation of life and the sacred Vesica Piscis is revealed. We theorize Leonardo da Vinci may well have created a *Vitruvian Woman.* which thus far has been lost to history.

W.A.M.: An acronym for Water-AM, or a tall glass of water in the morning, upon arising.

> *The secret of genius is to carry the spirit of the child into old age, which means never losing your enthusiasm.*
>
> **Aldous Huxley**

Recommended Websites

Anastasia Soare's Golden Ratio eyebrow products: www.AnastasiaBeverlyHills.com
Ann Louise Gittleman, Optimal Nutrition, Fat Flush & Parasite Removal pioneer: www.AnnLouise.com
www.unikeyhealth.com/parasite-flexi-test
ANDI Food Scale: www.EatRightAmerica.com
Blood Test for Omega Score™ from Life Extension Foundation: http://tinyurl.com/7p9d6gg
Blood Test for Vitamin D from Life Extension Foundation: http://tinyurl.com/6naey42
Blood Tests for health & longevity from Life Extension Foundation: 1-800-544-4440
Bob Cooley, the Genius of Flexibility/Resistance Stretching: www.TheGeniusOfFlexibility.com
Body Bridge: www.BodyBridge.com
Bruce Mandelbaum, Master Acupuncturist/Massage Therapist (NYC/CT): 203.733.5812
Cosmetic Toxicity check site: www.CosmeticsDataBase.com
Dave Asprey/Bullet Proof Coffee: www.BulletProof.com
Dave Scott (6-time Hawaiian Ironman Champion) Coaching: www.DaveScottInc.com
David Ison: Sound therapy pioneer. Beautiful, effective programs. www.TheIsonMethod.com
Dr. Barry Sears, Zone Diet pioneer: www.ZoneDiet.com
Dr. Joseph Mercola: One of the World's Leading Natural Health Websites: www.mercola.com
Dr. Richard Schulze, N.D.'s books/products (Detox, SuperFood, etc.): www.HerbDoc.com
Elaine Petrone's Miracle Medicine Ball Method™: www.ElainePetrone.com
Fashion Code, Sara & Ruth Levy: www.TheFashionCode.com
Food Babe: Vani Hari's fantastic truth in food & health site: www.foodbabe.com
Food Pesticide List: www.FoodNews.com
FreeWillAstrology: Rob Breszny's poetic, inspiring, funny & enlightening weekly forecasts.
Gary Null, health & natural healing champion: www.GaryNull.com
Golden Ratio Calipers: www.GoldenMeanCalipers.com
Golden Ratio video/Nature By Numbers: www.etereaestudios.com
Gurumarka, Master Yogi, Breathing, Lifestyle Coach: www.BreathIsLife.com
iPhone/iPad/iPod Upright System: www.apple.com/iphone/appstore/
Joe Cross' inspiring weight loss journey through fresh juice: www.fatsickandnearlydead.com
Juiceman Jay Kordich: www.Juiceman.com
LifeExtension: Resource for wellness, health supplements & anti-aging: www.LEF.org
Ma Back Roller: www.TheMaRoller.com
Mark Allen (6-time Hawaiian Ironman Champion) Coaching: www.MarkAllenOnline.com
Medicine Balls: www.SPRI.com
MedX Core Spinal Fitness System: www.CoreSpinalFitness.com
Mike Adams, the Health Ranger: www.NaturalNews.com
Radiation alerts: www.radiationnetwork.com • www.blackcatsystems.com/RadMap/map.html
Robert Kaehler, Master Posture/Flexibilty/Performance Coach: www.KaehlerCore.com
Sifu Rob Moses, PhysioStix Fitness Sticks: www.GoldenSpiralWellness.com
TC Fibonacci Water Bottles, Carafes & more: www.GoldenRatioProducts.com
Teeter Hang Ups DEX-II Spinal Decompression System: www.EnergyCenter.com
Wim Hof, The Iceman; wisdom & training: www.WimHofMethod.com
Xylitol toothcare/sweetener products: www.EpicDental.com www.XylitolUSA.com

Recommended Reading

GOLDEN RATIO

The Golden Ratio & Fibonacci Sequence: Golden Keys to Your Genius, Health, Wealth & Excellence, by Matthew Cross & Robert D. Friedman, M.D.

The Divine Code of Da Vinci, Fibonacci, Einstein & YOU, by Matthew Cross and Robert D. Friedman, M.D.

The Divine Code Genius Activation Quote Book, by Matthew Cross and Robert D. Friedman, M.D.

The DaVinci Code, by Dan Brown (esp. ch. 20)

The Wave Principle of Human Social Behavior and the New Science of Socionomics, by Robert R. Prechter, Jr.

The Elliott Wave Principle, by A.J. Frost & Robert R. Prechter, Jr.

The New View Over Atlantis, by John Michell

Taking Measure and *Tripartite*, by Scott Onstott

HOSHIN NORTH STAR

The Hoshin North Star Process, by Matthew Cross

BREATHING

Breathe, You Are Alive: The Sutra on the Full Awareness of Breathing, by Thich Nhat Hanh

Science of Breath, by Rama, Rudolph Ballentine and Alan Hymes

Breathing: The Master Key to Self Healing, by Andrew Weil (Audio CD)

Flood Your Body With Oxygen, by Ed McCabe

Breatheology: The Conscious Art of Breathing, by Stig Severinsen

The Wim Hof Method: Activate Your Full Human Potential, by Wim Hof. The definitive book authored by Wim Hof on his powerful method for realizing our physical and spiritual potential.

HYDRATION

Water for Health, Healing, Life: You're Not Sick, You're Thirsty, by Fereydoon Batmanghelidj, M.D.

NUTRITION

Mastering the Zone, by Barry Sears, Ph.D.

YOU: On A Diet Revised Edition: The Owner's Manual for Waist Management, by Michael Roizen, M.D., and Mehmet Oz, M.D.

The Fat Flush Plan, by Ann Louise Gittleman, Ph.D., C.N.S.

Dr. Schulze's 20 Steps to a Healthier Life, by Dr. Richard Schulze

The Omega Rx Zone, by Dr. Barry Sears

The Kind Diet, by Alicia Silverstone

Green For Life, by Victoria Boutenko

The Alternate Day Diet, by James Johnson, M.D.

The Joy of Juicing: Creative Cooking With Your Juicer, by Gary Null, Ph.D.

Diet For A New America, by John Robbins

Sugar Blues, by William Dufty

The Juiceman's Power of Juicing by Jay Kordich

Forks Over Knives: The Plant-Based Way To Health, by Gene Stone

User's Guide to Propolis, Royal Jelly, Honey, & Bee Pollen, by C. Leigh Broadhurst, Ph.D

Ratio: The Simple Codes Behind the Craft of Everyday Cooking, by Michael Ruhlman

Fat, Sick and Nearly Dead, by Joe Cross

POSTURE & EXERCISE

50 Pages To Peak Performance in Sports, Fitness & Life, by Dr. Ron Sandler, Matthew Cross & Robert Friedman, M.D.

Living Yoga, by Christy Turlington

Spiral Fitness (DVD), by Rob Moses

A.M./P.M. Yoga (DVD), by Rodney Yee

Consistent Winning, by Dr. Ron Sandler

Active Isolated Stretching: The Mattes Method, by Aaron L. Mattes

High Intensity Training The Mike Mentzer Way, by Mike Mentzer

The Genius of Flexibility: The smart way to stretch and strengthen your body and *Resistance Flexibility 1.0,* by Bob Cooley

ABCore Workout, (DVD) by Matthew Cross

Holographic Golf, by Larry Miller

DETOX

There Are No Incurable Diseases: Dr. Schulze's 30-Day Cleansing & Detoxification Program, by Dr. Richard Schulze, N.D.

The One-Minute Cure: The Secret to Healing Virtually All Diseases, by Madison Cavanaugh

Create Powerful Health Naturally with Dr. Schulze's 5-Day Liver Detox, by Dr. Richard Schulze, N.D.

The Cure for All Diseases, by Dr. Hulda Clark

The Miracle of Fasting, by Paul C. Bragg

Guess What Came to Dinner and *Zapped,* by Ann Louise Gittleman, Ph.D., C.N.S.

HAPPINESS

Happy For No Reason, by Marci Shimnoff

The How of Happiness, by Sonja Lyubomirsky

US: Transforming Ourselves and the Relationships that Matter Most, by Lisa Oz

The Millionaire's Map, by Matthew Cross

Live The Life You Love, by Barbara Sher

The 4-Hour Workweek, by Tim Ferriss

The Four Agreements, by Don Miguel Ruiz

Lessons of a Lakota, by Billy Mills

The Prophet, by Kahlil Gibran

The Astonishing Power of Emotions, by Esther & Jerry Hicks

Switch: How To Change Things When Change Is Hard, by Chip and Dan Heath

The Spontaneous Healing of Belief: Shattering the Paradigm of False Limits, by Greg Braden

Anatomy of An Illness, by Norman Cousins

The Stress of Life, by Hans Selye

The Politics of Happiness, by Derek Bok

Your Brain at Work, by David Rock

One Small Step Can Change Your Life: The Kaizen Way, by Robert Maurer, Ph.D

The 80/20 Principle, by Richard Koch

Order From Chaos, by Liz Davenport

What Color Is Your Parachute? A Practical Manual for Job-Hunters and Career-Changers by Richard N. Boles

The Sacred Earth, by Courtney Milne

Sacred Earth: Places of Peace and Power, by Martin Gray

Wholeliness: Embracing the Sacred Unity That Heals Our World, by Carmen Harra, Ph.D.

Journeys on the Edge: Living a Life that Matters, by Walt Hampton

Catching The Big Fish: Meditation, Consciousness & Creativity, by David Lynch

Transcendence: Healing and Transformation Through Transcendental Meditation, by Norman Rosenthal, M.D.

Ecstasy Is A New Frequency: Teachings of the Light Institute, by Chris Griscom

Chicken Soup for the Soul, by Jack Canfield and Mark Victor Hansen

The Alchemist, by Paulo Coelho

The Vortex: Where the Law of Attraction Assembles All Cooperative Relationships, by Esther and Jerry Hicks

No Matter What!: 9 Steps to Living the Life You Love, by Lisa Nichols

Design Your Life, by Dominick Quartuccio

BEAUTY

The Empress's Secret: The Natural Facelift at Your Fingertips, by Robert Klein, Ph.D.

YOU: Being Beautiful, by Michael Roizen, M.D., and Mehmet Oz, M.D.

How To Make People Like You in 90 Seconds Or Less, by Nicholas Boothman

The Function of The Orgasm, by Dr. Wilhelm Reich

Skeletal Types: Key to unraveling the mystery of facial beauty and its biologic significance, by Dr. Yosh Jefferson

Lindsay Wagner's New Beauty: The Acupressure Facelift, by Lindsay Wagner and Robert Klein, Ph.D.

Whole Body Dentistry, by Dr. Mark Briener

LONGEVITY

Counterclockwise: Mindful Health and the Power of Possibility, by Dr. Ellen Langer

Ending Aging: The Rejuvenation Breakthroughs That Could Reverse Human Aging in Our Lifetime, by Aubrey de Grey and Michael Rae

The Blue Zone: Lessons for Living Longer from the People Who've Lived the Longest, by Dan Buettner

RealAge: Are You As Young As You Can Be? by Dr. Michael Roizen

Relaxation Revolution: Enhancing Your Personal Health Through the Science and Genetics of Mind Body Healing, Herbert Benson, M.D.

The Divine Code of Life, Kazuo Murakami

Forever Young: Introducing the Metabolic Diet, Nicholas Perricone, M.D.

Healthy at 100: The Scientifically Proven Secrets of the World's Healthiest and Longest-Lived Peoples, by John Robbins

Younger Next Year: Live Strong, Fit, and Sexy - Until You're 80 and Beyond, by Chris Crowley and Henry S. Lodge

The Ageless Body, by Chris Griscom

Fantastic Voyage: Live Long Enough To Live Forever, by Ray Kurzweil

The Cure For All Diseases, by Hulda Clark, Ph.D. N.D.

Molecules of Emotion, by Candice Pert, Ph.D.

The Biology of Belief, by Bruce Lipton, Ph.D.

Become Younger, by Dr. Norman W. Walker

Whole Body Dentistry, by Dr. Mark Briener

Age Less, Live More, by Bernardo LaPallo

Secrets of the Superyoung, by Dr. David Weeks

GREAT ADD'L LEARNING

How To Think Like Leonardo da Vinci (especially the Da Vinci Diet section), by Michael J. Gelb

Fingerprints of the Gods and *Magicians of the Gods,* by Graham Hancock

The New View Over Atlantis, by John Michell

The New Economics of Business, Industry and Government, by Dr. W. Edwards Deming

Revitalizing Your Mouth, by Dr. David Frey

Awaken the Giant Within: How to Take Immediate Control of Your Destiny! by Anthony Robbins

The Path of Energy: Awaken Your Personal Power and Expand Your Consciousness, by Dr. Synthia Andrews, N.D.

Harmony: A New Way of Looking at Our World, by HRH Charles, The Prince of Wales, with Tony Juniper and Ian Skelly

Summerhill: A New View of Childhood, by A.S. Neill

Dumbing Us Down: The Hidden Curriculum of Compulsory Schooling, by John Taylor Gatto

Sounding the Inner Landscape: Music As Medicine, by Kay Gardner

Quality or Else!, by Clare Carwford-Mason and Lloyd Dobyns

The Late, Great Pennsylvania Station, by Lorraine B. Diehl

Rich Dad Poor Dad, by Robert T. Kiyosaki

The Art of Leading: 3 Principles for Predictable Performance Improvement, by Wally Hauck, Ph.D.

The Power of Alpha Thinking, by Jess Stearn

Ancient Aliens (*History Channel*; DVD set)

If You Love This Planet, by Dr. Helen Caldicott

Man 1, Bank 0, by Patrick Combs

Out of the Transylvania Night, by Aura Imbarus

Beekeeping For Dummies, by Howland Blackiston and Kim Flottum

The Joy Of Ritual: Spiritual Recipes to Celebrate Milestones, Ease Transitions, and Make Every Day Sacred, by Barbara Biziou

Biomimicry: Innovation Inspired by Nature, by Janine Benyus

The Shark's Paintbrush: Biomimicry and How Nature is Inspiring Innovation, by Jay Harman

Bibliography & Credits

Every effort has been made to assure complete & correct attribution; any omissions or errors will be corrected upon notification. Thank you to ALL sources for adding your genius to humanity's PEAK health, performance & longevity!

Authors' Notes, Introduction & Chapter 1

1618 Combination Lock, starfish, Einstein: wikipedia.org

Golden Ratio Pulse Graph, Parthenon: *The Golden Mean Book* (Stephen McIntosh), www.now-zen.com

Great Pyramid, Parthenon, wine glass, nautilus, wave,
galaxy,butterfly, tennis court, smoke spirals: iStockphoto.com

Skeleton, by T. Reczek after: http://upload.wikimedia.org/wikipedia/commons/2/21/Skelett-Mensch-drawing.jpg

Golden Ratio rectangular grid, pentagram with angles: T. Reczek

Golden Ratio Infographics: concept/design by M. Cross; input from R. D. Friedman, M.D.; rendered by T. Reczek; thumbnail pictures from/created by wikipedia.org, T. Reczek, author's collection, Steven McIntosh

Hoshin Kanri Japanese characters: T. Reczek

Deming Prize: Courtesy of JUSE/Japan

Hoshin North Star™ logo: Designed by M. Cross; rendered by T. Reczek

FAR Pyramid and FAR Flow Diagram: Designed by M. Cross; rendered by T. Reczek

Fibonacci statue by Robert Prechter, Sr., courtesy Robert Prechter, Jr., *The Elliott Wave Principle*

Lungs, bronchi, oxygen, phytoplankton, Houdini, Edison: www.wikipedia.org

http://en.wikipedia.org/wiki/File:Lungs_open.jpg

Lung volume graph: T. Reczek, after Vihsadas, http://en.wikipedia.org/wiki/File:LungVolume.jpg

Lungs: Gray's Anatomy, 1918 - public domain

Vital Capacity vs. age graph: from the Framingham Study, 1948-1968, adapted by T. Reczek,
(after Walford: Beyond the 120-Year Diet, originally from Kannel and Hubert, 1982.)

Biosphere 2: User: Gleam 8/9/99, http://en.wikipedia.org/wiki/File:Biosphere2_1.jpg

Birkel DA, Edgren L., *Hatha yoga: improved vital capacity of college students*,
Altern Ther Health Med. (2000) Nov.

Prechter, Robert R., Jr., *Pioneering Studies in Socionomics*, New Classics Library, pp. 278-293, (2003)

Walford, Roy, M.D., *Beyond the 120-Year Diet: How to Double Your Vital Years*, Da Capo Press, (2000)

http://thelongestlistofthelongeststuffatthelongestdomainnameatlonglast.com/long56.html

Lung graphic: Mariana Ruiz Villarreal "LadyofHats", e-mail: mrv_taur@gmx.net

David Blaine: MagicMama / https://commons.wikimedia.org/wiki/File:David_Blaine_Wikipedia.jpg

Harry Houdini: http://en.wikipedia.org/wiki/File:HarryHoudini1899.jpg

http://www.gallup.com/poll/166553/less-recommended-amount-sleep.aspx

60 Minutes: Stig Severinsen Can Hold His Breath For 22 Minutes;
https://www.youtube.com/watch?v=GI8-Ta2ujnw

https://www.breatheology.com/

https://en.wikipedia.org/wiki/Static_apnea

http://www.guinnessworldrecords.com/world-records/longest-swim-under-ice-breath-held

Stig Severinsen photo by Casper Tybjerg, from Træk Vejre and Breatheology.
https://commons.wikimedia.org/wikiFile:StigSeverinsenBlackWhitePortray.jpg

http://justonly.com/chemistry/pdfs/elemental_composition_human.pdf

http://web2.airmail.net/uthman/elements_of_body.html

Emsley, John, The Elements, 3rd ed., Clarendon Press, Oxford, 1998.

Haeckel Diatomea, https://commons.wikimedia.org/wiki/File:Haeckel_Diatomea_4.jpg

Zabel, Bernd, Construction and engineering of a created environment: Overview of the Biosphere 2closed system. Ecological Engineering, 13 (1999) 43 – 63.

Leaf 1: http://www.19thpsalm.org/Ch09/Algorithm-Topology.html

Leaf 2: http://www-plb.ucdavis.edu/labs/rost/virtual%20grape%20dreamweaver/Leaves%20Venation.htm

Lung branching: Patrick J. Lynch, medical illustrator; https://commons.m.wikimedia.org/wiki/File:Lungs_diagram_detailed.svg#mw-jump-to-license

Retina: https://upload.wikimedia.org/wikipedia/commons/2/26/Fundus_of_eye_normal.jpg

River: http://latindiscussion.com/forum/latin/study-finds-order-in-the-apparent-randomness-of-earths-evolving-landscape.21091/

Golden Ratio in Hexagon proof: http://www.cut-the-knot.org/do_you_know/Buratino3.shtml

Golden Spiral Ear Cochlea: Gray's Anatomy; contributed by Irina Florentina Dragoi, M.D.

J.Verguts, M.D., et.al., *Normative Data for Uterine Size According to Age and Gravidity and Possible Role of the Classical Golden Ratio; Ultrasound in Obstetrics & Gynecology*, Vol. 42, Issue 6, pages 713-717, December 2013.

Chapter 2

Stilles Mineralwasser, photographer: Walter J. Pilsak, Waldsassen, Germany. http://en.wikipedia.org/wiki/File:Stilles_Mineralwasser.jpg

Fatruvian man: Commisioned by the authors: ChloeHedden.com

Vitruvain man: www.lucnix.be, http://en.wikipedia.org/wiki/File:Da_Vinci_Vitruve_Luc_Viatour.jpg

Vitruvian Man body water compartments: by Matthew Cross; rendered by T. Reczek

Water drops: Emmanuel Torres. wwwFacebook.com/staticsolo

www.wikipedia.org/wiki/Alkahest

F. Batmanghelidj, *Your Body's Many Cries for Water*, Global Health Solutions, Inc.; 3rd Edition, 11/1/08

David Fleming, MD, Richard Jackson, MD, MPH, Jim Pirkle, MD, PhD, Second National Report on Human Exposure to Environmental Chemicals, CDC National Center for Environmental Health, January 2003

Giovanni Iazzetti, Enrico Rigutti, Atlas of Anatomy, Giunti Editorial Group, Taj Books, 1/05

Dracula cartoon: Shutterstock/illustrator KoMinx

Kordich, Jay, *The Juiceman's Power of Juicing: Delicious Juice Recipes for Energy, Health, Weight Loss, and Relief from Scores of Common Ailments*, William Morrow Cookbooks, (2007)

AP Probe Finds Drugs in Drinking Water, Associated Press, 3/9/08

Perricone, M.D., Nicholas, *The Perricone Weight-Loss Diet*, Ballantine Books (April 10, 2007)

Null, Ph.D., Gary, *The Joy of Juicing: Creative Cooking With Your Juicer*, Avery Trade; Rev Upd edition (5/31/01).

Miniverse Carafe, model with water bottle: www.GoldenRatioProducts.com

(Adapted from) Altman, PL., *Blood and Other Body Fluids. Federation of American Societies for Experimental Biology*, 1961. The Panel on Dietary Reference Intakes for Electrolytes and Water, The National Academies Press, Washington, D.C. February 11, 2004.

http://www.wired.com/2016/02/people-cross-antarctica-all-the-time-its-still-crazy-hard/

Jeukendrup, Asker and Gleeson, Michael, *Sport Nutrition-2nd Edition*, Human Kinetics; 2nd ed. ed. 12/31/09

5 to 3 clock: http://time.unitarium.com/utc/255

Uthman, Ed, M.D., *Elemental Composition of the Human Body*, http://web2.airmail.net/uthman/elements_of_body.html

Emsley, John, *The Elements*, 3rd ed., Clarendon Press, Oxford, 1998.

Metabolic Water graph adapted from Hoyt and Honig (1996). Copyright 1996 by CRC Press. Dietary Reference Intakes for Water, Sodium, Potassium and Sulphate. https://www.nap.edu/read/10925/chapter/6#85

Chapter 3

http://apod.nasa.gov/apod/ap001127.html

Moon phases: iStockphoto.com

Brainwave graph: M. Cross, rendered by Tom Reczek

Digital clock, pinecone: R. D. Friedman, M.D.

Chepesiuk, Ron: *Missing the Dark: Health Effects of Light Pollution*, 2/2/2009 www.medscape.com

Demas, TJ., Statland BE, *Serum caffeine half-lives*, Am J Clin Pathol. 1980 Mar;73(3):390-3

PN Prinz, et.al., *Higher plasma IGF-1 levels are associated with increased delta sleep in healthy older men*, Department of Psychiatry and Behavioral Sciences, University of Washington, Seattle, USA, Journals of Gerontology Series A: Biological Sciences and Medical Sciences, Vol 50, Issue 4 M222-M226

Stevens, Richard G. et.al., *The Role of Environmental Lighting and Circadian Disruption in Cancer and Other Diseases*, Environmental Health Perspectives, Volume 115, Number 9, September 2007

Trichopoulos, Dimitrios, MD, et.al., *Siesta in Healthy Adults and Coronary Mortality in the General Population*, Arch Intern Med. 2007;167(3):296-301

www.smh.com.au/news/National/Sleep-deprivation-is-torture Amnesty/2006/10/03/1159641317450.html

http://en.wikipedia.org/wiki/Sleep_deprivation

www.boston.com/business/globe/articles/2007/11/30/night_shift_a_probable_carcinogen/

http://www.sleepgrounded.com/

http://en.wikipedia.org/wiki/File:Die_H%C3%A4ngematte.jpg

"A light on at night can put you in a dark mood." Daily Mail. 11/18/10.http://www.dailymail.co.uk/health/article-1330721/A-light-night-dark-mood.html

Usain Bolt picture: Wikipedia.org, by Erik van Leeuwen

REM sleep data: www.webmd.com/sleep-disorders/excessive-sleepiness-10/sleep-101, www.sleepdex.org/

Mark Allen: Rich Cruse, courtesy of Mark Allen, MarkAllenOnline.com

Onen SH, Onen F, Bailly D, Parquet P. Prevention and treatment of sleep disorders through regulation of sleeping habits. Presse Med. 1994; Mar 12; 23(10): 485-9

Puhan Milo A, Suarez Alex, Cascio Christian Lo, Zahn Alfred, Heitz Markus, Braendli Otto et al. *Didgeridoo playing as alternative treatment for obstructive sleep apnoea syndrome: randomised controlled trial BMJ* 2006; 332 :266

Grimaldi, Daniela, et.al., Adverse Impact of Sleep Restriction and Circadian Misalignment on Autonomic Function in Healthy Young Adults, Hypertension, 2016;68:00-00.

Gallup sleep study, http://www.gallup.com/poll/166553/less-recommended-amount-sleep.aspx

http://www.answers.com/Q/What_is_in_between_the_tropic_of_cancer_and_the_tropic_of_Capricorn#slide=1

http://godplaysdice.blogspot.com/2007/12/how-much-land-is-in-tropics.htmls

https://en.wikipedia.org/wiki/Geographical_zone

https://www.bulletproofexec.com/why-bad-coffee-makes-you-weak/

http://www.coffeehabitat.com/2006/12/pesticides_used_2/

http://www.ncbi.nlm.nih.gov/pubmed/20182037

Maui Snares the Sun, by Matthew J. Norris; original commissioned work.

Sun Tarot Card, wikipedia; public domain.

John Ott: Author's collection.

All sun/solar/light/photosynthesis graphics: Tom Reczek, with input from R. D. Friedman, M.D. & M.K. Cross

Monkey w/ coffee cup: www.dreamstime.com/stock-illustration-monkey-drinking-tea-digital-illustration-red-shanked-douc-image48929068

Woman enjoying coffee at sunrise: www.istockphoto.com/photo/young-woman-drinking-coffee-on-the-pier-at-sunrise-gm472376630-63340795

Sphinx & Pyramid: www.istockphoto.com/photo/sphinx-gm173000545-7081248

Dr. Jack Kruse: courtesy of Jack Kruse, www.jackkruse.com

Allegory of the Cave drawing (Plato): by Veldkamp, Gabriele and Maurer, Markus; https://commons.wikimedia.org/wiki/File:Plato_-_Allegory_of_the_Cave.png

David, by Michelangelo: Photo by Jörg Bittner Unna; https://commons.wikimedia.org/wiki/File:%27David%27_by_Michelangelo_JBU03.JPG

Greek Sun God Helio, by Anton Raphael Mengs: Photograph by Steffi Roettgen, Anton Raphael Mengs 1728-1779, vol. 2: Leben und Wirken (Munich: Hirmer, 2003), plate 50; https://commons.wikimedia.org/wiki/File:Mengs,_Helios_als_Personifikation_des_Mittages.jpg

DNA courtesy Stephen McIntosh, *The Golden Mean Book*

DNA UV mutation.gif: www.wikepedia.org

Tropics of Cancer/Capricorn: www.worldatlas.com/ UV map of the world: www.earthobservatory.gov

Kuipers RS, et.al., Estimated macronutrient and fatty acid intakes from an East African Paleolithic diet.

Br J Nutr. 2010 Dec;104(11):1666-87

Dr. Joseph Mercola quote: http://www.mercola.com/article/vitamin-d-resources.htm

Dave Asprey Picture & BulletProof Coffee mug: www/BulletProof.com

The Golden Ratio Predicted: Vision, Cognition and Locomotion as a Single Design in Nature; Adrian Bejan J.A. Jones Distinguished Professor, Duke University, North Carolina, USA. *Adrian Bejan, Int. J. of Design & Nature and Ecodynamics. Vol. 4, No. 2 (2009) 97–104*

Golden Ratio in Hexagon proof: http://www.cut-the-knot.org/do_you_know/Buratino3.shtml

Chapter 4

http://en.wikipedia.org/wiki/File:C-reactive_protein.png

http://commons.wikimedia.org/wiki/File:Darwin_fish_ROF.svg

Image of the Buddha 2-3th century CE: British Museum. Personal photograph 2005. {GDFL} PHGCOM. http://commons.wikimedia.org/wiki/File:EmaciatedBuddha.JPG

http://commons.wikimedia.org/wiki/File:Grape_in_napa.jpg

Boyer, Jeanelle and Liu, Rui Hai, Apple Phytochemicals and their Health Benefits, Nutrition Journal, 2004, 3:5 doi:10.1186/1475-2891-3-5

apples, http://whfoods.org/genpage.php?tname=foodspice&dbid=15

Farzaneh-Far R; JAMA. 303(3):250-257;2010

Stomach 62% full by R. D. Friedman, M.D. after: http://commons.wikimedia.org/wiki/File:Gray1050-stomach.png.

Hands Cupped with Cherries: iStockPhoto.com

NSN Golden Ratio Zone Decoder graph: concept/design by M. Cross; input from R. D. Friedman, M.D.; rendered by T. Reczek

http://en.wikipedia.org/wiki/File:Cholesterol.svg; BorisTM

Plates/golden ratio: R. D. Friedman, M.D.

http://upload.wikimedia.org/wikipedia/commons/a/a2/Creation-of-adam.PNG

www.wellcorps.com/Explaining-The-Hidden-Meaning-Of-Michelangelos-Creation-of-Adam.html

Bougnoux, Philippe and Chajès, Veronique, *Omega–6/Omega–3 Polyunsaturated Fatty Acid Ratio and Cancer*, World review of nutrition and dietetics , 2003, vol. 92, pp. 133-151, Karger, Basel, SUISSE

Broadhurst, CL, Cunnane SC, Crawford MA., *Rift Valley lake fish and shellfish provided brain-specific nutrition for early Homo*, Br J Nutr. 1998 Jan;79(1):3-21

Hamazaki T, Okuyama H. *The Japan Society for Lipid Nutrition recommends to reduce the intake of linoleic acid. A review and critique of the scientific evidence.* World Rev Nutr Diet. 2003;92:109-132

Pasinetti GM, et.al., *Calorie restriction attenuates Alzheimer's disease type brain amyloidosis in Squirrel monkeys (Saimiri sciureus)*, J Alzheimers Dis. 2006 Dec;10(4):417-22

Pella, Daniel, et al., *Effects of an Indo-Mediterranean Diet on the Omega–6/Omega–3 Ratio in Patients at High Risk of Coronary Artery Disease: The Indian Paradox*, World review of nutrition and dietetics, 2003, vol. 92

Scholl, Johannes G., http://www.bmj.com/cgi/eletters/332/7544/752#130637

Simopoulos, AP, *The importance of the ratio of omega-6/omega-3 essential fatty acids*, Biomed Pharmacother. 2002 Oct;56(8):365-79

Linus Pauling Inst., Membrane Structure and Function,

http://lpi.oregonstate.edu/infocenter/othernuts/omega3fa/

http://www.smh.com.au/news/national/more-fat-people-in-world-than-there-are-starving-study-finds/2006/08/14/1155407741532.html

http://www.zonediet.com/EATING/HowtoMakeaZoneMeal/tabid/82/Default.aspx

http://www.chimphaven.org/chimps-facts.cfm

http://www.naturalnews.com/022792_food_raw_food_smoothies.html

http://www.sciencedaily.com/releases/2006/10/061013104633.htm

The George Mateljian Foundation/Kale: http://tinyurl.com/5d3auf

http://commons.wikimedia.org/wiki/File:Four_temperament.PNG

Jack Lalanne: http://en.wikipedia.org/wiki/File:Edjackfn.jpg

Bread loaf: http://commons.wikimedia.org/wiki/File:Boule_de_campagne_01.jpg by Zantastik

Meharban Singh, *Essential Fatty Acids and the Human Brain, The Indian Journal of Pediatrics*, Vol. 72., (3/05).

Pauwels, E. K.; Kostkiewicz, M (2008). "Fatty acid facts, Part III: Cardiovascular disease, or, a fish diet is not fishy". Drug news & perspectives 21 (10): 552–61.

Farzaneh-Far R et al., Association of Marine Omega-3 Fatty Acid Levels With Telomeric Aging in Patients With Coronary Heart Disease, JAMA. 2010;303(3):250-257.

Samieri, C; Lorrain, S; Buaud, B; Vaysse, C; Berr, C; Peuchant, E; Cunnane, S. C.; Barberger-Gateau, P, Relationship between diet and plasma long-chain n-3 PUFAs in older people: Impact of apolipoprotein E genotype. (2013)., The Journal of Lipid Research 54 (9): 2559–67.

Bazan, N. G.; Molina, M. F.; Gordon, W. C., Docohexaenoic acid signalolipidomics in nutrition: Significance in aging, neuroinflammation, macular degeneration, Alzheimer's and other neurodegenerative diseases., (2011)., Annual Review of Nutrition 31: 321–51.

Aline Hittle., "DHA in Slowing the Progression of AD." Baylor College of Medicine. http://www.bcm.edu/neurology/alzheimers/index.cfm?pmid=16413

Docosahexaenoic acid (DHA), http://en.wikipedia.org/wiki/Docosahexaenoic_acid

Longo, Valter D., et al., Prolonged Fasting Reduces IGF-1/PKA to Promote Hematopoietic-Stem-Cell-Based Regeneration and Reverse Immunosuppression, Cell Stem Cell, Volume 14, Issue 6, p. 810–823, 5 June, 2014.

Brandhorst et al., A Periodic Diet that Mimics Fasting Promotes Multi-System Regeneration, Enhanced Cognitive Performance and Healthspan.

Cell Metabolism, 22, 1–14, July 7, 2015. http://dx.doi.org/10.1016/j.cmet.2015.05.012

Lambert, Victoria, The new 'fake fast' diet may be easier and more effective than the 5:2, June 20 2015, http://tinyurl.com/qffrmrt

Cholesterol, Triglycerides, and Associated Lipoproteins - Clinical Methods - NCBI Bookshelf, http://www.ncbi.nlm.nih.gov/books/NBK351/#!po=23.7705

Partonen, T., et.al., Association of low serum total cholesterol with major depression and suicide. *The British Journal of Psychiatry*, Sep 1999, 175 (3) 259-262; DOI: 10.1192/bjp.175.3.259.

Bowden, J., Sinatra, M.D., S., *The Great Cholesterol Myth*, Fair Winds Press, 2012.

Ravnskov, Uffe, *The Cholesterol Myths: Exposing the Fallacy that Saturated Fat and Cholesterol Cause Heart Disease*, Newtrends Publishing, Inc., October 1, 2000.

Zhang C, et al. *Abdominal obesity and the risk of all-cause, cardiovascular, and cancer mortality: sixteen years of follow-up in US women. Circulation 2008;117(13):1658-1667.*

Engelsen O. and Kylling A. (2005), *Fast simulation tool for ultraviolet radiation at the Earth's surface. Optical Engineering,* 44 (4): 041012–041012-7.

https://upload.wikimedia.org/wikipedia/commons/1/18/UV_Index_NYC.png

Thomas J. Bruno, Paris D. N. Svoronos. *CRC Handbook of Fundamental Spectroscopic Correlation Charts.* CRC Press, 2005.

https://upload.wikimedia.org/wikipedia/commons/thumb/d/d9/Linear_visible_spectrum.svg/1280px-Linear_visible_spectrum.svg.png

Panda, S., et.al., *Time-Restricted Feeding Is a Preventative and Therapeutic Intervention against Diverse Nutritional Challenges.* Cell Metabolism. Volume 20, Issue 6, Dec. 2014, pp. 99101005.

Longo, Valter D., Panda, Satchidananda, *Fasting, Circadian Rhythms, and Time-Restricted Feeding in Healthy Lifespan*, Cell Metabolism 23, June 14, 2016

https://www.foundmyfitness.com/episodes/satchin-round-2

Chapter 5

Spine with Golden Ratios by T. Reczek after: http://en.wikipedia.org/wiki/File:Spinal_column_curvature.png

Skeleton, by T. Reczek after:
http://upload.wikimedia.org/wikipedia/commons/2/21/Skelett-Mensch-drawing.jpg

Pelvic, temporal, sphenoid bones with spirals by T. Reczek: after Mees, L.F.C.;
Secrets of the Skeleton: Form in Metamorphosis, Anthroposophic Press; September 1984

Forearm, Hand Golden Ratios: R. D. Friedman

David statue grids: T. Reczek after, http://en.wikipedia.org/wiki/File:Michelangelos_David.jpg

http://upload.wikimedia.org/wikipedia/commons/7/75/Posture_types_(vertebral_column).jpg,
V-Ugnivenko, author

Hartmann, O.J., *Dynamische Morphologie*; courtesy Scott Olsen, author of *The Golden Section: Nature's Greatest Secret*, (navel pic)

http://en.wikipedia.org/wiki/File:Computer_Workstation_Variables.jpg, Integrated Safety Management, Berkeley Lab

Poor posture/computer, osteoporosis, backbend: iStockphoto.com

Source: Briñol, Pablo, Petty, Richard E., Wagner, Benjamin; *Body posture effects on self-evaluation: A self-validation approach. European Journal of Social Psychology: Volume 39, Issue 6*, October 2009, Pages: 1053-1064.

No Sitting Zone graphic: by Matthew Cross; rendered by T. Reczek

Seated chakras, caduceus: www.wikipedia.org

Seated yoga figure with chakras and Golden Spirals: Scott Onstott: www.SecretsInPlainSight.com

Carpenter's level: http://commons.wikimedia.org/wiki/File:DetalleNivelDeBurbuja.jpg

Cuddy, Amy J.C., et.al., Power Posing: Brief Nonverbal Displays Affect Neuroendocrine Levels and Risk Tolerance, Psychological Science Online, http://tinyurl.com/2g5n6sw

https://en.wikipedia.org/wiki/Amy_Cuddy

http://www.ted.com/talks/amy_cuddy_your_body_language_shapes_who_you_are

Briñol, P., Petty, R. E. and Wagner, B. (2009), *Body posture effects on self-evaluation: A self-validation approach.* Eur. J. Soc. Psychol., 39: 1053–1064. doi: 10.1002/ejsp.607

https://upload.wikimedia.org/wikipedia/commons/thumb/4/49/Rod_of_asclepius_3d.svg/401px-

Mammalian Skull Dimensions and the Golden Ratio: Rafael J. Tamargo, MD and Jonathan A. Pindrik, MD; *The Journal of Craniofacial Surgery* Volume 30, Number 6, September 2019.

Chapter 6

Heart spiral muscle: J. Bell Pettigrew / The Bakken, Minneapolis, MN

Electrocardiogram Golden Ratios: T. Reczek after Agateller (Anthony Atkielski), http://en.wikipedia.org/wiki/File:SinusRhythmLabels.svg

Exercise reference - Dave Asprey interviews Dr. Richard Veech; YouTube episode #299 - https://www.youtube.com/watch?v=QO4WZlaoO7M&t=3582s

Nature's Energy Wave / N•E•W™ graph concept/design by M. K. Cross; input from R. D. Friedman, M.D., rendered by T. Reczek; inspired by Sandler, Dr. Ronald D.; Dennis D. Lobstein; *Consistent Winning: A Remarkable New Training System that Lets You Peak on Demand*, Rodale Press; October 1992

Bjorn Borg backhand: author's collection

Rob Moses, David Carradine, Shaolin Monk, PhysioStix: Courtesy of Rob Moses, GoldenSpiralWellness.com http://commons.wikimedia.org/wiki/File:Grade_I_hypertension.jpg; Author: Steven Fruitsmaak

Roger Federer, Wimbledon 2009: uploaded to wikipedia by Flickr member Squeaky Knees, Cornwall, UK; https://commons.wikimedia.org/wiki/File:Roger_Federer_(26_June_2009,_Wimbledon)_3_cropped.jpg

Speedometer (Saab 9-3): M. Cross, R. D. Friedman, M.D. and T. Reczek

Fahey, Thomas D., Swanson, George D., Medicina Sportiva, 12 (4): 124-128, 2008, *A Model for Defining the Optimal Amount of Exercise Contributing to Health and Avoiding Sudden Cardiac Death*

Jackicic, John M.; *Effects of Exercise Duration and Intensity on Weight Loss in Overweight, Sedentary Women: A Randomized Trial; JAMA* 290 (Sept. 10, 2003): 1,323-30

Sandler, Dr. Ronald D.; Dennis D. Lobstein; *Consistent Winning: A Remarkable New Training System that Lets You Peak on Demand*, Rodale Press; October 1992

Steinberg, Steve, *Men's Journal Magazine*, March 2004, on Baron Davis

Ulmer, Ph.D., Hanno, et al, George Clooney, the cauliflower, the cardiologist, and phi, the golden ratio., 13 December 2009, BMJ 2009;339:b4745

Heart graphic: Mariana Ruiz Villarreal "LadyofHats", e-mail: mrv_taur@gmx.net

Novak Djokovic picture from Wikipedia.org, by Wikipedia user Stefan1991

Yoga stretch: iStockphoto.com

Wright Balance, courtesy or Dr. David Wright: www.WrightBalance.com

McIntosh, Stephen; *The Golden Ratio Book*; Now & Zen, 1997.

Garber, Carol Ewing Ph.D., FACSM, et.al., *Quantity and Quality of Exercise for Developing and Maintaining Cardiorespiratory, Musculoskeletal, and Neuromotor Fitness in Apparently Healthy Adults: Guidance for Prescribing Exercise.* Medicine & Science in Sports & Exercise: July 2011, Vol.43, Issue 7, pp. 1334-1359.

White, Jr., J.W., and Doner, Landis, *Beekeeping in the United States, Agriculture Handbook*, No.335, Revised October 1980, p. 82-91.

Woodward, Mark, et. al., *The association between resting heart rate, cardiovascular disease and mortality: evidence from 112,680 men and women in 12 cohorts, European Journal of Preventive Cardiology*, 2014 21: 719

Levine, H.J. Rest heart rate and life expectancy. *J Am Coll Cardiol.* 1997;30:1104–1106.

The Lower the Heart Rate, the Longer the Life. http://hmatter.blogspot.com/2011/12/lower-heart-rate-longer-life.html

Hsia, Judith, et.al., Resting heart rate as a low tech predictor of coronary events in women: prospective cohort study, *BMJ*. 2009; 338: b219.

Heartrate of 62 BPM & mortality rate study: *Hsia, BMJ, 2/4/09.*

Roger Federer at Wimbledon 2009: Squeaky Knees, Cornwall, UK; uploaded by SpecialWindler: https://commons.wikimedia.org/wiki/File:Roger_Federer_(26_June_2009,_Wimbledon)_3_cropped.jpg

Chapter 7

Pulse-oximeter in Golden Ratio: Matthew Cross

http://en.wikipedia.org/wiki/File:Triathlon_pictogram.svg; Thadius856 (SVG conversion) & Parutakupiu (original image)

http://en.wikipedia.org/wiki/File:Badstuga,_efter_illustration_i_Acerbis_Travels,_Nordisk_familjebok.png

http://www.feinberg.northwestern.edu/nutrition/factsheets/fiber.html

www.HerbDoc.com: website of Dr. Richard Schulze

Mercola, J., *The No Grain Diet*, Plume, March 30, 2004

Sanjoaquin MA, Appleby PN, Spencer EA, Key TJ., *Nutrition and lifestyle in relation to bowel movement frequency: a cross-sectional study of 20630 men and women in EPIC-Oxford, Public Health Nutrition:* 7(1), 77–83, 2004.

Santana-Rios, Ph.D., Gilberto, Fiber Facts, http://lpi.oregonstate.edu/sp-su99/santana.html

Well Being Journal Vol. 7, No. 5 ~ September/October 1998

Data for calculating soluble/insoluble ratios was taken from the following two sources; in the event of conflicting measurements, the ratio closest to the Golden Ratio was the default selection: 1. Anderson JW. Plant Fiber in Foods. 2nd ed. HCF Nutrition Research Foundation Inc., 1990. 2. http://whfoods.org/

http://susandoreydesigns.com/insights/pasteur-recant.html

https://riordanclinic.org/2011/12/detox-natural-cleansing-to-remove-body-toxins/

Biologic EMF effects: www.jackkruse.com/emf-5-what-are-the-biologic-effects-of-emf/ L Marciani, et.al., *Effects of various food ingredients on gall bladder emptying.* Eur J Clin Nutr. 2013 Nov; 67(11): 1182–1187.

Kelder, Peter, [5 Tibetan Rites], *Ancient Secret of the Fountain of Youth*, Doubleday; Doubleday edition, 1/20/98

Dave Asprey picture and Bulletproof Coffee Mug: www.Bulletproof.com

Radiation reference - Dave Asprey interviews Dr. Richard Veech; YouTube episode #299 - https://www.youtube.com/watch?v=QO4WZlaoO7M&t=3582s

Radiation Definitions: *Gale Encyclopedia of Medicine & McGraw-Hill Concise Dictionary of Modern Medicine*

Chapter 8

Happiness pie graphs, Golden Ratio peace symbol, Golden Ratio work-reduction graph, 80/20 Principle graph, Order From Chaos Golden Ratio desk graph: T. Reczek

DNA molecule courtesy Stephen McIntosh, *The Golden Mean Book.*

New Jeruselem Golden Ratio sculpture: Andrew Rodgers, http://en.wikipedia.org/wiki/File:Golden_Ratio.jpg

The New Jerusalem (Tapestry of the Apocalypse): http://en.wikipedia.org/wiki/File:La_nouvelle_J%C3%A9rusalem.jpg

New Jerusalem painting: Michell, John, *The Dimensions of Paradise: The Proportions and Symbolic Numbers of Ancient Cosmology*; Adventures Unlimited Press (May 2, 2001)

Scott Onstott's Golden Ratio art: www.SecretsInPlainSight.com

Mona Lisa, Vitruvian Man, Leonardo da Vinci: www.wikepedia.org

DNA mandala: Computer Graphics Lab/UCSF

Ferriss, Timothy, *The 4-Hour Workweek: Escape 9-5, Live Anywhere, and Join the New Rich*; Crown, 4/24/07

www.gobankingrates.com/history-of-the-40-hour-work-week-and-its-effects-on-the-economy/

Lipton, Bruce H., Ph.D., *The Biology of Belief: Unleashing the Power of Consciousness, Matter, & Miracles*; Hay House; illustrated edition (September 15, 2008)

Lyubomirsky, Sonja, *The How of Happiness: A New Approach to Getting the Life You Want;* Penguin; Reprint edition, December 30, 2008

Murakami, Kazuo, *The Divine Code of Life: Awaken Your Genes and Discover Hidden Talents*; Atria Books/ Beyond Words (April 28, 2006)

Pert, Candace, Ph.D., *Molecules Of Emotion: The Science Between Mind-Body Medicine, Scribner* (1999)

Shimoff, Marci, *Happy for No Reason: 7 Steps to Being Happy from the Inside Out*; Free Press, (March 3, 2009)

What the Bleep Do We Know!?, 20th Century Fox film, (2004). http://en.wikipedia.org/wiki/Itzamna

en.wikipedia.org/wiki/Hot_chocolate

http://en.wikipedia.org/wiki/File:Cacao-pod-k4636-14.jpg

http://en.wikipedia.org/wiki/File:God_D_Itzamna.jpg

Drew Barrymore, by David Shankbone: http://en.wikipedia.org/wiki/File:Drew_Barrymore_2_by_David_Shankbone_cropped_2.jpg

Susan Sarandon: Tony Shek; http://commons.wikimedia.org/wiki/File:Susan_Sarandon_2005.jpg

Lefebvre, V.A., The Fundamental Structures of Human Reflexion. Journal of Social Biological Structure, Vol. 10, pp. 129-175. 1987, October.

http://upload.wikimedia.org/wikipedia/commons/a/a1/Semaphore_Delta.svg

http://upload.wikimedia.org/wikipedia/commons/1/1b/Semaphore_November.svg

https://en.wikipedia.org/wiki/Shaken,_not_stirred

Color therapy for sleep: http://decoratedlife.com/color-therapy-guarantee-sleep-life/

Yellow Brick Road Spiral: screen capture from *The Wizard of Oz* trailer; © Turner Entertainment Co.

Boy with dog: author's collection

Chapter 9

Sean Connery: Still from the public domain/copyright-free film trailer from the 1964 Hitchcock film *Marnie*
Marilyn Monroe: http://commons.wikimedia.org/wiki/File:Marilyn_Monroe_in_Niagara.jpg
Brad Pitt and Angelina Jolie: http://commons.wikimedia.org/wiki/File:Fcad3.jpg
Alexandra Popescu, Courtesy of and Copyright ©2019 Alexandra Popescu, www.DillyChilly.com
Christy Turlington: Courtesy of PETA; photo by Steven Klein
Golden Ratio Calipers: R. D. Friedman, M.D.
Anastasia Soare, Brow with Caliper Lines: Courtesy of Anastasia, www.anastasia.net/help.php?section=goldenratio
Michelangelo's David: modified by T. Reczek, after http://en.wikipedia.org/wiki/File:Michelangelos_David.jpg
Teeth with calipers: courtesy Dr. Eddie Levin: www.goldenmeangauge.co.uk
Golden Ratio Teeth, courtesy of Gary Meisner: www.PhiMatrix.com
Venus de Milo: http://en.wikipedia.org/wiki/File:Venus_de_Milo_Louvre_Ma399_n4.jpg
Adonis: http://en.wikipedia.org/wiki/File:Adonis3.jpg
Julia Roberts: http://en.wikipedia.org/wiki/File:Julia_Roberts_in_May_2002.jpg
George Clooney, by Nicolas Genin: http://en.wikipedia.org/wiki/File:George_Clooney_66ème_Festival_de_Venise_(Mostra)_3Alt1.jpg
Mona Lisa: http://en.wikipedia.org/wiki/File:Mona_Lisa.jpg
Khalil Gibran: http://en.wikipedia.org/wiki/File:Khalil_Gibran.jpg
Orgasm graph, Chocolate pie graph: T. Reczek
The Empress's Secret: www.TheEmpresssSecret.com
Roses, front and back: M. Cross
Buddha footprint: http://en.wikipedia.org/wiki/File:Buddha-Footprint.jpeg
Ackerman, Diane, *A Natural History of the Senses*, Vintage (September 10, 1991)
http://commons.wikimedia.org/wiki/File:Adonis_Mazarin_Louvre_MR239.jpg
Boothman, Nicholas, *How To Make People Like You in 90 Seconds or Less*, Workman Publishing Company; Reprint edition (July 2, 2008)
Breiter, Hans, Etcoff, Nancy et.al, *Beautiful Faces Have Variable Reward Value*, Neuron, Volume 32, Issue 3, 537-551, 8 November 2001
Cleese, John and Bates, Brian, *The Human Face*, DK ADULT; 1 edition (July 1, 2001)
Davis, Jeanie, *Men Who Dance Well May Be More Desirable As Mates*, WebMD.com, 12.21.05
Jefferson, Y., *Skeletal Types: Key to unraveling the mystery of facial beauty and its biologic significance.* J Gen Orthod. 1996 Jun;7(2):7-25
Mehrabian, Albert, *Nonverbal Communication*, Aldine Transaction (February 28, 2007)
http://en.wikipedia.org/wiki/Speculation_about_Mona_Lisa
www.oprah.com/article/oprahshow/20090304-tows-female-sex-study/6
http://en.wikipedia.org/wiki/File:Venus_de_Milo_Louvre_Ma399_n4.jpg
Reich, Wilhelm, Carfagno, Vincent R. *The Function of the Orgasm: Discovery of the Orgone (Discovery of the Orgone, Vol 1)*, Farrar, Straus and Giroux (May 1, 1986)

Chapter 10

Fountain of Youth: Lucas Cranach: http://en.wikipedia.org/wiki/File:Lucas_Cranach_d._%C3%84._007.jpg
Aquaporins: http://en.wikipedia.org/wiki/File:Aquaporin-Sideview.png
Jeanne Calment: http://en.wikipedia.org/wiki/File:JeanneCalmentaged40.jpg
Andersen, Helle R., et.al., *Low activity of superoxide dismutase and high activity of glutathione reductase in erythrocytes from centenarians, Age and Ageing*, 1998; 27: 643-648
Nautilus shell: iStockphoto.com

Census, www.census.gov/compendia/statab/cats/births_deaths_marriages_divorces/life_expectancy.html

Flanagan, Patrick, MD. (MA), *Hydrogen.... Longevity's Missing Link, Nexus* December, 1994-January 1995

Gavrilov, Leonid A. & Gavrilova, Natalia S. *The Biology of Life Span: A Quantitative Approach*; New York: Harwood Academic Publisher, (1991)

Human life expectancy, http://entomology.ucdavis.edu/courses/hde19/lecture3.html

Jeanne Calment, http://www.nytimes.com/2009/01/27/science/27agre.html?pagewanted=1&_r=1

Robbins, John, *Healthy at 100: The Scientifically Proven Secrets of the World's Healthiest and Longest-Lived Peoples*, Ballantine Books (August 28, 2007)

Walford, Roy L. M.D., *Beyond The 120-Year Diet*; Da Capo Press; Revised and Expanded edition (August 7, 2000).

Whitney, Craig R., Jeanne Calment, *World's Elder, Dies at 122, The New York Times*, 8/5/97

Buettner, Dan, *The Blue Zone: Lessons for Living Longer from the People Who've Lived the Longest*, National Geographic; Reprint edition (April 21, 2009).

Dean, Josh, *The Longevity Expedition*, National Geographic Adventure Magazine, June/July, 2009

Buettner, Dan, *Grecian Formula*, National Geographic Adventure Magazine, October, 2009

Casselman, Anne, *Long-Lived Costa Ricans Offer Secrets to Reaching 100*, National Geographic Adventure Magazine, April 2008

http://science.nasa.gov/headlines/y2006/images/telomeres/caps_med.jpg

Blackburn, Elizabeth and Epel, Elissa, *The Telomere Effect;* cover and excerpt *(2017)*

http://en.wikipedia.org/wiki/File:Telomere_caps.gif

Skloot, Rebecca, *The Immortal Life of Henrietta Lacks*, Crown; 1 edition, (February 2, 2010)

Benson, M.D., Herbert, *Relaxation Revolution: Enhancing Your Personal Health Through the Science and Genetics of Mind Body Healing*, Scribner; 1 edition (June 22, 2010).

http://en.wikipedia.org/wiki/Longevity_traditions#Biblical

http://commons.wikimedia.org/wiki/File:Foster_Bible_Pictures_0021-2.jpg

http://upload.wikimedia.org/wikipedia/commons/b/b8/Aubrey_de_Grey.jpg

http://en.wikipedia.org/wiki/Itzamna

http://en.wikipedia.org/wiki/Hot_chocolate

http://en.wikipedia.org/wiki/File:Cacao-pod-k4636-14.jpg

http://en.wikipedia.org/wiki/File:God_D_Itzamna.jpg

Eternal Clock, by Robbert van der Steeg, http://www.flickr.com/photos/robbie73/3387189144/

Farzneh-Far, Ramin, M.D., etal., *Association of Marine Omega-3 Fatty Acid Levels With Telomeric Aging in Patients With Coronary Heart Disease*. JAMA. 2010;303(3):250-257.

Williams S1, Tamburic S, Lally C., *Eating chocolate can significantly protect the skin from UV light.* J Cosmet Dermatol. 2009 Sep;8(3):169-73.

Food and Agriculture Organization of the United Nations, Chart: Cocoa Butter Fatty Acid Composition, Publisher, Rome: FAO, 1989., *Utilization of tropical foods: tropical oil-seeds, Series: FAO food & nutrition paper*, no. 47-5

Chocolate nutritional data and images courtesy of www.NutritionData.com.

Photo of co-author Matthew Cross running in the NYC Blizzard, Jan. 2016: Thank You Raquel Garcia!

SECTION III

21-Day Priority Coach™: Designed by & Copyright ©2017 by Matthew Cross

About the Authors, Hoshin Media/Products

- Robert D. Friedman, M.D.: Photo by Kim Jew • Matthew K. Cross: Photo by Diana Doroftei
- All Hoshin Media book covers: Designed by M. Cross; rendered by T. Reczek

The Authors

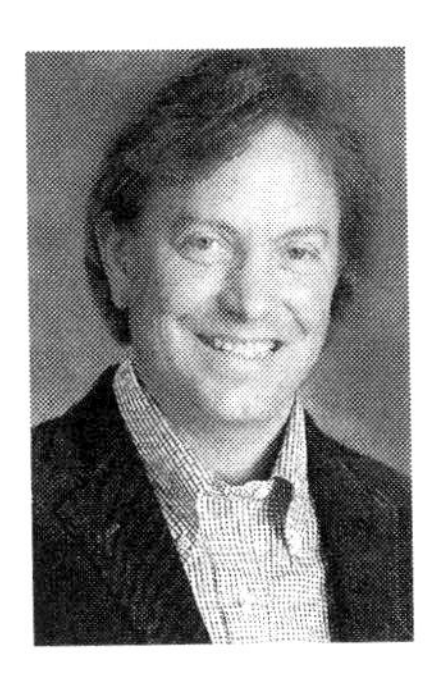

Robert D. Friedman, M.D.

is a visionary physician living in Santa Fe, New Mexico. He practiced medicine 25 years before turning his attention to the research and application of the Golden Ratio to support maximum health and longevity. His inspiration for Nature's Secret Nutrient/NSN comes from the original Latin root of the word *Physician: Physica—Things Relating to Nature,* along with his study and practice of Biomimicry Medicine. He co-authored with Matthew K. Cross *The Divine Code of Da Vinci, Fibonacci, Einstein & YOU,* a 660 page tour-de force on the Golden Ratio, which allows anyone to access the Code and apply it in their chosen field. That book's success inspired three other Golden Ratio-based books: *The Golden Ratio & Fibonacci Sequence, The Divine Code Genius Activation Quote Book* and *Nature's Secret Nutrient.* For timely Golden Ratio updates, link to Dr. Friedman's Twitter: **@BobFriedmanMD** Dr. Friedman can be reached at **DRrobert1618@gmail.com**

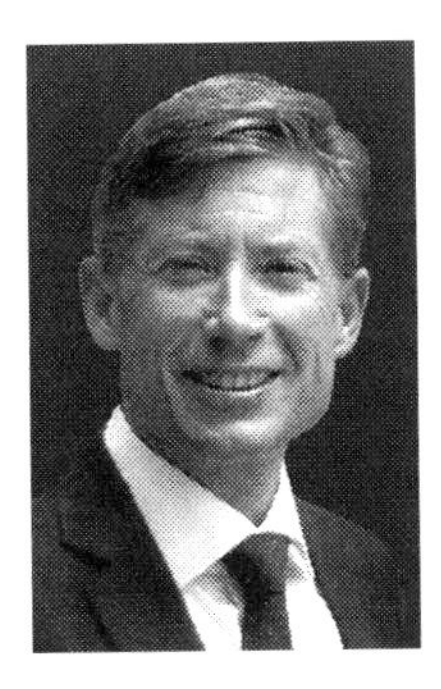

Matthew K. Cross

is Founder & CEO of Leadership Alliance, an international consulting firm providing breakthrough strategies for growth, genius and transformation. Matthew is the world's leading Priority Strategist, a Deming Quality Scholar, Hoshin Kanri strategic alignment specialist and speaker consulting with the Fortune 100 worldwide. Founder of The BioPerformance Institute, Matthew began his research into the life applications of the Golden Ratio at 13, which evolved into his pioneering work in Biomimicry Medicine and its integration into his athletic, business and life training systems for peak performance. In addition to co-authoring *The Golden Ratio & Fibonacci Sequence, Nature's Secret Nutrient, The Divine Code of Da Vinci, Fibonacci, Einstein & YOU* and *The Divine Code Genius Activation Quote Book* with Robert D. Friedman, M.D., Matthew is the author of *The Hoshin North Star Process, The Millionaire's MAP* and *Be Your Own President.* He's also an ancient history explorer and athlete (running, tennis), with a deep belief in everyone's unique genius. Reach Matthew at: **MC@LeadersAll.com** • Twitter: **@MatthewKCross**

The authors deliver engaging & informative interviews & presentations
Visit NSNpower.com for details.

Thank You

We are grateful to the many Geniuses of the Ratio, who have elucidated facets of the Golden Ratio diamond over time and made our road easier and more enjoyable to travel. The two Leonardo's, Fibonacci and Da Vinci, were of particular inspiration during this book's creation. We imagine we felt the same excitement they did when new Golden Ratio insights struck. There are also certain contemporary geniuses whose work kindled the activation and focus of the Nature's Secret Nutrient principles in us, in particular: John Michell, Dr. Ronald Sandler, Robert Prechter, Jr., Stephen McIntosh, Dr. W. Edwards Deming, Marshall Thurber, Barry Sears, Ph.D., Ann Louise Gittleman, M.S., C.N.S., Dr. Richard Schulze, Dr. Yosh Jefferson, Dr. Mehmet Oz, Dr. Michael Roizen, Dr. James O'Keefe, Hanno Ulmer, Ph.D., Ellen Langer, Ph.D., Elizabeth Blackburn, Ph.D., Elissa Epel, Ph.D., Janine Benyus, Jay Harman, Dr. Herbert Benson, Dr. Michael Holick, Dr. Jack Kruse, Anastasia Soare, Dr. Roy Walford, Aubrey de Gray, Ph.D., Dan Buettner, Gary Null, Michael J. Gelb, Michael Schneider, Scott Onstott, Graham & Santha Hancock, Wim Hof, Stig Severinsen, Michael Rossato-Bennett, Halsey Snow, Jean-claude Perez, Ph.D., Kazuo Murakami, Ph.D., Dan Brown, Robert Lawlor, Buckminster Fuller, Alan Watts, Bob Cooley, Robert Kaehler, Sonja Lyubomirsky, Marci Shimoff, Bruce Lipton, Ph.D., Amy Cuddy, Ph.D., Rob Moses, Dr. John Ott, Walt Disney, Dr. Joseph M. Juran; all being among the giants on whose shoulders we stand.

Among many people, places & products in the arena of bright inspiration, we gratefully acknowledge: Tim Ferriss, Anthony Robbins, Jack Canfield, Mark Victor Hansen, Peter Donovan, Jeff & Melissa Klepacki, Dick & Marci Bolles, Nathan & Lara MacPherson, Ted & Kelly Murphy, Clare Crawford & Robert Mason, Jan & Ron Jones, Michael Castine, Sonia, Jeffrey & Walter Ernstoff, Sam Sokol, Aura Imbarus and Lisa Carraway, Lars Bjork and Team Qlik. Two beautiful Vitruvian Women, Arihanto Luders and Diana Doroftei, also added their magic to this book's creation. Other Secret Nutrients which gave us added boosts include the following, key aspects of NSN among them: Iron Man Green Smoothies, DNA Power Fuel,™ Dagoba chocolate bars, green tea, JuicePress raw juices/NYC, Spiral~Chi, Golden Ratio breathing, hanging upside-down, running–and winning–5K races, midnight oil burning, sports massage at Paradise Spa/Stamford CT, Renew Body Wellness Spa NYC, Gong Fu Body Work Spa NYC (thanks Master Jimmy!), mountain hikes, Starbucks, Beatles music, Roger Federer, Zumbach's Coffee and Connecticut Muffin in New Canaan CT, The Roasting Plant Coffee House/NYC, Casey Neistat's vlogs, Saint Motel's music, NYC's Mansfield Hotel and Penn Club.

Special thanks to our simply brilliant graphic designer Tom Reczek. Thanks to artist Chloe Hedden for her great rendition of the commissioned ***Divine Code Vitruvian Woman***, which stands shoulder to shoulder (literally) with Da Vinci's ***Vitruvian Man***. We would also like to thank and acknowledge iStockPhoto.com & Wikipedia.org as sources for many of this book's high-quality illustrations. Wikipedia.org was also a key provider of copyright free material, which has greatly enhanced this work. A warm thank you to our contributing editors: Maxine "Eagle Eyes" Friedman, Diana Doroftei, Lou Savary, Vicki Melian-Morse and Chris Johnson.

In the spirit of saving the best for last, a heartfelt thank you to *you*, dear reader. The opportunity to share this life-transforming material with you is a great honor and delight. We look forward to meeting you on our site: **www.NSNpower.com**

Index

KEY NUMBERS & RATIOS

A

B

C

D

E

F

G

H

I

J

K

L

M

N

Q

R

S

T

U

V

W

X

Y

Z

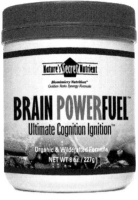

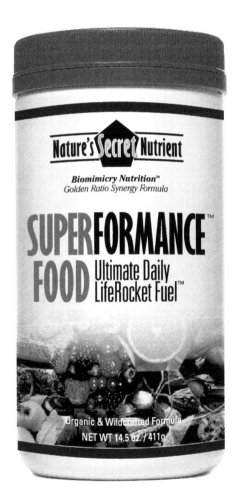

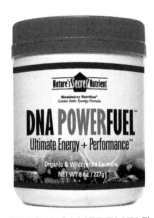

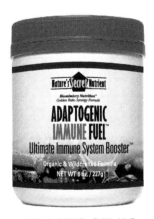

From Hoshin Media

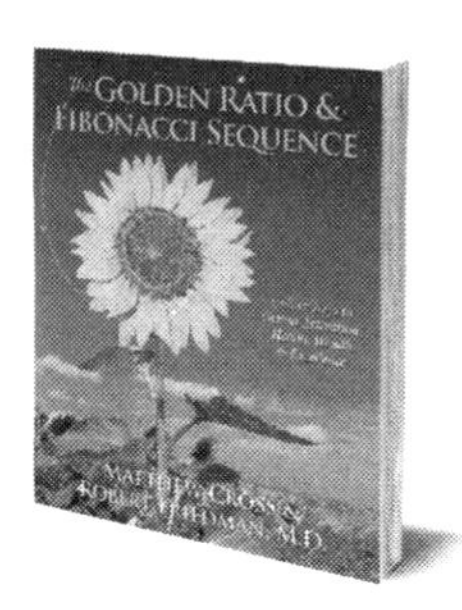

The Golden Ratio & Fibonacci Sequence

by Matthew K. Cross & Robert D. Friedman, M.D.

The world's first easily accessible, multi-facted portal to the Universal design and success code. A delightful introduction and primer to the golden keys to genius, health, wealth & excellence. 62 pages, richly illustrated in color with a fun and interactive approach. $16.18

> *The Golden Ratio is the Secret of the Universe.*
>
> Pythagoras

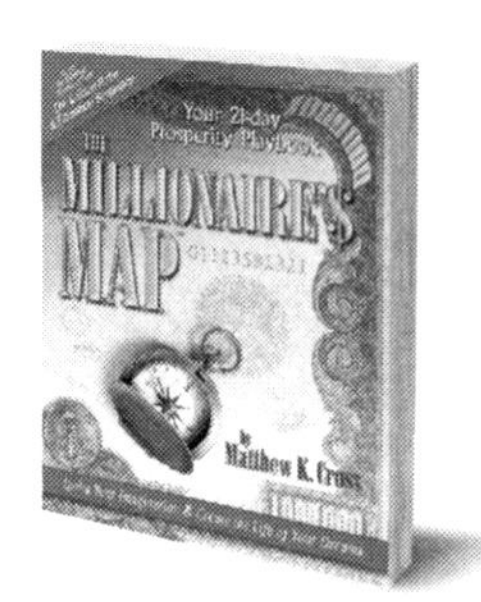

The Millionaire's MAP™

by Matthew K. Cross

Chart your way to abundance & wealth in life by tapping the power of your imagination with the Fibonacci Sequence, Nature's secret growth and transformation code. 144 page illustrated workbook. $24.95

> *The most powerful prosperity tool I've yet to encounter in 20 years of studying money and personal development.*
>
> Patrick Combs, bestselling author of *Major in Success* & *Man 1, Bank 0*

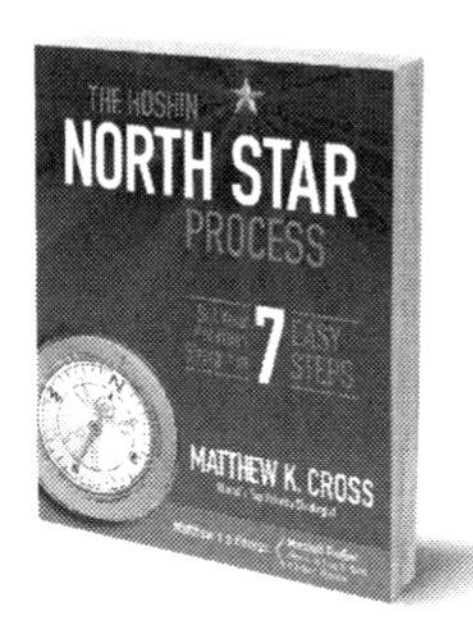

The Hoshin North Star Process™

by Matthew K. Cross

Chart your way to total success with the strategic alignment process of the world's greatest companies. 68 pages, illustrated workbook. $24.95

> *The odds of surviving the pace of the global investment banking environment have improved significantly, thanks to The Hoshin North Star Process.*
>
> Mark Mula, former Associate Director, UBS Global Strategy Development

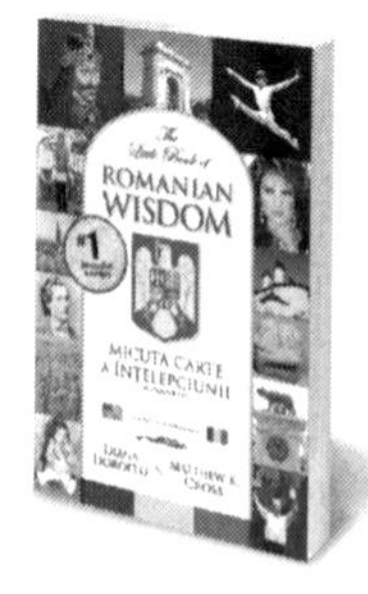

The Little Book of Romanian Wisdom

by Diana Doroftei & Matthew K. Cross

#1 Bestseller in Category

Discover the uniquely inspiring wisdom of Romania, through the words of its people. 184 pages, illustrated; in English & Romanian. $12.95

> *The ultimate guide for those interested in discovering themselves while learning about the mystical country of Romania.*
>
> Aura Imbarus, author of the Pulitzer Prize nominated *Out of the Transylvanian Night*

Available online at: **www.HoshinMedia.com**
For quantity purchases at discount, contact: Hoshin Media
P.O. Box 13 New Canaan, Connecticut 06840 USA

From Hoshin Media

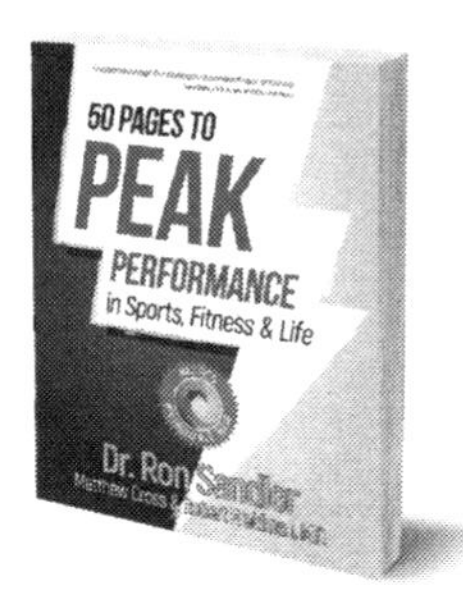

50 Pages to Peak Performance in Sports, Fitness & Life

By Dr. Ron Sandler, Matthew Cross & Robert Friedman, M.D.

This groundbreaking workbook equips performers in any arena with the golden key to access the greatest performance-on-demand-coach in history: Nature. 72 page illustrated workbook. $14.95

> *Fascinating concept that challenges conventional ideas of training.*
> Dave Scott, 6-time Ironman Triathlon Champion

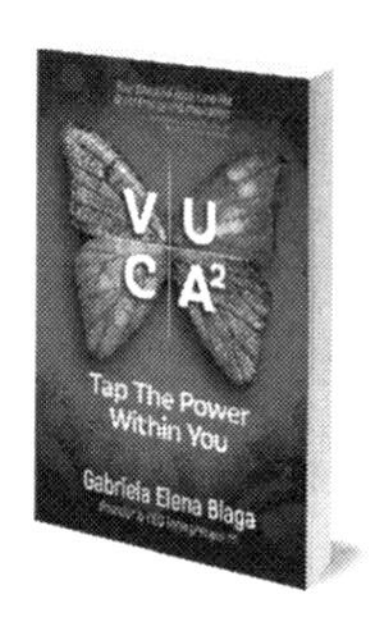

VUCA²: Tap the Power Within You

By Gabriela Elena Blaga

VUCA² = Vulnerability, Uniqueness, Courage and Authenticity.
A delightful workbook that clarifies your inner sight and strengths to step forward with greater confidence and success in relationships, work and life. 74 page illustrated workbook. $9.95

> *A practical and easy to implement guide that makes an extraordinary contribution to the world of wellness and wellbeing.*
> Walt Hampton, J.D., Founder & CEO, Summit Success, LLC; best selling author, *Journeys on the Edge: Living A Life That Matters*

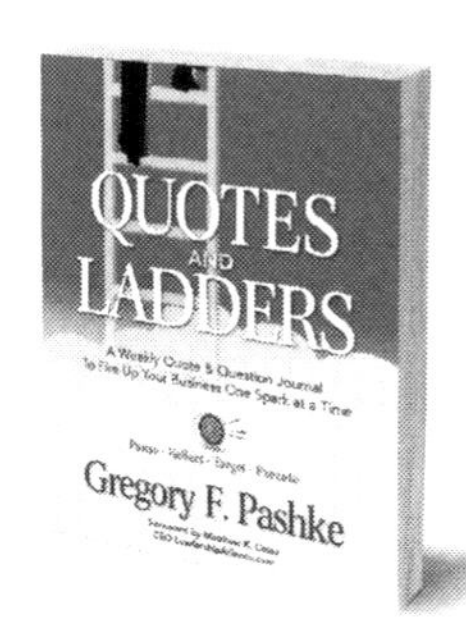

Quotes & Ladders Quotes and Ladders

A Weekly Quote & Question Journal to Fire Up Your Business One Spark at a Time

By Greg Pashke

A wonderfully simple, valuable and practical handbook that will elevate your perspective, grow your business—even transform your life. 70 pages. $16.95

> *A most valuable tool for weekly self-development; asks probing questions to stimulate thoughtful improvement. If you're looking for business and personal development tools–you have found your toolbox!*
> Jay Berkowitz, CEO, Ten Golden Rules

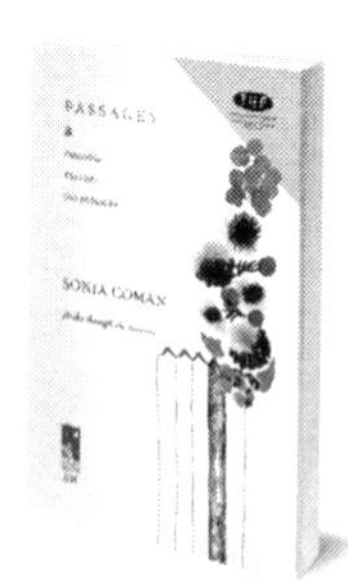

Passages: Haiku Through the Seasons

By Sonia Coman

Destined to become an instant favorite, *Passages: Haiku through the Seasons* is an enchanting collection in five languages. Invites you to explore the many facets of the diamond of the everyday and the beauty of life between heartache and promise. 132 pages with original illustrations by the author. $14.95

> *Pure poetry. Deeply moving. Reading PASSAGES fills my heart with joy.*
> Rev. Howard Lee Kilby, Former Secretary, The Haiku Society of America

Available online at: **www.HoshinMedia.com**
For quantity purchases at discount, contact: Hoshin Media
P.O. Box 13 New Canaan, Connecticut 06840 USA